KU-529-541

www.bma.org.uk/library

WITHDRAWN
FROM LIBRARY

BRITISH MEDICAL ASSOCIATION

0999067

Your *Case-Based* book includes free bonus access to RadCases online!

RadCases is an extensive online database of key cases for your rounds, rotations and exams.

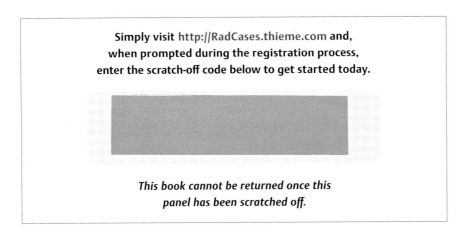

Simply visit http://RadCases.thieme.com and, when prompted during the registration process, enter the scratch-off code below to get started today.

This book cannot be returned once this panel has been scratched off.

Expand on **your *Case-Based* book with access to 250 core cases online.**

The scratch-off code above provides 12 months of access to an additional 250 neuro imaging cases via **RadCases.thieme.com**, our searchable online database of must-know cases.

You can also purchase e-subscriptions to key cases in other subspecialties by visiting **RadCases.thieme.com**.

Features of RadCases online include:

- A **user-friendly layout** that is ideal for self-study or quick reference
- Stress-free way to **study and review the most common and most critical cases**
- Clearly labeled, **high-quality radiographs** allow you to absorb key findings at-a-glance
- A **flexible search function** that lets you locate specific cases by age, differential diagnosis, modality, and more
- The ability to **bookmark cases** you want to revisit or 'hide' cases you've already learned

System requirements for optimal use of RadCases online

	WINDOWS	**MAC**
Recommended Browser(s)**	Microsoft Internet Explorer 7.0 or later, Firefox 2.x, Firefox 3.x	Firefox 2.x, Firefox 3.x, Safari 3.x, Safari 4.x
	** all browsers should have JavaScript enabled	
Flash Player Plug-in	Flash Player 8 or Higher*	
	* Mac users: ATI Rage 128 GPU does not support full-screen mode with hardware scaling	
Minimum Hardware Configurations	Intel® Pentium® II 450 MHz, AMD Athlon™ 600 MHz or faster processor (or equivalent)	PowerPC® G3 500 MHz or faster processor — Intel Core™ Duo 1.33 GHz or faster processor
	128 MB of RAM	128 MB of RAM
Recommended for optimal usage experience	Monitor resolutions: • Normal (4:3) 1024×768 or Higher • Widescreen (16:9) 1280×720 or Higher • Widescreen (16:10) 1440×900 or Higher DSL/Cable internet connection at a minimum speed of 384.0 Kbps or faster	

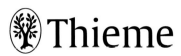

Differential Diagnosis in Pediatric Imaging

Rick R. van Rijn, MD, PhD
Pediatric Radiologist
Department of Radiology
Academic Medical Center Amsterdam
Amsterdam, The Netherlands

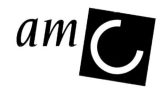

Johan G. Blickman, MD, PhD, FACR, FAAP
Professor and Associate Chairman
Department of Imaging Sciences URMC
Radiologist-in-Chief
Golisano Children's Hospital
University of Rochester Medical Center
Rochester, New York, USA

University Imaging

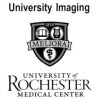

With 1506 illustrations

Thieme
Stuttgart · New York

Library of Congress Cataloging-in-Publication Data

Differentialdiagnostik in der p‰odiatrischen Radiologie. English.
Differential diagnosis in pediatric imaging / [edited by] Rick R.
van Rijn, MD, PhD, Paediatric radiologist, Department of Radiol-
ogy, Academic Medical Centre Amsterdam, Amsterdam, The
Netherlands, Johan G. Blickman, MD, PhD, FACR, Professor and
Associate Chairman, Department of Imaging Sciences URMC,
Director of Pediatric Radiology, Golisano Childrens Hospital,
Rochester, New York. -- Second Edition.

    p. ; cm.

  Includes bibliographical references and index.

  Summary: "Efficiency is the key word at the heart of the
concept for this diagnostic atlas - efficiency of presentation and
diagnostic efficiency achieved through its use. The contents
are arranged in chapters according to organ or body part. Each
chapter begins with a list of the radiographic findings referring
to the relevant table/page number for that finding. The text
within these tables is presented under three columns: possible diagnoses, radiographic findings, and general comments.
Corresponding sample images of the highest quality are then
provided for the more common conditions throughout. Rare
diseases are marked with asterisks and are illustrated where
appropriate. The hard-pressed radiologist will welcome this
work as an efficient and reliable guide to the interpretation of
pediatric images"--Provided by publisher.

  ISBN 978-3-13-143711-2 (hardback)

  1. Pediatric radiography. 2. Diagnostic ultrasonic imaging. 3.
Diagnosis, Differential. I. Rijn, Rick R. van, editor. II. Blickman,
Johan G., editor. III. Title.

  [DNLM: 1. Diagnostic Imaging. 2. Child. 3. Diagnosis, Differential. 4. Infant. WN 240]

  RJ51.R3D5413 2011

  616.07'54--dc22

                2010052679

Important note: Medicine is an ever-changing science undergoing continual development. Research and clinical experience are continually expanding our knowledge, in particular our knowledge of proper treatment and drug therapy. Insofar as this book mentions any dosage or application, readers may rest assured that the authors, editors, and publishers have made every effort to ensure that such references are in accordance with **the state of knowledge at the time of production of the book.** Nevertheless, this does not involve, imply, or express any guarantee or responsibility on the part of the publishers in respect to any dosage instructions and forms of applications stated in the book. **Every user is requested to examine carefully** the manufacturers' leaflets accompanying each drug and to check, if necessary in consultation with a physician or specialist, whether the dosage schedules mentioned therein or the contraindications stated by the manufacturers differ from the statements made in the present book. Such examination is particularly important with drugs that are either rarely used or have been newly released on the market. Every dosage schedule or every form of application used is entirely at the user's own risk and responsibility. The authors and publishers request every user to report to the publishers any discrepancies or inaccuracies noticed. If errors in this work are found after publication, errata will be posted at www.thieme.com on the product description page.

© 2011 Georg Thieme Verlag,
Rüdigerstrasse 14, 70469 Stuttgart, Germany
http://www.thieme.de
Thieme New York, 333 Seventh Avenue,
New York, NY 10001, USA
http://www.thieme.com

Cover design: Thieme Publishing Group
Typesetting by Maryland Composition, Maryland, USA

Printed by Everbest Printing Co Ltd., China

ISBN 978 3 13 143711 2   1 2 3 4 5 6

This book, including all parts thereof, is legally protected by copyright. Any use, exploitation, or commercialization outside the narrowlimits set by copyright legislation, without the publisher's consent, is illegal and liable to prosecution. This applies in particular to photostat reproduction, copying, mimeographing, preparation of microfilms, and electronic data processing and storage. Some of the product names, patents, and registered designs referred to in this book are in fact registered trademarks or proprietary names even though specific reference to this fact is not always made in the text. Therefore, the appearance of a name without designation as proprietary is not to be construed as a representation by the publisher that it is in the public domain.

Er bestaan geen ouders die niet heimelijk in hun kinderen iets bijzonders zien.
En ze hebben gelijk, de mogelijkheden zijn onbeperkt.

There are no parents who secretly don't see something special in their children.
Rightly so, their opportunities are endless.

Godfried Bomans, Dutch author (1913–1971)

Contents

Contributors

Jose C. Albillos Merino, MD
Pediatric Radiologist
Head of Radiology Department
Unidad Central de Radiodiagnóstico
Hospital Infanta Sofía
Madrid, Spain

Erik J. A. Beek, MD, PhD
Department of Pediatric Radiology
Wilhelmina Children's Hospital
University Hospital Utrecht
Utrecht, The Netherlands

Johan G. Blickman, MD, PhD, FACR, FAAP
Professor and Associate Chairman
Department of Imaging Sciences URMC
Radiologist-in-Chief
Golisano Children's Hospital
University of Rochester Medical Center
Rochester, New York, USA

Teresa Berrocal Frutos, MD, PhD
Department of Radiology
Pediatric Radiology Section
University Hospital La Paz
Madrid, Spain

Alistair D. Calder, FRCR
Department of Pediatric Radiology
Great Ormond Street Hospital for Children
London, United Kingdom

S. Murthy Chennapragada, MBBS, DMRD, DipNB, FRANZCR
Staff Specialist Radiologist
The Children's Hospital at Westmead
Clinical Senior Lecturer
University of Sydney
Sydney, Australia

Gloria del Pozo Garcia, MD, PhD
Associated Professor of Universidad Complutense
Department of Radiology
Pediatric Radiology Section
University Hospital
Madrid, Spain

Annick S. Devos, MD
Department of Pediatric Radiology
Erasmus Medical Center
Rotterdam, The Netherlands

Jeevish Kapur, MBBS, FRCR
Department of Diagnostic Imaging
National University Hospital
Singapore

Tracey Kilborn, MBChB, FRCR
Department of Radiology
Red Cross War Memorial Children's Hospital
Cape Town, South Africa

Albert H. Lam, MD, FRANZCR, DDU
Senior Staff Specialist Radiologist
Sydney Children's Hospital Networks
Clinical Professor
Sydney Medical School
University of Sydney
Sydney, Australia

Maarten H. Lequin, MD, PhD
Department of Pediatric Radiology
Erasmus Medical Center
Rotterdam, The Netherlands

Thomas H. J. MacDougall, MBBS, FRCR, FRANZCR
Staff Specialist Radiologist
John Hunter Hospital
Newcastle, Australia

John D. MacKenzie, MD
Assistant Professor and Chief, Pediatric Radiology
Department of Radiology and Biomedical Imaging
University of California, San Francisco
San Francisco, California, USA

Allan E. Oestreich, MD
Department of Radiology and Medical Imaging
Cincinnati Children's Hospital
Cincinnati, Ohio, USA

Catherine M. Owens, MRCP, FRCR
Department of Pediatric Radiology
Great Ormond Street Hospital for Children
London, United Kingdom

Simon G. F. Robben, MD, PhD
Department of Radiology
Academic Medical Center Maastricht
Maastricht, The Netherlands

Anje M. Spijkerboer, MD, PhD
Department of Radiology
Academic Medical Center Amsterdam
Amsterdam, The Netherlands

David A. Stringer, BSc, MBBS, FRCR, FRCPC
Department of Diagnostic Imaging and Intervention
KK Women's and Children's Hospital
Singapore

Harvey EL Teo, MBBS, FRCR
Department of Diagnostic Imaging and Intervention
KK Women's and Children's Hospital
Singapore

Rick R. van Rijn, MD, PhD
Pediatric Radiologist
Department of Radiology
Academic Medical Center Amsterdam
Amsterdam, The Netherlands

Navdeep Walia, MBBS, MD
Consultant Radiologist
Columbia Asia Hospital-Patiala
Patiala, Punjab, India

Nicky Wieselthaler, MBChB, FC Rad (D)
Department of Radiology
Red Cross War Memorial Children's Hospital
Cape Town, South Africa

Preface

Before you lies a new *Differential Diagnosis in Pediatric Imaging.*

In the last decades the field of pediatric radiology has changed tremendously, reflecting the adoption of digital imaging, workflow optimization, and the introduction of the electronic patient records. The acquisition, interpretation, and exchange of imaging data in the field of imaging have resulted in faster and timelier contribution to the diagnostic pathway. Imaging truly has become the "spider" in the diagnostic "web." Near-immediate imaging that aids in the care of children's illnesses is now the norm.

This evolution has occurred alongside the change in the realization that this escalating use of imaging modalities has a price, particularly a possible negative effect of ionizing radiation, particularly on children. Hence, the adoption of the widely accepted "image gently" campaign, which promotes the awareness of the potential harmful effects of ionizing radiation particularly in children.

Multislice computed tomography and magnetic resonance imaging—as well as the ever increasing use of ultrasound imaging—that once were available only to a handful of (university) hospitals are now are widely adopted throughout our exciting subspecialty and available everywhere. In contrast, the numbers of conventional fluoroscopic studies are steadily declining and the art of the barium studies will be lost on future generations of pediatric radiologists. All these modalities are being evaluated continuously so as to effectively, quickly, and safely image children.

All of these modalities need to be incorporated into the "online" knowledge base of imagers dealing with children, thus *Differential Diagnosis in Pediatric Imaging,* based on the Ebel et al. book *Differential Diagnosis in Pediatric Radiology* published in 1999.

Another, and perhaps even more, important change is the increasing impact of Internet on everything we do, both in our personal as well as in our professional lives. The Internet, which actually was launched in 1991 (August 6th is seen as the debut of the Web as a publicly available service on the Internet), has made the world a smaller place. As a result, international communication between pediatric radiologists has become as easy as walking down the hall to discuss a case with a colleague.

This virtually shrinking world is reflected in the way we worked together with all the contributing authors to this edition, without the need for face-to-face meetings or lengthy conference (video) calls—an impossible feat as recently as 20 years ago. The result: truly a collaboration of an international group of renowned authors on an internationally significant pediatric publication project.

We thank all the authors, without you this book work would not exist, without you the excellence would be impossible.

The editors have chosen to present the possible differential diagnostic possibilities of each imaging finding in the well-known three column format reflecting the diagnosis, imaging findings, and additional, hopefully useful, information concerning both.

The book is divided into six chapters, in which the first five chapters reflect the organ-based workflow commonly used today in modern imaging departments, whereas the sixth chapter is devoted to normal measurements, so important in assessing development in pediatric radiology.

The tables are illustrated with state-of-art imaging examples ranging from conventional radiography to advanced magnetic resonance techniques.

We hope that this book, intended for both radiologists (general and subspecialized pediatric ones) as well as those clinicians who request medical imaging studies in children, will find its way to many departmental libraries and, even more importantly, many workstations where imaging excellence is practiced in order to optimally care for sick kids!

On a final note, special thanks go to the editorial team at Thieme: Cliff Bergman, Annie Hollins, Stephan Konnry, and Heidi Grauel. A wonderful job to keep us engaged, relatively on time, and producing a wonderful result!

We are well aware that our achievement of today might well be the baseline of tomorrow, in fact, that is our profound wish, as our specialty evolves to ever better care of kids (after James Thrall, MD, Boston, MA, 1992).

Rick R. van Rijn, MD, PhD
Johan G. (Hans) Blickman, MD, PhD

Abbreviations

(123)I-MIBG	(123)I-metaiodobenzylguanidine	HU	Hounsfield units
99mTc	technetium-99m	IAC	internal auditory canal
AAIIMM	appendicitis, adhesions, intussusception, incarcerated hernia, Meckel diverticula, miscellanea	ICA	internal carotid artery
		ICP	intracranial pressure
AC	acromioclavicular	IHW	interhemispheric width
ADC	apparent diffusion coefficient	IT	intussusception
ADPKD	autosomal dominant polycystic kidney disease	IVC	inferior vena cava
AIDS	acquired immunodeficiency syndrome	IVU	intravenous urogram
ALL	acute lymphoblastic leukemia	JIA	juvenile idiopathic arthritis
AP	anteroposterior	LAD	left anterior descending
AR	autosomal recessive	LAMB	lentigines, atrial myxoma, mucocutaneous myxoma, blue naevi
ARDS	acute ("adult"-type) respiratory distress syndrome		
ARPKD	autosomal recessive polycystic kidney disease	LCH	Langerhans cell histiocytosis
ASD	atrial septal defect	LIP	lymphoid interstitial pneumonitis
ATRT	atypical teratoid/rhabdoid tumors	LSCC	lateral semicircular canal
AVN	avascular necrosis	LULs	left upper lobes
AVSD	atrioventricular septal defect	MAS	meconium aspiration syndrome
BPD	bronchopulmonary dysplasia	MCDK	multicystic dysplastic kidneys
BVWI	bladder volume wall thickness index	MMC	myelomeningocele
CCAM	congenital cystic adenomatoid malformation	MPS	mucopolysaccharidosis
CE	contrast enhancement	MRA	magnetic resonance angiography
CECT	contrast-enhanced CT	MRCP	magnetic resonance cholangiopancreatography
CF	cystic fibrosis	MRI	magnetic resonance imaging
CGD	chronic granulomatous disease	MRS	magnetic resonance spectroscopy
CLO	congenital lobar overinflation	NAA	N-acetylaspartate
CMV	cytomegalovirus	NAME	nevi, atrial myxoma, myxoid neurofibroma, epitheliodes
CNS	central nervous system		
CPP	choroid plexus papilloma	NEC	necrotizing enterocolitis
CSF	cerebrospinal fluid	NECT	non-contrast–enhanced CT
CT	computed tomography	NF	neurofibromatosis
CTA	CT-angiography	NG	nasogastric
CXR	chest X-ray	NHL	non-Hodgkin lymphoma
DD	differential diagnosis	NM	nuclear medicine
DESS	double echo steady state	NOF	nonosteogenic fibroma
DIP	desquamative interstitial pneumonitis	NSIP	nonspecific interstitial pneumonitis
DMSA	dimercaptosuccinic acid	OA	osteoarthritis
EBV	Epstein-Barr virus	PACS	picture archiving and communication system
ECMO	extracorporeal membrane oxygenation	PC	pelvicaliceal
ERCP	endoscopic retrograde pancreatography	PCT	pineal cell tumors
EU	excretory urography	PDA	patent ductus arteriosus
FD	fibrous dysplasia	PET	positron emission tomography
FLAIR	fluid-attenuated inversion recovery	PFFD	proximal focal femoral deficiency
GA	gestational age	PH	periventricular nodular heterotopia
GCT	germ cell tumor	PHPV	Persistent Hyperplastic Primary Vitreous
GD	gadolinium	PJP	Pneumocystis jiroveci pneumonia
GE	gastroenteritis	PNET	primitive neuroectodermal tumor
GER	gastroesophageal reflux	PPD	purified protein derivative
GFR	glomerular filtration rate	PSCC	posterior semicircular canal
GI	gastrointestinal	PTLD	posttransplant lymphoproliferative disorder
GLUT	glucose transporter	PVNS	pigmented villonodular synovitis
HASTE	half-Fourier acquisition single-shot turbo spin echo	RAD	reactive airway disease
		RCA	right coronary artery
HIV	human immunodeficiency virus	RDS	respiratory distress syndrome
HMD	hyaline membrane disease	RGU	retrograde urethrogram
HPS	hypertrophic pyloric stenosis	RI	resistive index
HRCT	high-resolution CT	RICH	rapidly involuting congenital hemangioma

RLQ	right lower quadrant	TAPVD	total anomalous pulmonary venous drainage
RML	right middle lobe	TAPVR	total anomalous pulmonary venous return
RSV	respiratory syncytial virus	TB	tuberculosis
RUL	right upper lobe	TORCH	toxoplasmosis, other infections, rubella,
RUQ	right upper quadrant		cytomegalovirus, and herpes simplex virus
SAPHO	synovitis, acne, palmoplantar pustulosis, hyper-	TTN	transient tachypnea of the newborn
	ostosis, and osteitis	UGI	upper gastrointestinal
SBO	small-bowel obstruction	UPJ	ureteropelvic junction
SCC	semicircular canal	US	ultrasound
SCIWORA	spinal cord injury without radiologic abnormality	VACTERL	vertebral defects, anal atresia, cardiac
SCM	sternocleidomastoid		malformations, tracheoesophageal fistula with
SCW	sinocortical width		esophageal atresia, radial or renal dysplasia,
SD	standard deviation		and limb anomalies
SDH	subdural hematomas	VCUG	voiding cystourethrogram
SSCC	superior semicircular canal	VP	ventriculoperitoneal
SSD	shaded surface display	VSD	ventricular septal defect
SSS	superior sagittal sinus	VUJ	vesicoureteral junction
STIR	short inversion time inversion recovery	VUR	vesicoureteral reflux

1 Thorax, Mediastinum, Heart, and Great Vessels

Thorax

The Lungs

Pleura and Diaphragms

→

Mediastinum

The Trachea

The Hilum

The Mediastinum

→

Heart and Great Vessels

Congenital Heart Disease

Cardiac Tumors

The Great Vessels

Cardiovascular Devices

Thorax

The Lungs

■ Diffuse Lung Disease

Lung Disease in the Neonate

The differential diagnosis for diffuse lung disease in the neonatal period is relatively narrow. The final diagnosis is reached by a combination of clinical and radiologic findings. Knowing the gestational age of the neonate is essential to constructing a sensible list of possibilities.

Table 1.1   Lung disease in the neonate

Diagnosis	Findings	Comments
Hyaline membrane disease (HMD)/ surfactant deficient disease/ respiratory distress syndrome ▷ *Fig. 1.1a, b*	On initial radiograph: Diffuse hypoaeration with small lung volumes, diffuse reticulogranular opacification with or without air bronchograms. Opacification may clear patchily following surfactant administration.	Occurs predominantly in neonates under 36–40-wk gestation. Appearances are due to diffuse alveolar microatelectasis owing to surfactant deficiency. This classic appearance is rare today owing to improved perinatal care, particularly the use of maternal glucocorticoids and direct tracheal instillation of exogeneous surfactant.
Transient tachypnea of the newborn ▷ *Fig. 1.2*	Normal or mildly increased lung volumes. Diffuse mild predominantly reticular opacification. Small pleural effusions common. May simulate HMD, meconium aspiration syndrome, or neonatal pneumonia, but unlike these clears rapidly (1–2 d).	Associated with cesarean delivery, rapid labor, and low birth weight.
Meconium aspiration syndrome (MAS) ▷ *Fig. 1.3*	Lung overinflation with radiating perihilar coarse opacities ("ropelike").	Radiologic features result from small airway obstruction and inflammation, resulting in alternating areas of overinflation and atelectasis. Occurs in term and postterm neonates following fetal distress. Highly susceptible to pneumothorax. Overall mortality up to 25%.
Neonatal pneumonia	Variable patterns. May simulate transient tachypnea of the newborn (TTN) or HMD. Pleural effusion present in two-thirds.	Group B *Streptococcus* most common agent. *Chlamydia pneumoniae* usually presents later (typically around 6 wk)
Neonatal heart failure ▷ *Fig. 1.8, p. 8*	May simulate TTN or HMD. Cardiomegaly may be present, but not usually in cases of abnormal pulmonary venous drainage (e.g., total anomalous pulmonary venous return [TAPVR]).	Common causes presenting in first week of life include left ventricular outflow obstruction, coarctation, aortic stenosis, hypoplastic left heart. Obstructed pulmonary venous return: TAPVR, stenosis of common pulmonary vein, mitral stenosis, cor triatrium. Myocardial disorders: myocardial ischemia, myocarditis, dysrhythmia. High output states: vein of Galen malformation, hepatic hemangioendothelioma.
Pulmonary lymphangiectasia ▷ *Fig. 1.4a, b, p. 6*	Coarse interstitial infiltrate. Occasional septal lines. Peribronchial thickening may result in air trapping. Large chylous effusion often present.	Rare. Indistinguishable from lymphangiomatosis radiologically.

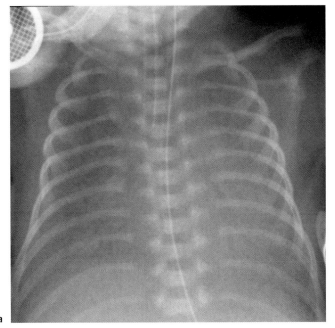

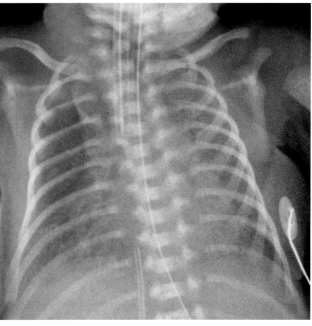

a

b

Fig. 1.1a, b   Hyaline membrane disease. (**a**) Chest radiograph in neonate born at 28 weeks' gestation with respiratory distress. The lungs are of small volume despite ventilation, with a diffuse infiltrate.

(**b**) Chest radiograph taken 48 hours later in the same child following endotracheal surfactant administration. There has been patchy clearing of the diffuse infiltrate.

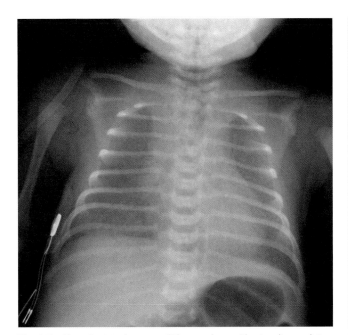

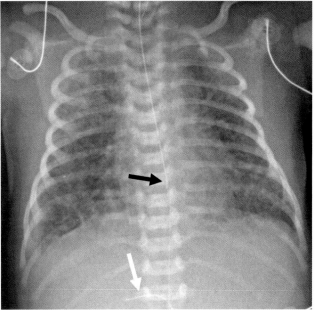

Fig. 1.2   Transient tachypnea of the newborn. Chest radiograph in a 38-week-gestation neonate delivered by emergency cesarean section. There is a diffuse fine interstitial infiltrate. The lung volumes are marginally increased with seven anterior ribs visible above the diaphragm. The child required overnight nasal positive pressure support only.

Fig. 1.3   Meconium aspiration syndrome. Chest radiograph in term neonate following emergency cesarean section. The lungs are overinflated with coarse opacities throughout the lungs. Note malposition of a nasogastric (NG) tube (black arrow) and umbilical venous catheter (white arrow).

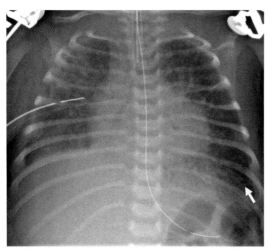
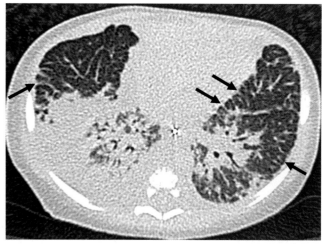

a   b

Fig. 1.4a, b   Pulmonary lymphangiectasia. (a) Chest radiograph in a neonate with a large right-sided pleural effusion at birth, now drained. There is diffuse lung reticulation with numerous interstitial lines (white arrow). **(b)** High-resolution CT (HRCT) in same child shows numerous linear opacities representing thickened interlobular septa (arrows). Biopsy confirmed pulmonary lymphangiectasia.

Diffuse Lung Disease Beyond the Neonatal Period

Characterizing diffuse lung disease requires a determination of the characteristics of the opacification, as discussed subsequently.

Bilateral Homogeneous Opacification: Bilateral Lung "White Out"

Increased vascular opacities

Diffuse airspace opacification

Diffuse peribronchial opacification

Reticulonodular opacification

Cystic lung disease

Nodular opacification: miliary pattern

Generalized patchy opacification

Diffuse hypertransradiancy/lung overinflation

Clearly, there is overlap between these groups.

Table 1.2   Bilateral homogeneous opacification: bilateral lung "white out"

Diagnosis	Findings	Comments
Deep expiration ▷ *Fig. 1.122, p. 72*	All contours obliterated. No air bronchograms. Degree of opacification does not relate to clinical status of child. Trachea often buckled, convex to the right (left if right aortic arch). Opacification may appear almost complete.	Exposure occurs at end of cry. Requires repeat film in inspiration.
Pulmonary hypoplasia	Small, opaque lungs may be present initially. Ribs may be short or downward sloping. Thorax may be bell-shaped. Evidence of secondary cause may be present (e.g., skeletal dysplasia).	Usually secondary to external thoracic compression of lungs in utero: mass (e.g., diaphragmatic hernia, large congenital cystic adenomatoid malformation [CCAM]), oligohydramnios usually due to renal failure [i.e., Potter sequence]) or rib cage abnormality (e.g., Jeune syndrome or in major abdominal wall defect). Idiopathic (primary) form rare, with frequent associated anomalies.
HMD (also known as respiratory distress syndrome [RDS], surfactant deficient disease) ▷ *Fig. 1.1, p. 5*	More commonly with reticulogranular pattern progressing to air space, but initial opacification may be homogeneous due to diffuse microatelectasis.	Occurs predominantly in neonates under 36–40-wk gestation. Appearances are due to diffuse alveolar microatelectasis owing to surfactant deficiency. This classic appearance is rare today owing to improved perinatal care, particularly the use of maternal glucocorticoids and exogeneous surfactant.
Bilateral large pleural effusions	Diffuse white out appearance on supine film.	
Underventilated lungs following intubation ▷ *Fig. 1.5*	Endotracheal tube (ETT) present: may be abnormally sited (e.g., in esophagus or bevel abutting tracheal wall).	This may be due to endotracheal tube obstruction or be intentional (e.g., when treating meconium aspiration with extracorporeal membrane oxygenation [ECMO]).
Severe diffuse pulmonary hemorrhage	Lung volumes often preserved.	Causes include bleeding diathesis, vasculitis, persistent pulmonary hypertension of the newborn. Occasionally following surfactant therapy.
Severe pulmonary edema	Cardiac enlargement often present.	

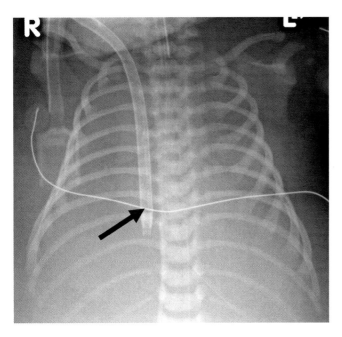

Fig. 1.5 Intentional hypoventilation. Chest radiograph of a neonate with severe meconium aspiration undergoing venovenous ECMO: the single ECMO cannula lies in the region of the right atrium (arrow). The lungs are completely opacified as a result of minimized ventilation parameters to protect them from barotrauma and rest the lungs for repair.

Increased Vascular Opacities

Distinction between pulmonary venous and arterial dilatation is not always straightforward, and the two may coexist. In venous dilatation, the enlarged vessels are less well defined than in arterial dilatation and have a vertical course in the upper zones with a horizontal course in the lower zones. In pulmonary arterial dilatation (pulmonary plethora), dilated arteries radiate from the hilum: the central pulmonary arteries and pulmonary outflow tract may also be dilated.

Table 1.3 Pulmonary venous dilatation

Diagnosis	Findings	Comments
Left ventricular outflow limitation	Cardiomegaly usually present.	Aortic coarctation, particularly in neonatal presentation, congenital aortic stenosis, hypoplastic left heart syndrome.
Left ventricular dysfunction ▷ *Fig. 1.32, p. 24*	Cardiomegaly usually present.	Myocarditis, anomalous coronary circulation, dilated cardiomyopathy.
Obstructed venous return ▷ *Fig. 1.6*	Heart size often normal.	Most commonly infracardiac total anomalous pulmonary venous drainage (TAPVD), also mitral valve disease.
High-output cardiac failure	Heart size may be normal or increased.	Consider if echocardiogram shows good left ventricle. Causes include vein of Galen malformation and hemangioendothelioma. Severe anemia in older child.

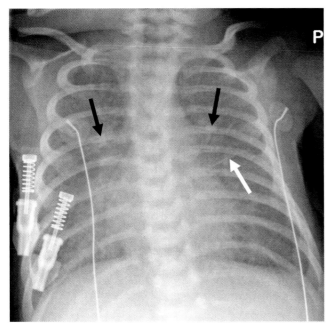

Fig. 1.6 Pulmonary venous hypertension. Chest radiograph in a neonate with obstructed infracardiac TAPVD. There are ill-defined enlarged central vessels (black arrows) with evidence of interstitial and alveolar pulmonary oedema (white arrow).

Table 1.4 Pulmonary arterial dilatation

Diagnosis	Findings	Comments
Left-to-right shunts ▷ *Fig. 1.7* ▷ *Fig. 1.153, p. 87*	Right atrial and ventricular enlargement in ASD, biatrial, and right ventricular enlargement in ventricular septal defect (VSD). Often just mild cardiomegaly and large pulmonary artery segment.	ASD, VSD, PDA, and atrioventricular septal defect (AVSD)/endocardial cushion defect most common lesions.
Admixture lesions ▷ *Fig. 1.8*	Pulmonary plethora in cyanotic child.	Causes include transposition of great arteries; truncus arteriosus; TAPVD; tricuspid atresia with VSD; double outlet right ventricle; single ventricle.
Pulmonary disease	Severe pulmonary disease resulting in pulmonary hypertension.	Cystic fibrosis (CF) most common cause in children. Also bronchiolitis obliterans.
Pulmonary hypertension: other causes ▷ *Fig. 1.16, p. 14*	Lungs often normal in appearance. May show dilated central arteries and "pruned" peripheral vasculature (see section on hilar enlargement).	Including primary pulmonary hypertension, pulmonary veno-occlusive disease, recurrent pulmonary embolism, partial anomalous pulmonary venous return.
Poststenotic ▷ *Fig. 1.159, p. 90*	Usually just pulmonary trunk ± proximal left pulmonary artery visibly dilated.	

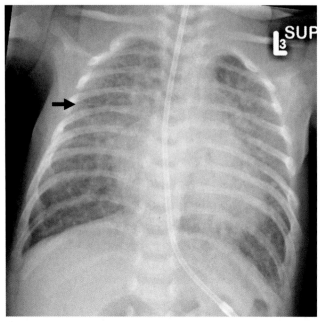

Fig. 1.7 Pulmonary overcirculation. Chest radiograph in an infant with a large atrioventricular septal defect, demonstrating marked pulmonary plethora with superadded pulmonary edema due to "overcirculation." Note the fissural fluid (arrow).

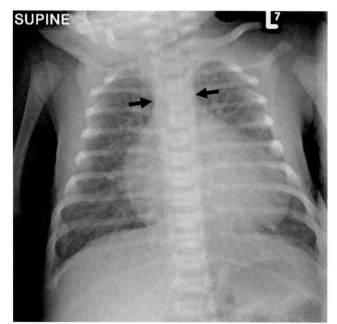

Fig. 1.8 Pulmonary plethora. Chest radiograph in an infant with dextro-transposition of the great arteries. There are well-defined enlarged vessels throughout the lungs. Note the narrow superior mediastinum (between arrows) due to superimposition of the aorta and main pulmonary artery, producing the "egg on a string" appearance.

Table 1.5 Mixed

Diagnosis	Findings	Comments
Left-to-right shunt with heart failure ▷ *Fig. 1.8*	Large heart with large pulmonary vessels and diffuse air-space/interstitial shadowing.	Heart failure may develop due to pulmonary overcirculation. Common with large septal defects, AVSD. May require pulmonary artery banding prior to definitive treatment.

Diffuse Airspace Opacification

Table 1.6   Diffuse air-space opacification

Diagnosis	Findings	Comments
Cardiogenic pulmonary edema ▷ *Fig. 1.8*	Heart usually but not always enlarged.	In the neonatal period, cardiogenic pulmonary edema is most commonly due to left-to-right shunts with pulmonary overcirculation. In later life, more common causes include myocarditis and dilated cardiomyopathy.
Acute ("adult"-type) respiratory distress syndrome (ARDS)	Diffuse bilateral air-space opacification within 24–48 h of precipitating event. Frequently associated with air leak phenomena in children (pneumomediastinum, pneumothorax, interstitial emphysema).	Common precipitating events are septicemia, neurologic disease, and near drowning.
Diffuse pulmonary hemorrhage ▷ *Fig. 1.9*	Usually normal lung volumes. May be diffuse or patchy air-space shadowing.	Causes include bleeding diathesis, vasculitis including Wegener granulomatosis, following surfactant therapy in neonates and idiopathic (acute idiopathic pulmonary hemosiderosis).
Near drowning ▷ *Fig. 1.10*	Appearance as ARDS.	May be considered a form of ARDS. Air-space shadowing may reflect aspiration of water resulting in permeability edema ("wet drowning") or negative pressure edema due to prolonged laryngospasm ("dry drowning"). Infective pneumonia may complicate.
HMD ▷ *Fig. 1.1, p. 5*	Low lung volumes due to microatelectasis, reticulogranular opacities: air bronchograms may be present.	In premature neonates (see previous sections).

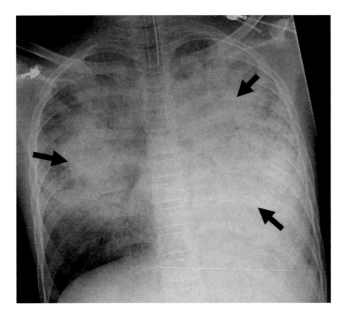

Fig. 1.9   Pulmonary hemorrhage. Chest radiograph in a 13-year-old girl requiring ventilation for atypical pneumonia who developed frank hemoptysis, with hemosiderin-laden macrophages on bronchoalveolar lavage. There is widespread, but patchy air-space shadowing (arrows) that is more extensive on the left.

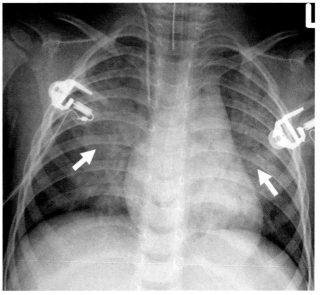

Fig. 1.10   Pulmonary edema in near drowning. Chest radiograph in a 2-year-old child found unconscious in a pond. There is bilateral central air-space shadowing (arrows).

Diffuse Peribronchial Opacification

Peribronchial opacification is a common finding in pediatric chest radiology, particularly in younger children. There appears to be a greater propensity for respiratory infections to involve small- and medium-sized airways in younger children. Smaller airway luminal size means peribronchial thickening often results in airway obstruction, usually manifest as air trapping.

Table 1.7 Diffuse peribronchial opacification

Diagnosis	Findings	Comments
Viral pneumonia/bronchiolitis ▷ *Fig. 1.11*	Peribronchial thickening particularly in hilar regions. Airway obstruction results in varying degrees of diffuse air trapping, patchy air trapping, and areas of atelectasis.	The distinctions between viral bronchitis, bronchiolitis, and bronchopneumonia are arbitrary. Common viral agents include respiratory syncytial virus (RSV), influenza, parainfluenza, adenoviruses, and enteroviruses. Recent evidence suggests that age is a better predictor of radiographic pattern than infecting organism: peribronchial opacities and lung hyperaeration are more common in infants, and alveolar opacities are more common in the older child.
Mycoplasma pneumonia	May mimic viral pneumonitis. The classic pattern is segmental or lobar interstitial changes (relatively specific feature) progressing to air-space shadowing. Hilar nodal enlargement in minority.	Common in school-aged children, accounts for up to 30% of childhood pneumonias.
Bronchial asthma	Seventy-five percent of radiographs in acute asthma will demonstrate peribronchial thickening and hyperaeration. Focal infiltrates and atelectasis in 25%. In chronic asthma, similar changes may be present in approximately 20%.	Be aware of asthma mimics. Conditions commonly mislabelled as asthma in children include CF, constrictive obliterative bronchiolitis, chronic foreign body aspiration, vascular ring, mediastinal mass, and tracheal mass lesion.
CF ▷ *Fig. 1.12a, b*	Milder cases may demonstrate peribronchial thickening as only abnormality and may simulate other conditions causing peribronchial thickening.	Should be considered in any child with recurrent respiratory problems.
Bronchiectasis ▷ *Fig. 1.12a, b* ▷ *Fig. 1.31, p. 24*	CXR: tram-track and ring shadows in areas of involvement on plain radiograph, with bronchial dilatation (airway larger than accompanying pulmonary artery). HRCT: for definitive diagnosis.	CF most common cause. Postinfectious causes now rare since pertussis and measles vaccination introduced. Primary immunodeficiencies, primary ciliary dyskinesia, allergic bronchopulmonary aspergillosis, amongst other causes.
Pulmonary venous hypertension ▷ *Fig. 1.6, p. 7* ▷ *Fig. 1.7, p. 8*	May simulate viral infection. Large heart may be present. Septal lines suggestive but rare. Small effusions, larger on the right, often present.	In neonate and infants, frequently due to large left-to-right shunts. In older children, consider myocarditis and dilated cardiomyopathy.
TTN ▷ *Fig. 1.2, p. 5*	Normal or mildly increased lung volumes. Diffuse mild predominantly reticular opacification. Small pleural effusions common. May simulate HMD, MAS, or neonatal pneumonia, but unlike these clears rapidly (1–2 d).	In neonates only.

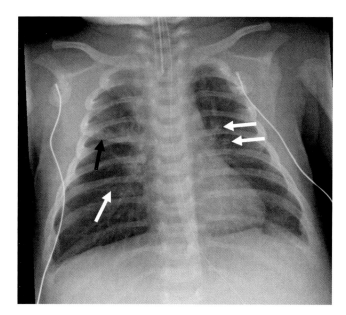

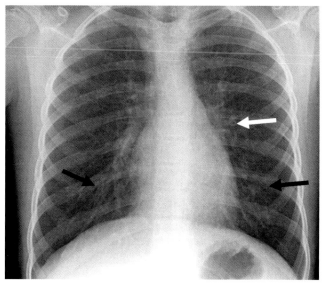

a

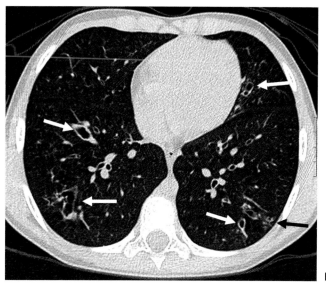

b

Fig. 1.11   RSV bronchiolitis. Chest radiograph of a 4-week-old girl with RSV-positive bronchiolitis. The lungs are overinflated. There is a diffuse peribronchial infiltrate (white arrows), with upward bowing of the horizontal fissure indicating early right upper lobe (RUL) collapse (black arrow)

Fig. 1.12a, b   Cystic fibrosis. (a) Chest radiograph in a 10-year-old girl with known CF. There is lung overinflation with diaphragmatic flattening. There is some mild central bronchial wall thickening (white arrow) and some subtle ring and tram-track opacities in the basal regions (black arrows). **(b)** HRCT in the same patient. There is diffuse mild bronchiectasis (white arrows). There are some subtle centrilobular nodularities (black arrow) representing areas of small airways mucus plugging.

Reticulonodular Opacification

A reticulonodular pattern (i.e., one consisting of discrete nodular and linear opacities) is typically due to disease of the pulmonary interstitium. The exact pattern depends on the distribution of changes. Thickening of the peribronchovascular interstitium results in peribronchial thickening centrally, but peripherally results in branching nodular opacities. Thickening of the interlobular septa results in septal lines: these may appear as vertically oriented lines in the upper zones, horizontally oriented lines in the lung periphery, or diffuse spidery lines throughout the lungs. Lung reticulation on a radiograph may also result from cystic change due to overlapping cyst walls, as in diffuse cystic lung diseases, from end-stage fibrotic changes ("honeycombing"), and from overlapping bronchial walls in severe bronchiectasis.

Table 1.8   Reticulonodular opacification

Diagnosis	Findings	Comments
HMD	(see section on diffuse neonatal lung disease)	
Neonatal pneumonia		
TTN		
Pulmonary lymphangiectasia ▷ *Fig. 1.4, p. 6*	Interstitial pattern often with septal lines. Pleural effusions very common and often large.	Primary pulmonary lymphangiectasia usually presents in neonatal period and is frequently fatal. May be secondary to congenital heart disease, particularly anomalous pulmonary venous connection, or following lymphatic injury, usually surgical. Also associated with Turner and Noonan syndromes.
Viral pneumonitis ▷ *Fig. 1.11, p. 11*	Peribronchial thickening the norm.	
Mycoplasma pneumonia	Patchy or unifocal interstitial infiltrate, often with hilar adenopathy.	
Pulmonary venous hypertension ▷ *Fig. 1.6, p. 7*	Transient appearance of interstitial pulmonary edema, with or without septal lines, often coexisting with central alveolar opacities.	
Bronchopulmonary dysplasia (BPD) ▷ *Fig. 1.13*	CXR: The classic form appears as "bubbly lungs" with an irregular pseudocystic appearance. In the "new" form, the chest radiograph may reveal only diffuse ground-glass opacity, a more uniform interstitial pattern, or a "bubbly" pattern with smaller, more uniformly sized bubbles. HRCT: Classic features include triangular subpleural and septal thickening and fibrosis, with patchy areas of air trapping. Changes may be more diffuse in "new" form.	A complication of prematurity. Two forms described: classic BPD occurs in children with prolonged positive pressure ventilation ± high inspired oxygen concentrations. "New" BPD probably reflects use of lower pressure ventilation strategies and surfactant therapy, and more reflects pulmonary immaturity in very-low-birth-weight infants rather than effects of barotrauma and oxygen toxicity. The previously described Mikity Wilson syndrome, whereby BPD-like changes developed in nonventilated premature infants, is probably the same condition as new-type BPD.
Langerhans cell histiocytosis (LCH) ▷ *Fig. 1.14* ▷ *Fig. 1.27, p. 21*	Nodular opacities ranging from 1 to 10 mm. Cystic changes may reflect pneumatocele formation due to bronchiolar involvement, or cystic degeneration of nodules. Pneumothorax common.	Lung involvement present in approximately 10% at presentation, and up to half with multiorgan involvement.
Interstitial lung disease: other	(see section on HRCT of interstitial lung disease)	
Leukemia	May be air-space or interstitial, diffuse, or localized.	Particularly with acute monocytic leukemia. May be first manifestation and may worsen with induction chemotherapy. Changes at least partly due to pulmonary hemorrhage.
Pulmonary fibrosis ▷ *Fig. 1.15*	"Honeycomb" pattern with volume loss.	The end stage of a variety of interstitial processes.
Pulmonary veno-occlusive disease ▷ *Fig. 1.16a, b, p. 14*	Pulmonary arterial dilatation with smooth interlobular septal thickening, small pleural effusions, and patchy ground-glass attenuation on CT. Hilar adenopathy may also be present. Combination of pulmonary arterial dilatation and smooth septal thickening is highly specific.	A postcapillary counterpart to primary pulmonary hypertension. Very poor prognosis.

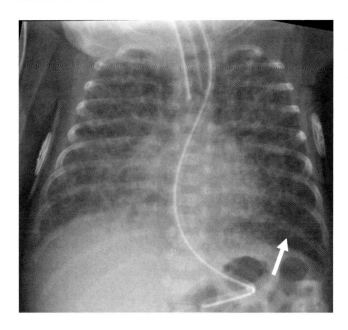

Fig. 1.13 Bronchopulmonary dysplasia. Chest radiograph in a 3-month-old infant born at 24 weeks' gestation, requiring prolonged ventilation. There is a diffuse "bubbly-lung" appearance due to summation of coarse interstitial opacities, and generalized lung overinflation with left basal hypertransradiancy (white arrow).

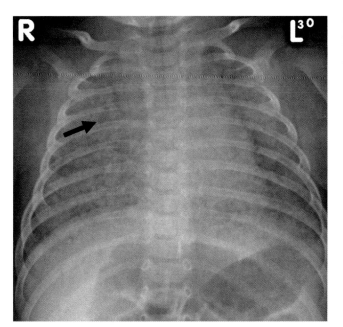

Fig. 1.14 Langerhans cell histiocytosis. Chest radiograph in a 3-month-old boy with lethargy and a lytic lesion in the left femur. There is a diffuse coarse reticulonodular infiltrate with one or two subtle areas of cavitation (arrow). (See also **Fig. 1.27**, a CT of the same child.)

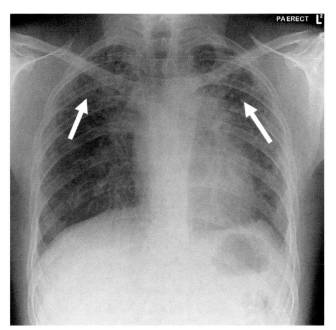

Fig. 1.15 Apical lung fibrosis due to drug reaction. Chest radiograph in an 8-year-old child who underwent conditioning with busulphan 5 years previously for BMT as treatment of relapsed acute myeloid leukaemia. There is apical lung reticulation (arrows) with volume loss evidenced by bilateral hilar elevation.

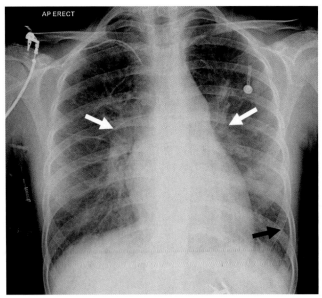

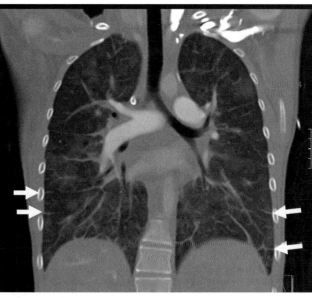

a

b

Fig. 1.16a, b   Pulmonary veno-occlusive disease. (a) Chest radiograph in a 12-year-old girl with progressive breathlessness, weight loss, and pulmonary hypertension. The central pulmonary arteries are enlarged (white arrows). There is extensive linear opacification with septal lines (black arrow). **(b)** Coronally reformatted CT image in the same patient demonstrates numerous thickened interlobular septa (white arrows). The diagnosis of pulmonary veno-occlusive disease was confirmed at postmortem examination.

Cystic Lung Disease

This category covers the radiographic appearance of diffuse rounded lucencies in the lungs: these may represent cysts or features that merely simulate a cystic appearance ("pseudocystic"; see also the section on focal lung lucencies).

Table 1.9   True cystic diseases

Diagnosis	Findings	Comments
LCH ▷ *Fig. 1.27, p. 21*	Nodules usually also present. Cysts reflect cavitation of nodules or pneumatocele formation.	Lung involvement present in approximately 10% at presentation, and up to half with multiorgan involvement.
Tuberous sclerosis	Multiple thin-walled cysts, usually small. Interstitial fibrosis in established cases. Chylothorax common.	Indistinguishable from lymphangioleiomyomatosis, with very similar pathogenesis of smooth muscle proliferation in bronchiolar walls.
Lymphangioleiomyomatosis	Thin-walled, randomly scattered cysts with normal intervening parenchyma. Associated chylothorax.	Females of childbearing age only. Exceedingly rare in children.
BPD ▷ *Fig. 1.13, p. 13*	Not true cysts, but areas of profound air trapping mixed with fibrotic bands producing "bubbly lungs."	In premature infants, usually those who required intubation and oxygen therapy.
Pulmonary interstitial emphysema ▷ *Fig. 1.52, p. 36*	Tubulocystic lucencies radiating from hilum. Not true cysts but areas of interstitial gas. Usually transient and diffuse, but may be localized, and may be persistent.	Usually occurs in premature neonates, usually in first week of life. Also occurs with increased frequency in hypoplastic lungs or in the presence of interstitial lung disease. Frequently associated with or precedes pnuemothorax or pneumomediastinum. Predicts development of BPD.
Bronchiectasis	Not true cysts, but saccular changes may simulate cysts.	CF most common cause. Postinfectious now rare since pertussis and measles vaccination introduced. Primary immunodeficiencies, primary ciliary dyskinesia, allergic bronchopulmonary aspergillosis, amongst other causes.
Multiple pneumatoceles	Usually localized, but occasionally multifocal, particularly following hydrocarbon ingestion (see section on focal lung lucencies).	
Multiple cavitating lesions	(see section on multiple cavitating lesions)	Such as granulomas or metastases.

Nodular Opacification: Miliary Pattern

A miliary pattern refers to diffuse small nodules that are 1 to 2 mm in size, named as such because they resemble millet seeds.

Table 1.10   Miliary patterns

Diagnosis	Findings	Comments
Miliary tuberculosis (TB) ▷ *Fig. 1.17a–c*	Discrete small nodules or "snowstorm" appearance, often with lymphadenopathy. Distinct appearance from endobronchially disseminated TB, which shows multiple centrilobular, tree-in-bud opacities.	Usually within 6 months of primary infection. Reflects hematogenous dissemination of primary infection. Liver, spleen, and brain may also be involved.
Histoplasmosis ▷ *Fig. 1.44, p. 31*	May simulate miliary TB. Resolves into multiple punctate calcifications after 9–24 mo.	Rare in nonendemic areas.
Metastatic disease	May exactly simulate miliary TB: may also have "snowstorm" appearance.	Usually thyroid carcinoma, most commonly papillary and follicular.
LCH ▷ *Fig. 1.14, p. 13*	Nodules often variable in size with coexistent cysts.	Lung involvement present in approximately 10% at presentation, and up to half with multiorgan involvement.

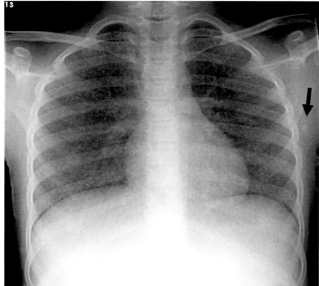

a

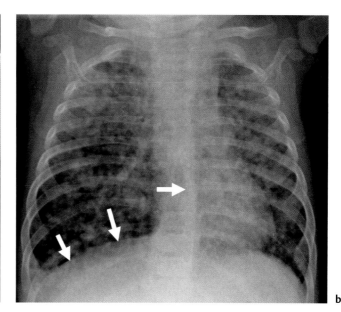

b

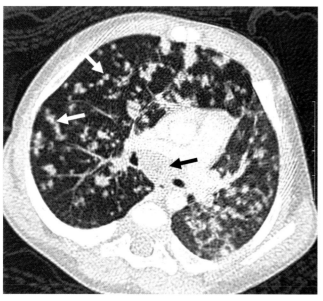

c

Fig. 1.17a–c   Disseminated TB. (a) Miliary TB. Chest radiograph in an 8-year-old child with TB meningitis. There are numerous small nodules throughout the lungs. Calcified lymph nodes are present in the left axilla (arrow). **(b)** Disseminated endobronchial TB with nodal partial obstruction of bronchus intermedius. Chest radiograph in a 6-month-old with prolonged fever and progressive respiratory distress. There is a diffuse, coarse nodular pattern throughout the lungs. The right middle and lower lobes are overinflated (arrows). **(c)** Disseminated TB with nodal partial obstruction of bronchus intermedius. CT of the same 6-month-old child shows numerous branching centrilobular nodules ("tree-in-bud" pattern, white arrows) with a large subcarinal nodal mass (black arrow) causing narrowing of the bronchus intermedius with air trapping. TB was isolated from gastric washings.

Generalized Patchy Opacification

Table 1.11   Generalized patchy opacification

Diagnosis	Findings	Comments
Bronchopneumonia ▷ *Fig. 1.18*	Irregularly distributed alveolar opacities. May be bilateral and diffuse or localized.	Unusual with pneumococcus. Occurs in staphylococcal, *Haemophilus influenzae*, pertussis, mycoplasma, and viral pneumonias.
Aspiration pneumonitis ▷ *Fig. 1.23, p. 20*	Opacities more commonly right-sided and in dependent lung regions: posterior segments upper lobes, apical, and posterior basal segments of lower lobes.	Aspiration may be from below (i.e., related to reflux) or from above (impaired swallow, tracheoesophageal fistula, meconium aspiration).
Pulmonary vasculitis ▷ *Fig. 1.24, p. 21*	Patchy or diffuse air-space opacification, occasionally ill-defined nodules. May develop cavitation.	Changes may reflect patchy pulmonary hemorrhage or inflammatory change. Examples include Wegener granulomatosis and Goodpasture syndrome.
Acute/subacute extrinsic allergic alveolitis	CXR: Acute: patchy, often subtle air-space opacities. Subacute: patchy often reticulonodular pattern. HRCT: centrilobular nodules and patchy ground-glass attenuation.	Known exposure to precipitating antigen and presence of serum precipitins to antigen make diagnosis,
LCH	Often with more discrete nodular densities and cyst formation.	
Hodgkin disease	Most commonly nodular, extending from mediastinum along peribronchovascular lymphatics. Pneumonic form shows patchy nonsegmental infiltrates. Usually with ipsilateral hilar/mediastinal nodal enlargement.	Non-Hodgkin lymphoma (NHL), where pulmonary involvement often occurs without nodal involvement.
Sarcoidosis	With or without bilateral hilar enlargement and right paratracheal lymphadenopathy. Variable pattern.	Lung involvement very rare in preteenaged children.
Idiopathic pulmonary hemosiderosis	Patchy alveolar opacities acutely during episodes of hemoptysis and pulmonary hemorrhage. Eventually develops reticular pattern followed in some by features of established fibrosis.	Clinical triad is of iron deficiency anemia, episodic hemoptysis, and patchy infiltrates on CXR.
Löffler syndrome	Rapidly changing "migratory" infiltrates.	An allergic reaction to a variety of insults, classically parasitic infection but also drugs.
Posttransplant lymphoproliferative disorder (PTLD)	Patchy air-space opacification a rarely reported pattern in PTLD. Hard to distinguish from rejection in lung transplant recipient.	Most common after thoracic (heart, lung, heart/lung) transplantation, but may occur with any transplant. Other thoracic manifestations include multiple nodules (most common), solitary pulmonary nodule, and mediastinal adenopathy.

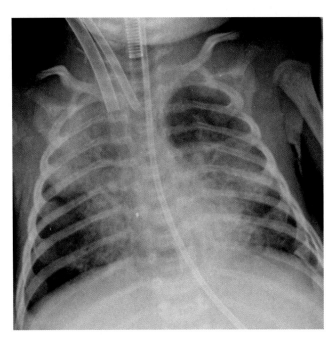

Fig. 1.18   Bronchopneumonia: pertussis. Chest radiograph in a 2-month-old infant with severe respiratory failure requiring venoarterial ECMO, later proven to be due to *Bordetella pertussis*. There are patchy coarse air-space infiltrates in the right middle lobe (RML), left lower lobe, lingula, and RUL.

Diffuse Hypertransradiancy

This is a relatively common pattern in children and generally implies diffuse air trapping due to valvelike obstruction of medium and small airways.

Table 1.12   Diffuse hypertransradiancy

Diagnosis	Findings	Comments
Bronchiolitis/viral lower respiratory tract infection ▷ *Fig. 1.11, p. 11*	Diffuse peribronchial opacities, large lung volumes with diaphragmatic flattening. There may be areas of subsegmental, segmental, or lobar atelectasis.	Common viral agents include RSV, influenza, parainfluenza, adenoviruses, and enteroviruses (see section on peribronchial opacification).
Bronchial asthma	In majority with acute asthma, minority with chronic steroid-maintained asthma.	Remember asthma mimics: CF, constrictive obliterative bronchiolitis, chronic foreign body aspiration, vascular ring, mediastinal mass, and tracheal mass lesion.
CF ▷ *Fig. 1.12, p. 11*	Evidence of bronchiectasis, relative volume loss in the upper lobes, and overall lung overinflation due to air trapping from small and large airway disease.	
Meconium aspiration syndrome ▷ *Fig. 1.3, p. 5*	Neonates only.	(see **Table 1.1**)
Cardiac failure (cardiac asthma) ▷ *Fig. 1.7, p. 8*	Peribronchial edema often results in air trapping. Heart may be enlarged.	
Pulmonary oligemia ▷ *Fig. 1.19*	Attenuated vessels, lung volumes usually normal. Cardiac contour may be abnormal.	In right heart congenital heart disease: tetralogy of Fallot, pulmonary atresia, Ebstein anomaly.

(continues on page 18)

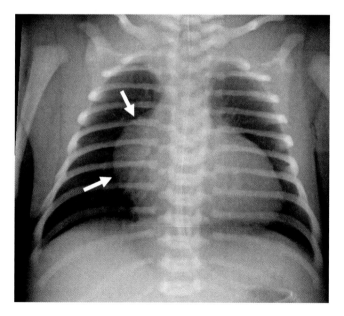

Fig. 1.19   Ebstein anomaly with pulmonary oligaemia. Chest radiograph in a neonate with cyanosis. The heart is enlarged, particularly the right atrial contour (arrows). The lungs are markedly oligemic with attenuated vasculature throughout. Echocardiography confirmed Ebstein anomaly.

Table 1.12   (Cont.) Diffuse hypertransradiancy

Diagnosis	Findings	Remarks
BPD ▷ *Fig. 1.13, p. 13*	Classic BPD: large lung volumes with multiple small, rounded, cystic lucencies, with intervening irregular opacity. CT findings: reticular opacities, areas of atelectasis, reduced bronchoarterial ratios, areas of hypertransradiancy, triangular subpleural opacities.	Pattern of BPD is changing with more effective treatment of RDS/HMD. "New" pattern BPD shows more diffuse interstitial changes with less pronounced cystic lucencies.
Chronic aspiration pneumonitis	Recurrent, migratory segmental opacities progressing to fibrotic changes. Peribronchial fibrosis may result in air trapping.	Aspiration either from above (unsafe swallow, tracheo-esophageal fistula) or below (reflux-related).
Constrictive obliterative bronchiolitis ▷ *Fig. 1.20a, b* ▷ *Fig. 1.68, p. 45*	CXR: May be normal. Diffuse overinflation with attenuated vascularity common. May be associated with large airway changes (bronchiectasis). Asymmetric involvement produces a relatively hyperlucent lung: the Swyer-James-Macleod syndrome. HRCT: Mosaic attenuation that is accentuated on expiratory sections. Centrilobular nodules with tree-in-bud pattern frequent.	Numerous causes: most common are postinfectious, particularly adenovirus and mycoplasma, connective tissue diseases, chronic lung transplant rejection, graft-versus-host disease following bone marrow transplant (BMT), post toxic fume inhalation, and idiopathic.
Extrinsic tracheobronchial compression ▷ *Fig. 1.21*	(see Table 1.51)	
Two lobe congenital lobar overinflation (CLO) ▷ *Fig. 1.22a–c*	Usually left upper and right middle lobe.	Up to 5% of CLO involves two lobes.
High ventilation pressures ▷ *Fig. 1.21*	Child intubated or on continuous positive airway pressure.	Position of diaphragms on radiograph may be used to guide pressure management, particularly with high-frequency oscillator therapy.

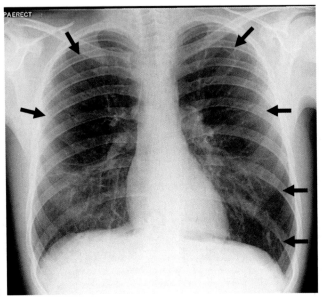

a

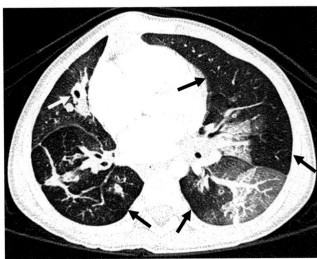

b

Fig. 1.20a, b   Constrictive obliterative bronchiolitis. (a) Chest radiograph in a 14-year-old boy with respiratory failure and prior adenovirus infection. There are extensive areas of hypertransradiancy with attenuated vessels in both lungs (arrows). **(b)** Expiratory CT section in same child demonstrates areas of hypertransradiancy (black arrows) indicating extensive air trapping. There are a few areas of mild bronchial dilatation (white arrow). This child underwent successful lung transplantation. Obliterative changes in bronchioles confirmed at histologic examination of explanted lungs.

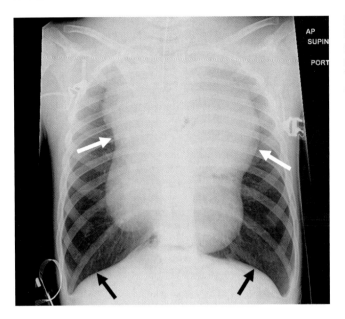

Fig. 1.21   Air trapping due to mediastinal mass. Chest radiograph in an 8-year-old boy requiring ventilation for respiratory distress. There is a large anterior mediastinal mass (white arrows). There is profound air trapping with very marked diaphragmatic flattening (black arrows). This improved with prone positioning. Histologic diagnosis was of T-cell type acute lymphoblastic leukemia.

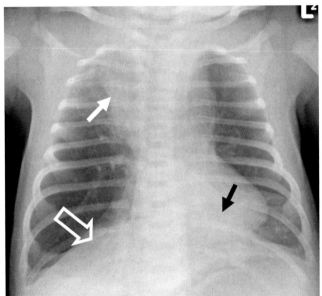

a

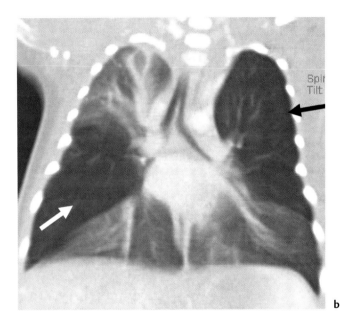

b

Fig. 1.22a–c   Congenital lobar overinflation involving two lobes. (**a**) Chest radiograph in an 8-week-old boy with progressive respiratory distress. There is overinflation of the right middle and left upper lobes (LULs), with compressive atelectasis of the RUL (white arrow), left lower lobe (black arrow), and right lower lobe (open arrow). (**b**) Coronally reformatted CT in the same patient showing hypertransradiancy of right middle (white arrow) and LULs (black arrow). The lingula was spared. (**c**) Ventilation (right) and perfusion (left) scintigrams in same patient showing nonventilated and perfused right middle (black arrows) and LULs (white arrows). The child had an excellent outcome following surgical resection of the overinflated lobes.

c

High-Resolution Computed Tomography of Diffuse Interstitial Lung Disease in Children

Interstitial lung disease in children is rare.

Table 1.13   HRCT of diffuse interstitial lung disease in children

Diagnosis	Findings	Comments
Aspiration pneumonitis ▷ *Fig. 1.23a, b*	Often nonspecific infiltrates progressing to established fibrosis and/or obliterative bronchiolitis. Typically involves dependent lung regions: apical and posterior basal segment so lower lobes.	Aspiration either from above (unsafe swallow, tracheo-esophageal fistula) or below (reflux-related).
Nonspecific interstitial pneumonitis (NSIP) ▷ *Fig. 1.24*	Share common CT appearances. Widespread ground-glass attenuation. In NSIP, upper zone honeycombing has been reported.	NSIP: probably underrecognized in children.
Desquamative interstitial pneumonitis (DIP)		DIP: Rare, usually In under-1-y-olds. Higher mortality than adult form.
Lymphoid interstitial pneumonitis (LIP)		LIP: strong association with immunodeficiency states and connective tissue diseases.
Chronic pneumonitis of infancy ▷ *Fig. 1.25*	Diffuse ground-glass change, interlobular septal thickening, and discrete centrilobular nodules described on HRCT.	Occurs exclusively in young infants. Children usually well at birth, with progressive respiratory symptoms starting from age 1–9 mo, resulting in death.
Systemic sclerosis/juvenile dermatomyositis ▷ *Fig. 1.26*	Features in order of decreasing frequency: ground-glass opacities, subpleural modularity, linear opacities, and honeycombing.	Lung involvement common in pediatric disease. Similar pattern to NSIP.
Alveolar proteinosis	Characteristic feature is diffuse ground glass with superimposed pattern of "crazy-paving" thickened interlobular septa. CT findings usually worse than clinical findings.	Congenital form is related to surfactant protein deficiencies and is usually fatal. Idiopathic form reflects disordered surfactant homeostasis: in children has onset from few months to several years of age.
Pulmonary lymphangiomatosis/ lymphangiectasia ▷ *Fig. 1.4, p. 6*	Smooth interlobular septal thickening, peribronchiolar thickening, patchy ground glass. Extrapleural and mediastinal fat shows increased attenuation. Chylous effusions frequent.	Radiologic distinction between lymphangiectasia and lymphangiomatosis usually not possible. Lymphangiectasia may be primary or secondary to cardiac disease or cardiac surgery.
Langerhan cell histiocytosis ▷ *Fig. 1.27*	Multiple nodules 1–3 mm, developing into thin-walled cysts ≤ 10 mm.	
Idiopathic pulmonary hemosiderosis ▷ *Fig. 1.28*	Acute phase: patchy ground glass and consolidation represents areas of hemorrhage. Subacute/chronic phase: Discrete uniform pulmonary nodules throughout the lungs with or without interlobular septal thickening. Occasionally progresses to established fibrotic change.	Unknown etiology. Onset usually before age of 3 y. Presentation with anemia and hemoptysis.

(continues on page 22)

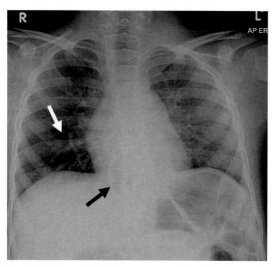
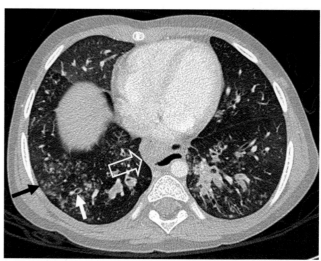

Fig. 1.23a, b   Aspiration pneumonitis. (**a**) Chest radiograph in a 9-year-old boy with cerebral palsy and previous Nissen fundoplication. There is hypertransradiancy in the right lower zone (white arrow). There is a gas-filled viscus above the diaphragm (black arrow). (**b**) Axial CT image in the same child demonstrates extensive hypertransradiancy in the lower lobes in keeping with air trapping, with areas of "tree-in-bud" nodularity indicating small airway plugging (black arrow) and some mild bronchial dilatation (white arrow). The Nissen fundoplication had "slipped" (open arrow), leading to recurrent reflux and aspiration.

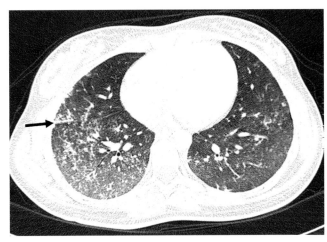

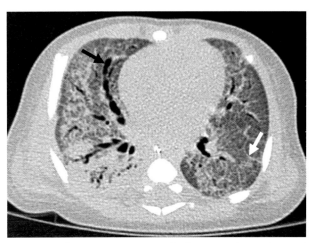

Fig. 1.24 Interstitial pneumonitis. Axial HRCT image in a 14-year-old boy with known Wegener granulomatosis. There are patchy areas of ground-glass attenuation (black arrow) with nodularity and septal thickening.

Fig. 1.25 Chronic pneumonitis of infancy. Axial HRCT image in a 6-week-old infant with progressive respiratory distress and pulmonary hypertension. There is diffuse ground-glass attenuation manifested by the "black bronchus" sign (black arrow) with areas of septal thickening (white arrow). Biopsy confirmed chronic pneumonitis of infancy and the child succumbed.

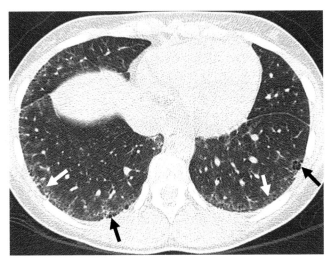

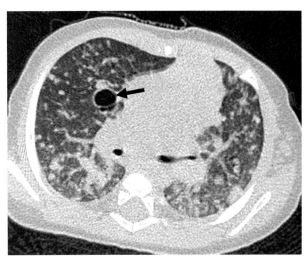

Fig. 1.26 Interstitial pneumonitis in juvenile dermatomyositis. Axial HRCT image in a 13-year-old girl with known juvenile dermatomyositis. There is diffuse basal subpleural ground glass and reticulation (white arrows) with areas of subpleural cyst formation or honeycombing (black arrows).

Fig. 1.27 Langerhans cell histiocytosis. Axial HRCT image in a 7-month-old child with a lytic lesion of the left femur and an abnormal chest radiograph (see **Fig. 1.14**). There are numerous lung nodules with a cavitating lesion in the RUL (arrow). The lung lesions resolved completely with chemotherapy for LCH.

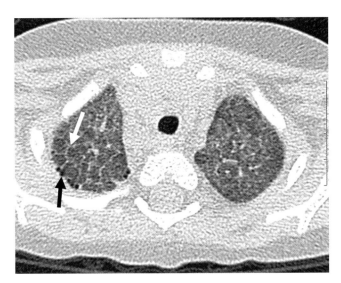

Fig. 1.28 Idiopathic pulmonary hemosiderosis. Axial CT image in a 2-year-old child with Down syndrome and recurrent hemoptysis. There is diffuse ground-glass attenuation, with areas of interlobular septal thickening (white arrow). There are subpleural cysts (black arrow) that may reflect fibrosis, although similar appearing dysplastic lung cysts are also a recognized feature of Down syndrome.

Table 1.13   (Cont.) HRCT of diffuse interstitial lung disease in children

Diagnosis	Findings	Comments
Pulmonary veno-occlusive disease ▷ *Fig. 1.16, p. 14*	Smooth interlobular septal thickening with patchy ground-glass change and effusions, with dilated central pulmonary arteries. Hilar adenopathy is frequently present. Normal appearing pulmonary veins, although transit through lung capillary bed may be prolonged.	Usually fatal without heart-lung transplantation. Unknown etiology, probably immune-mediated response to infection or drugs.
Extrinsic allergic alveolitis	Acute/subacute: diffuse patchy ground-glass attenuation with centrilobular nodules. Chronic: established fibrotic changes.	Most commonly due to inhalation of allergens from birds.
Sarcoidosis	Irregular septal thickening, perilymphatic nodularity resulting in beaded fissures. May progress to established fibrotic changes.	In teenaged children, similar to adults. Preschool form usually spares lungs.

■ Focal/Multifocal Lung Disease

Lobar Opacities

This category covers opacities confined to a lobar distribution, subdivided into lobar opacification without volume loss and lobar collapse.

Table 1.14   Lobar opacification: no volume loss

Diagnosis	Findings	Comments
Lobar pneumonia ▷ *Fig. 1.29*	Lobar opacification with air bronchograms.	Lobar pattern common in *Streptococcus pneumoniae* and *Klebsiella* infections. *Mycoplasma* typically produces lobar interstitial opacification.
Delayed clearance of lung fluid in congenital lobar emphysema.	On initial radiographs, followed by progressive overinflation.	May occur in other bronchpulmonary foregut malformations (e.g., bronchial atresia and CCAM).
Partial anomalous venous return (one lobe only)		Very rare.
Thymus simulating upper lobe consolidation or collapse ▷ *Fig. 1.30a, b*	Usually RUL, often when child rotated to the right. Can see lung markings through thymus. Horizontal lower border with notch at mediastinal border.	Commonly seen in infants. US useful in uncertain cases.

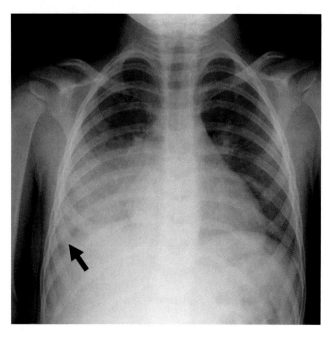

Fig. 1.29   Right lower lobe pneumonia. Chest radiograph in 4-year-old boy with cough, fever, and focal signs at the posterior right lung base. There is right basal consolidation, with preservation of the right heart border and the lateral diaphragmatic contour (arrow), suggesting right lower lobe involvement with sparing of the anterior and lateral basal segments. Blood cultures were positive for *S. pneumoniae*.

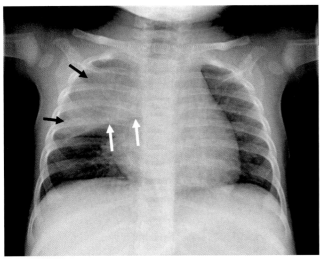
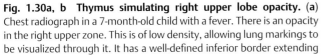
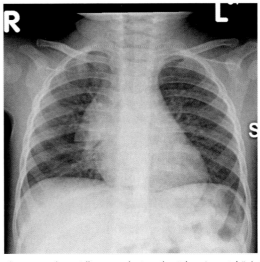

Fig. 1.30a, b Thymus simulating right upper lobe opacity. (a) Chest radiograph in a 7-month-old child with a fever. There is an opacity in the right upper zone. This is of low density, allowing lung markings to be visualized through it. It has a well-defined inferior border extending almost to the midline, producing the "thymic notch" (white arrows). Its lateral margin is undulating and does not quite reach the chest wall (black arrows). **(b)** Follow-up chest radiograph in same child 6 months later shows typical appearance of less enlarged right thymic lobe.

Table 1.15 Lobar collapse

Diagnosis	Findings	Comments
Mucus plugging ▷ *Fig. 1.31a, b, p. 24*	Mucus plugs themselves often not visible on chest radiography, often a diagnosis of exclusion.	In ventilated child, or spontaneously in child with asthma, CF, or other cause of bronchiectasis.
Foreign body aspiration	More typically results in overinflation, either of whole lung or lobe. Atelectasis suggests complete obstruction and may progress to bronchiectasis.	Typically between 6 mo and 3 y of age.
Malpositioned endotracheal tube	Most commonly intubates bronchus intermedius causing RUL and left lung collapse.	Particularly common in neonates as accurate tube placement is challenging.
Cardiomegaly ▷ *Fig. 1.32, p. 24*	Usually left lower lobe collapse due to left atrial enlargement, either isolated or as part of a dilated cardiomyopathy. Also seen following heart transplant when there is a relatively large graft.	Atelectasis may be compressive (i.e., due to direct compression of the lung) or obstructive (i.e., due to compression of lower lobe bronchus).
TB	Lobar or segmental collapse due either to extrinsic nodal compression or endobronchial infection: hilar and mediastinal adenopathy may be present.	Usually a feature of primary infection.
Vascular compression	Most lesions result in tracheal, carinal, or main bronchial compression. Dilated aorta occasionally causes LUL collapse.	
Bronchogenic cyst	Well-defined mass at apex of collapse.	Usually mediastinal and hence trachea, carina, or main bronchi involved.
Endobronchial neoplasm ▷ *Fig. 1.35, p. 26*	Lobulated mass with associated atelectasis, consolidation, or air trapping.	Most commonly bronchial carcinoid or adenoma.
Compressive atelectasis	Cause usually evident.	Due to diaphragmatic hernia, pleural effusion, pneumothroax, congenital lobar emphysema.

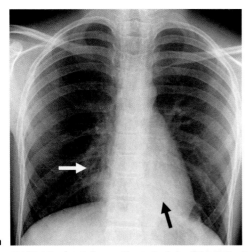
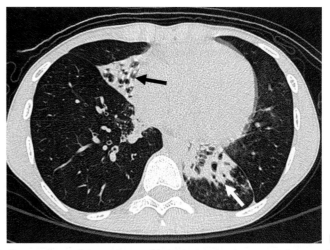

a   b

Fig. 1.31a, b   Lobar collapse in bronchiectasis. (a) Chest radiograph in a 14-year-old child with developmental delay and cough. There is increased retrocardiac density (black arrow) in keeping with segmental collapse of the left lower lobe. The right heart border is effaced in keeping with middle lobe collapse, with ring opacities in this region (white arrow). **(b)** Axial HRCT image in same child demonstrating collapse with bronchial dilatation in the RML (black arrow) and apical segment of the left lower lobe (white arrow).

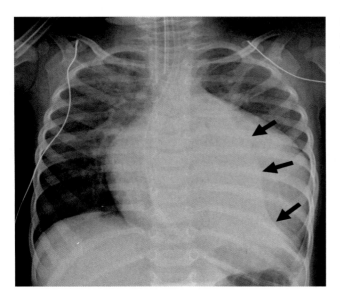

Fig. 1.32   Massive cardiomegaly causing left lower lobe collapse. Chest radiograph in a 14-month-old child with dilated cardiomyopathy. There is gross cardiomegaly with collapse of the left lower lobe (black arrows) due to compression of the left lower lobe bronchus.

Solitary Pulmonary Mass/Masslike Lesion

Solitary pulmonary masses in children are more frequently benign or developmental in origin than in adults. Primary lung malignancy in particular is very rare. Many pulmonary "masses" are not true mass lesions.

Table 1.16   Non-neoplastic mass lesions

Diagnosis	Findings	Comments
Intralobar bronchopulmonary sequestration ▷ *Fig. 1.33*	CXR: solid rounded or triangular opacity at medial lung base, left more commonly than right. CT/MRI: Arterial supply from thoracic aorta, venous drainage usually to pulmonary veins. May be partially air-containing, suggesting previous infection.	No separate pleural covering. Presentation with recurrent infection.
Extralobar bronchopulmonary sequestration ▷ *Fig. 1.34a, b, p. 26*	CXR: solid rounded or triangular opacity in left medial lung base (very rare on right). CT/MRI: Arterial supply from abdominal aorta or branches, venous drainage often systemic (azygous/hemiazygous). Solid appearing in most cases: presence of air suggests esophageal communication.	Antenatal or early postnatal diagnosis in 90%. Separate pleural covering. May occur below diaphragm. Frequent associated anomalies: diaphragmatic hernia, congenital heart disease, other bronchopulmonary foregut malformations.
Intrapulmonary bronchogenic cyst	Usually rounded, fluid density lesion, 1–6 cm in size. Air-fluid level usually implies current or recent infection. May cause airway obstruction resulting in collapse or air trapping.	Two to twenty percent of bronchogenic cysts are intrapulmonary: may reflect migration of mediastinal cyst.
Lung abscess	CXR: Appearances often of discrete consolidation. May develop air-fluid level. CT: shows a thick, well-defined, enhancing wall.	When air-filled, may simulate pneumatocele or cavitary necrosis: these lack a well-defined enhancing wall, however.
Inflammatory pseudotumor ▷ *Fig. 1.35a, b, p. 26*	Variably sized, often peripheral lesion. Up to 25% calcified. Occasionally causes airway obstruction.	Synonyms include plasma cell granuloma, inflammatory myofibroblastic pseudotumor, fibrous histiocytoma, and xanthogranuloma. Usually children older than 5 y. May be locally invasive but does not metastasize.
Granuloma	Often centrally calcified nodules < 3 cm in size. Show no growth over time.	Usually infective in origin: primary TB, histoplasmosis. Other causes: chronic foreign body (e.g., talc), sarcoidosis.
Hydatid cyst	Usually lower lobes. Typically well-defined rounded mass, ≤ 20 cm in diameter, with rapid increase in size. Communication with bronchial tree results in various patterns of cyst collapse.	Solitary lesions in 75%. Often asymptomatic. Casoni test positive in only 60%.
Pulmonary arteriovenous malformation	Usually lower lobes. Usually well-defined rounded or lobulated mass. Feeding/draining vessels may appear as cordlike bands radiating from hilum to mass. CT accurate in diagnosis.	Solitary in one-third. Only 10% manifest in childhood.

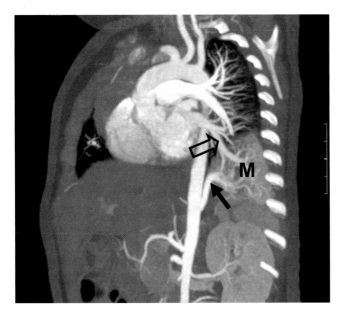

Fig. 1.33   Interloper bronchopulmonary sequestration. Sagittal oblique maximal intensity projection image from CT dataset in neonate with antenatal diagnosis of congenital cystic adenomatoid malformation. There is a left lower lobe mass (M) with systemic arterial supply from the abdominal aorta (black arrow) and venous drainage via the inferior pulmonary vein (open arrow).

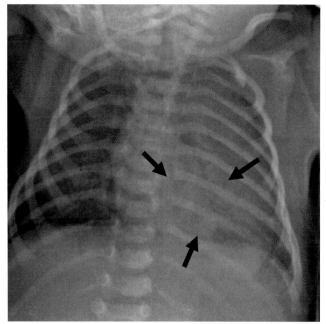

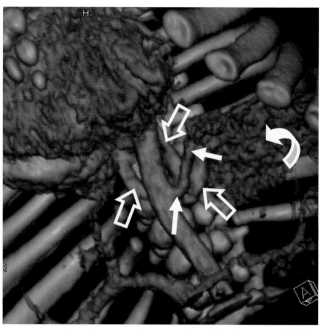

a

b

Fig. 1.34a, b Extralobar bronchopulmonary sequestration. (a) Chest radiograph in a neonate with antenatally diagnosed lung malformation. There is an ill-defined mass in the retrocardiac region (arrows). (b) Volume-rendered tomographic image from CT dataset in same neonate shows a left lower lobe mass (curved arrow) with arterial supply from the lower thoracic aorta (white arrows) and systemic venous drainage via the azygous system (open arrows).

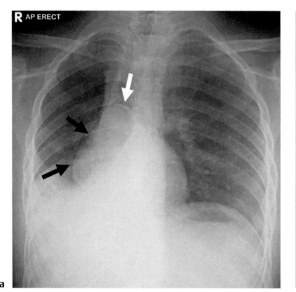

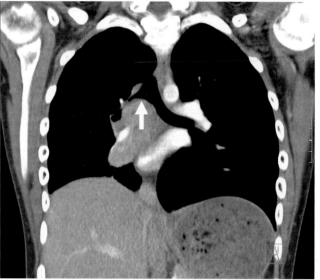

a

b

Fig. 1.35a, b Inflammatory pseudotumor. (a) Chest radiograph in a 15-year-old boy with breathlessness. There is a large soft-tissue mass (black arrows) that abuts the carina and right main bronchus (white arrow). This is causing right lower lobe collapse. (b) Coronally reformatted CT image in same child shows the mass bulging into carina (arrow) and occluding the right main bronchus.

Table 1.17   Neoplastic pulmonary lesions

Diagnosis	Findings	Comments
Solitary pulmonary metastasis ▷ *Fig. 1.36a, b*	Usually well-defined, rounded or lobulated, and soft-tissue attenuation on CT. Distinction from benign nodules difficult and may require biopsy.	Common primaries include Wilms tumor, osteo-sarcoma, germ cell tumor (GCT), Ewing sarcoma, hepatoblastoma.
Bronchial carcinoid	Often central, endobronchial mass causing airway obstruction. Seventy-five percent in lobar bronchi, 10% in mainstem bronchi, and 15% peripheral. Twenty-five percent calcified, particularly central lesions.	Rarely causes carcinoid syndrome.
Bronchogenic carcinoma	Central mass with bronchial obstruction. Occasionally peripheral lesion.	Very rare. Undifferentiated carcinoma, bronchoalveolar carcinoma, and squamous cell carcinoma are most common histologic types. Poor prognosis: median survival 7 mo.
Pleuropulmonary blastoma ▷ *Fig. 1.37, p. 28*	Mixed solid and cystic lesion often in subpleural location.	Possible relationship to congenital cystic lung lesions in some cases. Aggressive with poor prognosis.
Hamartoma	Usually smooth lobulated mass < 4 cm in lung periphery. Calcification present in up to 20%: "popcorn" pattern specific. Fifty percent contain areas of fat density on CT, a diagnostic feature. Central lesions may be endobronchial and cause airway obstruction.	Most common benign tumor of lung. Usually asymptomatic unless endobronchial (3%–20% of lesions).
Post-transplant lymphoproliferative disorder (PTLD) ▷ *Fig. 1.38a, b, p. 28*	Well-circumscribed nodule 3–5 cm in diameter, often without mediastinal/hilar nodal enlargement.	Most common after thoracic (heart, lung, heart/lung) transplantation, but may complicate any transplant. Other thoracic manifestations include multiple nodules (most common), patchy air-space opacification, and mediastinal adenopathy.

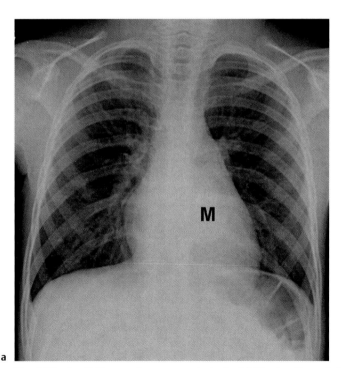
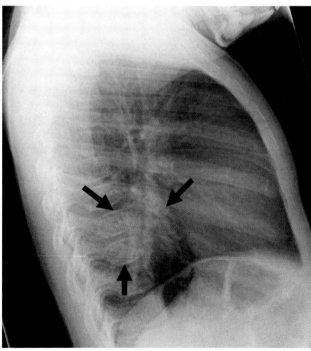

a   b

Fig. 1.36a, b   Solitary pulmonary metastasis. (**a**) Chest radiograph in a 6-year-old girl with relapsed stage 4 Wilms tumor. There is a large retrocardiac mass (M). (**b**) Lateral view in same child shows subtle mass in left lower lobe (black arrows).

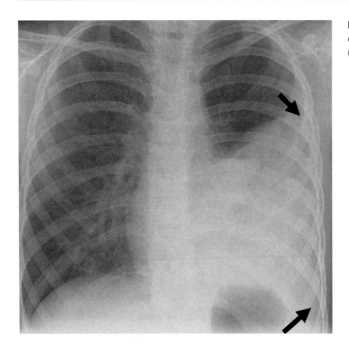

Fig. 1.37 Pleuropulmonary blastema. Chest radiograph in a 7-year-old girl demonstrating a large left basal mass with a broad pleural base (arrows). Biopsy demonstrated pleuropulmonary blastema.

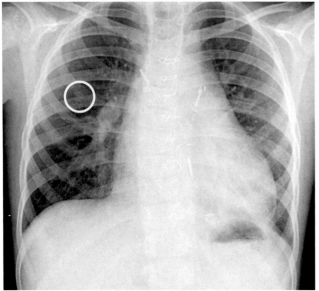

a

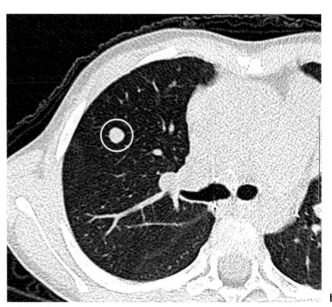

b

Fig. 1.38a, b Post (lung) transplant lymphoproliferative disorder. (a) Routine chest radiograph in a 7-year-old girl 26 months following heart-lung transplant for primary pulmonary hypertension. There is a solitary pulmonary nodule (circled). **(b)** Axial CT image obtained in the same patient, confirming the presence of a solitary pulmonary nodule. The serum Epstein–Barr virus load was elevated, and the lesion disappeared after modulation of the immunosuppressive regime.

Table 1.18   Extrapulmonary thoracic neoplasms

Diagnosis	Findings	Comments
Thoracic neuroblastoma ▷ Fig. 1.39a, b	Posterior/paraspinal mass. May cause rib splaying and destruction with or without intraspinal extension.	Younger age group than adrenal site, with better prognosis.
Ewing sarcoma ▷ Fig. 1.40	Mass centered on and expanding/destroying rib.	Seven percent in older children, but 30% in children younger than 10 y. May simulate fracture, osteomyelitis.
Rhabdomyosarcoma	May be sclerotic or destructive rib lesion.	Older children/adolescents.
Askin tumor	Rib destruction with pleural effusion.	Primitive neuroectodermal tumor (PNET) arising from intercostal nerves (as opposed to Ewing sarcoma, which is a PNET of bone). Usually young Caucasian females.
Metastases		Leukemia and neuroblastoma most common primaries.

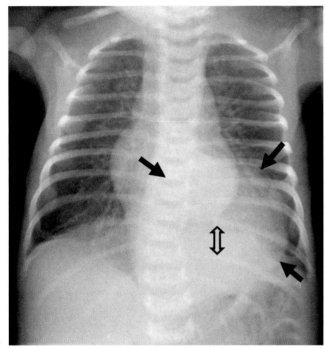

a

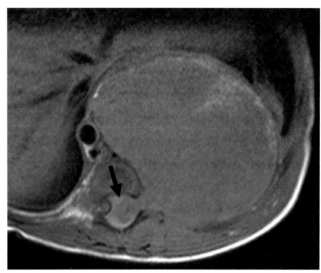

b

Fig. 1.39a, b   Thoracic neuroblastoma. (a) Chest radiograph in a 5-month-old boy demonstrating a large lower thoracic mass (black arrows), which is causing widening of posterior rib spacing (double arrow). **(b)** Thoracic neuroblastoma. Axial T1-weighted MRI in same child demonstrates posterior mediastinal mass with intraspinal extension (arrow).

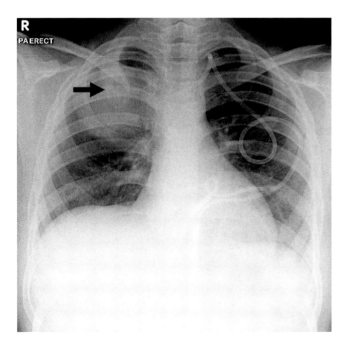

Fig. 1.40   Ewing sarcoma/primitive neuroectodermal tumor (PNET) of the rib. Chest radiograph in a 13-year-old girl with a chest wall mass. There is a soft-tissue mass arising from and expanding the right first rib. Histologic examination showed a PNET.

Table 1.19 "Pseudomass" lesions

Diagnosis	Findings	Comments
Round pneumonia ▷ *Fig. 1.41*	Rounded area of opacification, with or without air bronchograms.	Commonly due to *S. pneumoniae*, occurs in children younger than 8 y. Probably occurs due to immaturity of collateral lung ventilation limiting spread of infection.
Encysted pleural effusion	Elliptical opacity usually in right midzone. Lateral view confirms fissural location.	
Round atelectasis	Rounded area of collapse adjacent to area of pleural abnormality, with characteristic distortion of surrounding vessels.	Rare in children.
Hematoma	A blood-filled traumatic cavity, may persist for months after injury.	
Large mucus plugs in CF ▷ *Fig. 1.42a, b*	Occasionally simulate a mass.	Diagnosis usually known.
Ectopic kidney	Mass anteroinferiorly with rounded upper border, with or without diaphragmatic hernia. More common on the left.	Rare form of ectopia. May also occur with diaphragmatic hernia or following traumatic diaphragmatic injury.

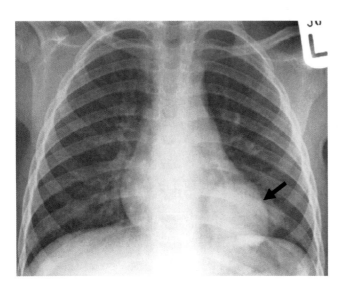

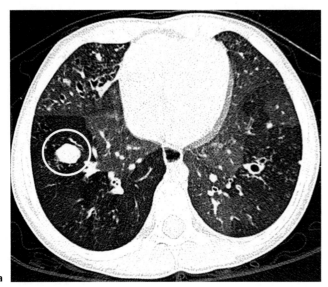

a

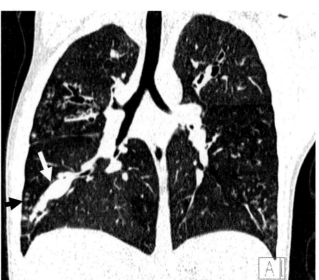

b

Fig. 1.41   Round pneumonia. Chest radiograph in a 4-year-old boy with cough and fever. There is a rounded opacity in the left lower lobe (arrow). This resolved completely following antibiotic therapy.

Fig. 1.42a, b   Mucus plugs in cystic fibrosis. (a) Conventional HRCT image in a 6-year-old girl with known CF. There is a nodular opacity in the right lower lobe within an area of air trapping (arrows). **(b)** Reformatted oblique coronal image from contiguous thin-section multidetector CT in same patient a few weeks later. The nodule is shown to be a large mucus plug within a segmental lower lobe bronchus (white arrow). There are small branching nodules peripheral to this, in keeping with small airway plugging (black arrow).

Multiple Pulmonary Masses

See **Table 1.2**.

Table 1.20   Multiple pulmonary masses

Diagnosis	Findings	Comments
Septic emboli ▷ *Fig. 1.43a, b*	Multiple, often ill-defined round or wedge-shaped opacities, variable size and may cavitate. Nodules may show central poor enhancement prior to cavitation.	Common causes: infected venous catheter, endocarditis, occasionally from staphylococcal osteomyelitis.
LCH ▷ *Fig. 1.14, p. 13* ▷ *Fig. 1.27, p. 21*	Multiple nodules 1–3 mm, developing into thin-walled cysts ≤ 10 mm.	Lung involvement present in approximately 10% at presentation, and up to half with multiorgan involvement.
Granulomatous infection ▷ *Fig. 1.44*	Often a miliary pattern.	Histoplasmosis and TB most common.

(continues on page 32)

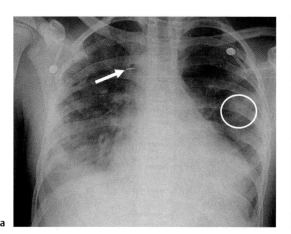 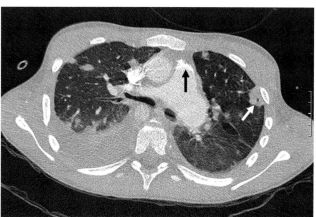

a   b

Fig. 1.43a, b   Septic emboli. (a) Chest radiograph in a 12-year-old boy with a history of treated Fallot tetralogy and fever. There is a right pleural effusion and multifocal consolidation, with a more nodular area in the left midzone (circled). A surgical clip (arrow) is from a previous modified Blalock-Taussig shunt. **(b)** Axial CT image in same patient shows multiple nodules, one showing cavitation (white arrow), and a large right-sided pleural effusion. Note the heavily calcified pulmonary artery homograft (black arrow). This was identified as the source of sepsis.

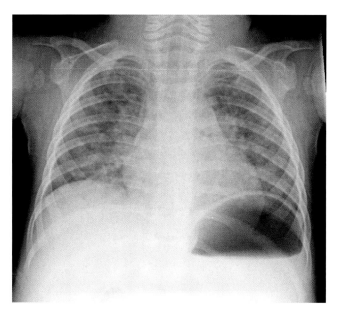

Fig. 1.44   Histoplasmosis. Chest radiograph in a 3-year-old boy from the Philippines with a mild febrile illness, demonstrating multiple, ill-defined pulmonary nodules. Histoplasmosis serology was positive.

Table 1.20 (Cont.) Multiple pulmonary masses

Diagnosis	Findings	Comments
Pulmonary metastases ▷ *Fig. 1.45*	Typically rounded and well defined, randomly distributed in lung periphery, basal predominance. Well-defined lesions more likely to be metastatic than ill-defined or spiculated lesions.	Distribution reflects hematogeneous spread. Distinction from benign causes, even when multiple, not entirely reliable. Wilms tumor and osteosarcoma most common primaries.
Multiple arteriovenous malformations	Multiple round or lobulated masses often with visible feeding/draining vessels radiating from hilum. Lower lobe predominance.	Two-thirds associated with Osler-Weber-Rendu syndrome (hereditary hemorrhagic telangiectasia).
Wegener granulomatosis ▷ *Fig. 1.46*	Multiple often irregular masses of varying sizes, lower lobe predominance. Cavitation frequent with thick walls. May also develop diffuse pulmonary hemorrhage.	Upper respiratory tract involvement present in majority: rhinitis, sinusitis, otitis media, and tracheitis.
Respiratory papillomatosis ▷ *Fig. 1.47a, b*	Usually mixed solid and cystic pulmonary nodules, predominantly in peripheral dependent regions of lungs. Often with associated bronchiectasis.	Human papillomavirus infection of respiratory mucosa. Only 1% of laryngeal papillomatosis spreads to lungs, but prognosis for pulmonary involvement is poor. Malignant degeneration rare but recognized.

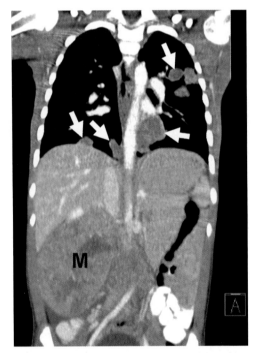

Fig. 1.45 Wilms tumor with pulmonary metastases. Coronally reformatted CT image demonstrating large right renal mass (M) and multiple soft-tissue–dense pulmonary nodules (arrows).

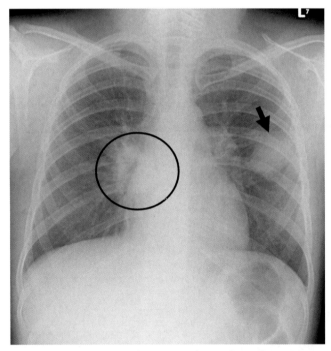

Fig. 1.46 Wegener granulomatosis. Chest radiograph in a 12-year-old girl with known cytoplasmic antineutrophil cytoplasmic antibody–positive vasculitis. There is an obvious nodule in the left midzone (arrow) and a more subtle but large nodule in the right hilar region (circled).

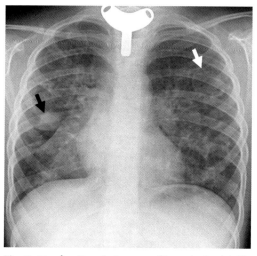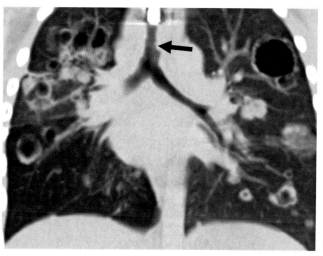

a   b

Fig. 1.47a, b   Respiratory papillomatosis. (a) Chest radiograph in a child with known respiratory papillomatosis. Note the tracheostomy present for laryngeal disease. There are multiple lung lesions, some of which are solid appearing (black arrow) but many of which have cavitated (white arrow). **(b)** Coronally reformatted CT image in same patient demonstrates multiple nodules in varying stages of cavitation. Note the irregularity of tracheal lumen (arrow).

Multiple Cavitating Lesions

Table 1.21   Multiple cavitating lesions

Diagnosis	Findings	Comments
Septic pulmonary emboli ▷ *Fig. 1.43, p. 31*	Multiple nodules with varying degrees of cavitation.	Common causes: infected venous catheter, endocarditis, occasionally from staphylococcal osteomyelitis.
Invasive pulmonary aspergillosis ▷ *Fig. 1.48*	Inflammatory/hemorrhagic nodules progressing to cavitation over 1–2 wk.	Occurs in neutropenic patients, particularly following lung transplantation. Progression to cavitation appears to be relatively rare in children.
Wegener granulomatosis ▷ *Fig. 1.46*	(see **Table 1.20**)	
Laryngotracheobronchial papillomatosis ▷ *Fig. 1.47a, b*	(see **Table 1.20**)	
Cavitating pulmonary metastases		Osteosarcoma metastases most frequently cavitate.
LCH ▷ *Fig. 1.14, p. 13* ▷ *Fig. 1.27, p. 21*	(see previous discussion)	

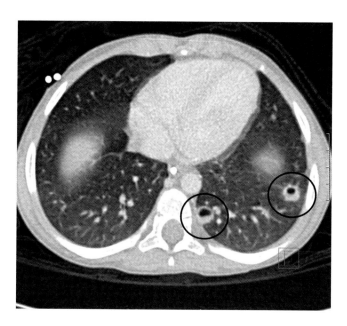

Fig. 1.48   Invasive pulmonary aspergillosis. Axial HRCT image in a 4-year-old child 3 weeks following BMT for primary immunodeficiency. A CT 5 days earlier demonstrated inflammatory nodules with perilesional haloes. The nodules have now cavitated (circled).

Focal Lung Lucencies

Table 1.22 Lobar pattern

Diagnosis	Findings	Comments
Congenital lobar emphysema ▷ *Fig. 1.49a, b*	Progressively overinflated lobe with mass effect, herniates across midline. Attenuated vessels within affected lobe.	LUL in 43%, RML in 35%, RUL in 20%. Two lobes involved in up to 5%. Rare in lower lobes. Most causes due to localized bronchomalacia within lobar bronchus. Occasionally due to extrinsic compression by PDA, dilated pulmonary artery in absent pulmonary valve syndrome, bronchogenic cyst.
Foreign body aspiration ▷ *Fig. 1.65, p. 43*	Lobar overinflation or atelectasis may occur, or even coexist in the same lobe. Foreign body itself rarely radiopaque.	Most common inhaled foreign body is peanut.
Bronchiolitis obliterans	May appear on CXR to involve only one or two lobes; however, CT usually reveals more diffuse abnormality.	
Congenital bronchial atresia ▷ *Fig. 1.50a, b*	Overinflated lobe with opacity at apex of lobe: this represents a fluid-filled bronchocoele distal to the atretic segment.	Asymptomatic in 50%. May simulate congenital lobar inflation.

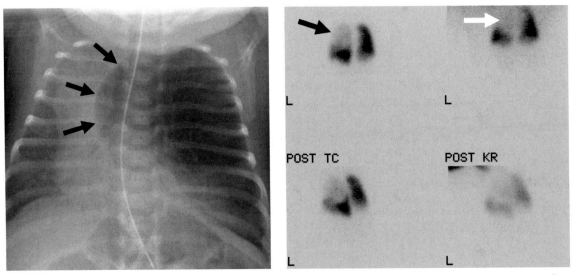

Fig. 1.49a, b   Congenital lobar overinflation. (a) Chest radiograph in a 3-week-old infant with progressive respiratory distress. There is massive overinflation of the LUL, which herniates across the midline (black arrows). The lung markings within the LUL are distorted and attenuated. **(b) Congenital lobar emphysema.** Ventilation/perfusion scintigram in a different child also with LUL congenital lobar emphysema: there is absent perfusion (black arrow) and ventilation (white arrow) of the LUL.

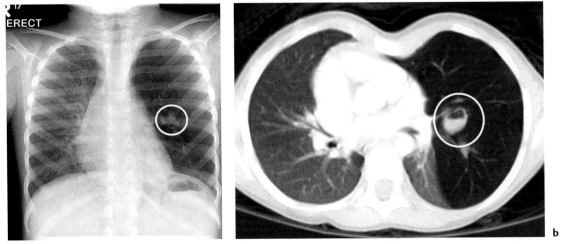

Fig. 1.50a, b   Congenital bronchial atresia. (a) Chest radiograph in a 5-year-old child with mild breathlessness. There is marked hypertransradiancy of the LUL, with a nodular opacity lateral to the hilum (circled). **(b)** Axial CT image in the same child demonstrates hypertransradiancy of the LUL with a rounded structure containing an air-fluid level at the origin of the upper lobe bronchus: this is a bronchocoele, which results from mucoid impaction distal to the atretic segment of bronchus.

Table 1.23   Nonlobar pattern

Diagnosis	Findings	Comments
Congenital cystic adenomatoid malformation ▷ *Fig. 1.51a, b*	Single or multiple usually thin-walled cysts, may have solid components. Larger lesions may exert mass effect. Occasionally show progressive overinflation similar to CLO if a bronchial communication is present.	Stocker classification: Type 1: one cyst larger than 2 cm plus other cysts (75% of cases, good prognosis). Type 2: multiple macrocysts < 2 cm in size. Type 3: microcystic with solid appearance (poor prognosis).
Congenital diaphragmatic hernia ▷ *Fig. 1.83, p. 54*	Multiple lucencies in continuity with abdominal bowel gas, often marked contralateral mediastinal shift. Scaphoid abdomen. The NG tube may or may not pass into the chest. Umbilical vein catheter displaced upwards. If doubt, contrast via NG tube may confirm bowel in hernia. US may also be useful.	
Air-filled bronchopulmonary sequestration	Medially in lower lobes, more commonly on left.	Intralobar form may contain air due to collateral air drift, although presence of air often thought to be due to infection. Air in extralobar form implies an esophageal connection.
Persistent localized pulmonary interstitial emphysema ▷ *Fig. 1.52a, b, p. 36*	Multiple tubulocystic lucencies radiating from the hilum, usually localized rather than diffuse (e.g., acute pulmonary interstitial emphysema). On CT lucencies may show a central dot or stripe, representing the bronchovascular bundle.	Small minority of cases of interstitial emphysema will persist. Cystic spaces may continue to expand, generating mass effect and requiring resection.
Pneumatoceles ▷ *Fig. 1.53a, b, p. 36*	CXR and CT: Localized, often multiple tubular lucencies within area of consolidation. May contain an air-fluid level. Usually no enhancing wall (e.g., lung abscess).	May represent interstitial air due to necrosis of bronchiolar walls or localized air trapping due to bronchiolar obstruction. Most common with *Staphylococcus aureus* and *S. pneumonia*. Usually occur at time of recovery. Most spontaneously and often rapidly resolve.
Air-filled intrapulmonary/ parenchymal bronchogenic cyst ▷ *Fig. 1.54, p. 36*		Ten to twenty percent are intrapulmonary or parenchymal. Air in bronchogenic cyst implies infection.
Cavitary necrosis ▷ *Fig. 1.79, p. 52*	CT: Ill-defined air spaces within areas of nonenhancing lung parenchyma.	Although in adults considered a grave sign and an indication for surgery, not such a poor prognostic sign in children. May progress to abscess formation.
Draining pulmonary abscess	Air-fluid level within cavity with thick enhancing wall.	Usually associated with persistent fever.

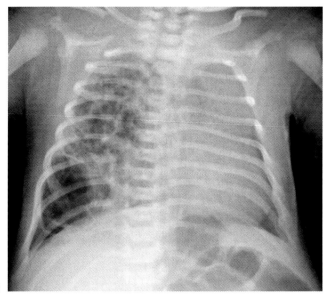

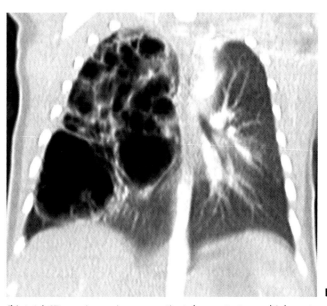

a

b

Fig. 1.51a, b Congenital cystic adenomatoid malformation.
(**a**) Chest radiograph in a neonate with an antenatally diagnosed lung malformation. There are multiple cystic lucencies occupying the entire right hemithorax, with contralateral mediastinal displacement.

(**b**) Axial CT scan image in same patient demonstrates multiple cysts of varying sizes in the right lower lobe, the largest in excess of a centimeter in size, in keeping with a type 1 congenital cystic adenomatoid malformation, which was confirmed on histology.

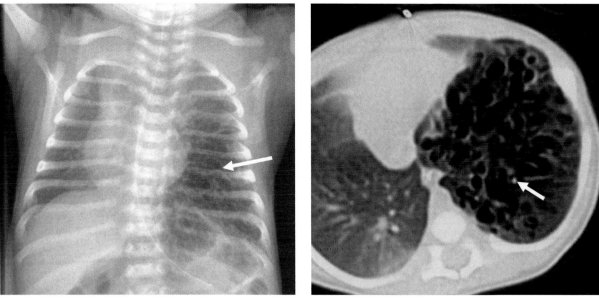

a

b

Fig. 1.52a, b Persistent pulmonary interstitial emphysema. (a) Chest radiograph in a 4-week-old premature neonate ventilated since birth. There is a collection of cystic structures in the left lower zone (arrow). These were not present at birth. **(b)** Axial CT image in the same patient demonstrates multiple tubulocystic lucencies, some of which contain a central bronchovascular dot (arrow). The lucencies resolved with conservative management over 6 weeks.

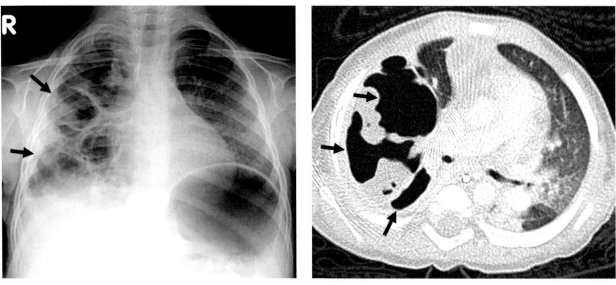

a

b

Fig. 1.53a, b Pneumatocoeles. (a) Chest radiograph in an 18-month-old child recovering from right lower lobe pneumonia and empyema. There are multiple lucencies throughout the right lower lobe. There is residual pleural thickening (arrows). **(b)** Axial CT image in the same patient. There are multiple tubulocystic lucencies radiating from the hilum within the consolidated right lower lobe (arrows).

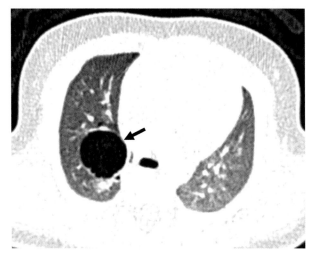

Fig. 1.54 Parenchymal bronchogenic cyst. Axial CT image in a 2-month-old boy with antenatally diagnosed lung malformation. There is a single air-filled cyst in the right lower lobe (arrow). This could represent a type 1 CCAM, but on histologic examination was a bronchogenic cyst.

■ Pulmonary Disease in the Immunocompromised Child

Immunodeficiency in children may be primary or acquired. The primary immunodeficiency states are a heterogeneous group of disorders including disorders of antibody production (e.g., immunoglobulin A deficiency, hypogammaglobulinemia), T-cell function (e.g., common variable immunodeficiency, severe combined immunodeficiency), granulocyte function (e.g., chronic granulomatous disease), and various other disorders (e.g., Wiskott-Aldrich syndrome, ataxia telangiectasia, DiGeorge syndrome). Worldwide, the most common acquired immunodeficiency state is due to human immunodeficiency virus (HIV) infection. Immunodeficiency is also commonly iatrogenic, typically following myeloablative chemotherapy and conditioning for BMT, or with immunosuppresive drug regimens for rheumatologic disorders and following solid organ transplantation. Most pulmonary complications relate to opportunistic infection. Infecting organisms are determined by which arm of the immune system is compromised: for example, most fungal infections occur in the neutropenic patient, whilst *Pneumocystis jiroveci* pneumonia (PJP) and cytomegalovirus (CMV) pneumonitis occur in the setting of T-cell dysfunction and lymphopenia. Neoplastic disease has an increased frequency in immunodeficient states. Finally, there are some pulmonary complications that are specific patients following BMT.

Table 1.24 Infective complications

Diagnosis	Findings	Comments
Invasive pulmonary aspergillosis ▷ *Fig. 1.48, p. 33* ▷ *Fig. 1.55*	Angioinvasive aspergillosis: classic early finding is of inflammatory nodules with perilesional ground-glass attenuation reflecting hemorrhage and/or exudates. These may show poor enchancement centrally, and progress to necrotic cavitation over 14 d, often with "air-crescent" formation. These features are relatively specific but rare in children. Airways invasive aspergillosis: small centrilobular nodules with or without tree-in-bud configuration, or areas of peribronchovascular consolidation.	Occurs in neutropenic patients, usually following myeloablative chemotherapy, in first 100 d following BMT. Occasionally also seen in chronic granulomatous disease (CGD), where it behaves more indolently.
Pneumocystis jirovecii pneumonia (PJP)	CXR: hyperinflation with diffuse interstitial infiltrate progressing to alveolar shadowing. HRCT: Classic finding of diffuse ground-glass attenuation with areas of segmental or lobular sparing producing a geographic pattern of opacification. Often nonspecific appearances. A minority develop cysts/pneumatoceles.	Occurs in children with HIV, primary immunodeficiency, and in early postneutropenic phase following BMT. Now rare due to effective prophylaxis in these patients: most commonly found at presentation in HIV/primary immunodeficiency.

(continues on page 38)

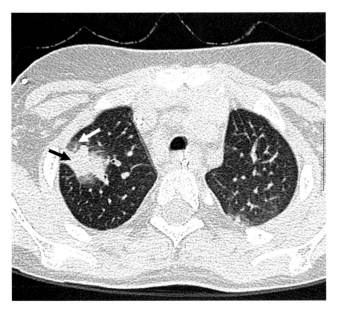

Fig. 1.55 Invasive pulmonary aspergillosis. Axial HRCT image of chest in an 11-year-old girl who is neutropenic and septic following BMT. There is an area of nodular consolidation in the RUL (black arrow), with perilesional ground-glass attenuation ("halo" sign: white arrow): this represents areas of perilesional hemorrhage and/or inflammatory change and is a typical, although not entirely specific, feature of invasive pulmonary aspergillosis.

Table 1.24   (Cont.) Infective complications

Diagnosis	Findings	Comments
CMV pneumonitis ▷ *Fig. 1.56a, b*	HRCT: multiple small, often ill-defined or ground-glass attenuation nodules.	Most commonly following BMT.
Varicella zoster pneumonitis ▷ *Fig. 1.74, p. 48*	Acute: multiple small to medium size nodules ± diffuse infiltrate. Chronic: heals with calcification.	Primary illness often more prolonged and severe in immunodeficient children with more complications.
TB	Similar patterns to infection in immunocompetent children, with lymphadenopathy a common feature. Cavitation rare.	Common in HIV, and may occur at any stage of infection.
Other fungal infections	Variable patterns: cavitation common.	Include histoplasmosis, cryptococcosis (in HIV), *Nocardia, Candida*.

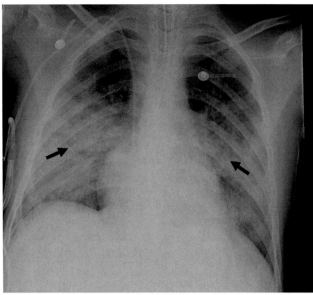
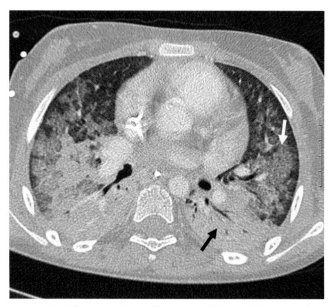

a   b

Fig. 1.56a, b   CMV pneumonitis. (a) Chest radiograph in the same child as in **Fig. 1.55**, taken 4 weeks later in the early postengraftment phase, presenting with sepsis and respiratory failure. There is a bilateral central lung infiltrate (arrows). **(b)** Axial CT image in the same patient demonstrates confluent consolidation in the dependent regions of the lung (black arrow), with extensive ground-glass change more anteriorly (white arrow). Bronchoalveolar lavage identified the presence of a high titer of CMV.

Table 1.25   Noninfectious complications

Diagnosis	Findings	Comments
Lymphoid interstitial pneumonitis	CXR: Diffuse reticulonodular infiltrate, ± patchy airspace opacities. Lymphadenopathy common. HRCT: centrilobular nodules, ground-glass opacities, septal and peribronchovascular thickening.	Occurs in one-third of children with HIV. Probably reflects a disordered immune response to HIV itself or Epstein-Barr virus. Associated with slower progression of HIV infection.
Kaposi sarcoma		Very rare in children with HIV.
Lymphoma	Similar patterns to NHL in immunocompetent children.	NHL occurs with 60× frequency of normal population in patients with HIV.
PTLD ▷ *Fig. 1.38, p. 28*	Multiple well-defined nodules of varying size, or single well-circumscribed nodule 3–5 cm in diameter. Occasionally patchy air-space opacification and mediastinal adenopathy.	Most common after thoracic (heart, lung, heart/lung) transplantation, but may occur with any transplant.

Table 1.26 Complications specific to BMT

Diagnosis	Findings	Comments
Diffuse alveolar hemorrhage	CXR: patchy/multifocal air-space shadowing. HRCT: patchy areas of ground glass and consolidation.	Occurs early after engraftment in 10%–20% of autologous BMTs. Associated with infectious complications and poor outcome.
Drug toxicity ▷ *Fig. 1.15, p. 13*	Variable patterns, may progress to fibrosis.	Bleomycin, busulphan, and methotrexate most commonly implicated.
Idiopathic interstitial pneumonia	Nonspecific and variable features, including diffuse air-space and interstitial infiltrates.	A diagnosis of exclusion: probably caused by conditioning regimen. Usually occurs 6–8 wk post-BMT.
Constrictive obliterative bronchiolitis	CXR: hyperinflation, peribronchial thickening. HRCT: patchy air trapping with or without associated bronchial dilatation.	Occurs in late phase (> 3 m post-BMT). A manifestation of chronic graft-versus-host disease.
Bronchiolitis obliterans organizing pneumonia	HRCT: patchy consolidation in subpleural or peribronchial distribution.	Late complication. Fever and cough. Responds well to steroids.
Graft-versus-host disease	May manifest as obliterative bronchiolitis, occasionally as LIP-like pattern.	Often evidence of graft-versus-host disease elsewhere (in skin, liver, gastrointestinal [GI] tract).

■ Differential Transradiancy

Lungs that appear of different density to each other present a common challenge to the pediatric radiologist. After assessing technical factors that may account for the appearances, particularly patient rotation and lateral decentering, the first task is to identify which side is abnormal. The most useful factor here is assessment of the bronchovascular markings in each lung: a lung of abnormally reduced density usually demonstrates attenuated or distorted vessels. If the lung markings are normal in both lungs, suspect a chest wall abnormality or technical factors.

Unilateral Increased Density

Table 1.27 Unilateral increased density with ipsilateral mediastinal displacement (volume loss)

Diagnosis	Findings	Comments
Total lung collapse ▷ *Fig. 1.57*	Opaque hemithorax of reduced volume.	Most common: misplaced endotracheal tube, mucus plugging, main bronchial foreign body, mediastinal mass (see section on lobar atelectasis for causes).
LUL collapse	Veil-like opacity over left lung, with or without loss of mediastinal contours. Usually some sparing in lower zone and costophrenic angle.	(see section on lobar collapse)

(continues on page 40)

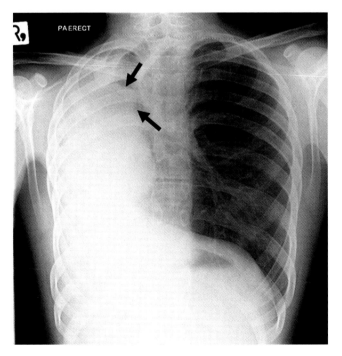

Fig. 1.57 Total lung collapse due to bronchial obstruction. Chest radiograph in a child with inflammatory myofibroblastic tumor. There is a soft-tissue mass encroaching on the carina (arrows). There is total collapse of the right lung. The left lung is overinflated.

Table 1.27   (Cont.) Unilateral increased density with ipsilateral mediastinal displacement (volume loss)

Diagnosis	Findings	Comments
Pulmonary agenesis/aplasia ▷ *Fig. 1.58a, b* ▷ *Fig. 1.144, p. 31*	Marked shift of heart and mediastinum. Herniation of contralateral lung across midline.	Pulmonary agenesis: absent lung parenchyma, vasculature and main bronchus. Pulmonary aplasia: rudimentary bronchus present.
Unilateral hypoplastic lung	Similar to aplasia, but with a small, often unaerated lung present; interrupted pulmonary artery and small bronchus may be present on cross-sectional imaging.	Extreme pulmonary hypoplasia may simulate agenesis/aplasia.
Pulmonary venolobar syndrome (scimitar syndrome, hypogenetic lung syndrome) ▷ *Fig. 1.59a, b*	Hypoplastic right lung with anomalous venous drainage, often visualized as scimitar-shaped tubular structure passing from hilum toward intrahepatic inferior vena cava (IVC).	Associated with right-sided diaphragmatic anomalies, hemivertebrae, and congenital heart disease (CHD) particularly ASD and VSD.

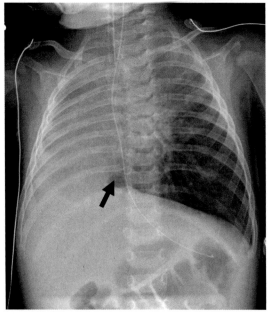
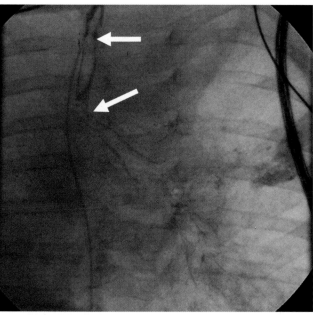

a   b

Fig. 1.58a, b   Pulmonary aplasia in congenital tracheal stenosis. (a) Chest radiograph in a 5-month-old girl with known congenital tracheal stenosis. There is overinflation of the left lung which crosses the midline (arrow). No aerated right lung is demonstrated. **(b)** Contrast bronchogram in the same child demonstrates absent right main bronchus and narrowed trachea (arrows). A rudimentary RUL tracheal bronchus was also present.

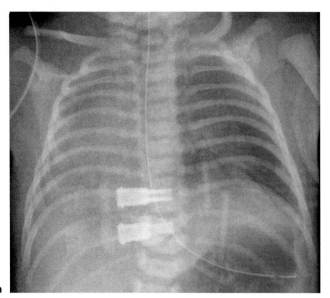
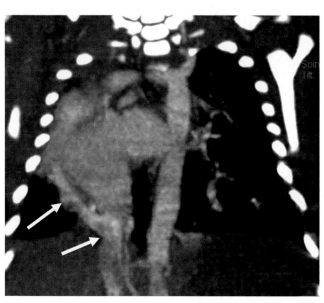

a   b

Fig. 1.59a, b   Pulmonary hypoplasia in scimitar syndrome. (a) Chest radiograph in a neonate with mild respiratory distress. There is opacification of the right hemithorax with ipsilateral mediastinal displacement. **(b)** Coronally reformatted CT image demonstrates anomalous venous drainage of the hypoplastic right lung, with the scimitar vein draining into the IVC (arrows).

Table 1.28   Unilateral increased density with contralateral mediastinal displacement

Diagnosis	Findings	Comments
Massive pleural effusion ▷ *Fig. 1.60*	Confirmed by US.	(see section on pleura)
Congenital diaphragmatic hernia ▷ *Fig. 1.61*	Early films or following decompression with NG tube may show little aeration of herniated bowel: right-sided Bochdalek hernias may show herniation of liver only, appearing as white out.	(see section on diaphragm)
Cystic adenomatoid malformation ▷ *Fig. 1.62*	Large type 3 lesions, or large lesions on early films before clearance of lung fluid may give white out appearance.	

(continues on page 42)

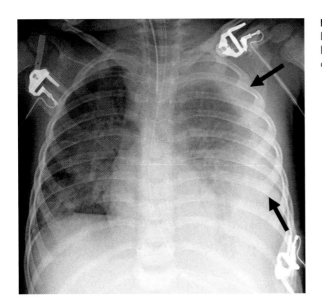

Fig. 1.60   Massive pleural effusion. Chest radiograph in an 18-month-old boy with pneumococcal sepsis and hemolytic uremic syndrome. There is a large left-sided pleural effusion (arrows) with mass effect manifested by mild contralateral mediastinal shift.

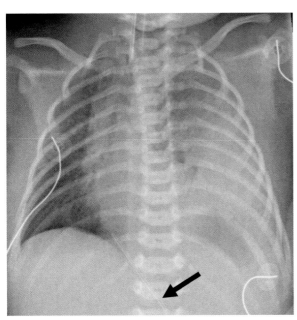

Fig. 1.61   Congenital diaphragmatic hernia. Chest radiograph in a neonate with antenatally diagnosed left congenital diaphragmatic hernia. There is an opacity occupying most of the left hemithorax with mass effect. There is a paucity of bowel gas within this. The umbilical venous catheter is displaced toward the hernia (arrow).

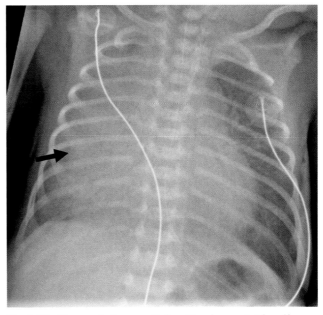

Fig. 1.62   Nonaerated congenital cystic adenomatoid malformation. Chest radiograph in a 5-day-old boy with antenatally diagnosed CCAM. There is a homogeneously dense mass lesion in the right mid-zone with an ill-defined lateral margin (arrow). This had the appearance of multiple cystic spaces on CT with some spaces filled with air. The chest radiograph appearance reflects retained fetal lung fluid.

Table 1.28   (Cont.) Unilateral increased density with contralateral mediastinal displacement

Diagnosis	Findings	Comments
Expansile pneumonia	Usually lobar rather than whole lung.	Classically, *Klebsiella pneumoniae* has mass effect.
Large pleural or pulmonary mass ▷ *Fig. 1.63a, b*	Pleurally based mass may show rib changes.	(see **Tables 1.16** and **1.17**)
Thoracic neuroblastoma ▷ *Fig. 1.64a, b*	Posterior mediastinal mass, often with spinal and rib changes.	Thoracic lesions tend to have better prognosis and occur in younger children.

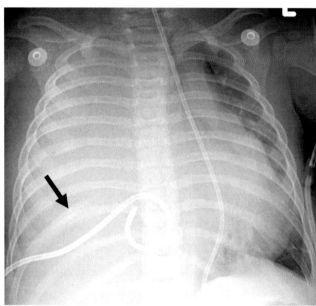

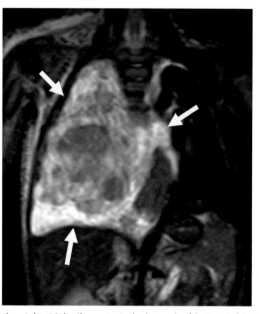

a   b

Fig. 1.63a, b   Pleurally based mass. (a) Chest radiograph in a 9-month-old boy with progressive respiratory distress. There is complete opacification of the right hemithorax with contralateral mediastinal displacement. There is destruction and periosteal reaction of the right 10th rib posteriorly (arrow). **(b)** Coronal STIR MRI in the same child demonstrates a large mixed signal intensity mass occupying the entire right hemithorax (arrows). This was a rhabdoid tumor.

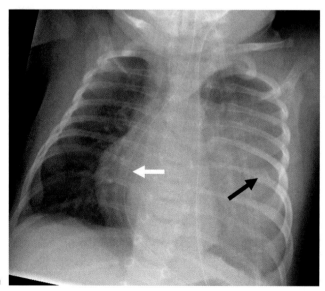

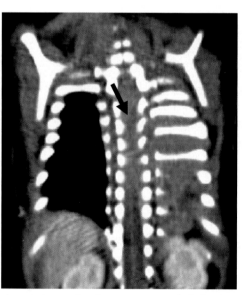

a   b

Fig. 1.64a, b   Neuroblastoma. (a) Chest radiograph in a 7-month-old child with failure to thrive. There is an ill-defined mass in the left hemithorax, causing esophageal displacement (white arrow), abnormal posterior rib separation, and rib destruction with a pathologic fracture (black arrow). **(b)** Coronally reformatted CT in the same patient shows marked intraspinal extension of tumor (arrow).

Table 1.29 Unilateral increased density with neutral mediastinum

Diagnosis	Findings	Comments
Supine pleural effusion	May result in diffuse increase in opacification as only sign. Unusual in children, and usually some evidence of fluid in lateral pleural space. US confirms.	Larger effusions result in mass effect.
Bronchopulmonary sequestration	Very large lesions occasionally occupy entire thorax.	

Unilateral Increased Transradiancy

Table 1.30 Unilateral increased transradiancy with contralateral mediastinal displacement

Diagnosis	Findings	Comments
Foreign body aspiration into main bronchus ▷ *Fig. 1.65*	Hyperlucent lung with increased volume. Right lung slightly more common than left. May look normal in film in full inspiration. Expiratory films essential if inspiratory film normal: decubitus film or film following manual abdominal compression, if these are not possible.	Sensitivity of plain radiography 68%–74%, specificity 45%–67%. Bronchoscopy or CT utilized in equivocal cases.
Mucus plugging of main bronchus	Mucus plug itself usually not visible on radiography.	In ventilated child, or in child with asthma or CF.

(continues on page 44)

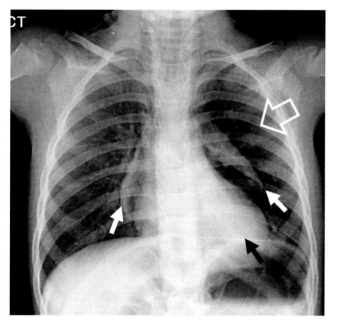

Fig. 1.65 Foreign body aspiration. Chest radiograph in a 3-year-old girl with progressive respiratory distress after choking on peanuts. There is thymic elevation (white arrows) indicating a pneumomediastinum. There is partial left lower lobe collapse (black arrow) with hypertransradiancy of the LUL (open arrow). A peanut was retrieved from the left main bronchus at bronchoscopy.

Table 1.30   (Cont.) Unilateral increased transradiancy with contralateral mediastinal displacement

Diagnosis	Findings	Comments
Extrinsic bronchial compression ▷ *Fig. 1.66a, b*	Evidence of extrinsic lesion often present (e.g., mediastinal mass).	Lymphadenopathy, bronchogenic cyst, vascular abnormality.
Bronchial stenosis/ bronchomalacia	Bronchomalacia requires bronchogram to demonstrate.	Often as part of extensive tracheobronchial stenosis (see section on tracheal pathology).
Endobronchial lesion	Lobulated central mass.	Bronchial carcinoid commonest primary lesion.
Congenital lobar emphysema ▷ *Fig. 1.49, p. 34*	Overinflated lobe may occupy entire hemithorax, compressing lower lobes.	LUL in 43%, RML in 35%, RUL in 20%. Two lobes involved in up to 5%. Rare in lower lobes. Most causes due to localized bronchomalacia within lobar bronchus. Occasionally due to extrinsic compression by PDA, dilated pulmonary artery in absent pulmonary valve syndrome, bronchogenic cyst.
Tension pneumothorax ▷ *Fig. 1.67*	Absent lung markings with mediastinal shift, and eversion of the diaphragm.	Requires emergency decompression.

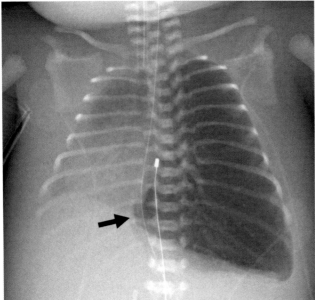

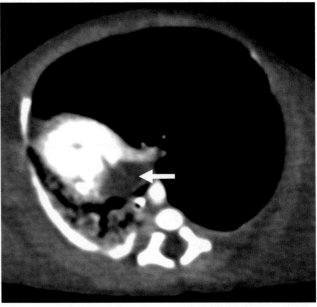

a
b

Fig. 1.66a, b   Mediastinal bronchogenic cyst. (a) Chest radiograph in a 1-week-old infant with respiratory distress. There is marked overinflation of the left lung, which herniates across the midline (arrow). The right lung is collapsed. **(b)** Axial CT image in the same patient demonstrates a mediastinal mass lesion of fluid density at the level of the carina (arrow), causing collapse of the right lung and air trapping in the left lung. Histologic examination confirmed a bronchogenic cyst.

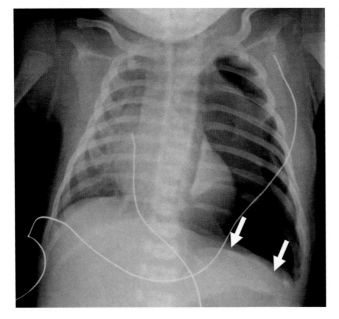

Fig. 1.67   Tension pneumothorax. Chest radiograph in a 1-month-old infant following chest drain removal after surgery for aortic coarctation. There is a large left-sided pneumothorax causing diaphragmatic eversion (arrows) and contralateral mediastinal shift, indicating tension.

Table 1.31   Unilateral increased transradiancy with neutral mediastinum

Diagnosis	Findings	Comments
Swyer-James-MacLeod syndrome ▷ *Fig. 1.68a, b*	May be small or normal volume lung, with poor perfusion and small hilum. Air trapping on expiration. CT shows evidence of small airway disease involving both lungs.	This is a variant of constrictive obliterative bronchiolitis with asymmetrical involvement.
Ventral pneumothorax ▷ *Fig. 1.69*	Lucency most striking anteromedially. Deep costophrenic sulcus ipsilaterally.	Patient usually supine.
Bronchial atresia ▷ *Fig. 1.50, p. 34*	Usually lobar hyperlucency with tubular/nodular opacity at apex of lucency representing bronchocele.	Fifty percent are asymptomatic/incidental.
Asymmetric lung perfusion	Vessels attenuated on hypoperfused side.	Causes include pulmonary embolism, postcardiac surgery (e.g., unilateral Blalock-Taussig shunt, failed pulmonary artery anastomosis).

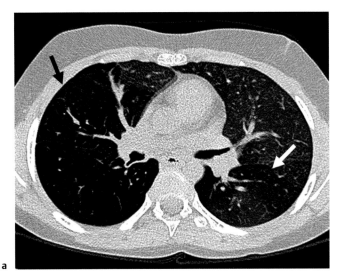

a

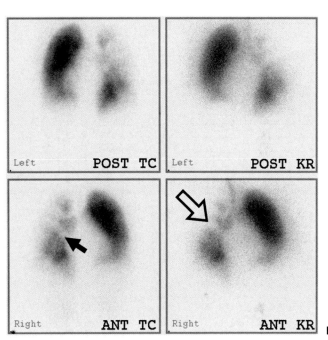

b

Fig. 1.68a, b   Asymmetric bronchiolitis obliterans (Swyer-James-Mcleod syndrome). (a) Axial expiratory HRCT image in a 10-year-old girl with cough and dyspnea. There is extensive right-sided air trapping indicated by hypertransradiancy (black arrow). There is some patchy air trapping in the left lung (white arrow). **(b)** Ventilation and perfusion scintigram in the same patient shows profoundly reduced and patchy ventilation (open arrow) and perfusion (arrow) of the right lung, and some more subtle defects in the left lung.

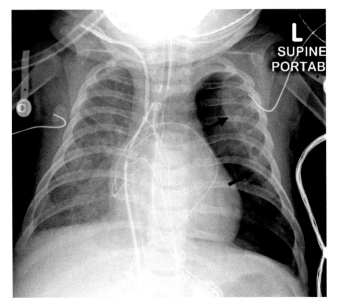

Fig. 1.69   Ventral pneumothorax. Chest radiograph in a 5-month-old child following chest drain removal after cardiac surgery. There is extensive lucency in the left hemithorax with a sharply defined heart border. The medial lung edge is shown (arrows).

Table 1.32   Unilateral increased transradiancy with ipsilateral mediastinal displacement

Diagnosis	Findings	Comments
Unilateral hypoplastic lung	Small volume lung with reduced vascularity.	May be primary in association with abnormal vascular supply (atretic/interrupted pulmonary artery, anomalous venous drainage), or secondary, most commonly due to congenital diaphragmatic hernia.
Pulmonary venolobar syndrome (scimitar syndrome, hypogenetic lung syndrome)	Hypoplastic right lung with anomalous venous drainage, often visualized as scimitar-shaped tubular structure passing from hilum toward intrahepatic IVC. Hypoplastic lung may be of increased or decreased density.	Associated with right-sided diaphragmatic anomalies, hemivertebrae, and CHD, particularly ASD and VSD.

Table 1.33   Pseudohyperlucency

Diagnosis	Findings	Comments
Patient rotation ▷ *Fig. 1.70*	Hyperlucency usually on side to which patient is rotated (regardless of projection).	Assess rotation in small children by rib morphology, in older children by position of clavicles.
Lateral decentering	All tissues toward one side of film are of reduced density.	
Chest wall abnormality ▷ *Fig. 1.71*	Normal pulmonary parenchymal appearances. Asymmetrical axillary folds may suggest pectoralis asymmetry.	Examples include scoliosis, Poland syndrome (absent pectoralis muscle associated with ipsilateral syndactyly), mammary hypoplasia (e.g., secondary to Blalock-Taussig shunt), following amputation.

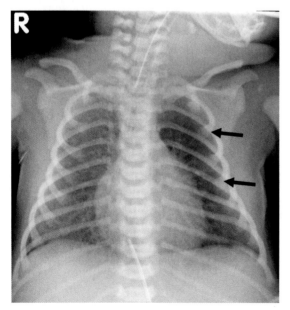

Fig. 1.70   Patient rotation. Chest radiograph in a 2-day-old neonate with persistent pulmonary hypertension of the newborn. There is relative hypertransradiancy of the left hemithorax: the child is rotated to the left as indicated by relatively short appearance of anterior ribs on the left (arrows).

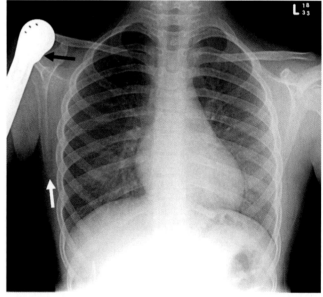

Fig. 1.71   Chest wall asymmetry. Chest radiograph in a 10-year-old girl with previous osteosarcoma of the right humerus that was resected 2 years previously. There is relative increased hypertransradiancy of the right hemithorax due to loss of right pectoral muscle bulk. Note humeral prosthesis (black arrow) and reduced bulk of muscles projected in right axilla (white arrow).

■ Pulmonary Calcifications

Table 1.34   Solitary/focal pulmonary calcifications

Diagnosis	Findings	Comments
TB ▷ *Fig. 1.72*	Usually single nodular focus anywhere in parenchyma (no lobar predominance) ± calcified draining lymph nodes.	Represents healed primary complex: appears 6 mo to 2 y after primary infection.
Histoplasmosis	May be indistinguishable from TB. Disseminated calcifications also occur.	Coccidioidomycosis may have similar appearances.
Calcified metastasis ▷ *Fig. 1.73*	Lower lobe predominant, peripheral usually well defined.	Osteosarcoma, occasionally papillary thyroid carcinoma. Treated metastases of any origin may also calcify.
Hamartoma	"Popcorn" chondroid calcification. Fat present in lesion is pathognomonic, but only occurs in half.	Rare, but more often symptomatic in children than in adults, and may be large.
Bronchial carcinoid	Occasionally calcified. Usually central, endobronchial lesion with airway obstruction.	Carcinoid syndrome rare but has been described.

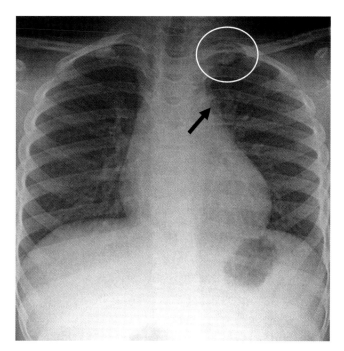

Fig. 1.72   Healed TB (Ghon focus/Rhanke complex). Chest radiograph in a 6-year-old girl presenting with tuberculous spondylitis. There is a calcified granuloma in the left lung apex (circled), with a calcified node in the aortopulmonary window region (arrow).

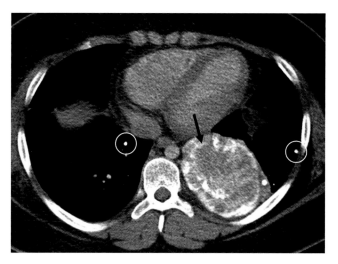

Fig. 1.73   Metastastic osteosarcoma. Axial CT image in a 15-year-old boy with known metastatic osteosarcoma. There are multiple small, calcified nodules (circled) in addition to a large, ossified mass in the left lower lobe (arrow) with peripheral calcification and a trabecular pattern of central calcification.

Table 1.35 Multifocal/disseminated/diffuse pulmonary calcifications

Diagnosis	Findings	Comments
Granulomas	Calcified miliary nodules.	Particularly histoplasmosis. Also coccidioidomycosis.
Healed varicella pneumonitis ▷ Fig. 1.74	Numerous tiny calcifications.	Rare in younger children: occurs in immunocompromised.
Metastatic pulmonary calcification	Occurs in anterior portions of lungs.	Occurs in acute and chronic renal failure, post-renal transplantation, post-cardiac surgery. Reflects abnormal calcium metabolism.
Multiple calcified metastases ▷ Fig. 1.73, p. 47	Lower lobe predominant, peripheral, usually well-defined nodules.	This is not the same as metastatic pulmonary calcification. Osteosarcoma, occasionally papillary thyroid carcinoma. Treated metastases of any origin may also calcify.
Alveolar microlithiasis	CXR: ground-glass or established fibrosis. HRCT: Tiny sandlike calcifications. Lungs may be avid on bone scintigraphy.	Very rare in children, presentation usually in adult life. Unknown etiology. Often asymptomatic.
Mitral stenosis	Varying from pulmonary hemosiderosis with small ill-defined nodules through to pulmonary ossification with 5-mm nodules showing cortex and trabeculation.	Rare.

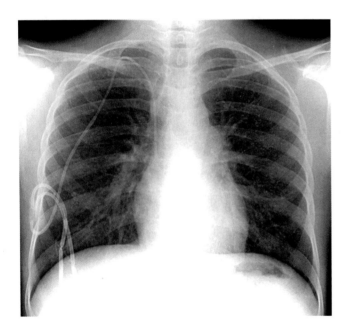

Fig. 1.74 Healed varicella pneumonitis. Chest radiograph in a 16-year-old boy with CD40 ligand deficiency (a primary immunodeficiency state), and history of previous varicella pneumonitis. There are numerous punctuate pulmonary calcifications.

Pleura and Diaphragms

■ Pneumothorax

Table 1.36 Pneumothorax patterns

Diagnosis	Findings	Comments
Lateral pneumothorax	Clear lung edge visible with thin pleural line.	Erect or semierect.
Apical pneumothorax	Clear lung edge visible with thin pleural line.	Usually erect film.
Subpulmonary pneumothorax ▷ *Fig. 1.75*	Lucency mirrors diaphragmatic surface, often with deep costophrenic sulcus. Lung edge and pleural line not necessarily visible.	Common patterns in neonates and infants in intensive care unit.
Anteromedial pneumothorax ▷ *Fig. 1.76*	Crisply defined heart border with lucent area adjacent. Lung edge and pleural line not necessarily visible.	
Tension pneumothorax ▷ *Fig. 1.67, p. 44*	Diaphragmatic eversion and contralateral mediastinal displacement.	Requires emergency needle thoracotomy.
Hydropneumothorax	Air-fluid level with horizontal interface on horizontal beam film.	
Pseudopneumothorax	Most commonly due to overlying skin fold. No pleural line visible. Interface between densities may fade out or extend beyond the chest wall.	Repeat film with corrected rotation may be required.

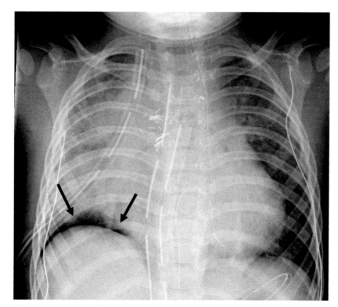

Fig. 1.75 Subpulmonary pneumothorax. Chest radiograph in an 18-month-old boy following surgery for pulmonary atresia. There is a lucency below the right lung whose lower margin is crisply defined (arrows). This is not drained by the apically placed pleural drain.

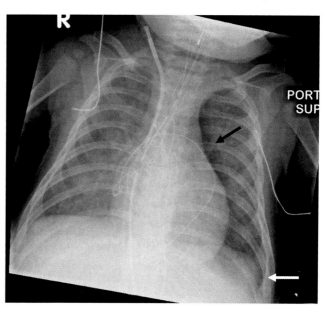

Fig. 1.76 Anteromedial pneumothorax. Chest radiograph in a 5-month-old child following cardiac surgery. There is a medial lucency on the left with crisp definition of the heart border. The medial lung edge is visualized (black arrow). There is deepening of the left costophrenic sulcus (white arrow).

Table 1.37   Pneumothorax cases

Diagnosis	Findings	Comments
Barotrauma	Often preceded by or coexisting with pulmonary interstitial emphysema.	Common in ventilated neonates, particularly those with HMD and meconium aspiration syndrome. Hypoplastic lungs are also prone to barotrauma.
Trauma		Iatrogenic, penetrating injury, blunt trauma to chest.
Airway disease ▷ *Fig. 1.77*	Evidence of underlying disease (e.g., peribronchial thickening). Blebs/bullae rarely visualized.	Particularly CF and asthma: rupture of blebs and bullae, or overdistended acini in areas of air trapping. In CF, lung may not collapse completely owing to reduced compliance.
Infection	Cavitating pneumonia occasionally spreads to pleural space. Often complicated by bronchopleural fistula.	Particularly with TB.
Interstitial lung disease	Evidence of underlying disease. Usually cystic change or established fibrosis present.	In children, LCH is the most common interstitial lung disease to cause pneumothorax.
Malignant disease	Subpleural pulmonary metastases.	Usually sarcoma, particularly osteosarcoma.
Spontaneous	Normal underlying lungs: very occasionally visualize bleb.	Rare in young children. Typically in tall athletic males. Occasionally in Marfan syndrome.

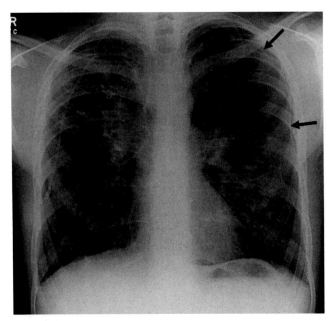

Fig. 1.77   Pneumothorax in cystic fibrosis. Chest radiograph in a 15-year-old with known CF and chest pain. There is a small left-sided pneumothorax; the lung edge and pleura clearly visible (arrows). The lung does not collapse owing to reduced compliance.

■ Pleural Effusion

Table 1.38 Pleural effusion patterns

Diagnosis	Findings	Comments
Lateral/lamellar ▷ *Fig. 1.80, p. 52*	Parallels chest wall. Common pattern in children.	
Fissural ▷ *Fig. 1.7, p. 8*	May simulate mass. Lateral radiograph often confirms position in fissure.	
Loculated	Medially convex collection produces lentiform shape, may simulate pulmonary abscess. Fluid does not shift with change of posture.	Usually in empyema or occasionally hemothorax.
Subpulmonic ▷ *Fig. 1.78a, b*	Diaphragm appears to be peaked laterally. US used to confirm.	
Pseudoeffusion	Usually due to skin fold from overlying arm.	

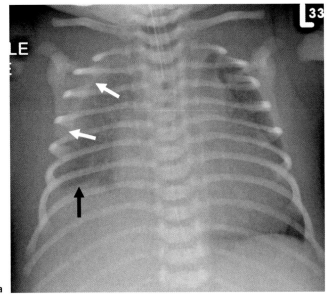
a

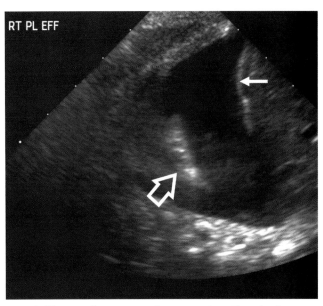
b

Fig. 1.78a, b Subpulmonic effusion. (a) Chest radiograph in a 3-day-old boy with congenital heart disease. The right hemidiaphragm appears elevated and flattened (black arrow). There is pleural fluid laterally (white arrows). **(b)** Coronal US image in the same patient. There is a large predominantly subpulmonary effusion. The white arrow indicates the diaphragm, and the open arrow indicates the lung.

Table 1.39 Pleural effusion causes

Diagnosis	Findings	Comments
Parapneumonic	Underlying lung consolidation. US may show minor septation or simple anechoic effusion.	Distinction from empyema frequently requires aspiration.
Empyema ▷ *Fig. 1.79*	Difficult to distinguish from simple parapneumonic effusion on radiograph. May be lobulated. US: echoic fluid, thin or thick septations or even solid appearing collection. CT: pleural enhancement, thickening of extrapleural fat, lobulated appearing collection.	Commonly following streptococcal or staphylococcal pneumonia. Incidence may be rising in children. Treated with either tube thoracostomy with fibrinolytics or surgically (usually video-assisted thoracoscopy).
Tuberculous	Primary complex often not visible.	Rare prior to school age. Ten percent of primary TB.
Neoplastic	CXR: may visualize lobulated pleural mass. CT: irregular/nodular pleural thickening.	Common causes: leukemia/lymphoma. Metastatic disease particularly Wilms tumor, and sarcoma, primary tumors including PNET, Askin disease, mesothelioma.
Chylothorax ▷ *Fig. 1.80*	May be evidence of lymphangiectasia.	Fluid milky after feeding. May be idiopathic, secondary to lymphatic injury (e.g., birth trauma, cardiac surgery), or associated with lymphangiectasia.
Pancreatitis	Usually left-sided and small.	
Subphrenic abscess	Usually small, sympathetic effusion.	
Transudative	Often larger on the right.	In low albumin states, cardiac failure, "third spacing" in sepsis.
Hemothorax	Hyperdense on CT examination: density measures 30–80 Hounsfield units (HU) depending on age of blood.	Usually following trauma or iatrogenic.

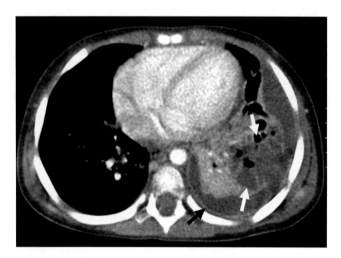

Fig. 1.79 Empyema. Axial contrast-enhanced CT image in a 3-year-old boy with empyema referred for surgical drainage. There is an irregular left pleural collection with pleural thickening and enhancement and widening of the subcostal fat space (black arrow). The underlying lung demonstrates an area of cavitary necrosis (white arrows), which has a recognized association with empyema.

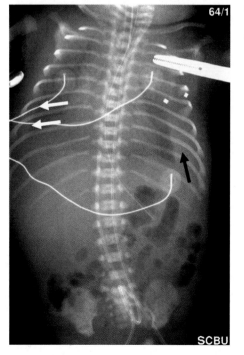

Fig. 1.80 Neonatal chylous pleural effusion. Thoracoabdominal radiograph in a neonate. There is a large left-sided pleural effusion (black arrow) and a smaller right-sided effusion (white arrows). Fluid was chylous on aspiration.

Table 1.40 Pleural thickening and masses

Diagnosis	Findings	Comments
Postempyema ▷ *Fig. 1.81*	"Rind" of pleural thickening along lateral margin.	
Associated rib lesion ▷ *Fig. 1.38, p. 28*	Rib abnormal.	Fracture or neoplasm (primary lesions: PNET, Askin tumor).
Pleural metastasis ▷ *Fig. 1.82a, b*	Solid pleural thickening.	Leukemia, neuroblastoma, and Wilms tumor most common primary lesions.
Ipsilateral pulmonary vascular anomaly	Pleural companion shadows due to collateral vessels in pleural space. Occurs in pulmonary artery or vein atresia.	
Primary pleural neoplasm	Lipoma: fat density areas. Liposarcoma: nonspecific infiltrative mass. Mesothelioma: Not asbestos-related: occasionally following radiotherapy. Similar to adult form.	All rare.

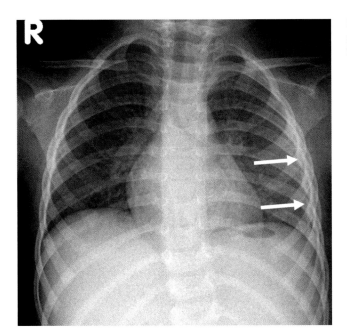

Fig. 1.81 Pleural thickening following empyema. Chest radiograph in an 18-month-old girl 1 month following tube thoracostomy for empyema. There is residual irregular pleural thickening (arrows).

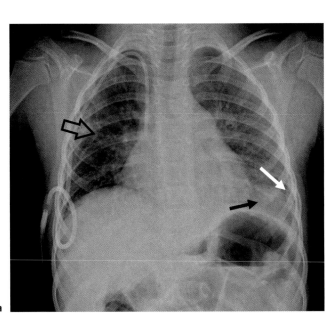

a

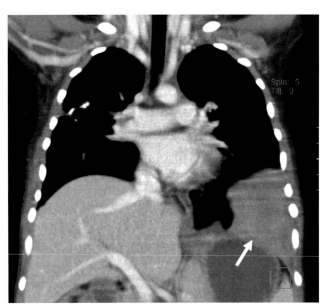

b

Fig. 1.82a, b Pleural metastasis. (a) Chest radiograph in a 5-year-old girl with previous stage 4 Wilms tumor: note lung sutures in right lung from previous nodule resection (open arrow). There is an ill-defined mass in the left lower zone with a broad diaphragmatic pleural base (black arrow) and some lobulated lateral pleural thickening (white arrow). **(b)** Coronally reformatted CT image in the same patient confirms presence of large pleurally based mass in left costophrenic angle: biopsy confirmed relapsed Wilms tumor.

■ Diaphragmatic Defects

Table 1.41   Diaphragmatic hernias and congenital diaphragmatic defects

Diagnosis	Findings	Comments
Bochdalek hernia ▷ *Fig. 1.83* ▷ *Fig. 1.61, p. 41*	More commonly left-sided. Usually contains bowel ± solid viscera. NG tube and umbilical catheters may deviate toward defect. Gas in hernia in continuity with abdominal bowel gas, which is sparse. Compresses ipsilateral ± contralateral lung, resulting in hypoplasia.	Large defects almost invariably presenting in neonatal period.
Morgagni hernia ▷ *Fig. 1.84a, b* ▷ *Fig. 1.85a, b*	Predominantly right-sided (10:1). Hepatic lobe(s), stomach, duodenum, small and large bowel, as well as spleen and omentum may all herniate. Chest and abdomen radiograph: soft-tissue density projected over the costophrenic and cardiophrenic angles. Lateral view: only the posterior portion of the diaphragm is discernable, the hernia is retrosternal density. The plain radiograph is often sufficient, especially when the hernia contains aerated bowel. US, possibly CT. Scintigraphy if hemorrhaging.	Rare approximately 7% of congenital hernias; very rarely bilateral. Early childhood, adulthood. Associated anomalies: scimitar syndrome, unilobar lungs, Hirschsprung disease. Complications: incarceration, gastric volvulus. Many are asymptomatic.
Hiatus hernia	May be sliding or rolling.	May be component of Bochdalek hernia.
Diaphragmatic eventration ▷ *Fig. 1.86a, b, p. 56*	More commonly right sided. Diaphragm shows reduced excursion and lobulated contour with upward displacement.	Due to a congenitally thin diaphragm. Unilateral associated with trisomies 13, 15, and 18, and Beckwith-Wiedemann syndrome. Bilateral in congenital CMV infection and toxoplasmosis.
Hiatus hernia	Widening of the esophageal hiatus. Central supradiaphragmatic hernia, mainly consisting of a small section of the cardia, varying from a small nubbin to several centimeters. Lateral view: middle mediastinum. Sliding hernia seen only in inspiration. Gastroesophageal overdistention may be required to demonstrate gastroesophageal reflux. Danger of reflux esophagitis, even peptic esophageal stricture. US, endoscopy.	Gastroesophageal reflux and vomiting from birth, failure to thrive, iron deficiency anemia, melena, and hematemesis indicate reflux esophagitis. Infants are most commonly affected.
Paraesophageal hernia ▷ *Fig. 1.87, p. 56*	Cardia in normal position part of stomach herniates alongside the esophagus through the esophageal hiatus. Right more common than left. Plain radiograph: circular "cyst" in the cardiophrenic angle. Lateral view: central in position. Confirmation with a contrast study.	Mainly in older infants and school age children. Seldom symptoms, occasionally vomiting.
Bochdalek hernia (lumbocostal and pleuroperitoneal canals) ▷ *Fig. 1.88a, b, p. 56*		Mnemonic: BBBB, Bochdalek, Back, Big, Babies

(continues on page 57)

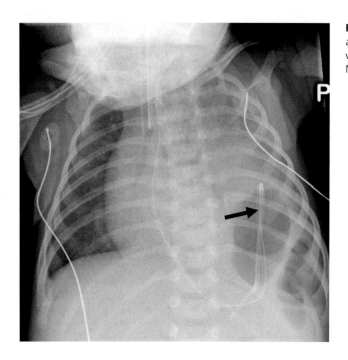

Fig. 1.83   Bochdalek hernia. Chest radiograph in a neonate with antenatally diagnosed diaphragmatic hernia. There are bowel loops within the left hemithorax, including the stomach which contains an NG tube (arrow).

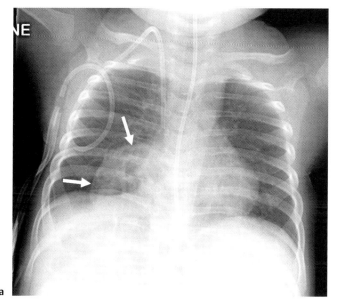 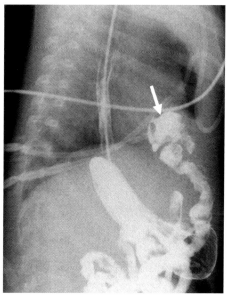

a   b

Fig. 1.84a, b   Morgagni hernia. (**a**) Chest radiograph in an infant with antenatally diagnosed diaphragmatic defect. There is a soft-tissue–dense opacity in the right medial lower zone (arrows) obscuring the right heart border. (**b**) Lateral screen grab image from fluoroscopic examination of the same child following barium administration via NG tube. A loop of bowel herniates into the chest via an anterior diaphragmatic defect (arrow).

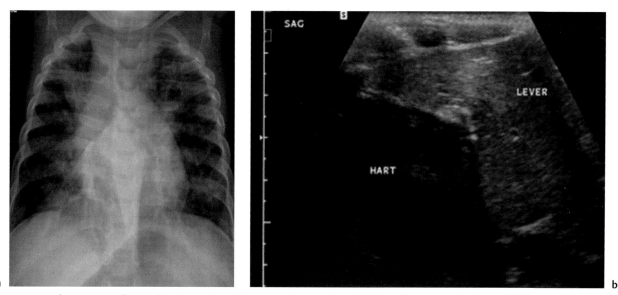

a   b

Fig. 1.85a, b   Morgagni hernia. (**a**) Chest radiograph shows a Morgagni hernia. (**b**) US of the same patient shows herniation of the left liver lobe.

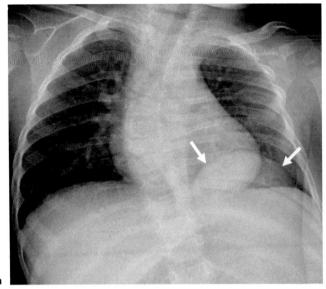

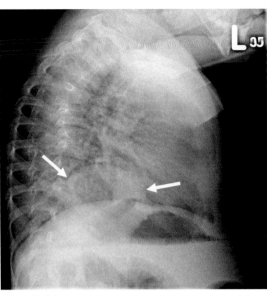

a

b

Fig. 1.86a, b   Diaphragmatic eventration. (a) Chest radiograph in an 11-month-old boy with the VATER association (*v*ertebral anomalies, *a*nal atresia, *t*racheoesophageal fistula, *e*sophagel atresia, *r*enal and/or *r*adial anomalies). There is a focal bulge to the left hemidiaphragm (arrows). **(b)** Lateral chest radiograph in the same child confirms focal diaphragmatic bulging in the midportion, containing some bowel gas within (arrows).

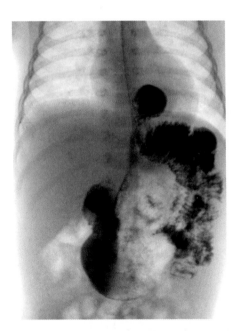

Fig. 1.87   Barium follow-through of a paraesophageal hernia with jejunal involvement in a 2-month-old girl.

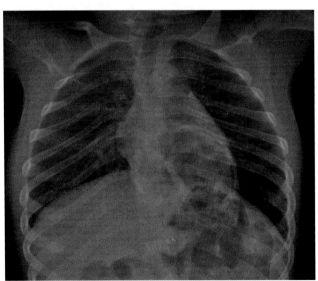

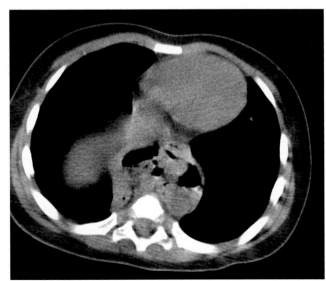

a

b

Fig. 1.88a, b   Bochdalek hernia. (a) Bochdalek hernia in an 8-year-old boy. **(b)** CT of the same patient shows the posterior paravertebral location of the herniation.

Table 1.41   (Cont.) Diaphragmatic hernias and congenital diphragmatic defects

Diagnosis	Findings	Comments
Bochdalek hernia: larger neonatal diaphragmatic defect ▷ *Fig. 1.89* ▷ *Fig. 1.90* ▷ *Fig. 1.91a, b*	Predominantly left-sided. Herniation of stomach, spleen, and bowel; liver when right-sided. Kidney position high. The hemithorax is initially dense after birth, becoming cystic or honeycombed when the bowel fills with air. The diaphragm is not identified. Mediastinum deviated to the contralateral side. Small scaphoid abdomen with no air, absent liver shadow. US (prenatal and postnatal).	Most common true diaphragmatic defect, rarely with a hernial sac. Severe illness. Decisive for the prognosis: degree of ipsilateral and contralateral pulmonary hypoplasia. Commonly associated with other anomalies (cardiovascular, malrotation, skeletal, etc). Requires immediate surgical repair and/ or ECMO until the lungs mature. Prognosis: still only 45% survival rate.
Bochdalek hernia: less severe forms, diagnosed later	Left more common than right. Dense homogeneous or cystic honeycombing appearance caused by air-containing bowel loops. Lateral view posterolateral herniation.	In neonates or in older infants. Milder clinical symptoms than with the larger defect, occasionally even an incidental finding. Associated with other anomalies.
Bochdalek hernia: late type, delayed presentation	Radiographic findings only after the first or second week of life, occasionally even later. Initially normal chest radiograph, with sudden onset of density and mediastinal shift. When right-sided: "absent liver" sign, as the liver is displaced into the thorax, and air-containing bowel loops fill the right upper quadrant of the abdomen.	Origin is unclear; it is thought that the liver and spleen prevent herniation in infancy. Clinical symptoms occur simultaneously with the radiographic changes.

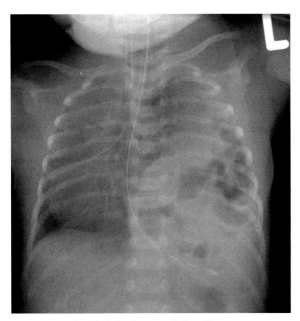

Fig. 1.89   **Left-sided diaphragmatic hernia.**

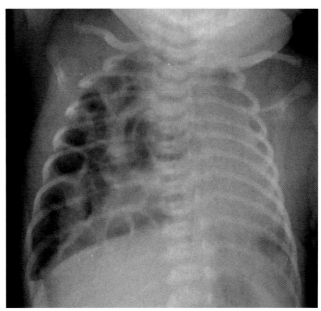

Fig. 1.90   **Right-sided diaphragmatic hernia.**

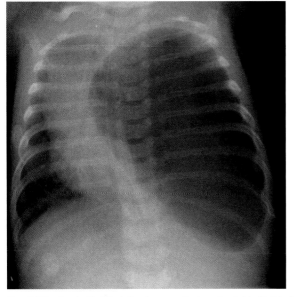

a

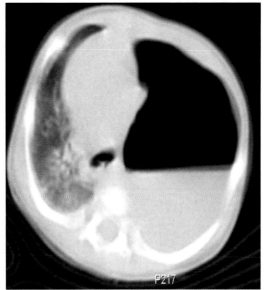

b

Fig. 1.91a, b   **Left-sided diaphragmatic hernia.** (**a**) Left-sided diaphragmatic hernia with an intrathoracic stomach. (**b**) CT of the same patient shows a dilated intrathoracic stomach.

■ Elevation of the Hemidiaphragms

Table 1.42 Bilateral elevation of the diaphragms

Diagnosis	Findings	Comments
Expiratory film ▷ *Fig. 1.92*	Clinical status of patient belies radiographic appearance. Buckling of trachea to the right (if left aortic arch).	Repeat film usually required. Often occurs at end of cry.
Any cause of increased abdominal volume/pressure ▷ *Fig. 1.93a, b*	Clue usually provided by abdominal appearances.	Examples include extreme aerophagy, ascites, bowel obstruction, large abdominopelvic mass, hepatosplenomegaly.
Bilateral lung atelectasis		Examples include intentional underventilation on ECMO, blocked ETT, mucus plugging, severe surfactant deficiency.
Neuromuscular abnormalities	Paralytic chest deformity may be present: steeply angled, narrowed ribs, narrow intercostal spaces.	
Bilateral phrenic nerve palsy	Absent motion of diaphragms on fluoroscopy or US.	Severe respiratory distress/arrest on lying flat.
Bilateral diaphragmatic defects		Rare and very poor prognosis.

(continues on page 59)

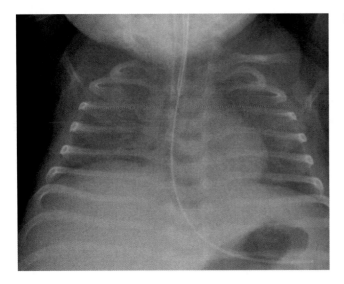

Fig. 1.92 Expiratory chest radiograph in a 3-week-old girl.

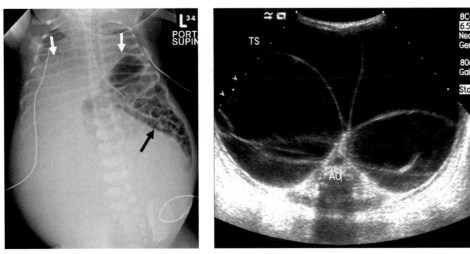

a

b

Fig. 1.93a, b Abdominal mass causing diaphragmatic elevation.
(**a**) Thoracoabdominal radiograph in a female neonate with respiratory distress and abdominal distension. There is a large abdominopelvic mass causing displacement of bowel loops (black arrow) and elevation of both hemidiaphragms (white arrows). (**b**) Transverse abdominal US image in same neonate shows a huge multicystic mass occupying almost entire abdomen. At surgery, it was revealed that massive follicular ovarian cysts were present.

Table 1.42 (Cont.) Bilateral elevation of the diaphragms

Diagnosis	Findings	Comments
Aerophagia	Air-distended stomach and loops of bowel on the radiograph.	Physiologic in infants; with mental retardation, in habitual swallowing of air, and in tracheoesophageal fistula.
Ascites, peritonitis, chyloperitoneum or hemoperitoneum, urinary Ascites ▷ *Fig. 1.94*	Ascending colon displaced medially, "floating" bowel loops are anterior and medial in the abdomen. Bowel loops are centralized on the anteroposterior radiograph. Commonly, simultaneous small pleural effusions.	Multiple causes: hepatic disease, renal failure with edema, peritonitis (secondary to necrotizing enterocolitis), urinary ascites in male neonates with posterior urethral valves. Chylous after trauma to lymphatic duct.
Ileus ▷ *Fig. 1.95*	Multiple air-fluid levels in nondistended or mildly distended bowel loops, or, in paralytic ileus, generalized bowel distention.	Acute abdominal symptoms.
Hirschsprung disease	Distended bowel loops, absence of bowel.	In infants; distended abdomen, infrequent bowel movements.
Bilateral atelectasis	Bilateral increased interstitial markings, underinflation or absent aeration of the lungs.	Predominantly in young infants with HMD; mucus plugging after surgery or in CF.
Hepatosplenomegaly	Suggested on US and radiography (displaced gastric bubble).	In leukemia, lymphoma, storage diseases, etc.
Abdominal cavity expansion ▷ *Fig. 1.96, p. 60* ▷ *Fig. 1.97, p. 60*	Large cystic and solid abdominal tumors.	Visible and palpable masses, especially in infants.
Infantile spinal atrophy, chronic form, and congenital myotonic dystrophy	Paralytic chest deformity, kyphoscoliosis club feet.	Pareses, atrophy, or hypotonia of all muscles with onset in the first year of life. Affects the intercoastal muscles with severe resultant respiratory insufficiency.
Bilateral phrenic nerve paralysis ▷ *Fig. 1.98a, b, p. 60*	No motion of the hemidiaphragms (may include eventration) on fluoroscopy, US. Risk of aspiration pneumonia. Also seen with cervical spine injury.	Clinically: Severe respiratory distress. Causes include birth trauma, poliomyelitis, Werdnig-Hoffman disease, Guillain-Barré syndrome, or may be idiopathic. Most commonly unilateral.
Eventration of the diaphragm	Exaggerated curvature of both hemidiaphragms into the thoracic cavity.	Unilateral more common than bilateral. Malformation of the diaphragm muscles, presents in infancy.
Bilateral diaphragmatic hernias and agenesis of the diaphragms	Abdominal viscera herniated into the chest. Resultant pulmonary hypoplasia, pneumothoraces develop with ventilation.	Severe respiratory distress at birth, associated phrenic nerve paralysis.

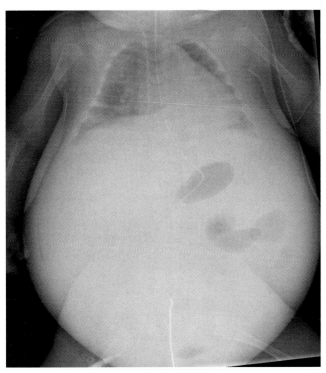

Fig. 1.94 Massive ascites in a 12-week-old neonate.

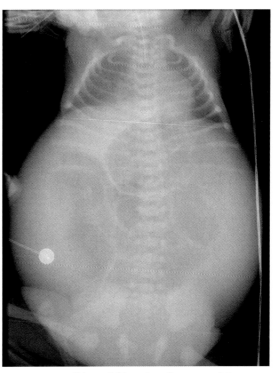

Fig. 1.95 Small bowel dilatation after necrotizing enterocolitis.

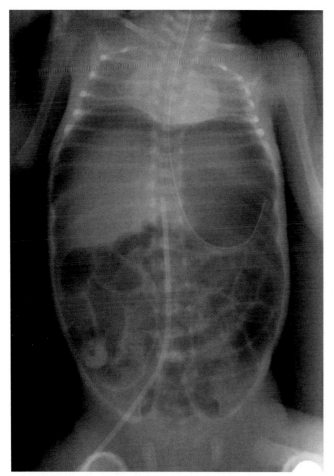

Fig. 1.96 **Pneumoperitoneum in a neonate with necrotizing enterocolitis.**

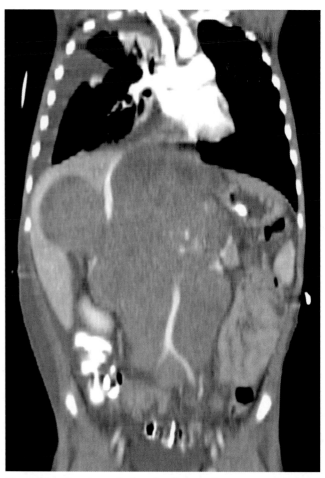

Fig. 1.97 **Elevation of the diaphragm due to an abdominal neuroblastoma.**

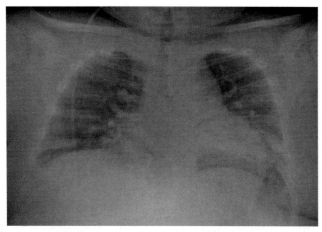

a

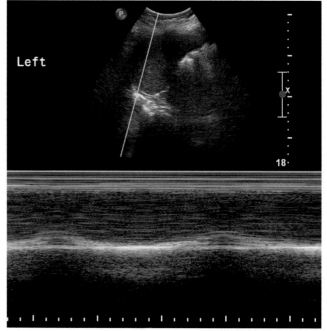

b

Fig. 1.98a, b   **Bilateral phrenic nerve paralysis.** (**a**) Bilateral phrenic nerve paralysis in a 12-month-old girl. (**b**) B-mode US shows paralysis of the diaphragm.

Table 1.43   Unilateral elevation of the hemidiaphragm

Diagnosis	Findings	Comments
Normal finding ▷ *Fig. 1.99*	Right hemidiaphragm projects "higher" due to the underlying liver.	In situs inversus, the left hemidiaphragm is elevated.
Chilaiditi	Gas-distended colon interposed between liver and diaphragm.	Normal variant.
Gastric distension	Dilated stomach and elevated left hemidiaphragm.	After prolonged crying. Occasionally reflects acute gastroparesis.
Unilateral pulmonary atelectasis ▷ *Fig. 1.100*	Segmental/subsegmental atelectasis may cause "tenting." Underinflation, even opacification, of the ipsilateral lung. Mediastinal shift to the involved side due to volume loss. Hilar reaction of lymphadenopathy.	Foreign body aspiration, atelectasis associated with pneumonia, mucus plugs, malpositioned endoctracheal tube.

(continues on page 62)

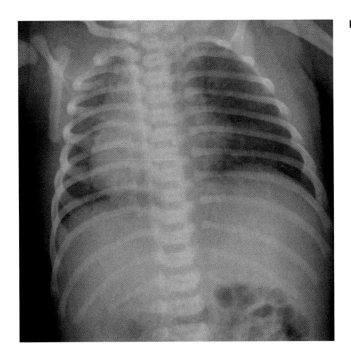

Fig. 1.99   Elevation of the the left hemidiaphragm in situs inversus.

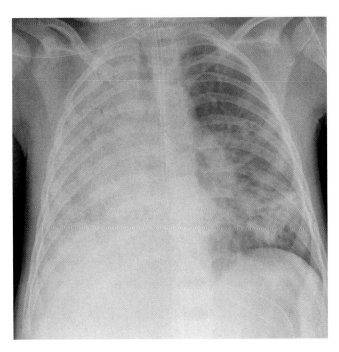

Fig. 1.100   Right-sided atelectasis in a 6-year-old boy with H1N1 pneumonia.

Table 1.43   (Cont.) Unilateral elevation of the hemidiaphragm

Diagnosis	Findings	Comments
Subpulmonary effusion ▷ *Fig. 1.78, p. 51* ▷ *Fig. 1.101a, b* ▷ *Fig. 1.102a, b* ▷ *Fig. 1.103a, b*	Chest radiograph: Hemidiaphragm appears elevated with flattening of the medial diaphragmatic angle. Decubitus view: diagnostic in the case of free flow of the effusion. Lateral view: obliquely oriented posterior density with a meniscus sign in the posterior costophrenic angle. US is very useful. Diaphragm is typically laterally peaked.	More common in older children with pneumonia, with CHD, ascites (in lymphoma), and in renal disease (nephritic syndrome or acute glomerulonephritis). US confirms.
Abdominal mass ▷ *Fig. 1.104a, b*	Mass may be evident on plain radiograph. US usually required in first instance.	For example, Wilms tumor, neuroblastoma, hepatoblastoma, large ovarian cyst.

(continues on page 64)

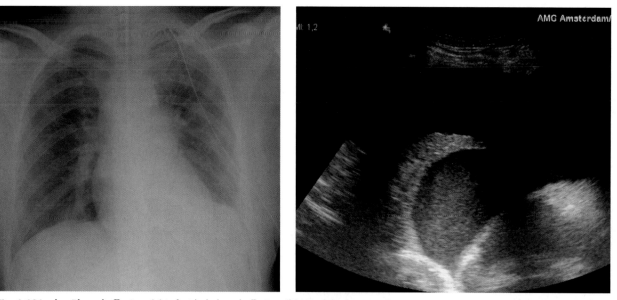

Fig. 1.101a, b   **Pleural effusion. (a)** Left-sided pleural effusion. (**b**) US of the same patient.

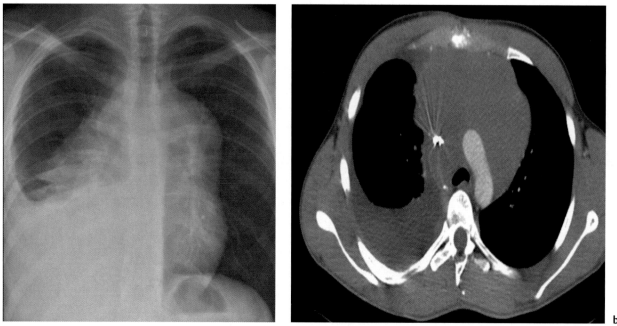

Fig. 1.102a, b   **Pleural effusion. (a)** Right-sided pleural effusion in an 8-year-old boy with T-cell lymphoma. (**b**) CT of the same patient shows a pleural effusion and the T-cell lymphoma in the anterosuperior mediastinum.

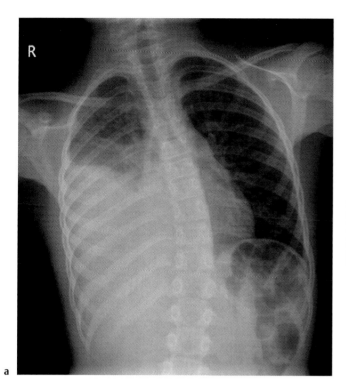

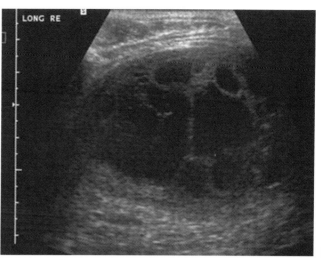

Fig. 1.103a, b Empyema. (a) Right-sided empyema in a 6-year-old girl. (b) US of the same patient shows a loculated effusion.

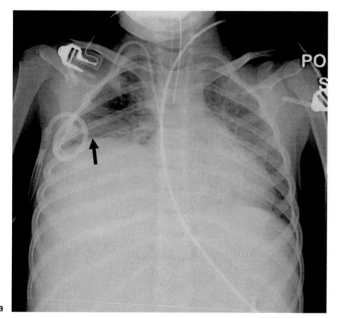

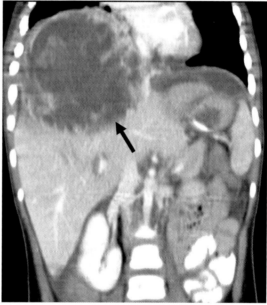

Fig. 1.104a, b Elevation of diaphragm due to hepatic mass. (a) Chest radiograph in a 3-year-old girl with known hepatic yolk sac tumor: there is marked elevation of the right hemidiaphragm (arrow) with some compressive atelectasis at the right lung base. (b) Coronally reformatted image from abdominal CT in the same child demonstrates a large heterogeneous mass in the superior liver segments (arrow), elevating the right hemidiaphragm.

Table 1.43   (Cont.) Unilateral elevation of the hemidiaphragm

Diagnosis	Findings	Comments
Phrenic nerve palsy ▷ *Fig. 1.105*	Elevated diaphragm showing paradoxical motion on US or fluoroscopy.	After thoracic surgery or with large mediastinal mass.
Eventration of the diaphragm ▷ *Fig. 1.86a, b, p. 56*	Elevated, lobulated diaphragm, may show paradoxical motion.	Due to a congenitally thin diaphragm. Unilaterally associated with trisomies 13, 15, and 18, and Beckwith-Wiedemann syndrome.
Pulmonary hypoplasia/aplasia ▷ *Fig. 1.106*	Globally small lung, may be hyper- or hypotransradiant.	
Gastric distension ▷ *Fig. 1.107* ▷ *Fig. 1.108*	Due to large amounts of air and fluid in the stomach (e.g., in pyloric stenosis), malrotation.	Aerophagia is common in infants and is of no consequence. In other children, it is associated with vomiting, epigastric pain, and bloating.

(continues on page 65)

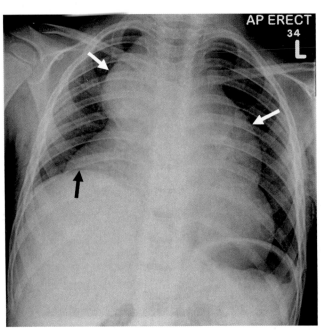

Fig. 1.105   Phrenic nerve palsy. Chest radiograph in an 8-year-old boy with acute lymphoblastic leukemia and mediastinal mass (white arrows). There is elevation of the right hemidiaphragm (black arrow): dynamic US demonstrated paradoxical motion of the right hemidiaphragm, strongly suggestive of a right phrenic nerve palsy.

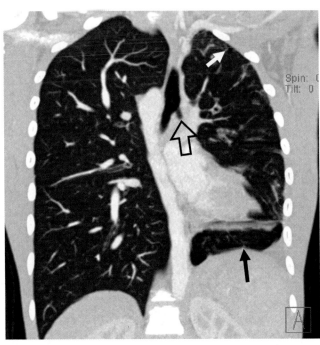

Fig. 1.106   Hypoplastic left lung. Coronally reformatted CT image in a 7-year-old boy with a previous double aortic arch. The left hemidiaphragm is elevated (black arrow). There are pulmonary dysplastic changes including a small subpleural cyst (white arrow). The left main bronchus is small (open arrow). Other images showed absence of the left main pulmonary artery.

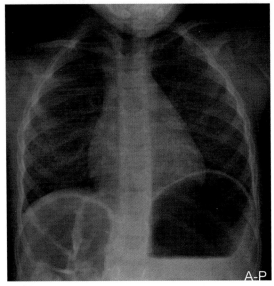

Fig. 1.107   Aerophagia.

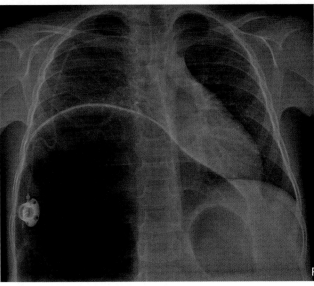

Fig. 1.108   Postsurgical ileus in an 8-year-old boy.

Table 1.43   (Cont.) Unilateral elevation of the hemidiaphragm

Diagnosis	Findings	Comments
Contralateral emphysema (check-valve mechanism, congenital lobar emphysema)	Hyperlucent contralateral lung. Depressed hemidiaphragm on that side. Ventilation-perfusion scan: diminished perfusion of the contralateral lung.	Distant breath sounds on the contralateral side. Must exclude aspirated foreign body.
Abdominal or diaphragmatic tumor ▷ *Fig. 1.109a, b* ▷ *Fig. 1.110a, b*	Liver tumor, splenic cysts, trauma. Also abdominal neoplasms.	Distended abdomen.

(continues on page 66)

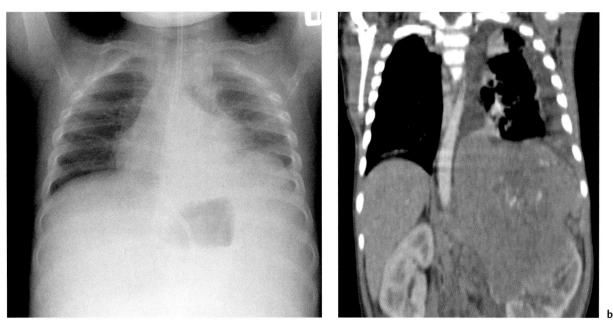

Fig. 1.109a, b   Neuroblastoma. (**a**) Elevated left hemidiaphragm in a 2-year-old boy. (**b**) Coronal CT reconstruction of the same patient shows a large intra-abdominal neuroblastoma causing the elevation.

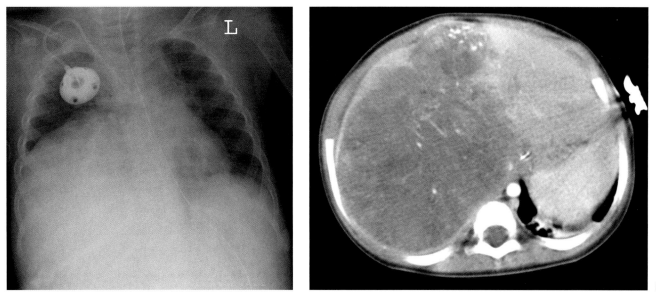

Fig. 1.110a, b   Hepatoblastoma. (**a**) Elevated right hemidiaphragm. (**b**) CT of the same patient shows a large, PRETEXT stage 3 hepatoblastoma.

Table 1.43   (Cont.) Unilateral elevation of the hemidiaphragm

Diagnosis	Findings	Comments
Subphrenic abscess	Blunting of the costophrenic angle due to air effusion. Occasionally, a crescent of air may be visible under the diaphragm with or without an air-fluid level. Signs of ascites. US or CT: complex cystic mass with air.	Occurs after perforation of a hollow viscus, after pancreatitis, or after previous abdominal surgery.
Phrenic nerve paralysis ▷ *Fig. 1.111a–c*	More commonly right-sided. Mediastinum deviated to the opposite side. Compression atelectasis of the right lower lobe above the high diaphragm. In left-sided paralysis: stomach (and bowel loops) may be displaced superiorly. Caution: fractures of the ribs, clavicle, or cervical vertebrae! Paradoxical diaphragmatic motion on fluoroscopy.	Causes: Trauma, including birth trauma, after thoracotomy, with complications of endotracheal intubation, mediastinal tumor. In neonates, may be associated with Erb palsy.
Eventration of the diaphragm ▷ *Fig. 1.112*	Very marked superior bowing of the hemidiaphragm, either partial or complete. Radiographic appearance same as in paralysis, fluoroscopy can differentiate between the two. In eventration, there is diminished diaphragmatic motion. Compression atelectasis occurs in the lower lobes in severe cases. Left side more common than right.	Mostly asymptomatic, rarely bilateral. Generally an incidental finding in the first year of life. Congenital anomaly of diaphragm muscle with poor function. In severe cases: dyspnea, cyanosis, nasal flaring. May be associated with pulmonary hypoplasia, chromosomal abnormalities, in utero infections.
Pulmonary hypoplasia or agenesis ▷ *Fig. 1.113*	Mediastinal shift to the ipsilateral side, small pulmonary vessels; small-sized lung, or underaerated to the extent that it may only appear as a hazy density in the involved hemithorax. Lateral view: band of increased restrosternal soft tissue. Scintigraphy, angiography.	Depending on the size, may be asymptomatic or present with respiratory symptoms. Associated with partial anomalous pulmonary return (scimitar syndrome).
Postsurgical ▷ *Fig. 1.114*	Mediastinal shift to the ipsilateral side.	In most cases, a temporary effect as a result of pulmonary atelectasis.

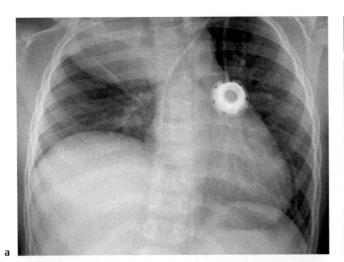
a

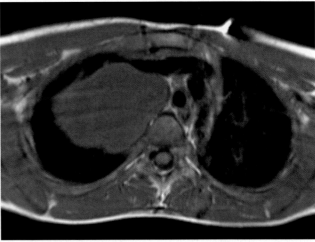
b

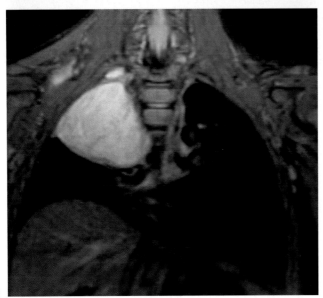
c

Fig. 1.111a–c   Neuroblastoma. (a) Elevated left hemidiaphragm in a 2-year-old boy with a neuroblastoma. **(b)** Axial T1-weighted MRI of the same patient shows the extent of the tumor. **(c)** Coronal T1-weighted postcontrast MRI shows homogeneous contrast enhancement.

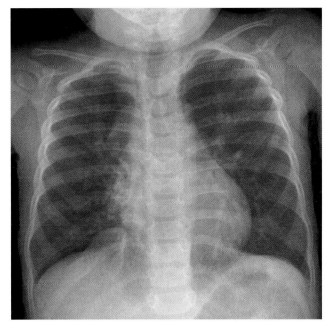

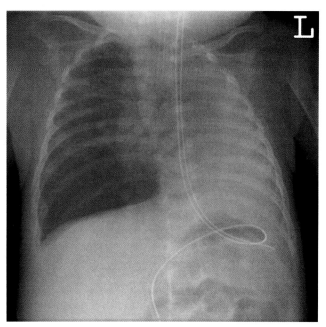

Fig. 1.112 Eventration of the right hemidiaphragm in an 18-month-old girl.

Fig. 1.113 Left-sided pulmonary agenesis in an 8-week-old boy.

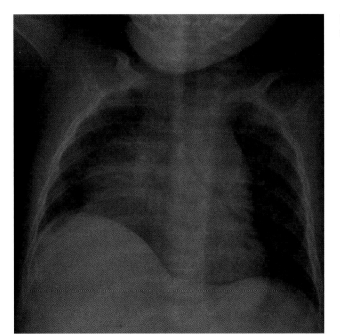

Fig. 1.114 Thymic cyst. Postsurgical chest radiograph after drainage of thymic cyst (see **Figs. 1.180** and **1.198**).

■ Diaphragmatic Flattening

Diaphragmatic flattening may be bilateral or unilateral, depending on the cause.

Table 1.44   Bilateral flattening of the hemidiaphragms

Diagnosis	Findings	Comments
Obstructive pulmonary emphysema, CF, bronchiolitis, RAD ▷ *Fig. 1.115* ▷ *Fig. 1.116*	Market flattening and depression of the hemidiaphragms, increased pulmonary lucency, decreased or suspended diaphragmatic motion (under fluoroscopy). Narrow mediastinum, small cardiac silhouette barrel chest. Radiography, fluoroscopy, US.	Viral infections, CF, α-1 antitrypsin deficiency. Congenital cutis laxa, aspirated foreign body in the trachea or in both bronchi, vascular rings, other cardiovascular anomalies, paratracheal masses. Any time the diameter of the airway is narrowed, the work of breathing must be increased for the same air exchange: flattened diaphragms.
Acidosis, dehydration	Hypovolemia, decreased pulmonary vascular markings, marked flattening of the hemidiaphragms, mildly decreased diaphragmatic motion.	Dyspnea. Diagnosis is clinical and with laboratory results in pyloric stenosis and storage disease (in infancy).
Bilateral pleural effusion ▷ *Fig. 1.117*	Bilateral blunt costophrenic angles, if large lung-field opacification. Diaphragmatic borders are generally obscured. US confirms.	Trauma, hemothorax, or chylothorax. Severe renal disease.
Bilateral tension pneumothorax	Chest radiograph is diagnostic. Pulmonary markings are absent. In most cases, the lungs are well demarcated and often collapsed.	Many causes: occurs in cavitating pneumonia, trauma, and in mechanically ventilated neonates.

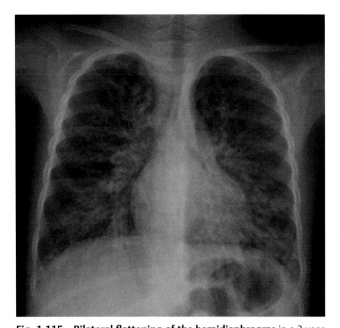

Fig. 1.115   Bilateral flattening of the hemidiaphragms in a 3-year-old girl with CF.

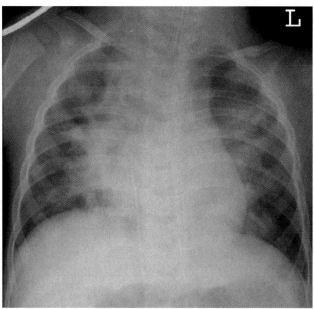

Fig. 1.116   Bilateral flattening of the hemidiaphragms in a 20-month-old boy with RSV infection.

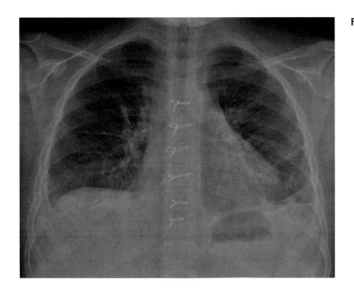

Fig. 1.117 Bilateral pleural effusion in a 12-year-old girl.

Table 1.45 Unilateral flat hemidiaphragm

Diagnosis	Findings	Comments
Exudative pleural effusion, empyema	Unilateral, partial, or total silhouette sign. Diaphragmatic contour possibly obscured, diaphragmatic motion may be decreased or absent on fluoroscopy, US.	Hematologic changes, signs of inflammation. TB must be excluded.
Unilateral check-valve mechanism (foreign-body aspiration)	Decreased pulmonary vascular markings, hilar prominence, narrow mediastinum, small cardiac silhouette.	Clinical signs with gasping, expiratory dyspnea, more marked than in inspiration. Inspiratory intercostal retraction. Foreign bodies mainly in 2–3 y olds.
Diseases with a unilateral lucent lung, including cysts, pneumatoceles, etc. ▷ *Fig. 1.118a, b*	May be normal radiographs. Fluroscopy: suspended or decreased diaphragmatic motion and flattening of the ipsilateral hemidiaphragm.	The symptoms depend on the primary disease, patient may be asymptomatic.
Unilateral tension pneumothorax ▷ *Fig. 1.119, p. 70*	Increased lucency of the affected hemithorax, absent lung markings. Progressive mediastinal displacement to the contralateral side leading to mediastinal herniation. Diaphragmatic motion decreased to absent.	Occurs in cavitating pneumonia, trauma, foreign body aspiration. Dyspnea.

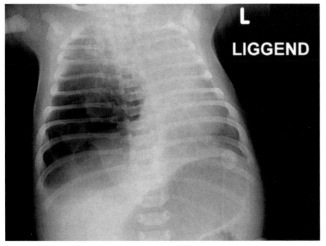

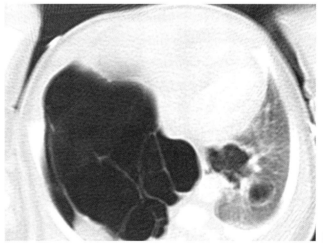

a   b

Fig. 1.118a, b Pulmonary blastoma. (**a**) Unilateral flat diaphragm in a child with pulmonary blastoma. (**b**) Coronal CT of the same patient depicts the extent of the disease.

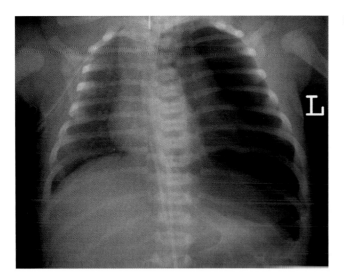

Fig. 1.119   Left-sided tension pneumothorax in a neonate.

Table 1.46   Diaphragmatic hump (unilateral)

Diagnosis	Findings	Comments
Partial eventration ▷ *Fig. 1.112, p. 67*	Most commonly as anteromedial hump due to a localized weakness in the muscle of the diaphragm, right more common than left. Lateral radiograph confirms the diagnosis.	Harmless incidental finding, especially in infants. Most are asymptomatic. DD: diaphragmatic hernia.
Tumors of the diaphragm ▷ *Fig. 1.120a, b*	Localized total elevation of the affected hemidiaphragm.	Very rare in children.

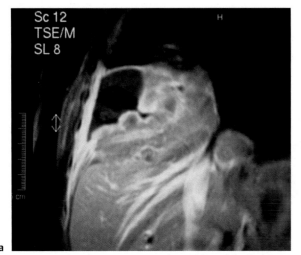

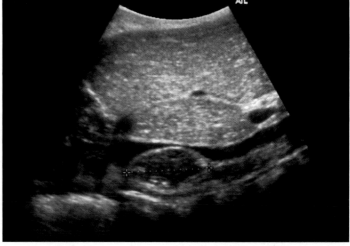

a   b

Fig. 1.120a, b   Rhabdomyosarcoma. (a) Coronal T1-weighted postcontrast MRI in a child with a rhabdomyosarcoma of the diaphragm. **(b)** US of the same patient displays the versatility of this modality in children.

Mediastinum

The Trachea

■ Fixed Tracheal Stenosis and Tracheomalacia

Tracheal pathology in children generally consists of tracheal narrowing that may be fixed (tracheal stenosis), this can be subdivided in long and short segmental stenosis, or variable (tracheomalacia). Presentation is typically with stridor, which is inspiratory with extrathoracic upper airway problems and biphasic with intrathoracic tracheal narrowing. Expiratory wheeze suggests more distal airway narrowing. Tracheal stenosis is frequently due to extrinsic compression and obstruction, and consequently dysphagia due to coexistent esophageal compression (particularly in the older child eating solids) may be present. In babies, the tracheal diameter is dependent on the respiratory phase, and a decrease in caliber of up to 50% is considered to be normal. This can make the interpretation of the trachea on a conventional radiograph difficult for the inexperienced radiologist.

■ Tracheal Displacement

Displacement of the trachea as visualized on plain radiographs or other imaging modalities may provide an important clue to pathology in related structures.

Table 1.47 Displacement and anterior buckling on the lateral radiograph

Diagnosis	Findings	Comments
Normal ▷ *Fig. 1.121* ▷ *Fig. 1.122*	Buckling in expiration.	More common in younger children, when radiograph taken at end of cry.
Esophageal dilatation ▷ *Fig. 1.123, p. 72* ▷ *Fig. 1.124, p. 72*		Achalasia, foreign body obstruction, esophageal atresia before and after surgery.
Esophageal duplication ▷ *Fig. 1.125, p. 72*	Can present with or without communication to the esophageal lumen.	Can remain undiagnosed for a prolonged period.
Cystic hygroma (cavernous lymphangioma) ▷ *Fig. 1.126, p. 72*	Cervical mass, with possible intrathoracic extension. Narrowed airway (larynx, trachea). Cystic components of variable size; optimal delineation of extend with MRI.	Most common site: neck and flanks. Mostly large and growing tumor. Patients may present with stridor. Diagnosis usually antenatal/clinical.
Bronchogenic cyst ▷ *Fig. 1.127a, b, p. 73*	Mainly near the carina; also in posterior (seldom anterior) mediastinum with narrowing or displacement of the trachea, main bronchi, or esophagus. CT and MRI	Origin: tracheobronchial tree. Content: clear fluid, seldom air (communication with the airway). Growth of the cyst is possible.
Neurogenic tumors ▷ *Fig. 1.128a–c, p. 73*	Posterior mediastinum. Anteriorly displaced esophagus. Calcifications can be seen.	Vanillylmandelic acid elevated in most cases, bone marrow can be involved. Opsoclonus, ataxia ("dancing eyes and feet") metaiodobenzylguanidine (MIBG) scintigraphy and MRI.
Anomalous vessels with tracheal displacement		(see **Table 1.100**)
Pharyngeal diverticulum	Lateral outpouching on upper gastrointestinal (UGI) study	Patients may present with swallowing difficulty.
Foregut duplication cyst	May communicate with esophageal lumen.	

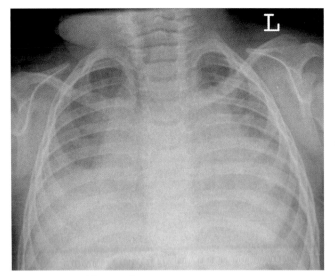

Fig. 1.121   Buckling trachea in expiration.

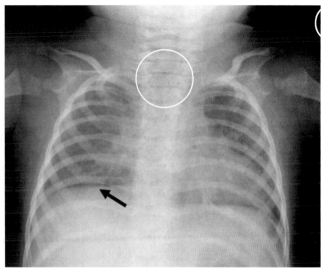

Fig. 1.122   Normal tracheal buckling in expiration. Chest radiograph obtained in an uncooperative 18-month-old boy. The diaphragm is at the level of the fourth anterior rib (arrow). The trachea is markedly buckled (circled).

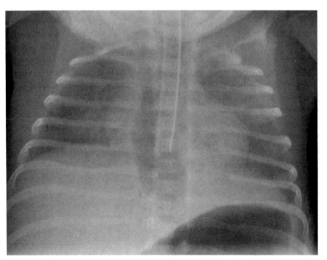

Fig. 1.123   Tube erroneously positioned in esophagus.

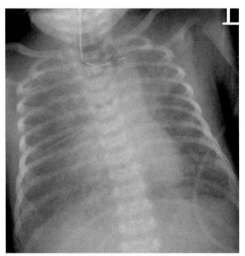

Fig. 1.124   Esophageal atresia. Note the curved NG tube in the proximal blind-ending esophagus.

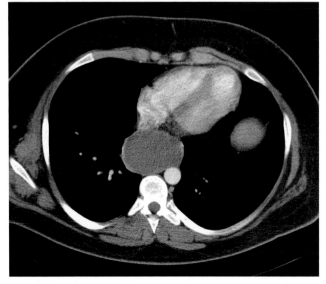

Fig. 1.125   Esophageal duplication in a 15-year-old girl presenting with dysphagia.

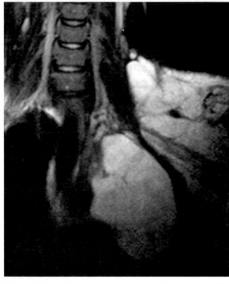

Fig. 1.126   Cystic hygroma in a 14-year-old girl.

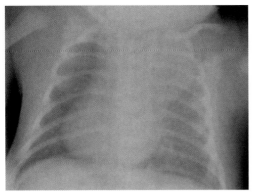
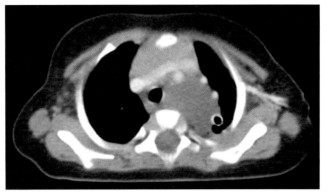

Fig. 1.127a, b   Bronchogenic cyst. (**a**) Chest radiograph showing a bronchogenic cyst in a 5-month-old boy. (**b**) Chest CT of the same patient.

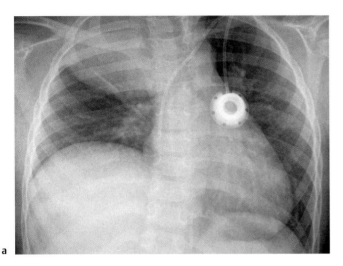
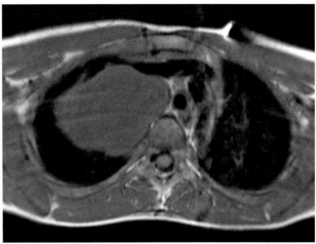

Fig. 1.128a–c   Neurogenic tumor. (**a**) Thoracic neuroblastoma in a 5-year-old boy. Note the elevation of the diaphragm as a result of vagus involvement. (**b**) Axial T1-weighted MRI of the same patient. (**c**) Coronal T1-weighted contrast-enhanced MRI of the same patient shows intense homogeneous enhancement.

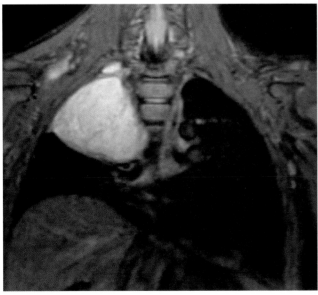

Table 1.48   Posterior displacement and buckling (anterior impression)

Diagnosis	Findings	Comments
Enlarged thyroid gland	Posterior displacement of the esophagus. Scout radiograph, barium swallow. US. Thyroid scintigraphy	Anterior swelling in the midcervical region. Mainly prepubertal and pubertal females.
Innominate artery syndrome ▷ *Fig. 1.129*		(see **Table 1.100**)
Widened ascending aorta		(see **Table 1.96**)
Lymphoma ▷ *Fig. 1.130a, b*	Tumor mass (lymphadenopathy) in superior, anterior, and middle mediastinum. Also pleural effusion, lung parenchyma, and skeletal involvement may be seen. CXR, MRI, and fludeoxyglucose-positron emission tomography (PET)-CT.	External cervical lymph adenopathy, visible or palpable. Splenomegaly, nephromegaly possible at any stage.
Bronchogenic cyst ▷ *Fig. 1.127, p. 73*	Small solitary space-occupying mass may disrupt lung aeration: local overinflation due to air trapping or atelectasis. Air-fluid level in the cyst. CT or MRI for diagnosis.	Asymptomatic or expectoration of fluid contents; stridor to severe dyspnea.
Sternal osteomyelitis or sternal tumor	Osteolysis, periostitis, soft-tissue tumor. US, CT, MRI.	Localized swelling over the sternum, pain, fever.
Teratoma, dermoid mesenchymoma, thymic tumor or cyst ▷ *Fig. 1.131a, b*	Solitary or multicystic. Teratoma may contain teeth, bone, calcification, fat. Pleural effusion suggests malignancy.	Tracheal displacement does not occur with a normal or hyperplastic thymus.
Thymic tumor		Thymic neoplasms all rare in childhood, including thymoma, lymphosarcoma, and primary carcinoma. Large thymic cysts are rare.

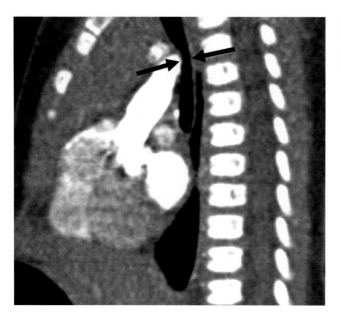

Fig. 1.129   Innominate artery compression. Sagittal reformat of thoracic CT in infant with stridor and pulsatile compression of the trachea on bronchoscopy. The trachea is significantly narrowed (between arrows) at the level of the innominate artery.

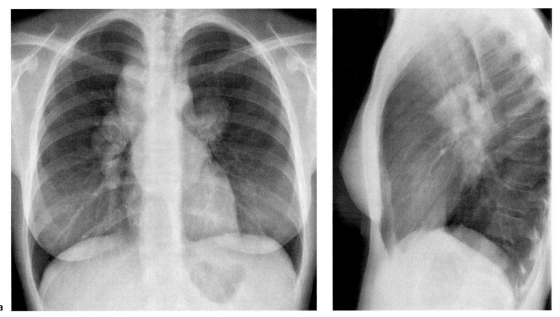

Fig. 1.130a, b   Lymphoma. (a) Lymphoma in a 14-year-old girl. (b) Note the anterior compression of the trachea by enlarged lymph nodes.

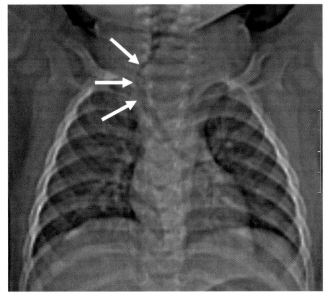

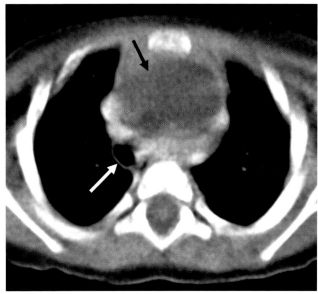

Fig. 1.131a, b   Posterolateral tracheal displacement by teratoma. (a) CT scout view in an 8-month-old boy with stridor. The trachea is narrowed and markedly displaced laterally (arrows) by an upper mediastinal mass. (b) Axial CT section in same patient demonstrates marked posterior and lateral displacement of the trachea (white arrow) by a cystic mass (black arrow). Histologic examination demonstrated a mature cystic teratoma.

Table 1.49 Lateral displacement and buckling on the anteroposterior radiograph

Diagnosis	Findings	Comments
Normal finding: left aortic arch	Deviation and displacement of the trachea to the right and anteriorly.	(see **Table 1.95**)
Right aortic arch ▷ *Fig. 1.132* ▷ *Fig. 1.133*	Trachea displaced to the left. Left-sided indentation of the trachea	(see **Table 1.100**)
Aberrant left pulmonary artery ("pulmonary sling") ▷ *Fig. 1.134a, b*	Displacement of the lower trachea to the left.	(see **Table 1.100**)
Mass effect of volume loss	Common imaging findings: displacement of trachea and mediastinum. Upper lobe collapse particularly on right may result in lateral tracheal displacement. Paratracheal mass may displace trachea. If vessels pass behind the esophagus, then the tracheal diameter is unaffected.	Causes: trauma, foreign-body aspiration, postoperative. Differential diagnosis: TB, lymphoma, cysts, tumors, and hygromas. Aberrant vessels may be isolated or associated with congenital heart disease.

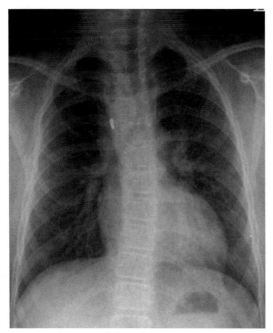

Fig. 1.132 **Right aortic arch.** Note the Botallian duct clip on the right side of the mediastinum instead of the left.

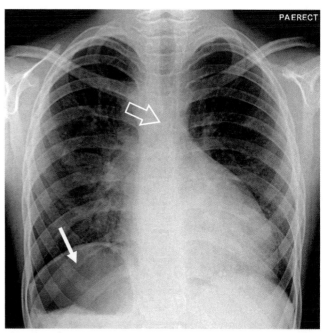

Fig. 1.133 **Leftward displacement of trachea by right aortic arch.** Chest radiograph in a 13-year-old boy with history of complex congenital heart disease. The lower trachea is displaced to the left due to a right aortic arch (open arrow). Note dextrogastria (white arrow).

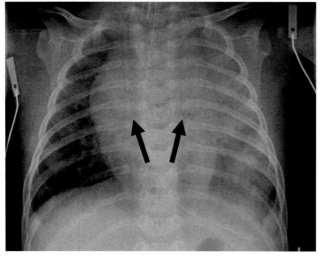

Fig. 1.134a, b **Pulmonary artery sling. (a)** Chest radiograph in neonate with stridor. The tracheal angle is wide (arrows). There is diffuse increased opacification in the left hemithorax. **(b)** Axial CT

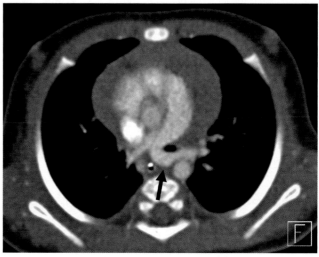

image in same patient demonstrates retrotracheal course of left pulmonary artery (arrow) with associated tracheal stenosis.

Table 1.50 Long-segment tracheal stenosis

Diagnosis	Findings	Comments
Normal finding: expiratory collapse ("floppy trachea") ▷ *Fig. 1.135*	Caliber fluctuations up to 50% are physiologic.	With or without stridor. Physiologic in first year of life and an example of the softness of the immature tracheal cartilage.
Elastic tracheal stenosis (tracheomalacia)	Mostly associated with hyperlucent lung. Fluoroscopy, bronchography and spot films, bronchoscopy.	Abnormally soft tracheal cartilage (past infancy). Late sequela of endotracheal intubation, tracheostomy, and surgical repair of esophageal atresia (even without dilatation).
(Laryngo-)tracheitis DD: epiglottitis	CXR is unnecessary and possibly dangerous; this is a clinical diagnosis. In epiglottitis, there is marked swelling of the epiglottis, occasionally with subglottic tracheal narrowing.	All the signs of infection. Inspiratory stridor, severe respiratory distress, barking cough, hoarseness, gasping, fever. Epiglottitis is rare today due to inoculation.
Primary tracheal stenosis (intramural) ▷ *Fig. 1.136*	Mainly in combination with unilateral or bilateral pulmonary hypoplasia. Preoperative CT with virtual bronchoscopy.	Congenitally malformed small and nonelastic cartilage rings and absent dorsal membrane. Rigid tracheal wall. Severe respiratory distress. Ninety percent diagnosed in first year of life.
Intramural tracheal tumors	Long-segment narrowing occurs only in papillomatosis as it spreads from the larynx to the trachea. Wartlike excrescences from the tracheal mucosa can be delineated on CXR and CT, proven at endoscopy.	Varying degrees of inspiratory and expiratory stridor.

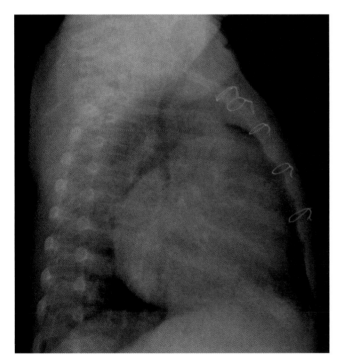

Fig. 1.135 Expiratory collapse/buckling of the trachea on a lateral chest radiograph.

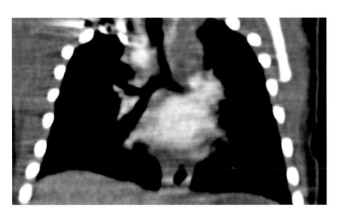

Fig. 1.136 Tracheal stenosis on coronal CT.

Table 1.51   Short-segment tracheal stenosis

Diagnosis	Findings	Comments
Right aortic arch (also with aberrant left subclavian artery); sometimes caused by asymmetric double aortic arch ▷ *Fig. 1.137*	Tracheal impression on the right, deviated to the left, above the bifurcation at the level of the left aortic arch. CXR: Trachea deviated to left at level of arch and narrowed. Associated oesophageal narrowing. CT/MRI and/or echocardiogram: definitive evaluation.	Vascular ring more common with right arch with aberrant left subclavian than with right arch and mirror image branching. Ductus may be patent or merely a ligamentous remnant (see **Table 1.96**).
Double aortic arch ▷ *Fig. 1.138* ▷ *Fig. 1.139a, b*	Chest X-ray (CXR): Narrowing of trachea at level of double arch. The right arch is usually dominant, and radiographic appearance may simulate a right arch (i.e., trachea deviates to left). Obstructive overinflation frequent. Associated esophageal narrowing. CT/magnetic resonance imaging (MRI) and/or echocardiogram: definitive evaluation. Bilateral tracheal and esophageal impression above the bifurcation. Impression is ventral on the lateral view (dorsal impressions of the esophagus). MRI.	A segment of either arch may be atretic: this can make distinction from other vascular rings challenging. For example, a double arch with atresia of the distal left arch may be very similar in appearance to a right arch with mirror image branching (see **Table 1.100**).
Left brachiocephalic and common carotid artery (left innominate artery; "innominate artery compression syndrome") ▷ *Fig. 1.129, p. 74*	Defined by >50% narrowing of trachea at level of innominate artery. The innominate artery may be anatomically normal, be dilated or aneurysmal, or have a distal origin from the arch with an abnormally horizontal course of innominate artery across trachea. Ventral tracheal compression just below the level of the clavicle.	A controversial entity: In many cases, the primary abnormality is tracheomalacia, which allows the innominate artery to take the apparently abnormal course. Mild narrowing of the airway at the level of the innominate artery is a normal finding in many infants. Aortopexy may be beneficial in some symptomatic cases, however (see **Table 1.100**).
Aberrant left pulmonary artery ("pulmonary sling") ▷ *Fig. 1.134, p. 76*	CXR: The lower trachea is displaced to the left. The carina is often widely splayed and may appear almost horizontal. There may be overinflation, more commonly of the right lung, due to main bronchial compression. CT/MRI: left pulmonary artery arises anomalously from distal pulmonary trunk or right pulmonary artery, and runs between trachea and esophagus.	There is frequently (~50%) associated long-segment congenital tracheal stenosis and an abnormal tracheal branching pattern. Also associated with patent ductus arteriosus (PDA), atrial septal defect (ASD), tetralogy of Fallot, and persistent left-sided superior vena cava.
Tracheal foreign body aspiration	Mimics a stenosis, especially if radiolucent. Mobile foreign bodies can occur. Normal findings on radiography are common. Endoscopy. Fluoroscopy may show asymmetric diaphragmatic motion.	Acute onset. Stridor, especially in young children ("virtual vacuum cleaners"). Localization hint: coins project en face in the esophagus, only laterally as trachea too narrow.
Swallowed foreign bodies (radiopaque or radiolucent) ▷ *Fig. 1.140*	Impacted foreign bodies may compress the trachea dorsally (secondary to edema).	Acute onset of stridor or mild respiratory symptoms in small children. Difficulty in swallowing.
Stenosis after surgical repair of esophageal atresia, compression by the dilated proximal esophagus	Findings resemble those of left-sided brachiocephalic trunk. Stenosis at the height of the anastomosis. UGI with caution.	Typically barking cough, stridor caused by localized tracheomalacia.
Postintubation, tracheostomy, and surgery ▷ *Fig. 1.141*		Usually caused by too large a tube, resulting in pressure ischemia of respiratory mucosa. Accounts for 90% of mature acquired laryngotracheal stenoses. Develops in 1%–5% of patients undergoing prolonged endotracheal intubation. Postesophageal atresia, late sequelae of mucosal granulomas, scarring, or strictures. Stridor following extubation may require reintubation.

(continues on page 80)

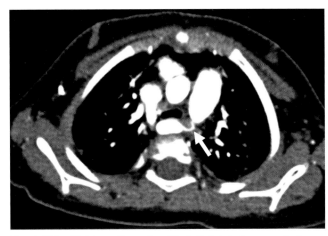

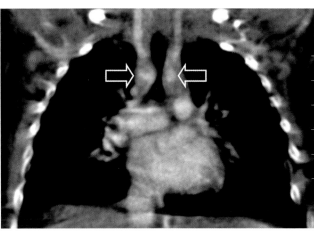

Fig. 1.137 Right aortic arch with left-sided ductus arteriosus. Axial CT image in an infant with stridor: the descending aorta lies posterior to the trachea. A right arch was present (not shown). The ductus arteriosus is patent (arrow), connecting the descending aorta to the left pulmonary artery, completing a vascular ring.

Fig. 1.138 Double aortic arch (arrows) on coronal contrast-enhanced CT.

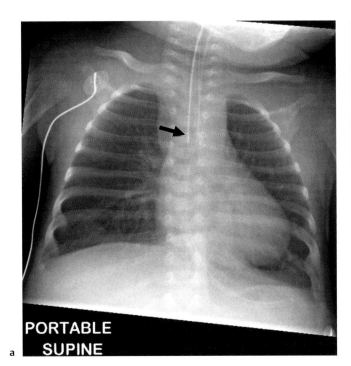

a

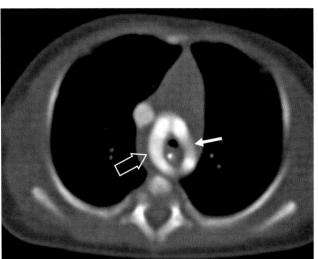

b

Fig. 1.139a, b Double aortic arch. (a) Chest radiograph in an infant with stridor requiring ventilation. The lower trachea deviates slightly to the left (arrow). **(b)** Axial CT image in same patient following intravenous contrast demonstrates a double aortic arch: the right arch (open arrow) is slightly larger than the left arch (white arrow).

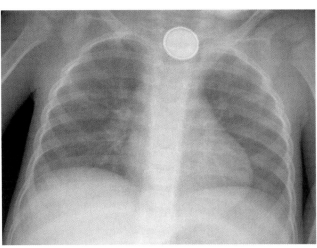

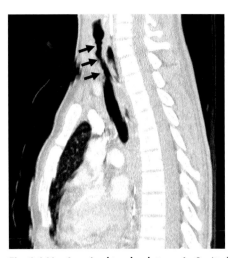

Fig. 1.140 Coin battery ingestion. Note the beveled edge that is pathognomonic for a coin battery. This is an indication for emergency bronchoesophagoscopy.

Fig. 1.141 Acquired tracheal stenosis. Sagittal reformat of thoracic computed tomography (CT) demonstrating acquired tracheal stenosis (arrows) in a 13-year-old girl following prolonged intubation on an adult intensive care unit after a road traffic accident.

Table 1.51   (Cont.) Short-segment tracheal stenosis

Diagnosis	Findings	Comments
Masses—extramural: paratracheal or bronchogenic cysts, goiter, lymphadenopathy, lymphoma, and localized retropharyngeal abscess ▷ *Fig. 1.142a–c*	Tracheal lumen narrowed at the level of the lesion. US, CT, MRI are most useful. Variable appearance according to lesion.	Respiratory symptoms vary with the mass size: stridor, gasping, labored breathing, chronic recurrent infections. Need for endoscopy usually based on clinical findings. Common lesions include lymphoma, bronchogenic cyst, esophageal duplication cyst, neuroenteric cyst, mediastinal teratoma, lymphadenopathy, thymic lesions, lymphatic malformation, and hemangioma.
Masses—intramural: hemangioma, polypoid hemangioendothelioma, lymphangioma, cysts, ectopic goiter (subglottic) ▷ *Fig. 1.143*	Endoscopy; CXR, CT, MRI. Soft-tissue density may be visible on CXR. There may be generalized air trapping.	Rare: more common causes include subglottic hemangioma, Wegener granulomatosis, and laryngotracheal papillomatosis.
Segmental tracheal stenosis, segmental tracheomalacia	Seldom an isolated lesion, more commonly in combination with tracheoesophageal fistula or after surgical repair of esophageal atresia, at the site of the anastomosis and fistula repair.	
Traumatic		Occasionally occurs following blunt trauma to larynx and trachea. Also occasionally following caustic ingestion and inhalational and thermal injuries.
Congenital tracheal stenosis ▷ *Fig. 1.144a, b*	May be short-segment, long-segment, or even extend into the main bronchi. Often features complete cartilaginous rings, producing an abnormally rounded appearance of the airway on cross-section. Diagnosis usually made at endoscopy ± contrast bronchography. Echocardiography and CT performed to identify extrinsic compression.	Up to 1% of all laryngotracheal stenoses. Frequently associated with cardiac defects, particularly pulmonary artery sling. Also associated with pulmonary agenesis and aplasia.

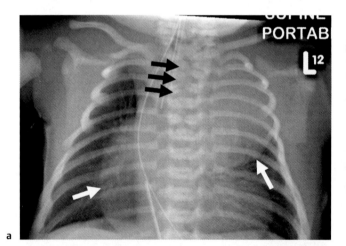

a

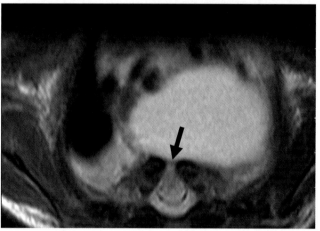

b

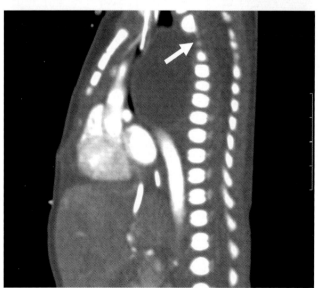

c

Fig. 1.142a–c Tracheal compression by neuroenteric cyst.
(**a**) Chest radiograph in neonate with antenatal diagnosis of congenital lung malformation and respiratory distress. There is a mass extending from the left apex to the right lower zone (white arrows). There are associated midline segmentation defects in the upper thoracic spine (black arrows). The trachea is displaced to the right. (**b**) Axial short inversion-time inversion-recovery (STIR) MRI in same patient demonstrates water dense structure arising from midline segmentation defect (arrow). (**c**) Sagittal reformat of CT in same patient. The cystic structure is again demonstrated arising from the region of the segmentation defect (arrow).

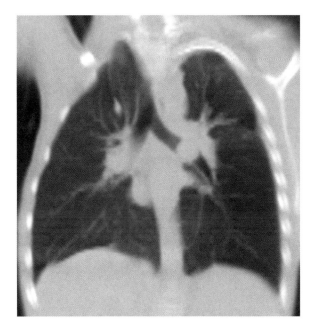

Fig. 1.143   Carcinoid in the left mainstem bronchus in a 13-year-old boy.

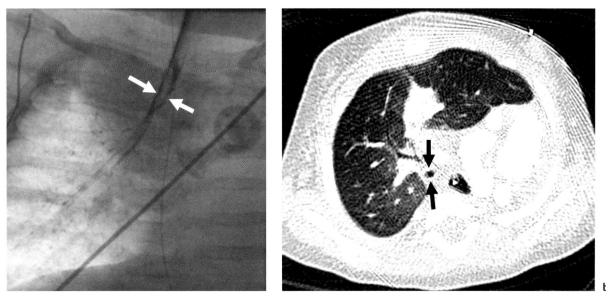

a

b

Fig. 1.144a, b   Congenital tracheal stenosis with agenesis of left lung. (a) Contrast bronchogram in neonate with stridor demonstrates tracheal narrowing with focal narrowing due to complete cartilaginous rings (between arrows). The left main bronchus is absent. **(b)** Axial CT image in same patient demonstrates absent left lung with herniation of right lung across the midline. The trachea has an unusually rounded morphology (between arrows), in keeping with complete cartilaginous rings.

Table 1.52 Tracheomalacia

Diagnosis	Findings	Comments
Primary ▷ **Fig. 1.145a, b**	Diagnosis is based on identifying expiratory collapse of the involved airway. This may be achieved with bronchoscopy, bronchography, or occasionally with dynamic (inspiratory and expiratory) CT.	Most commonly in association with prematurity. May be due to primary cartilage disorders such as polychondritis, chondromalacia, or with metabolic disorders including the mucopolysaccharidoses. Also in association with tracheoesophageal fistula.
Secondary	As primary, but may also have indication of secondary cause.	Most commonly iatrogenic following intubation or tracheostomy. Also following infective tracheobronchitis or due to extrinsic compression: any cause of fixed stenosis due to extrinsic compression may also cause tracheomalacia, particularly those involving vascular compression.
Tracheobronchomegaly (Mounier-Kuhn syndrome)	Marked dilatation of trachea and main bronchi in inspiration, with expiratory airway collapse. Recurrent respiratory infections result in bronchiectasis and lung fibrosis.	Rare. Deficiency of elastin in tracheal walls.

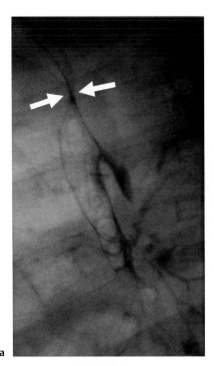
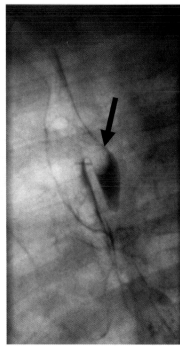

Fig. 1.145a, b Tracheomalacia following esophageal atresia/tracheoesophageal fistula. (a) Contrast bronchogram in a 4-year-old boy with persistent stridor following neonatal repair of esophageal atresia with tracheoesophageal fistula. At atmospheric pressure in expiration, there is complete collapse of the upper trachea (between arrows). **(b)** Contrast bronchogram at positive end expiratory pressure of 20 mm Hg. The airway narrowing is overcome. Note the remnant of the tracheoesophageal fistula (arrow).

a

b

Table 1.53 Widened caliber of the trachea and bronchi

Diagnosis	Findings	Comments
Previous intubation and suction	Dilatation occurs in the upper trachea above the bifurcation.	In neonates and young infants with chronic disease.
Tracheomegaly, bronchomegaly (Mounier-Kuhn syndrome)	Abnormal width of the trachea and bronchi, later sacklike bronchiectasis. Expiratory collapse of the tracheal wall (trachea dilates in inspiration). Bronchoscopy: abnormal mobility of the posterior tracheal wall, occasionally with mucosal changes (membranous atrophy of the posterior wall), anterior bowing of the intercartilaginous sections.	Congenital malformation with hypoplasia of elastic fibers of the smooth muscle. Predominantly in young and schoolaged children (2–14 y). Noisy bitonal cough, recurrent infections, fever sputum production, pneumonias. May also be asymptomatic. Complication: pneumothorax.

The Hilum

The hilum encompasses the root of the lung and consists of the major pulmonary vessels, bronchial walls, and lymph nodes. Hilar enlargement in children may be due to a general increase in hilar markings, usually reflecting peribronchial thickening such as occurs in viral lower respiratory tract infection, CF, and asthma. True hilar enlargement represents either hilar lymphadenopathy or hilar pulmonary arterial enlargement. Adenopathy is characterized by a lobulated outline to the hilum, often with filling in of the hilar point at the junction of the superior pulmonary vein with pulmonary artery. Arterial enlargement demonstrates retained vascular contours, often with a dilated main pulmonary artery. Distinction between arterial enlargement and adenopathy is best achieved with cross-sectional imaging.

In children, the lymph nodes will only be seen if they are enlarged and thus pathologic in size. For a detailed evaluation of the hilum, contrast-enhanced CT or MRI should be used.

Although the hilum can be visualized on the lateral film, it is not common practice to obtain routine lateral films in children; as radiation protection, this is essential (image gently).

Table 1.54 Bilateral hilar enlargement due to lymphadenopathy

Diagnosis	Findings	Comments
Bronchiolitis, reactive airway disease (RAD), viral infections of the lower airways ▷ *Fig. 1.146a, b*	Minimal interstitial prominence, peribronchial thickening, hyperinflation (especially in viral infections). The hilar lymph nodes are increased in size rather than density; the outline is hazy.	Episodes of coughing, possibly febrile, signs of infection. Seasonal occurrence of RSV infections, mainly in autumn and winter.
Measles	Hila are dense, with prominent bronchovascular markings. In the exanthematous phase of measles pneumonia, the hila are widened and more dense, and lung markings are increased; miliary nodules are also present adjacent to the hila.	Nowadays rare as a result of vaccination programs.
Pertussis	The increased dense hilar markings and perihilar signs ("shaggy heart") reflect bronchitis in the cartarrhal stage. Increased pulmonary density occurs mainly in the basal segments.	Diagnosed by the typical episodes of coughing in the convulsive stage, previously known as "catarrhal bronchitis."

(continues on page 84)

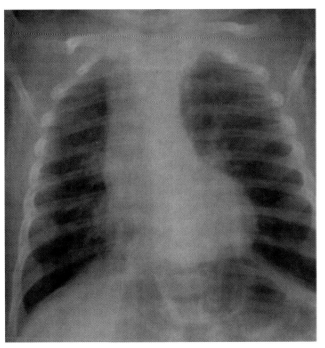
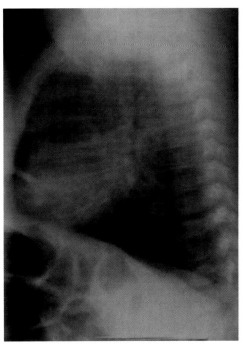

a   b

Fig. 1.146a, b   Bronchiolitis. (a) Bronchiolitis in a 20-month-old boy. **(b)** Lateral chest radiograph shows flattening of the diaphragm.

Table 1.54 (Cont.) Bilateral hilar enlargement due to lymphadenopathy

Diagnosis	Findings	Comments
CF ▷ *Fig. 1.147*	Densely enlarged hila, initially moderate and increasing over ensuing years. Increasing pulmonary involvement with chronic infiltrative changes. Secondary hyperinflation and barrel chest deformity. Late findings resemble bronchiectasis.	Onset in infancy, Increasing and progressing in childhood. All signs of chronic infection with dyspnea and cough.
Malignant lymphoma/leukemia ▷ *Fig. 1.148a–c* ▷ *Fig. 1.149a–c, p. 86* ▷ *Fig. 1.150, p. 86*	Neoplastic mediastinal enlargement is mostly due to bilateral lymph node enlargement, particularly the paratracheal nodes.	Diagnosed on bone marrow biopsy. Hematologic changes. Peripheral lymphadenopathy, hepatosplenomegaly. Bruises. Hilar involvement in Hodgkin disease in 50%, more common than in NHL.
Mycoplasma infection	Hilar enlargement accompanied by segmental pneumonia, particularly in the lower lobes (may even be unilateral). Radiographic appearance commonly resembles TB.	Mild leucocytosis or normal white cell count. Organism must be positively proven. Bronchoalveolar lavage.
LCH, malignant histiocytosis	Mild, rarely marked hilar enlargement with sharp outlines. Evolves into interstitial pulmonary changes with small patches and confluent densities mainly in the bases. Emphysematous blebs, honeycomb lungs.	
Chronic aspiration	Combination of bilateral hilar enlargement with multiple disseminated small patchy pulmonary densities.	
Fungal infection	May be unilateral. Perihilar and occasional mediastinal lymph node involvement. Caution: air-space disease.	
TB ▷ *Fig. 1.151, p. 86*	Nodular density to increasing hilar width. Primary complex in the lungs. Loss of the mediastinal contour.	Small children to young school age. Gradual onset, with or without cough. Rarely febrile. Purified protein derivative (PPD) positive. May also be asymptomatic. Increasingly seen in the western world after a period of relevant low incidence.
Bacterial pneumonia	In association with bilateral air space disease. Unlikely under 18–24 mo as mother's antibodies still present.	Clinical signs of pneumonia.
Castlemann disease	May involve single or multiple mediastinal compartments, including the hila.	A group of rare lymphoproliferative disorders that are more common in adults.
Sarcoidosis ▷ *Fig. 1.152a, b, p. 87*	Characteristically symmetric lobulated lymph nodes; no pulmonary changes in stage 1, later (stage 2) there are small patchy densities in the lungs. Other lymph nodes can also become involved (tracheobronchial, paratracheal).	This classic adult presentation is extremely rare in preteenaged children.
Vascular causes: increased hilar and pulmonary vascular markings—active: left-to-right shunt	Enlarged hila with enlarged vessel caliber.	(see **Table 1.75**)
Specific type: pulmonary hypertension	Pulmonary arteries are significantly enlarged close to the hilum, and constricted peripherally ("arterial pruning").	
Vascular causes: increased hilar and pulmonary vascular markings—passive: cardiac failure	Enlarged hila and increased caliber of the vessels that are hazy in outline.	
Vascular causes: increased hilar and pulmonary vascular markings—pulmonary valve failure	Massively enlarged hila, with decreased peripheral pulmonary vascular markings.	Rare, most commonly in tetralogy of Fallot (see **Table 1.78**).
Metastases	Neoplastic in nature, lobulated or egg-shaped lymph nodes.	
Granulomatous infections	More usually unilateral.	TB, histoplasmosis.
Other infections	Milder hilar enlargement can occur in many acute and chronic pulmonary infections.	Examples include RSV (often more right-sided), pertussis (now rare), chicken pox, measles, mycoplasma, bacterial pneumonia.

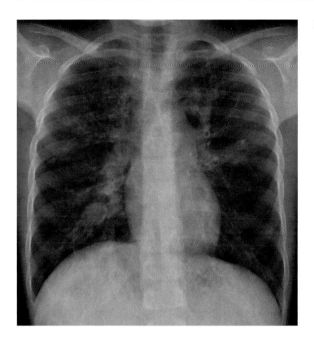

Fig. 1.147   Bilateral hilar enlargement in cystic fibrosis.

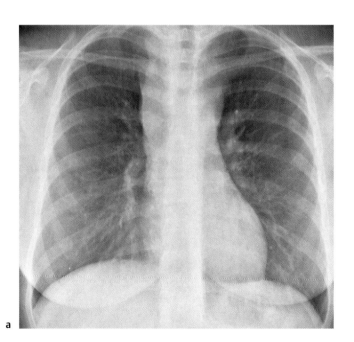

a

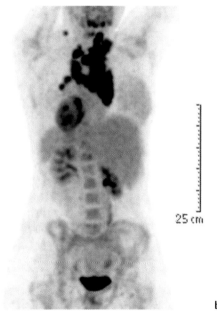

b

Fig. 1.148a–c   Lymphoma. (a) Bilateral hilar enlargement in a 16-year-old girl with lymphoma. (**b**) PET-CT of the same patient shows the extent of disease. (**c**) PET-CT of the same patient.

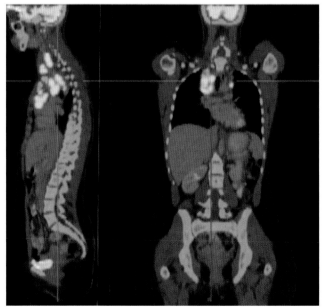

c

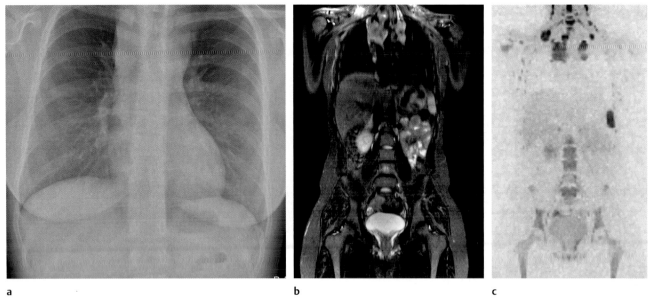

a   b   c

Fig. 1.149a–c   Lymphoma. (a) Bilateral hilar enlargement in a 16-year-old girl with lymphoma. **(b)** Whole-body STIR MRI shows pathologic lymph node enlargement. **(c)** Diffusion-weighted whole body imaging with background signal suppression, a new diffusion-weighted imaging technique for whole body imaging that produces PET-like images.

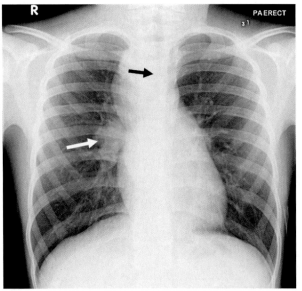

a

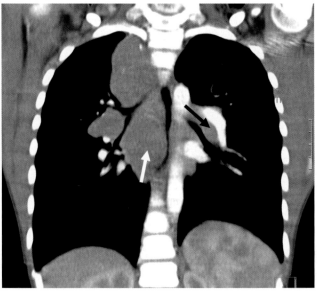

b

Fig. 1.150a, b   Hodgkin disease. (a) Chest radiograph in an 8-year-old boy with cervical lymphadenopathy and night sweats. There is right paratracheal lymphadenopathy causing some tracheal displacement (black arrow). There is also right hilar enlargement (white arrow).

(b) Coronally reformatted CT in the same patient demonstrates adenopathy as described, but with further lymph node enlargement in the subcarinal (white arrow) and left hilar stations (black arrow). Lymph node biopsy confirmed Hodgkin disease.

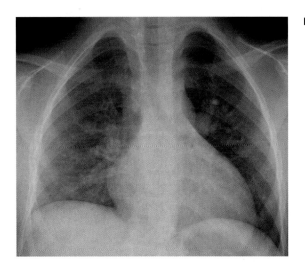

Fig. 1.151   Bilateral hilar enlargement in a 16-year-old boy.

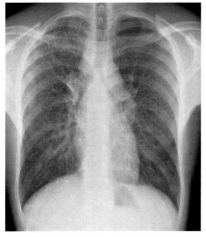
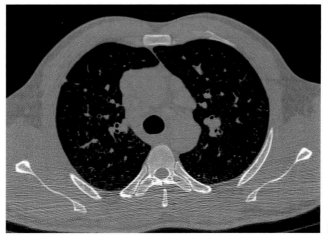

a   b

Fig. 1.152a, b   Sarcoidosis. (**a**) Stage 2 sarcoidosis. (**b**) CT of the same patient shows interstitial abnormalities.

Table 1.55   Bilateral hilar enlargement due to pulmonary arterial dilatation

Diagnosis	Findings	Comments
Left-to-right shunt ▷ *Fig. 1.153*	Cardiac enlargement with VSD and PDA. Right atrial enlargement only in ASD.	ASD, VSD, PDA, AVSD.
Primary pulmonary hypertension	Large central vessels, "pruned" peripheral vessels.	Rare, idiopathic condition with poor prognosis. Familial and sporadic forms. Presentation with dyspnea and chest pain.
Chronic pulmonary disease	Usually evidence of underlying lung disease.	CF most common. Also BPD, interstitial fibrosis, pulmonary hypoplasia.
Pulmonary valve regurgitation	Often massive pulmonary arterial dilatation, may cause airway obstruction.	Usually as a variant of tetralogy of Fallot ("absent pulmonary valve syndrome").
Recurrent pulmonary emboli		Rare in children. Usually line associated (e.g., children on total parenteral nutrition).
Pulmonary venous abnormality ▷ *Fig. 1.16, p. 14*	Mixed arterial and venous dilatation, with or without frank pulmonary edema.	Examples include anomalous venous return, pulmonary vein stenosis, pulmonary veno-occlusive disease, left atrial obstruction.

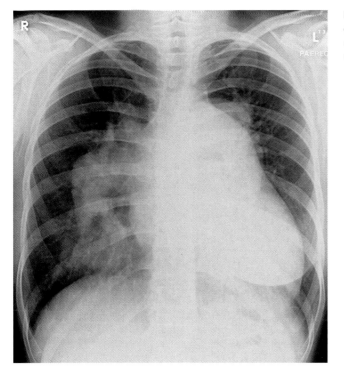

Fig. 1.153   Massive pulmonary arterial dilatation. Chest radiograph in a 14-year-old female with Eisenmenger syndrome. There is massive dilatation of the main and central pulmonary arteries, with relatively oligemic lung periphery.

Table 1.56 Unilateral hilar enlargement due to lymphadenopathy

Diagnosis	Findings	Comments
Nonspecific upper or lower respiratory tract infection (bronchiolitis) ▷ *Fig. 1.154* ▷ *Fig. 1.155*	Peribronchial thickening, increased pulmonary vascular markings. Effacement of the mediastinal contour at the level of the hilum, more commonly bilateral.	Fever, cough, wheezin
TB (primary infection)	Nodular density leads to increasing hilar size. Primary complex in the lungs. Loss of the mediastinal contour. Usually right-sided. Often associated subcarinal ± paratracheal lymphadenopathy. May cause air trapping or collapse (see **Fig. 1.17c**). Rim enhancement with low central density on CT. Calcification rare in primary infection. Primary focus may or may not be visible.	Small children to young school age. Gradual onset, with or without cough. Rarely febrile. PPD positive. May also be asymptomatic.
Other granulomatous infection		Histoplasmosis, coccidioidomycosis.
Bacterial, mycoplasma, and fungal pneumonias	Disease correlates with the radiographic appearance. Unilateral more common than bilateral.	Signs of acute infection, cough, moderate dyspnea.
Viral pneumonia ▷ *Fig. 1.156*	Pulmonary changes are the same as described with bilateral viral pneumonia. Rarely unilateral.	Cough, signs of infection.
Metastases	Unilateral, moderately well defined, hilar lymphadenopathy; confirmed on the lateral radiograph.	
Malignant lymphoma/leukemia ▷ *Fig. 1.157*	Mostly with other signs of lymphoma (mediastinal, paratracheal, bronchial), effusions. Bilateral hilar enlargement far more common.	Signs of systemic illness.
Infectious mononucleosis ▷ *Fig. 1.158*	Unilateral or bilateral. No pulmonary changes.	Serologic proof of the specific Epstein-Barr viral antibodies.
Pertussis		(see **Table 1.50**)
Vascular causes: unilateral enlargement of the pulmonary artery		
Absent pulmonary valve with unilateral agenesis of the pulmonary artery	Marked widening of one hilum, mainly the right, with a very small left hilum. Very rare variant of tetralogy of Fallot.	
Valvular pulmonary stenosis	Widened left hilum and pulmonary artery segment.	(see **Table 1.76**)

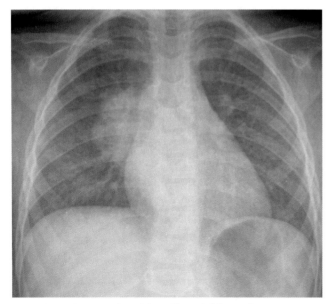

Fig. 1.154 Pneumonia with unilateral hilar enlargement in a 9-year-old girl.

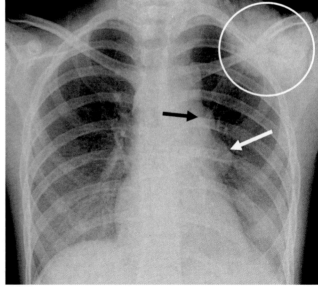

Fig. 1.155 Unilateral hilar adenopathy in TB. Chest radiograph in a 14-year-old Arabic girl with TB isolated from a lymph node biopsy. There is left hilar (white arrow) and aortopulmonary (black arrow) lymphadenopathy. There is some ill-defined left lower lobe opacification and a small left-sided pleural effusion. An apparent lobulated mass overlying the left clavicle (circled) was a hair braid artifact.

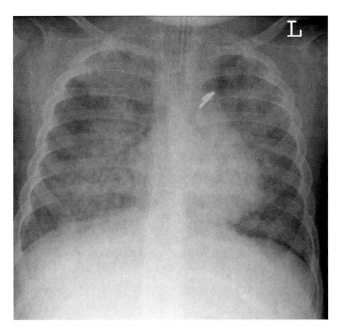

Fig. 1.156 **RSV pneumonia** in a 20-month-old boy.

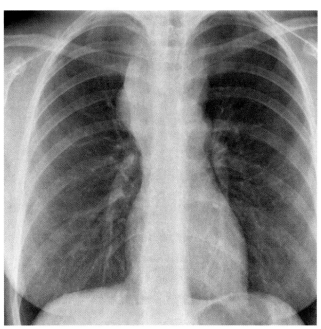

Fig. 1.157 **Stage 2 Hodgkin lymphoma** in a 16-year-old girl.

Fig. 1.158 **Epstein-Barr virus** in a 16-year-old boy.

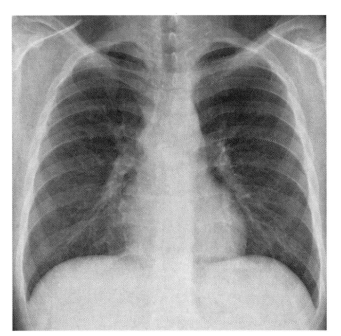

Table 1.57 **Unilateral hilar enlargement due to arterial enlargement**

Diagnosis	Findings	Comments
Poststenotic dilatation ▷ *Fig. 1.159, p. 90*	Enlarged main pulmonary segment and apparent enlargement of proximal left pulmonary artery. Proximal right pulmonary artery dilatation concealed on frontal radiograph.	
Pulmonary hypertension with absent contralateral pulmonary artery	Small, oligemic contralateral lung.	For example, in unilateral pulmonary hypoplasia.

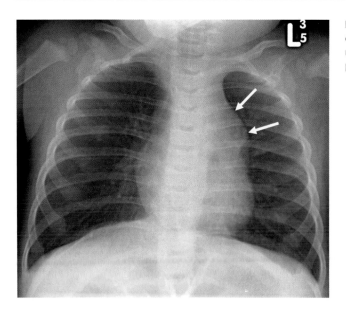

Fig. 1.159 Poststenotic dilatation. Chest radiograph in a 10-month-old girl with known severe pulmonary valvular stenosis. There is enlargement of the left hilum due to poststenotic dilatation of the main and left pulmonary arteries (arrows).

■ Simulated Hilar Enlargement

Apparent hilar enlargement, and particularly an increase in hilar density without enlargement, may be due to superimposed densities on the frontal projection. This is usually clarified by a lateral projection or CT examination.

Table 1.58   Pitfalls with unilateral hilar enlargement or density

Diagnosis	Findings	Comments
Segmental pneumonia in the superior segments of the lower lobes	Frontal view: projects over the hilar region. Lateral view: posterior in position. Hilum unremarkable.	Signs of pneumonia.
Atelectasis of the RUL, one of the segments, or partial atelectasis of the middle lobe	Diagnosis on the lateral view, hilum unremarkable	Clinical symptoms (e.g., dyspnea).
Metastases ▷ *Fig. 1.160a, b*	Round densities that project outside of the hilum on the lateral radiograph.	
Mass posterior to hilum		For example, metastasis, intrapulmonary bronchogenic cyst.

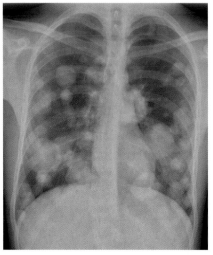

a

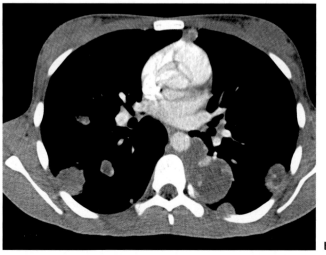

b

Fig. 1.160a, b   Metastases. (a) Multiple pulmonary metastases in a 17-year-old. **(b)** Chest CT shows that the enlarged hilum actually is a pulmonary metastasis.

The Mediastinum

The mediastinum is the central space of the thorax located between the two pleuropulmonary cavities to the right and left, the cervicothoracic inlet above, and the interdiaphragmatic thoracoabdominal outlet inferiorly. It contains the heart and great vessels, the thymus, the esophagus, the trachea and main bronchi, lymph nodes, and mediastinal pleural reflections, as well as the vagus and phrenic nerves.

On the lateral thoracic radiographs, the mediastinum is divided into the anterior, middle, and posterior compartments (**Fig. 1.161a**). The anterior mediastinum is located between the sternum and the pulmonary root, and the posterior mediastinal space extends posteriorly from a line connecting the anterior surfaces of the thoracic vertebral bodies. The middle mediastinum is the remaining portion.

On the frontal thoracic radiograph, the mediastinum is divided in the superior, middle, and inferior mediastinum (**Fig. 1.161b**). The superior mediastinum extends from the thoracic inlet to the superior aspect of the hila. The middle mediastinum comprises the hilar region. The inferior mediastinum is bordered by the lower aspect of the hila and the diaphragm.

This division of the mediastinal space is used for putting together a differential diagnosis. Keep in mind, however, that lesions arising in one mediastinal compartment often involve an adjacent one, which makes it sometimes difficult to define the originating site.

Neonates and Infants

The superior and often the middle mediastinum are physiologically widened because of the presence of the thymus. When the thymus shrinks or disappears, as a consequence of stress, the mediastinum will appear narrow. The thymus rebounds after relief of the stress. The shape and size of both the normal as well as the rebounding thymus is highly variable from patient to patient.

Older Children

The thymus gradually involutes. By the age of 3 years, the thymus is usually not border-forming on the frontal chest radiograph.

School-aged Children

The mediastinum assumes the size and contours as in adults.

■ Imaging Techniques

This space can be examined using anteroposterior and lateral thoracic radiographs (**Fig. 1.162**), US (**Fig. 1.163**), CT (**Fig. 1.164**), and MRI (**Fig. 1.165**).

In early childhood, the mediastinum does lend itself to US examination. There are three main approaches to the mediastinum: (1) suprasternal approach allows examination of the superior mediastinum; (2) right and left parasternal approach, with the patient in lateral decubitus, explores the anterior mediastinal compartment and the heart; (3) subcostal abdominal approach allows transdiaphragmatic investigation, which is useful for masses of the cardiophrenic angles.

MRI is superior to CT for evaluating extension of lesions, in particular of tumors invading the spinal canal and those in contact with the heart or the cervicothoracic or thoracoabdominal junction.

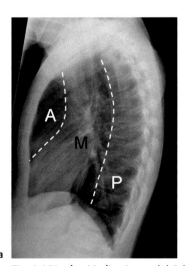
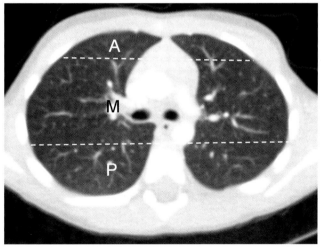

a   b

Fig. 1.161a, b   Mediastinum. (a) Schematic representation of the mediastinum on a lateral chest radiograph. **(b)** Schematic representation of the mediastinum on a contrast-enhanced chest CT.
A Anterior
M Middle
P Posterior

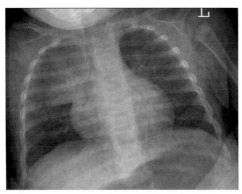

Fig. 1.162   Normal thymus on conventional radiograph.

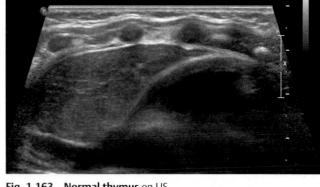

Fig. 1.163   Normal thymus on US.

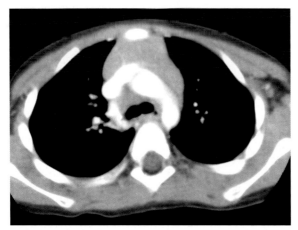

Fig. 1.164   Normal thymus on CT.

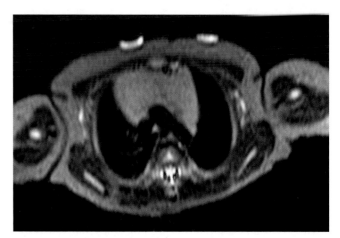

Fig. 1.165   Normal thymus on MRI.

Table 1.59   Widening (fullness) of the anterior mediastinum

Diagnosis	Findings	Comments
Thymus ▷ *Fig. 1.166a–f*	Extremely variable in its radiographic appearance. May mimic cardiomegaly, upper lobe consolidation. Its outline can be convex, concave, wavy, or notched (indentation from anterior ribs). Similar to cardiac silhouette in density. On a lateral view, retrosternal clear space is filled in. US, CT, MRI.	Normal finding. Prominent soft-tissue density until the age of 3 y. A normal thymus has no mass effect on the trachea. Atrophies with stress of acute illness and on steroid therapy. Regenerates (rebounds) after the illness has cleared or the steroid therapy is terminated. Shape and size varies patient to patient, both normally and after rebound.
Thymoma	Commonly unilateral upper mediastinal mass. Calcifications and cysts may be detected in the thymoma. Can cause displacement or compression of the trachea.	Very rarely occurs in children. Encapsulated, noninvasive, or invasive. Round or ovoid epithelial cell mass may be lobulated. Symptoms present late.

(continues on page 94)

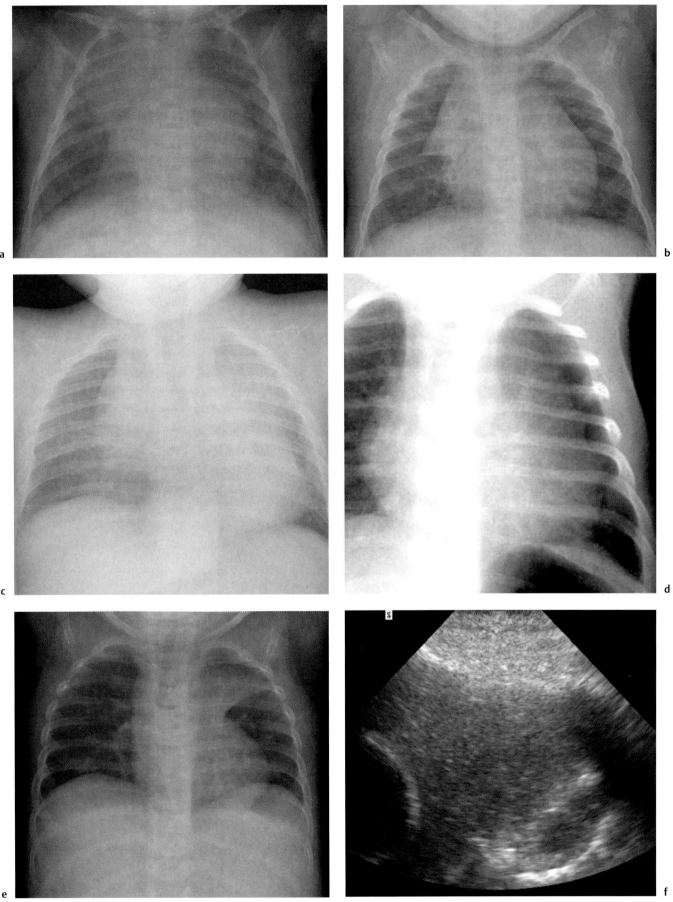

Fig. 1.166a–f   Thymus. (a) Normal thymus. **(b)** Thymic "sail" sign. **(c)** Normal thymus. Note the hypoplastic claviculae in cleidocranial dysostosis. **(d)** "Wavy" sign. **(e)** Asymmetric thymus, which can lead to an erroneous diagnosis of RUL pneumonia. **(f)** US of the same patient clearly shows a normal thymus.

Table 1.59   (Cont.) Widening (fullness) of the anterior mediastinum

Diagnosis	Findings	Comments
Mediastinitis		
T-cell leukemia/NHL (with thymic infiltration) ▷ *Fig. 1.167a, b* ▷ *Fig. 1.168*	Lymphoma cells infiltrate the thymus, causing enlargement and lobular lateral borders. Paratracheal, parabronchial, perihilar neoplastic lymphadenopathy. CXR usually shows a widening of the anterior mediastinum that may extend into the middle or posterior mediastinum. Contrast-enhanced CT or MRI defines the extent of the disease and will also detect lung parenchymal involvement, pleural effusions, chest wall disease, and complications caused by impingement on vital structures, most commonly the airway. The lesion is often heterogeneous and the low attenuation areas represent necrosis. Rebound enlargement of the thymus often occurs following treatment. The thymus is then usually homogeneously enlarged without associated lymphadenopathy.	Very high peripheral white-cell count. Most common cause of a mediastinal mass in the pediatric age group, accounting for 46%–56% of all mediastinal masses and over 80% of the malignant ones. Frequently affects children under the age of 5 y. Boys are more often affected than girls. Gradual onset of cough, respiratory distress, dysphagia, and even cardiac failure may be presenting symptoms. Central nervous system and gonadal involvement can also occur. Usually presents as abdominal, thoracic, or head and neck mass. Lymphoblastic or T-cell NHL is the most common type and can be indistinguishable from acute lymphoblastic leukemia. Over one-third of NHLs have their primary site in the mediastinum.
LCH	Mediastinal adenopathy, as part of generalized lymphadenopathy. Involvement of the thymus may be seen on CT, showing a low-attenuation masslike enlargement of the thymus with enhancing septa and presence of thymic calcifications. Cannot be differentiated on a chest film from the normal thymus until they have become very large or if the trachea is displaced.	Group of idiopathic disorders characterized by the proliferation of specialized bone marrow–derived Langerhans cells and mature eosinophils. The pathogenesis is unknown. Often combined with T-cell immunodeficiency. Fever, hepatosplenomegaly, generalized lymphadenopathy are present. A rare disease.
Thyroid, retrosternal goiter, thyroid carcinoma ▷ *Fig. 1.169a, b*	Retrosternal soft-tissue density that often projects above the clavicles and moves with swallowing. Larger masses often displace and may narrow the esophagus and trachea. Can best be diagnosed by radionuclide thyroid scan but can also be recognized on US, CT, and MRI.	Ectopic thyroid tissue, may occur anywhere in the midline from the base of the tongue to the mediastinum. Locations outside the midline (e.g., neck) have been described. Predominantly in prepubertal girls.
Teratoma	A mass lesion of which 97% occur in the anterior mediastinum, either within or near the thymus gland. It can extend from the anterior to the middle mediastinum. Only 3% occur in the posterior mediastinum. Larger tumors are often bilateral and asymmetric. Can "splay" the carina Contains soft tissue, fat, fluid, or calcium; the latter two findings are pathognomonic. Could be predominantly cystic. Their outlines are sharp, wavy, or rounded. Pleural fluid may occur. CXR may show calcifications. CT and MRI can define the extent and internal characteristics of the mass(es) better than CXR.	Derive from multipotential cells that arise from an early event in embryogenesis. Because of this multipotential nature, different tissues may be found within the mass, and these may be well differentiated or immature. They comprise 10%–25% of anterior mediastinal tumors in children, and teratoma is the most common mediastinal GCT. Teratomas can be mature (benign), immature, and mixed malignant types. Mature (benign) teratomas account for approximately 75% of all mediastinal GCTs. They can occur at any age but there are two peaks of incidence: at 2 y of age and in adolescence. Large tumors tend to produce respiratory symptoms due to tracheobroncheal compression. In older children, often very large asymptomatic masses are found.

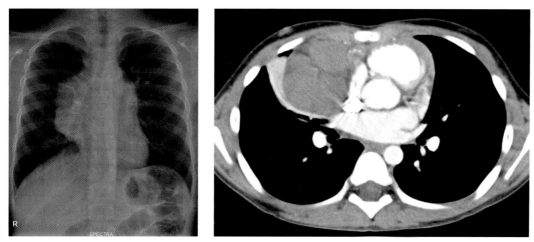

Fig. 1.167a, b   Hodgkin lymphoma. (a) Hodgkin lymphoma in an 8-year-old boy. (**b**) Contrast-enhanced CT of the same patient.

Fig. 1.168   Hodgkin lymphoma in a teenager.

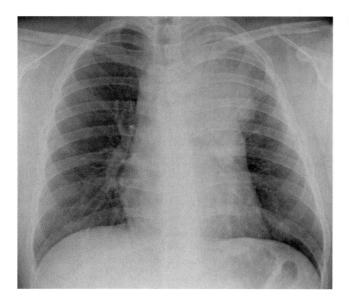

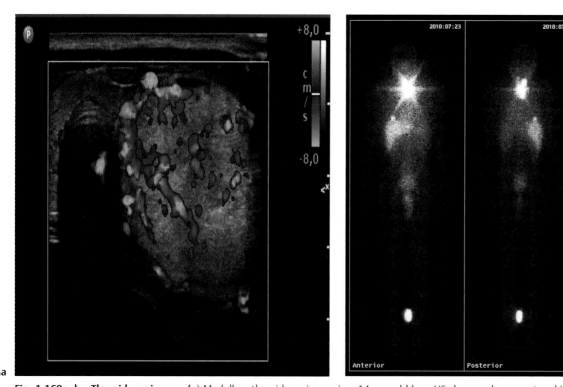

Fig. 1.169a, b   Thyroid carcinoma. (a) Medullary thyroid carcinoma in a 14-year-old boy. US shows enlargement and increased vascularity. (**b**) Radionuclide thyroid scan of the same patient.

Table 1.60   Widening (fullness) of the middle mediastinum

Diagnosis	Findings	Comments
Lymphoma (NHL), (T-cell) leukemia ▷ *Fig. 1.170* ▷ *Fig. 1.171*	Paratracheal, parabronchial, and perihilar lymphadenopathy may extend into the anterior mediastinum. Lymphoma cells may infiltrate and enlarge the thymus. Pleural effusion and tracheal narrowing may also occur. CXR usually shows lymph node enlargement and a widened, dense, and sharply defined anterior mediastinal lesion. Contrast-enhanced CT or MRI defines the extent of the lesion better.	NHL frequently affects children under the age of 5 y. Hodgkin lymphoma is rare in children < 5 y but its incidence increases in later childhood and in the teenage years. Pediatric NHL usually presents as abdominal, thoracic, or head and neck masses. Lymphoblastic or T-cell NHL is the most common type and can be indistinguishable from acute lymphoblastic leukemia. Over one-third of NHLs have their primary site in the mediastinum. Pediatric Hodgkin disease is more likely to present as asymptomatic cervical or supraclavicular lymphadenopathy; systemic symptoms such as fever being more common with Hodgkin disease. Two-thirds of patients with Hodgkin disease will have mediastinal lymphadenopathy.
Mediastinitis, mediastinal effusion ▷ *Fig. 1.172a, b*	Localized (abscess) or diffuse (cellulitis) pus. CXR shows superior mediastinal widening and obliteration of normal mediastinal contours. Trachea may be displaced or narrowed. Pleural effusion often present. CT shows obliterated mediastinal fat, low attenuation mediastinal fluid collection, air collections, abscess, pleural and pericardial fluid, and adenopathy. Early postoperative changes and mediastinitis are difficult to differentiate. Contrast study with a water-soluble contrast medium is indicated to check for perforation, stenosis, or displacement.	Mostly results from perforation of the esophagus or trachea; spontaneously or secondary to malposition of catheters or tubes, foreign body aspiration or ingestion, after open chest surgery, leakage at sites of surgical anastomoses, tumor, and infection.
Mediastinal fat deposition	CT: exquisite delineation of the excess fat, more common in anterior and posterior mediastinum.	Most often seen as a complication of steroid therapy. Seen in obesity, Cushing syndrome.
Sarcoidosis ▷ *Fig. 1.173*		(see **Table 1.11**)
TAPVD		(see **Table 1.85**)
Nephrotic syndrome	Symmetric widening of the middle mediastinum, enlarged cardiac silhouette with a normal lateral view.	Due to fluid retention in the mediastinum.
Traumatic aortic dissection	Widening of the middle mediastinum as a result of mediastinal hemorrhage.	Rare in children.

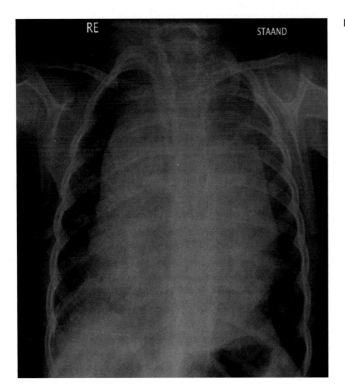

Fig. 1.170   T-cell lymphoma.

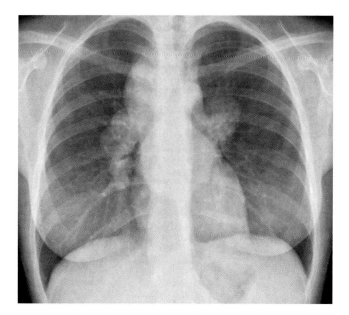

Fig. 1.171   T-cell lymphoma in a 14-year-old girl.

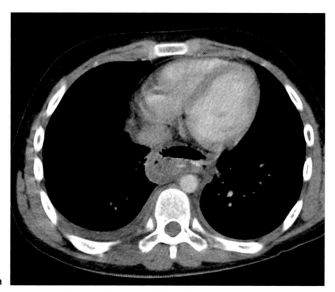

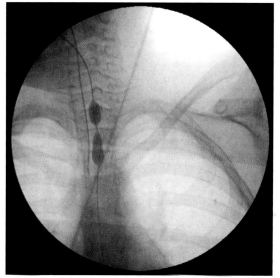

a   b

Fig. 1.172a, b   Mediastinitis. (a) Mediastinitis in a 15-year-old boy after lye ingestion. **(b)** Pneumodilatation of the esophagus of the same patient; the balloon shows a waist at the level of the stenosis.

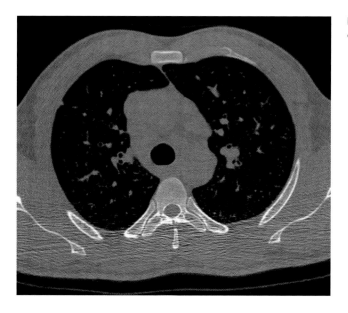

Fig. 1.173   Sarcoidosis. Chest HRCT in a patient with stage 2 sarcoidosis. Note the bilateral hilar enlargement.

Table 1.61   Widening (fullness) of the posterior mediastinum

Diagnosis	Findings	Comments
Vertebral lesions	Paravertebral soft-tissue mass. CT demonstrates vertebral destruction. MRI better for the soft-tissue component and extent.	(see **Table 4.116**)
Neurogenic tumor (neuroblastoma, ganglioneuroma) ▷ *Fig. 1.174a, b* ▷ *Fig. 1.175* ▷ *Fig. 1.176a, b*	Well-circumscribed paraspinal soft-tissue mass, round to ovoid, in the posterior mediastinum that contains calcifications in 50%–75%. Can be bilateral and asymmetric. Often widening of intercostal spaces. Erosion or destruction of ribs is possible. CT and MRI to delineate the extent of the mass. MRI is excellent to assess extension into the vertebral canal.	Originates from the sympathetic ganglia. Neuroblastoma is the most common posterior mediastinal mass in young children. Approximately 16% of all neuroblastomas are of mediastinal origin. Neuroblastoma is a highly malignant tumor. It occurs mostly in children < 3 y. Children may present with a variety of signs and symptoms (fever, malaise, bony metastasis, cord compression, paraneoplastic syndromes, skin metastases, opsomyoclonus, etc.). Ganglioneuromas are benign tumors that may represent matured neuroblastoma. They are often an incidental finding.
Neurenteric cyst	Well-defined mass, tubular or rounded, in the posterior mediastinum, preferentially on the right side, may be bilateral. Frequently associated with vertebral dysraphism including hemivertebrae and anterior spina bifida. Lower cervical and upper thoracic vertebrae are usually affected. Frequently attached to the vertebra by a fibrous band and may extend intraspinally through the spinal defect. MRI is imaging modality of choice.	Cysts lined with GI mucosa, most are mucus-filled. Sixty-five percent are diagnosed in the first year of life. Represent a failure of complete separation of the notochord from the foregut during the third week of embryogenesis. In a third of the patients, these cysts are associated with malformations of central nervous system (tethering, syringohydromyelia, or an intradural cyst) and/or GI tract.
Hematoma associated with vertebral fracture	Widened mediastinum and flattened, fractured vertebral body on CXR and CT. CT will demonstrate the posterior mediastinal hematoma.	(see **Table 4.70**)
Mediastinal echinococcosis	A smooth, round, dense opacity on CXR. CT and MRI may show cystic masses, their exact location, and may demonstrate if there are daughter cysts. The germinative membrane may be visible. Calcifications are well visualized on CT and sometimes on CXR.	Mediastinal localization is rare.

(continues on page 100)

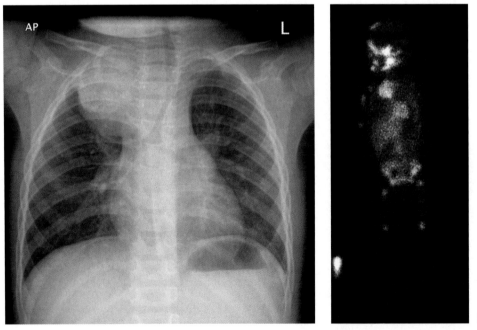

a   b

Fig. 1.174a, b   Neuroblastoma. (a) Neuroblastoma in a 1-year-old girl. **(b)** Iodine-123 MIBG shows intense uptake in the tumor.

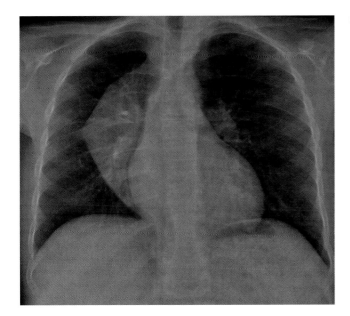

Fig. 1.175   Ganglioneuroma in a 12-year-old girl.

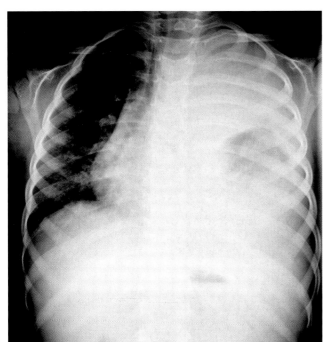

a

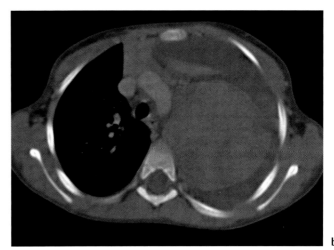

b

Fig. 1.176a, b   Ganglioneuroma. (a) Ganglioneuroma in a 3-year-old boy. (**b**) MRI of the same patient.

Table 1.61   (Cont.) Widening (fullness) of the posterior mediastinum

Diagnosis	Findings	Comments
Paraspinal abscess (so-called migrating abscess) ▷ *Fig. 1.177a–d*	Typical radiographic findings are not detectable until 2–4 wk after the onset of symptoms. CXR shows a paravertebral density; more common bilateral (TB), collapse of the intervertebral disk and destruction of the adjacent vertebral bodies. MRI is the investigational tool of choice in diagnosing spondylodiscitis, particularly in the early stages of the disease when other investigations still yield negative results.	Possible clinical signs are limping, refusal to sit or walk, increased irritability, neurologic or abdominal symptoms. Etiology in children includes both infectious and inflammatory causes. *S. aureus* is the most common bacterium isolated.

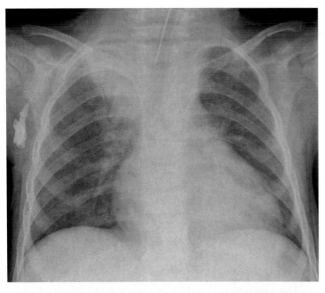

a

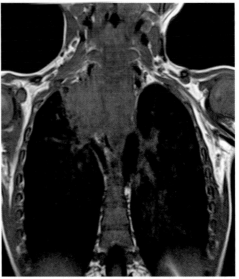

b

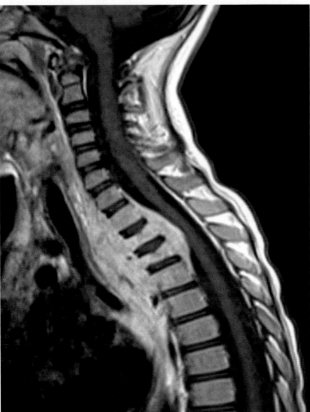

c

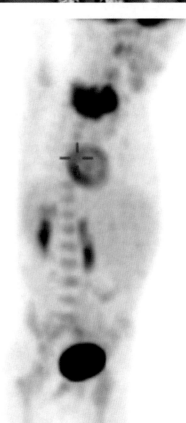

d

Fig. 1.177a–d   Spondylodiscitis. (a) Spondylodiscitis in a 4-month-old boy with CGD. **(b)** Coronal T1-weighted MRI of the same patient shows a paraspinal mass extending into the RUL. **(c)** Sagittal contrast-enhanced T1-weighted sagittal MRI of the same patient. The lesion shows intense homogenous enhancement. **(d)** PET-CT shows intense uptake around the cervical spine.

Table 1.62   Unilateral widening of the anterior mediastinum—right or left

Diagnosis	Findings	Comments
Thymus ▷ *Fig. 1.178a, b*		Normal finding. Most common cause in infancy, less common in older children (> 3 y) (see **Table 1.59**).
Thymoma, thymolipoma	Thymoma: (see **Table 1.59**). Thymolipoma: Superior and middle compartments of the anterior mediastinum, substernal in location. Linear calcification occurs in 7.5%–20% of cases. Often grows to a very large size and may cause displacement of the trachea. On CXR, occasionally the diagnosis of a fatty lesion can be entertained when the periphery of the mass appears more radiolucent than its bulky center. On CT and MRI, the mass is sharply defined and predominantly fatty.	Thymolipomas are benign hamartomas containing fat. Lobulated and encapsulated. Half of the cases are asymptomatic and discovered incidentally.
Teratoma, dermoid		(see **Table 1.59**)
Cervicomediastinal lymphangioma or hemangioma ▷ *Fig. 1.179, p. 102*	The diagnostic modalities of choice are US and MRI. On US, macrocystic lesions appear as a multiloculated or septated cystic mass, sometimes with fluid–fluid levels. On Doppler US, flow can be demonstrated only within the septa. Microcystic lesions are hyperechoic ("bright") without any flow on Doppler. On MRI, lymphatic malformations are septated masses with a low signal intensity on T1-weighted and a high signal intensity on T2-weighted sequences. The presence of proteinaceous fluid or hemorrhage within the lesion can cause variable signal intensity on both T1- and T2-weighted sequences.	The majority of vascular anomalies involving the mediastinum are actually lymphatic malformations. Typically, they involve the anterior mediastinum but are not restricted to any particular mediastinal compartment; other locations include the axilla, superior mediastinum, mesentery, retroperitoneum, and lower limbs. Often discovered at birth and usually asymptomatic. Spontaneous shrinkage can occur but sudden enlargement is an indication of bleeding or inflammation. In symptomatic patients, sclerosing therapy with the aid of interventional radiology can be useful.
Morgagni hernia		
Thymic cysts ▷ *Fig. 1.180, p. 102*	Soft-tissue masses, which may be unilateral or bilateral, if border forming, on CXR. Calcifications are rare. DD: cystic teratoma.	One percent of all mediastinal masses. Girls/boys: 2/1. Two-thirds diagnosed in the first year of life. Large cysts in neonates may cause respiratory distress, recurrent respiratory tract infections, cough, dyspnea, dysphagia.

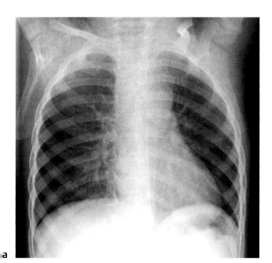
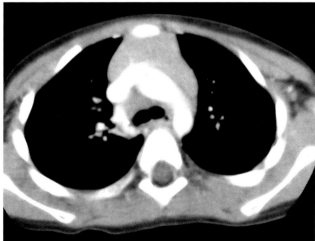

Fig. 1.178a, b   Thymus. (a) Asymmetric widening of the mediastinum in a 17-month-old girl. **(b)** CT of the same patient shows that the thymus causes the physiologic asymmetric widening (in this case, US could have been the technique of choice).

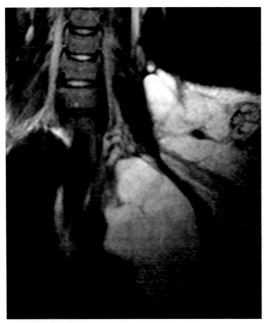

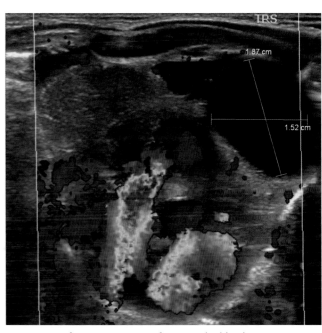

Fig. 1.179 Cervicomediastinal lymphangioma on T2-weighted coronal MRI of a 14-year-old girl.

Fig. 1.180 Thymic cyst on US of a 3-month-old girl.

Table 1.63 Unilateral widening of the middle mediastinum—right, superior compartment

Diagnosis	Findings	Comments
Paratracheal lymphadenopathy ▷ *Fig. 1.181*	Increased distance between the right mediastinal border and the lucent stripe of the trachea. Hilar lymph nodes may or may not be enlarged. To visualize lymph nodes on CT, intravenous contrast should be used.	TB and in older school-aged children Hodgkin disease.
Azygos fissure ▷ *Fig. 1.182*	On CXR, a mass or curvilinear density in the right upper lungfield or paramediastinally, ending with a teardrop density, the azygos vein.	An accessory fissure caused by the azygos vein being "caught" by the budding lung tissue of the RUL.
Anomalies of the aortic arch, (e.g., high right aorta), poststenotic dilatation in aortic stenosis, or coarctation of the aorta		(see **Table 1.83**)

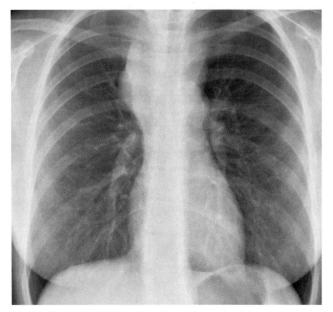

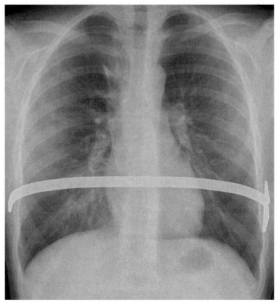

Fig. 1.181 Hodgkin lymphoma in a 17-year-old girl.

Fig. 1.182 Azygos fissure in a patient with pectus excavatum treated with a Nuss bar.

Table 1.64   Unilateral widening of the middle mediastinum—right, middle compartment

Diagnosis	Findings	Comments
Achalasia (so-called megaesophagus)	The flattened lateral border of the dilated esophagus overlaps the right mediastinum, causing widening of the middle mediastinum. Air-fluid level in the esophagus, or heterogeneous density caused by food content, or only air. Small or absent stomach bubble. Confirmation with esophagram.	(see **Table 2.31**)

Table 1.65   Unilateral widening of the middle mediastinum—left, superior compartment

Diagnosis	Findings	Comments
Para-aortic lymphoma	Soft-tissue density, sharply demarcated at the level of the aortic arch. Projected over the great vessels on the lateral CXR. CT.	Most are tuberculous in origin.
High-riding aortic arch		(see **Table 1.83**)
Aortic aneurysm		(see **Table 1.83**)

Table 1.66   Unilateral widening of the mediastinum—right or left, superior compartment

Diagnosis	Findings	Comments
Bronchogenic cyst ▷ *Fig. 1.183a, b*	Usually unilocular, round or oval, fluid-filled density. May be air-filled when there is communication with the tracheobronchial tree (rare). CXR may demonstrate a discrete rounded mass near to the carina (often subcarinal) or in the paratracheal region, sometimes displacing or compressing the trachea, bronchi, or esophagus. There may also be hyperinflation, atelectasis, or consolidation associated. CT and MRI are helpful to determine nature and extent. Enhancement on CT is minimal and peripheral, on T2 sequences the cyst "lights up like a lightbulb."	Congenital abnormality of division of the embryonic primitive foregut. Five percent of all pediatric mediastinal masses. The most common of the bronchopulmonary malformations. Most occur in the middle mediastinum (85%), at or near the carina, but localization may be in the posterior mediastinum, intrapulmonary, or more rarely in the neck, pericardium, or abdominal cavity. There is usually no communication with the airways. Most commonly mediastinal (85%). Patients are asymptomatic or cyst can cause persistent cough, progressive dyspnea, wheeze, stridor, and cyanosis.
Ectopic thymus (retrocaval thymus)	Thymic tissue posterior to the superior vena cava. May extend into the posterior mediastinum. Characteristic imaging features on CT and MRI.	In normal infants. Most cases in children 2 y of age or younger. Mostly an incidental finding, no biopsy is needed.
Hemihypertrophy	Increase in the extrathoracic soft tissues, ipsilateral skeletal enlargement.	Apparent external differences in size between the two halves of the body.

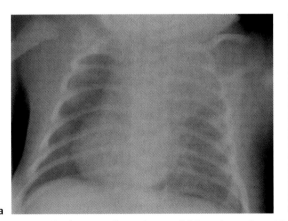
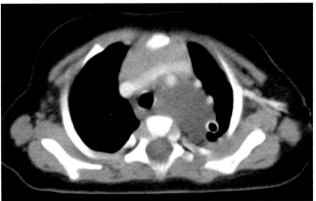

a   b

Fig. 1.183a, b   **Bronchogenic cyst.** (**a**) Bronchogenic cyst in a neonate. (**b**) CT of the same patient.

Table 1.67 Unilateral widening of the middle mediastinum—right or left, inferior compartment

Diagnosis	Findings	Comments
Diaphragmatic hernias and defects		(see **Table 1.86**)
Mediastinal pancreatic pseudocyst	Air-fluid or fluid-containing mass in the middle to lower mediastinum. Convex expansion of the affected side of the mediastinum or of the heart border. Pleural effusion is present in majority of cases. CT demonstrates the presence of thin- or thick-walled cystic lesion.	Rare complication of acute or chronic pancreatitis. May have no specific symptoms or may be associated with back pain, dysphagia, or esophageal reflux.

Table 1.68 Unilateral widening of the posterior mediastinum—right or left

Diagnosis	Findings	Comments
Neurogenic tumors (neuroblastoma, ganglioneuroma, ganglioneuroblastoma, neurofibroma) ▷ *Fig. 1.184a, b*		(see **Table 1.61**)
Neurenteric cysts		(see **Table 1.61**)
Esophageal duplications, tumors, and cysts ▷ *Fig. 1.185*	On chest radiographs, benign mediastinal cysts may appear as a sharply marginated, round or oval area of increased opacity. UGI contrast examination will show extrinsic or intramural mass effect. Their appearance at CT or MRI imaging mimics that of bronchogenic cysts. The CT features of such a benign mediastinal cystic structure ranges from (a) a smooth, oval, or tubular mass with a well-defined thin wall that usually enhances after intravenous contrast administration; (b) homogeneous low attenuation (0–20 HU); (c) no enhancement of cyst contents; and (d) no infiltration of adjacent mediastinal structures. Masses that show most or all of these features are invariably benign. MRI can be useful in showing the cystic nature of these masses because these cysts "light up" when imaged with T2-weighted sequences.	Developmental in origin; may result from failure of the solid esophageal tube to vacuolate completely to form a hollow tube or from abnormal budding of the dorsal foregut. Uncommon. Many are asymptomatic, but they may cause dysphagia, pain, or other symptoms owing to compression of adjacent structures. The majority are detected in infants or children, usually adjacent to or within the esophageal wall. Ectopic gastric mucosa in the cyst may cause hemorrhage or perforation of the cyst or infection.
Bronchogenic cysts ▷ *Fig. 1.186,a–c, p. 106*		(see **Table 1.66**)
Paraspinal hematoma		(see **Table 4.116**)
Superiorly located paravertebral meningocele	Round, smooth, or lobulated homogeneous mass in the upper, posterior mediastinum sometimes associated with multiple vertebral segmentation anomalies and widening of the spinal canal. CT and MRI are essential, not only for the diagnosis, but also for the depiction of relationship to surrounding structures and the exclusion of other possible accompanying lesion such as neuroma in the setting of neurofibromatosis type I.	Herniation of leptomeninges through an intervertebral foramen or a defect in the vertebral body to form a cerebrospinal fluid–filled sac. Intrathoracic meningocele is rare and is usually associated with neurofibromatosis type I or Marfan syndrome. Rarely as an isolated defect. Most of the reported thoracic meningoceles are not strictly anterior in location, but also lateral or anterolateral. Clinical manifestations are closely related with its size and its relationship to surrounding structures. Back pain, paraparesis from insult to the spinal cord, shortness of breath, coughing, and palpitation by compression of the lung and mediastinal structures but also progressive hydrothorax caused by rupture of meningoceles all has been reported in the literature. Small meningoceles may be incidentally diagnosed on a routine chest radiograph.
Ectopic thymus		(see **Table 1.66**)
Paraspinal abscess (so-called migrating abscess)		(see **Table 1.61**)
Teratoma		(see **Table 1.61**)

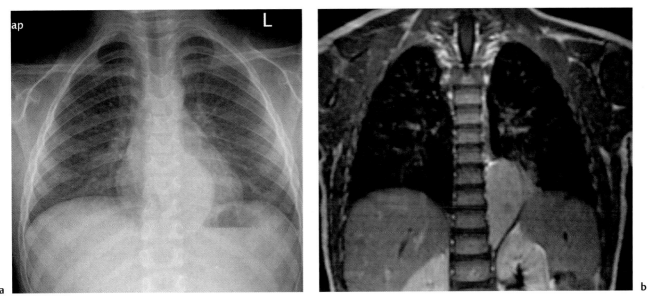

a   b

Fig. 1.184a, b   Neuroblastoma. (**a**) Neuroblastoma in a 5-year-old girl. (**b**) T1-weighted coronal MRI of the same patient.

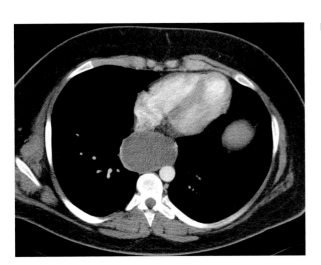

Fig. 1.185   Esophageal duplication in a 15-year-old girl.

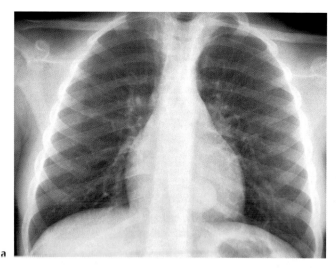

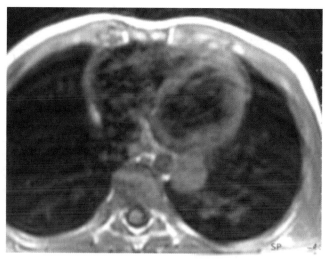

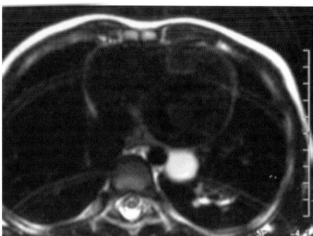

Fig. 1.186a–c   Bronchogenic cyst. (a) Bronchogenic cyst. **(b)** T1-weighted MRI of the same patient. **(c)** T2- weighted MRI of the same patient.

Table 1.69   Unilateral widening of the posterior mediastinum—inferior compartment

Diagnosis	Findings	Comments
Inferior pulmonary ligament/ accessory lung	Radiographically similar to extralobar pulmonary sequestration; however, there is a connection between the esophagus or bronchi by a supernumerary bronchus.	Accessory lung buds or extensions. Clinically and histologically identical to pulmonary sequestration. Is found incidentally.
Chylothorax and other mediastinal effusions	Unilateral, very rare (< 10%) bilateral. Paramediastinal effusion, often in combination with a pleural effusion.	Lymphatic fluid in the pleural space secondary to leakage from the thoracic duct or one of its main tributaries. Results from birth trauma or is "idiopathic" in neonates; traumatic in older children. May also occur with lymphangectasia and after cardiac surgery. Milky fluid after eating.
Pulmonary sequestration (intralobar or extralobar) ▷ *Fig. 1.187a–c*		(see **Table 1.21**)
Bochdalek hernia		
Neuroblastoma/ganglioneuroma		(see **Table 1.61**)
Very rare tumors		
Lipoma **Lipomatosis**	CT and MRI to determine location and extent of the disease. Low attenuation of fat content on CT. High signal on T1-spin echo weighted imaging.	Very rare tumors.
Mediastinal pheochromocytoma	Chest film shows a rounded or oval density. The salt-and-pepper appearance on MRI is characteristic, with the pepper representing flow voids of vessels and the salt representing the T1-bright tumor parenchyma. MIBG scintigraphy.	Vascularized chromaffin cell neoplasms that secrete catecholamines and, in some cases, other active peptides. Classic symptoms are hypertension, headache, palpitation, and excessive sweating.
Metastatic tumors	Paravertebral, adjacent to the mediastinum; rounded or ovoid densities. Mostly occurring with a known primary tumor.	

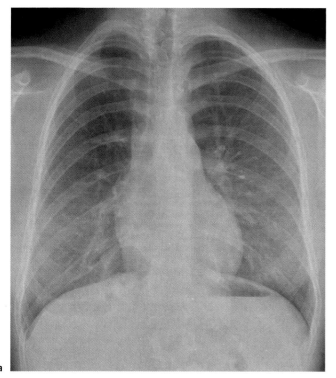

a

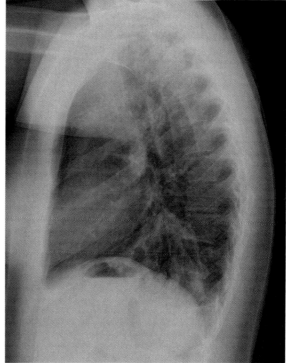

b

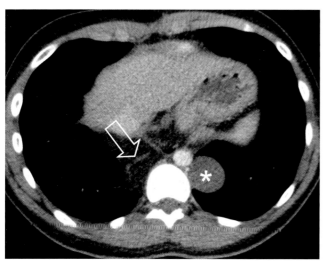

c

Fig. 1.187a–c Pulmonary sequestration. (**a**) A 15-year-old girl with an extralobar pulmonary sequestration and a Bochdalek hernia. (**b**) Lateral radiograph of the same patient. (**c**) Contrast-enhanced CT depicting both the extralobar pulmonary sequestration (arrow shows the feeding artery) and the Bochdalek hernia (asterisk).

Table 1.70 The "empty" or narrow mediastinum

Diagnosis	Findings	Comments
Immune deficiency states (DiGeorge syndrome, Bruton agammaglobulinemia, congenital hypogammaglobulinemia), lymphopenic agammaglobulinemia, Nezelof syndrome	A very narrow superior mediastinum due to absence of the thymus on CXR.	MRI to confirm absence of thymus.
Transposition of the great vessels		(see **Tables 1.76** and **1.83**)
Ebstein anomaly		(see **Table 1.78**)
Thymic stress atrophy ▷ *Fig. 1.188, p. 108*	For example, due to infection, infant respiratory distress syndrome, steroids.	

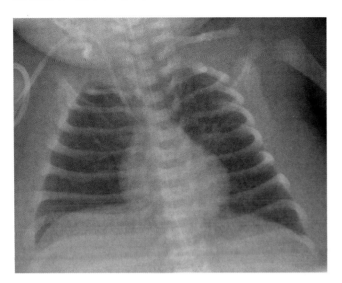

Fig. 1.188   Neonatal stress depicted by a narrow mediastinum.

Table 1.71   Mediastinal air

Diagnosis	Findings	Comments
Esophagus		
Eructation	Coincidental timing of the radiograph during burping.	Normal finding, especially in infants.
Incompetent lower esophageal sphincter	Air outlines the esophagus, bowed slightly convex to the right.	(see **Table 2.31**)
Achalasia		(see **Table 2.31**)
Esophageal stenosis or stricture	Air or heterogeneous lucency in the dilated portion proximal to the narrowing.	(see **Table 2.31**)
Hiatus hernia and paraesophageal hernia ▷ *Fig. 1.187, p. 107*	Cystic lucency in the cardiophrenic angle of the mediastinum or overlying the cardiac silhouette. On the lateral view in the middle mediastinum.	(see **Table 2.31**)
Tracheoesophageal fistula ▷ *Fig. 1.189*	Passage of air into the esophagus via the fistula.	(see **Table 2.33**)
Trachea		
RDS and birth trauma	The lucency of the wide air-filled trachea and the main bronchi is enhanced by the surrounding density of the air space disease (HMD, RSD).	In neonates with dyspnea, tachypnea, cyanosis.
Mediastinum		
Cysts	Pericardial cyst, bronchogenic cyst.	
Abscess, mediastinitis ▷ *Fig. 1.190a, b*	Irregular air collection scattered throughout the mediastinum; small cysts or "string of pearls" appearance.	(see **Table 1.60**)

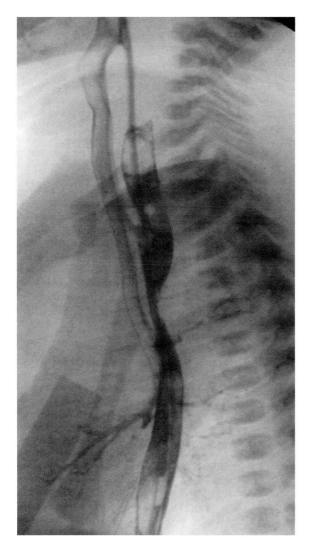

Fig. 1.189 Tracheoesophageal fistula or a so-called H-fistula.

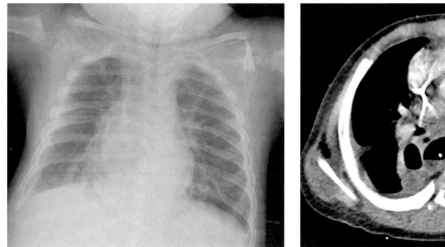

a

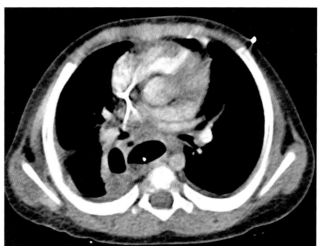

b

Fig. 1.190a, b Mediastinitis. (a) Mediastinitis due to iatrogenic esophageal perforation after balloon dilatation of an esophageal stricture. **(b)** Contrast-enhanced CT of the same patient.

Table 1.72   Pneumo(thorax) mediastinum

Diagnosis	Findings	Comments
Pneumomediastinum (mediastinal emphysema) ▷ *Fig. 1.191a–c*	Linear or bubbly air collections in the mediastinum. In infants, the air can outline both lobes of the thymus, "butterfly" sign. Large collections of air may elevate the thymus on both the frontal and lateral radiographs to produce a "spinnaker sail" sign. Air outlines the aortic arch and trachea and extends into neck and subcutaneous tissues. Occasionally causes a pneumothorax or even pneumoperitoneum.	In infants on mechanical ventilation; in neonates may be spontaneous in origin, a complication of increased intra-alveolar pressure (even coughing, vomiting) causing alveolar rupture. Air then passes into the interstitium of the lung and travels along the perivascular space to the hilum and into the mediastinum. In older children most commonly seen in asthma, unless there is history of trauma. Rarely the consequence of aspirated foreign body or rupture of the trachea/bronchus.
Medial pneumothorax ▷ *Fig. 1.192*	The "sharp mediastinum" sign on a supine view; an apical lucency on an upright view.	To differentiate from pneumomediastinum by a lateral decubitus (horizontal beam) film. The air in the pleural space "rises," where mediastinal air does not move.
Mach effect, mimicking pneumomediastinum ▷ *Fig. 1.193*	A thin band of lucency immediately adjacent to the mediastinum.	"Artifact"; the appearance is caused by the transition between two very different densities (air in lung, mediastinal soft tissue).
Rotation ▷ *Fig. 1.194*	When the lateral chest radiograph is slightly rotated in infants, a retrosternal thin band of lucency is seen.	Projectional: represents the anterior lung on the side away from the table.

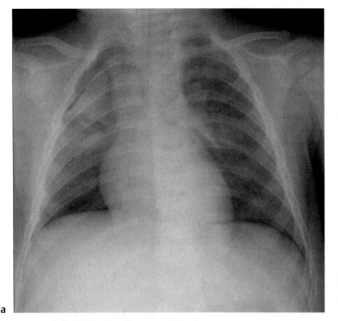

a

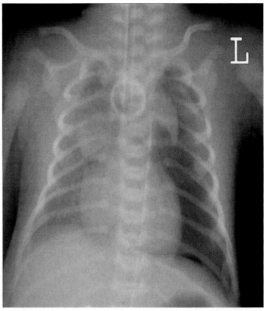

b

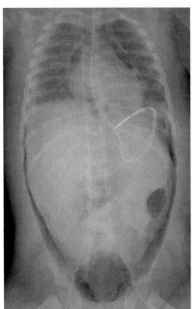

c

Fig. 1.191a–c   Pneumomediastinum. (a) Pneumomediastinum and right-sided pneumothorax in a 2-year-old boy. **(b)** Pneumomediastinum and left-sided pneumothorax in a neonate. **(c)** Retroperitoneal pneumoperitoneum and pneumomediastinum in a neonate.

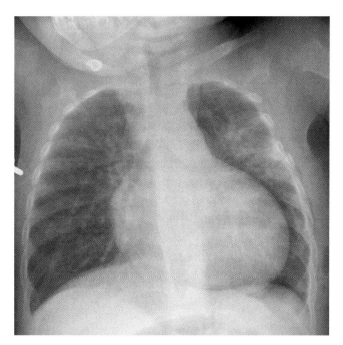

Fig. 1.192   Medial pneumothorax in a 1-year-old boy.

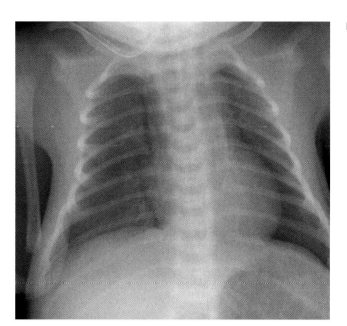

Fig. 1.193   Mach effect.

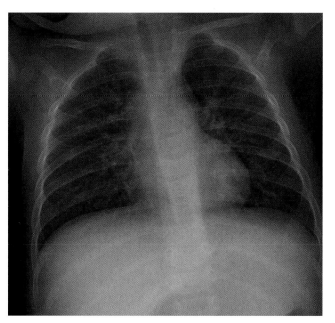

Fig. 1.194   Rotation effect. A retrosternal thin band of lucency is seen.

Table 1.73   Mediastinal displacement

Diagnosis	Findings	Comments
Due to volume loss: unilateral pulmonary atelectasis, pulmonary hypoplasia, pulmonary agenesis, postlobectomy and pneumonectomy ▷ *Fig. 1.195a, b*	Mediastinal shift to the abnormal side. Contralateral compensatory overinflation. Elevation of the hemidiaphragm of the involved side with often contralateral diaphragmatic depression. Narrowed intercostal spaces on the abnormal side.	
Due to overexpansion: congenital lobar emphysema, tension pneumothorax, airtrapping with foreign body aspiration, cysts, bullae, unilateral pleural effusion, pectus excavatum, tumor, lung sequester ▷ *Fig. 1.196a, b* ▷ *Fig. 1.197* ▷ *Fig. 1.198*	Mediastinal shift away from the lesion. Depression of the diaphragm of the hyperinflated side.	

(continues on page 114)

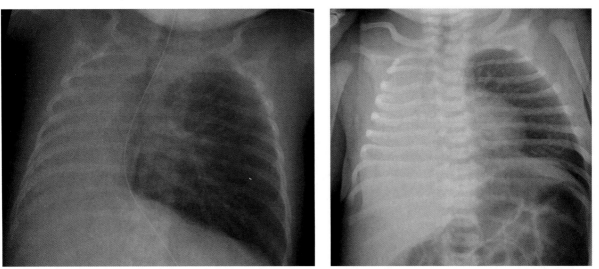

a   b

Fig. 1.195a, b   Mediastinal shift. (a) Postpneumonectomy mediastinal shift in a neonate. **(b)** Right-sided pulmonary agenesis.

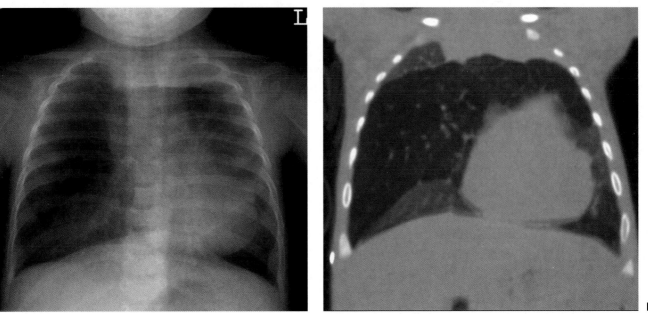

a   b

Fig. 1.196a, b   Congenital lobar emphysema. (a) Congenital lobar emphysema in a 3-month-old boy. **(b)** Coronal reconstruction of a CT of the same patient clearly shows congenital lobar emphysema of the right middle lobe.

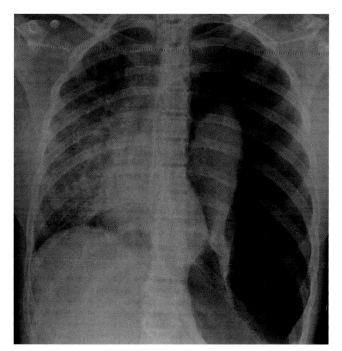

Fig. 1.197   Left-sided tension pneumothorax in a 13-year-old girl.

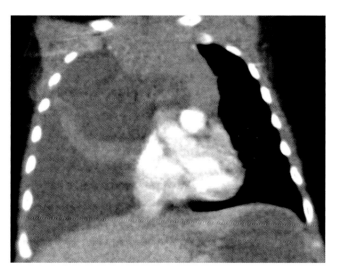

Fig. 1.198   Mediastinal shift due to hemorrhage in a thymic cyst (see **Fig. 1.180**).

Table 1.73   (Cont.) Mediastinal displacement

Diagnosis	Findings	Comments
Diaphragmatic causes: eventration of the diaphragm		(see **Table 1.46**)
Congenital diaphragmatic hernia		
Foreign body aspiration ▷ *Fig. 1.199a, b*	In inspiration, both lungs may be equally aerated, the mediastinum is central. In expiration, only the uninvolved healthy side will decrease in size; the involved side retains more air due to air trapping. The mediastinum shifts to the healthy side.	Air trapping in expiration due to bronchial narrowing or check-valve mechanism. Dynamic mediastinal motion. Common cause of respiratory distress in children between 6 mo and 3 y of age.
Chest deformation ▷ *Fig. 1.200a, b*	Especially seen in patients with pectus excavatum in whom the mediastinum is shifted (in nearly all cases to the left side).	

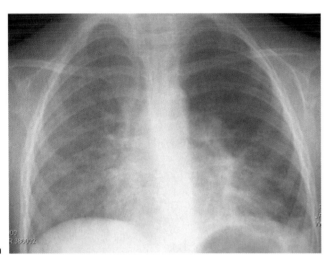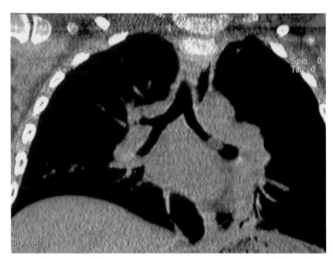

a   b

Fig. 1.199a, b   Foreign body aspiration. (**a**) A 2-year-old boy with persistent airway infection and hyperinflation of the left lung. (**b**) CT of the same patient shows a foreign body, a peanut, lodged in the left mainstem bronchus.

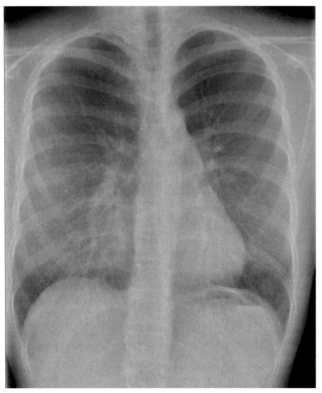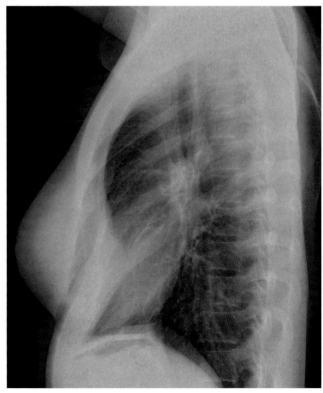

a   b

Fig. 1.200a, b   Pectus excavatum. (**a**) Pectus excavatum in a 13-year-old girl. The right cardiac shadow is obliterated. (**b**) Lateral radiograph of the same patient shows the extent of the pectus excavatum.

Heart and Great Vessels

Congenital Heart Disease

CHD has an incidence of approximately 8 per 1000 live births; the 10 most common entities account for 80% of all cases (**Table 1.74**).

Historically, the conventional chest radiograph has played a significant role in the work-up of children with CHD. There have been numerous descriptions that were so-called diagnostic for CHD; one could think of the "egg on string" sign in case of transposition of the great vessels. However, as the presentation of CHD on the chest radiograph depends on a multitude of factors, these signs are not diagnostic (for completeness, we will present them in the tables of this chapter).

A study in 128 children with suspected CHD showed that conventional chest radiograph has a sensitivity of 26%–59% for structural heart disease and an equally poor positive predictive value of 46%–52%. It is important to note that there is no evidence that conventional radiographs can serve as a screening test for CHD.

Currently, the most widely adopted diagnostic strategy is primary imaging with cardiac US. Based on the US findings, either CT, if anatomy needs to be depicted, or MRI, if functional imaging or depiction of intracardiac anatomy is needed, will be performed. Diagnostic angiography is now rarely performed and only in those cases where CT and/or MRI are not diagnostic or if pressure measurements are necessary.

It is also important to note that cardiac imaging is a "team sport" in which a close collaboration between the cardiologists and radiologists is essential.

Table 1.74 Incidence of top 10 CHD

	Condition	Incidence (%)
Cyanotic CHD	Transposition of great vessels	4
	Tetralogy of Fallot	4
Obstructive CHD	Pulmonary stenosis	9
	Aortic stenosis	5
	Coarctation	5
	Hypoplastic left heart syndrome	4
CHD with left-to-right shunt	Ventricular septal defect	36
	Patent ductus arteriosus	9
	Atrial septal defect	5
	Arterioventricular septal defect	4

Table 1.75 Dynamically increased pulmonary vascularity (left-to-right shunt) without cyanosis

Diagnosis	Findings	Comments
VSD ▷ *Fig. 1.201, p. 116*	In case of a small defect, the cardiac silhouette and vessels have a normal appearance. If the defect is large they enlarge. With a large defect and high right ventricular and pulmonary pressure (Eisenmenger syndrome), the hilar vessels become enlarged and in contrast the lung markings become diminished towards the periphery.	Twenty-five percent of all congenital cardiac anomalies. Clinical symptoms are dependent on the size of the VSD.
ASD II (patent foramen secundum) ▷ *Fig. 1.202, p. 116*	Cardiomegaly and prominent pulmonary artery. On the lateral chest radiograph an increased contact area between the sternum and the heart is seen (infundibular expansion).	May present later in life.
PDA ▷ *Fig. 1.203, p. 116*	In the neonatal period, the lung fields may become dense over time due to pulmonary edema. Cardiomegaly and increased pulmonary flow may occur in infants.	In neonates, the Botallian duct may remain patent or reopen.

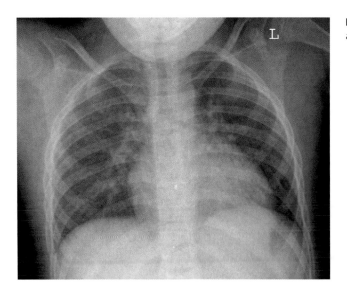

Fig. 1.201 Chest radiograph with increased vascular markings in a 5-year-old girl.

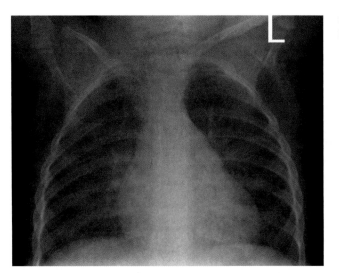

Fig. 1.202 Anteroposterior chest radiograph of a 16-month-old boy with ASD.

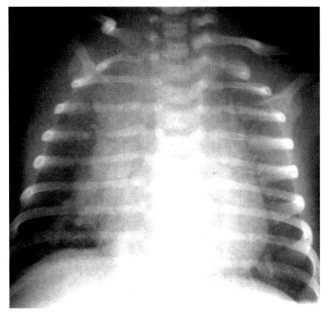

Fig. 1.203 PDA. Chest radiograph in a premature neonate with increased vascular markings and a large cardiac shadow indicative of a persistent Botallian duct.

Table 1.76 Dynamically increased pulmonary vascularity with cyanosis

Diagnosis	Findings	Comments
TAPVD ▷ *Fig. 1.204a–c*	Cardiomegaly. In Type I, a "figure of eight" or "snowman" configuration may be depicted on PF.	Type I: Supracardiac TAPVD—The pulmonary veins drain to the right atrium via the superior vena cava. Type II. Cardiac TAPVD—The pulmonary veins come together behind the heart and then drain to the right atrium through the coronary sinus. Type III. Infracardiac TAPVD—The pulmonary veins drain to the right atrium via the hepatic (liver) veins and inferior vena cava.

(continues on page 118)

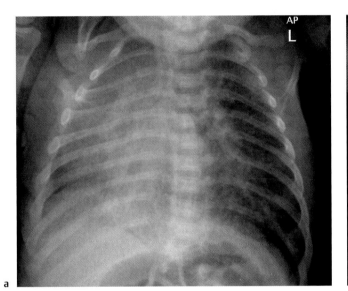

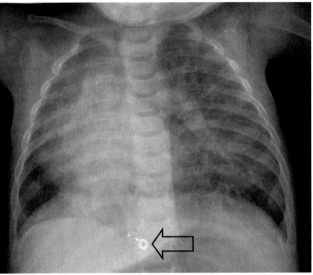

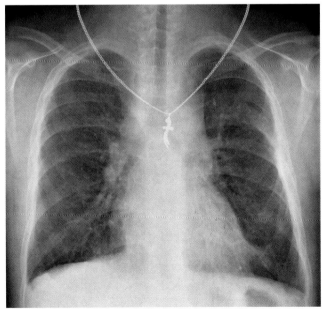

Fig. 1.204a–c Pulmonary venous drainage. (a) Type III TAPVR in a 1-month-old boy shows increased vascularity in the right lung. The draining vein is not visible. (**b**) Radiograph of the same patient after closure of the aberrant pulmonary vein, at the age of 5 months, using an amplatzer device (arrow). (**c**) Posteroanterior chest radiograph of a 14-year-old boy with CGD wearing a scimitar on a necklace.

Table 1.76   (Cont.) Dynamically increased pulmonary vascularity with cyanosis

Diagnosis	Findings	Comments
Transposition of the great vessels ▷ *Fig. 1.205*	Enlarged cardiac silhouette where the heart is oval in shape and the cardiac apex is upturned. There is a narrow vascular pedicle (slender mediastinum). Classic sign: "egg-on-a-string."	The systemic and pulmonary circulations are transposed and therefore separated; an ASD or VSD is obligatory for survival.
Truncus arteriosus ▷ *Fig. 1.206*	Cardiomegaly and increased pulmonary vascularity.	Type I: Origin of a single pulmonary trunk from the left lateral aspect of the common arterial trunk, with branching of the left and right pulmonary arteries from the pulmonary trunk. Type II: Separate but proximal origins of the left and right pulmonary arterial branches from the posterolateral aspect of the common arterial trunk. Type III: Branch pulmonary arteries originate independently from the common arterial trunk or aortic arch, most often from the left and right lateral aspects of the trunk.
AVSD: endocardial cushion defect, septum primum defect, ASD I ▷ *Fig. 1.207*	Cardiomegaly with mild increase of pulmonary vascularity.	Common in trisomy 21.

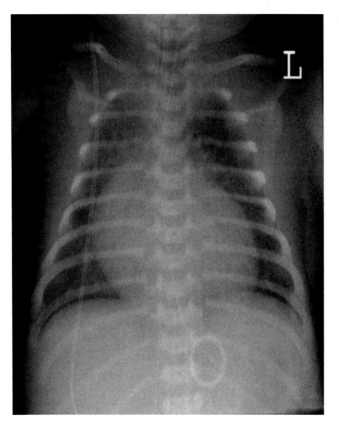

Fig. 1.205   Classic "egg-on-a-string" sign in a 1-day-old boy.

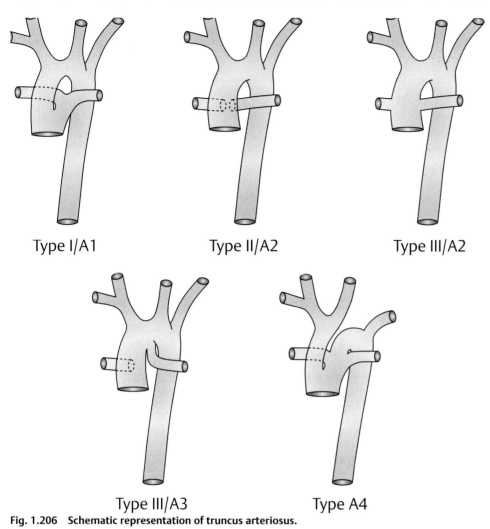

Type I/A1   Type II/A2   Type III/A2

Type III/A3   Type A4

Fig. 1.206   Schematic representation of truncus arteriosus.

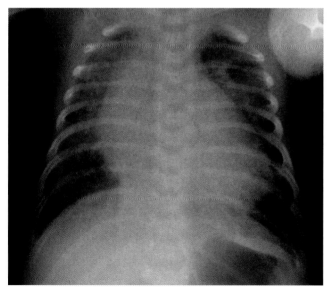

Fig. 1.207   AVSD in a 6-week-old girl with Down syndrome. Note the cardiomegaly and increased vascularity.

Table 1.77   Congenital cardiac anomalies with passively increased vascular markings (engorgement)

Diagnosis	Findings	Comments
TAPVD, type III	Diffuse bilateral opacification of the lungs; the heart initially has a normal size but may enlarge later in life.	The imaging findings mimic pneumonia and overhydration.

Table 1.78   Congenital cardiac anomalies with decreased pulmonary vascular markings (flow): obstruction at the level of the right heart, with right-to-left shunting and cyanosis

Diagnosis	Findings	Comments
Tetralogy of Fallot ▷ *Fig. 1.208*	As a result of decreased pulmonary vascularity, the lungs are hyperlucent. The cardiac silhouette is normally not enlarged. The heart may assume a "boot" shape (coeur en sabot).	Right-sided aortic arch in 25% of cases. Tetralogy of Fallot consists of pulmonary stenosis, right ventricular hypertrophy, VSD, and overriding aorta.
Pulmonary valve anomaly	Poststenotic dilatation of the pulmonary outflow tract.	
Ebstein anomaly ▷ *Fig. 1.209*	Significant cardiomegaly in combination with a slender vascular pedicle.	In most cases, a right-to-left shunt with cyanosis is present.

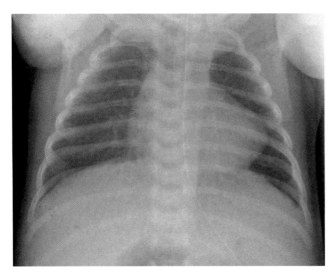

Fig. 1.208   Chest radiograph of a 5-week-old boy with tetralogy of Fallot. Note the uplifted apex leading to a boot-shaped heart.

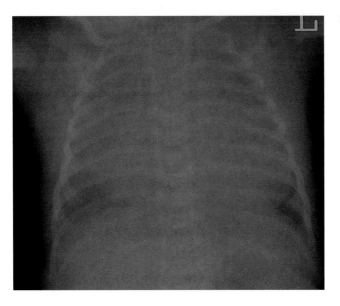

Fig. 1.209   A 1-day-old boy with Ebstein anomaly.

■ Cardiac Positional Anomalies

On chest radiographs, the position of the heart can be defined as dextrocardia, mesocardia, and levocardia. However, as the position of the heart is defined by the position of the atria, where the right atrium lies on the right side and the left atrium on the left side, plain radiographs cannot rule out positional anomalies in all cases. For this, cardiac US is the diagnostic modality of choice.

The tracheobronchial tree morphology is, in general, in keeping with the position of the atria and thus can serve as a guide in deciding the cardiac situs on chest radiographs.

Table 1.79 Cardiac positional anomalies

Diagnosis	Findings	Comments
Levocardia		
Physiologi	Normal anatomic position of the heart.	
Isolated	The heart is left-sided, but there is an abdominal situs inversus.	Often in combination with congenital cardiac anomalies.
Dextrocardia		
Isolated ▷ *Fig. 1.210*	The heart is right-sided, but the abdominal organs have a normal position. In the majority of cases, the anatomy of the heart is otherwise normal.	

Situs inversus totalis
   ▷ *Fig. 1.211*
   ▷ *Fig. 1.212a, b, p. 122*
	Right-sided heart with abdominal situs inversus.	Kartagener syndrome (also known as immotile cilia syndrome); combination of situs inversus totalis, bronchiectasia, and chronic sinusitis.

Ivemark syndrome	Dextroisomerism in which both lungs have three lobes and an epiarterial bronchus. There is asplenia and in up to 33% of cases there is dextrocardia.	Commonly associated with severe congenital cyanotic heart disease.
Isomerism		
Isomerism	Midline position of the heart, liver, and stomach. Both sides of the body may have a more or less left- or right-sided morphologic layout.	Commonly associated with CHD.

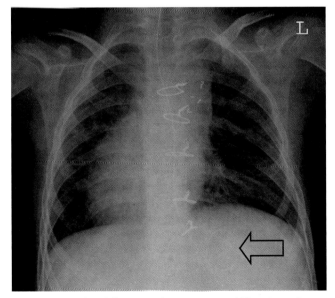

Fig. 1.210 Isolated dextrocardia in an 8-year-old boy. Note the position of the NG tube in the normally positioned stomach (arrow).

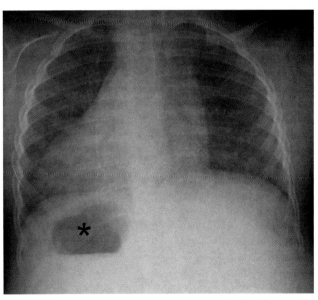

Fig. 1.211 Situs inversus totalis in a 21-month-old girl. Note the right-sided gas bubble in the stomach (asterisk).

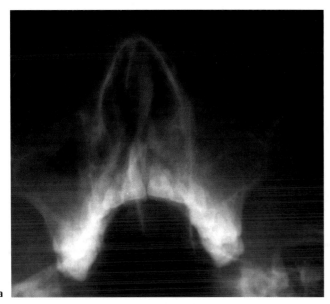
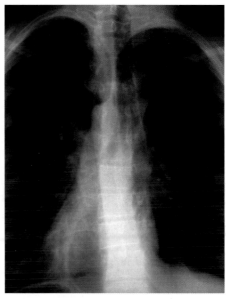

a   b

Fig. 1.212a, b   Situs inversus totalis. (**a**) Watersview of a male teenager showing opacification of the the maxillary sinus, in keeping with sinusitis. (**b**) Posteranterior chest radiograph of the same patient as in (**a**) shows dextrocardia. The diagnosis Karthagener syndrome was made.

Cardiac Tumors

In the pediatric age group, primary cardiac tumors are extremely rare; a prevalence of 0.0017 to 0.28% in autopsy series has been reported. However, with the increasing use of CT and MRI, they may be identified more often, and radiologists should be familiar with their imaging findings.

The majority of primary cardiac tumors are benign, and less then 10% are malignant. However, the majority of cases will be secondary tumors and/or metastatic disease.

Table 1.80   Cardiac tumors—septal/myocardial tumor

Diagnosis	Findings	Comments
Benign tumors		
Fibroma	Solitary tumor. Primary location ventricular septum. Calcifications are common. Low attenuation on CT. Isointense on T1-weighted and hypointense on T2-weighted images. Little to no enhancement after gadolinium.	Can extend into the ventricular conduction system and cause arrhythmia. Can be associated with Gorlin syndrome.
Teratoma	Atrial and ventricular wall. Heterogeneous, encapsulated cystic masses.	Rare tumor, most often arising from the pericardial space.
Hemangioma	Can be found anywhere in the heart. Subendocardial nodules (2–4 cm diameter).	Exceedingly rare cardiac tumor.
Histiocytic nodule	Nodular deposits on the valves or ventricular endocardium on US.	Also known as infantile histiocytic cardiomyopathy, oncocytic cardiomyopathy, histiocytic cardiomyopathy, Purkinje cell tumor, focal lipid cardiomyopathy, and idiopathic infantile cardiomyopathy.
Malignant tumors		
Intrapericardial pheochromocytoma	Vascular tumor arising from the autonomic paraganglia. Predominantly in atrial septum.	
Metastatic cardiac tumors	Multiple discrete firm epicardial nodules on autopsy.	Melanoma has a tendency to spread to the heart. Estimated to be 20 times more common than primary cardiac tumors.

Table 1.81   Cardiac tumors—intracardiac tumor

Diagnosis	Findings	Comments
Benign tumors		
Rhabdomyoma	Bright intramural mass on cardiac US. Predominantly in the ventricular myocardium. Often multiple lesions. Can protrude into the cardiac cavity.	Most common benign primary cardiac tumor (> 60%). Preferential cardiac location intraventricular. Strongly related to tuberous sclerosis, present in 43%–72% of patients.
Myxoma	Primary location in left atrium (90%), but also found in right atrium. Mostly a solitary tumor. Pediculated mass with irregular nonhomogeneous small lucencies on US. Heterogeneous mass with low attenuation on CT. Heterogeneous mass, bright on T2-weighted imaging with heterogeneous enhancement after gadolinium.	Most common primary cardiac tumor in adults. Can be associated with Carney complex (autosomal dominant syndrome of cardiac myxomas and hyperpigmented skin lesions), LAMB (*l*entigines, *a*trial myxoma, *m*ucocutaneous myxoma, *b*lue nevi), and NAME (*n*aevi, *a*trial myxoma, *m*yxoid neurofibroma, *e*pithelides).
Hemangioma	Can be found anywhere in the heart. Subendocardial nodules (2–4 cm diameter).	Exceedingly rare cardiac tumor.
Malignant tumors		
Angiosarcoma	Most common malignant tumor in adults. Primary location right atrium. Broad-based mass with epicardial, endocardial, and/or intracavitary extension. Areas of high signal intensity on T1-weighted images, focal or linear along pericardium.	Pulmonary metastatic disease is a common finding.
Rhabdomyosarcoma ▷ *Fig. 1.213a, b*	Can occur in any heart chamber. More likely to involve valves. Variable appearance from completely solid to mostly cystic/necrotic.	Poor prognosis.
Fibrosarcoma	Can occur in any heart chamber, with preference for the left atrium. Mostly multifocal. Often lobulated mass.	Poor prognosis, death within 1 y after diagnosis.
Metastatic cardiac tumors ▷ *Fig. 1.214, p. 124*	Can be seen as an extension of tumor thrombus (e.g., Wilms tumor). Hematologic spread most common.	

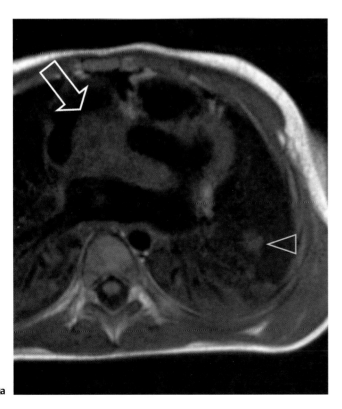
a

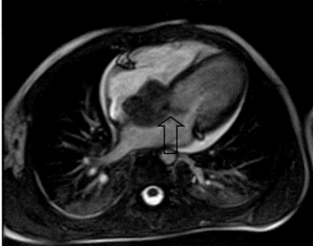
b

Fig. 1.213a, b   Rhabdomyosarcoma. (a) Axial T1-weighted postcontrast. Note the presence of lung metastases (arrowhead). Biopsy proved primary, maliganant cardiac rhabdomyosarcoma in atrial septum (arrow). (Courtesy of A. Taylor, MD, FRCP, FRCR, Cardiorespiratory Unit, UCL Institute of Child Health & Great Ormond Street Hospital for Children, London, United Kingdom.) **(b)** Balanced steady-state free precession cine image (systolic frame) of the same patient shows extension into the anterior leaflet of the mitral valve (arrow), which is a finding suggestive of malignancy.

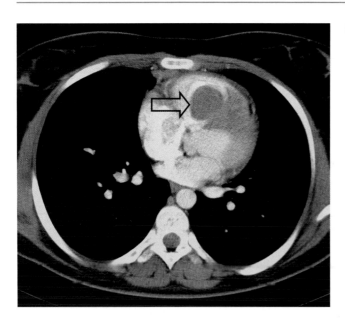

Fig. 1.214   Metastatic osteosarcoma to the right ventricle in a 17-year-old girl (arrow).

The Great Vessels

In young children, the great vessels, on conventional radiographs, are or can be obscured by the shadow of the thymus. As the thymus diminishes in size, the great vessels become more and more visible.

Imaging of the great vessels will mostly be done using CT and/or MRI. The use of diagnostic angiography should be considered to be obsolete.

Table 1.82   The great vessels, normal appearance

Diagnosis	Findings	Comments
Normal aorta and pulmonary artery	Left-sided aorta.	In young children, the aorta is not always visible due to overlying thymic tissue. The diameter of the aorta is influenced by respiration. In expiration, the aorta can enlarge and mimic a pathologic situation.
Normal superior vena cava	In children, the outline can be obscured by the thymus.	

Table 1.83   The great vessels, pathologic changes of the aorta (size, shape, position)

Diagnosis	Findings	Comments
Dilatation (aneurysm) of the ascending aorta	Dilated right-sided aorta shadow. Displacement of the superior border leads to an aortic knuckle.	The ascending aorta should not form a distinct shadow (i.e., be border-forming) below the age of 10 y. Causes include congenital valvular aortic stenosis, aortic insufficiency, truncus arteriosus, and aneurysms.
PDA ▷ *Fig. 1.215a, b* ▷ *Fig. 1.216a, b*	Dilatation of the ascending aorta and main pulmonary artery.	Endovascular treatment with plugs (e.g., Amplatzer device) is a widely used technique. The device is visible on conventional radiographs. Dislocation, into the pulmonary circulation, may occur. Other techniques are endovascular coiling or transthoracic clipping.
Narrow vascular pedicle in transposition of the great vessels ▷ *Fig. 1.205, p. 118*	A result of the ascending aorta projecting over the pulmonary trunk. Seen in transposition of the great vessels.	
Right-sided aortic arch (high right aorta) ▷ *Fig. 1.217*	Right aortic arch in the right superior mediastinum.	Can be seen as a solitary anomaly. However, mostly seen in combination with tetralogy of Fallot (25%) or truncus arteriosus (35%).

(continues on page 126)

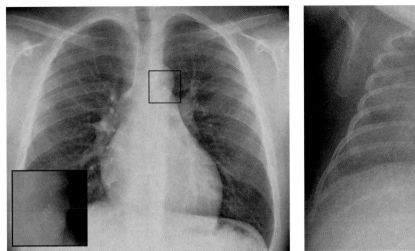
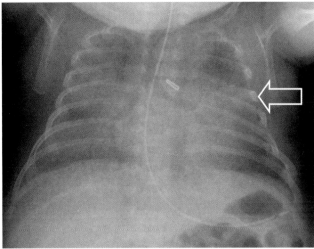

a   b

Fig. 1.215a, b   PDA. (**a**) A 14-year-old boy with a coil in the Botallian duct (see insert). (**b**) A 2-week-old boy after clipping of the Botallian duct. Note the dislocated rib as a result of the left thoracotomy (arrow).

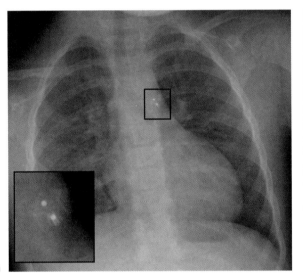
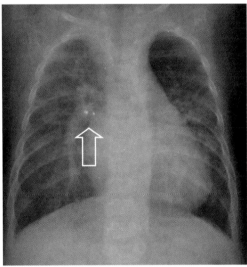

a   b

Fig. 1.216a, b   PDA. (**a**) A 2-year-old girl after endovascular treatment for a persistent Botallian duct using an Amplatzer device (see insert). (**b**) Posteroanterior radiograph of the same child as in (**a**) shows dislocation of the Amplatzer plug into to the pulmonary artery (arrow).

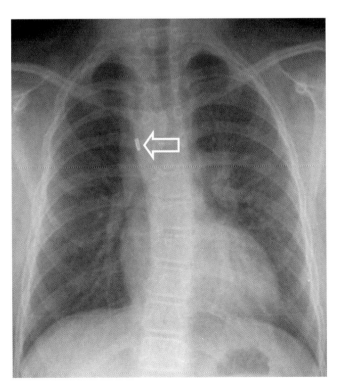

Fig. 1.217   Right-sided aortic arch in a 12-year-old girl. Note the clip on the Botallian duct, which is situated in the right side of the mediastinum (arrow).

Table 1.83   (Cont.) The great vessels, pathologic changes of the aorta (size, shape, position)

Diagnosis	Findings	Comments
Coarctation of the aorta ▷ *Fig. 1.218a, b* ▷ *Fig. 1.219*	Slight predominance of the left-sided aortic arch. On the conventional radiograph a "figure of 3" can be seen. Hypertrophy of the intercostal vessels can lead to rib-notching. If present, the positive predictive value is 50%	
Aortic aneurysm	In the majority of cases, dilatation of the ascending aorta.	Rare in children, mostly the result of trauma or infection.
Aneurysmal dilatation of the ductus arteriosus ▷ *Fig. 1.220*	Visible on cardiac US or MRI. Extremely rare.	May calcify later in life.

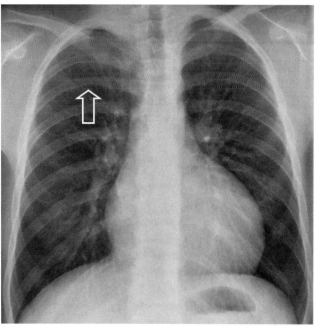

a

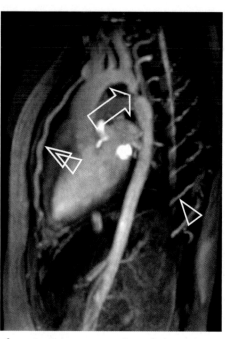

b

Fig. 1.218a, b   Coarctation of the aorta. (a) A 14-year-old boy with coarctation of the aorta. As a result of hypertrophy of the intercostal arteries, inferior rib notching is seen (arrow). **(b)** Maximum intensity projection of a magnetic resonance angiography in another patient shows the coarctation of the aorta (arrow), hypertrophy of the intercostal arteries (arrowhead), and hypertrophy of the mammarian arteries (double arrowhead).

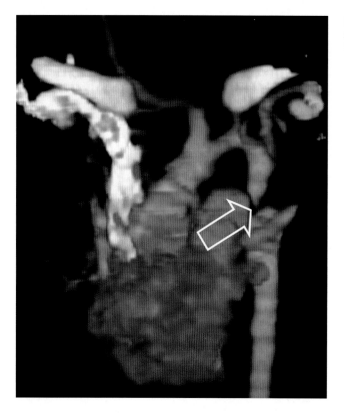

Fig. 1.219   Coarctation of the aorta. CT angiography surface-shaded three-dimensional rendered image of coarctation of the aorta in a 1-month-old boy.

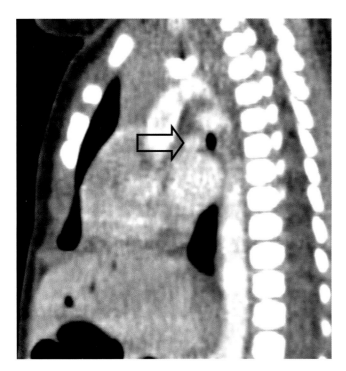

Fig. 1.220 Aneurysmal dilatation of the Botallian duct (arrow). (Courtesy of J.I.L.M. Verbeke, Pediatric Radiologist, VU Medical Centre Amsterdam, the Netherlands.)

Table 1.84 The large vessels, changes in contour of the pulmonary artery

Diagnosis	Findings	Comments
Enlarged main pulmonary segment	Convex dilatation of the pulmonary vasculature.	Seen in pulmonary stenosis with poststenotic dilatation.
Small pulmonary artery (e.g., in tetralogy of Fallot)	The contour of the pulmonary artery is flat or concave.	

Table 1.85 The great vessels, changes in contour of the superior mediastinal veins

Diagnosis	Findings	Comments
Absent silhouette of the superior vena cava	"Empty" superior vena cava contour.	Due to "rotation" of the heart due to the enlarging right atrium.
Persistent left superior vena cava and duplicated superior vena cava	Widening of the left superior mediastinum.	Can be seen as an isolated anomaly.
TAPVD (type I)	Bilateral widening of the mediastinum superior.	

■ Coronary Artery Disease

Compared to adults, coronary artery disease in children is a rare finding; however, with the advent of modern imaging techniques, the pediatric radiologist should be aware of the pathology of coronary arteries.

Table 1.86 Coronary artery disease

Diagnosis	Findings	Comments
Congenital anomalies	Abnormal origin and course of coronary arteries: 1. Absent left main trunk (split origination of left coronary artery) 2. Anomalous location of coronary ostium within aortic root or near proper aortic sinus 3. Anomalous location of coronary ostium outside normal aortic sinuses 4. Anomalous origination of the coronary ostium from opposite, facing "coronary" sinus 5. Single coronary artery.	The most common anomaly is an aberrant origin of the main left or right coronary artery from the wrong sinus of Valsalva. Often an incidental finding during coronary angiography, with an estimated incidence of 0.3%–0.8%.
	Anomalies of coronary arterial anatomy: 1. Congenital ostial stenosis or atresia (left coronary artery, left anterior descencing [LAD] artery, right coronary artery [RCA], circumflex coronary artery [Cx] 2. Coronary ectasia or aneurysm 3. Coronary hypoplasia 4. Intramural coronary artery (muscular bridge) 5. Subendocardial coronary course 6. Coronary crossing 7. Anomalous origination of posterior descending artery from anterior descending branch or septal penetrating branch 8. Absent posterior descending branch (PD) (split RCA) 9. Absent LAD (split LAD) 10. Ectopic origination of first septal branch.	
	Anomalies of coronary termination: 1. Inadequate arteriolar/capillary ramifications 2. Abnormal communication of coronary arteries.	Congenital coronary artery fistula is a relatively rare anomaly defined as an abnormal direct communication between any coronary artery and any of the cardiac chambers. Coronary arteriovenous fistulas: an anomaly in which the coronary arteries have a direct communication with the pulmonary veins.
Stenosis	Narrowing of the lumen of the vessel. Unlike in adults, almost never based on atherosclerosis.	Can be seen in patients with Takayasu arteritis.
Dilatation ▷ *Fig. 1.221* ▷ *Fig. 1.222*	Dilation, regional or over a longer trajectory, of the coronary arteries.	Can be seen in Kawasaki disease, LEOPARD syndrome (extremely rare).

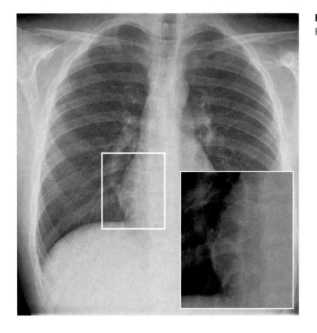

Fig. 1.221   Calcified coronary artery aneurysms in a 17-year-old boy with Kawasaki disease.

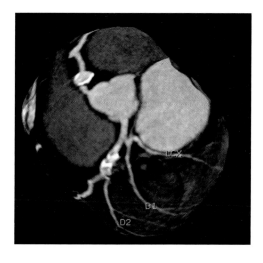

Fig. 1.222 Electrocardiography-gated CT angiography shows aneurysms of the RCA and LAD artery in a 13-year-old boy with Kawasaki disease.
D1 First diagonal branch of LAD
D2 Second diagonal branch of LAD
LCX Left circumflex artery

Rings and Slings

A vascular ring is the result of anomalous development of the aortic arch. In the embryologic stage, the aorta forms a ring around the primitive foregut, and anomalous development leads to an aortic ring or sling.

Historically, the primary diagnostic tool was the contrast (barium) swallow; however, with the advent of CT and MRI, this technique has been superseded and should be considered obsolete.

In young children, the main presenting symptom may be stridor, often the result of concomittant tracheomalacia. Later in life, dysphagia is the most common symptom.

Table 1.87 Aberrant arteries and vascular rings

Diagnosis	Findings	Comments
Anomalous vessels with posterior esophageal and anterior tracheal impression ▷ Fig. 1.223a, b	Most commonly caused by double aortic arch.	In rare cases, seen in combined right aortic arch, left ductus arteriosus, and abberant subclavian artery.
Anomalous vessels with anterior tracheal impression and normal esophagus ▷ Fig. 1.224	Most commonly caused by an innominate artery or a single arterial trunk combining the innominate artery and the left common carotid artery.	

(continues on page 130)

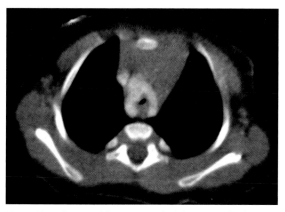 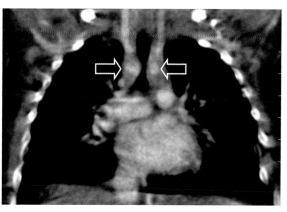

b

Fig. 1.223a, b Double aortic arch. (a) A 3-month-old girl with a double aortic arch. **(b)** Coronal reconstruction clearly shows the relation of the double aortic arch to the trachea (arrows). The trachea is compressed as a result of the double aortic arch.

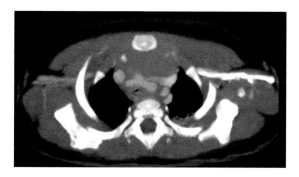

Fig. 1.224 Inspiratory stridor in a 9-month-old boy. Contrast-enhanced CT shows an innomate artery compressing the trachea.

Table 1.87 (Cont.) Aberrant arteries and vascular rings

Diagnosis	Findings	Comments
Anomalous vessels with a small oblique esophageal impression and a normal trachea ▷ *Fig. 1.225a–c*	Most commonly caused by an aberrant right subclavian artery (lusorian artery).	
Anomalous vessels with anterior esophageal impression and posterior tracheal narrowing ▷ *Fig. 1.226a, b*	Most commonly caused by a pulmonary sling or anomalous left pulmonary artery arising from the right pulmonary artery.	

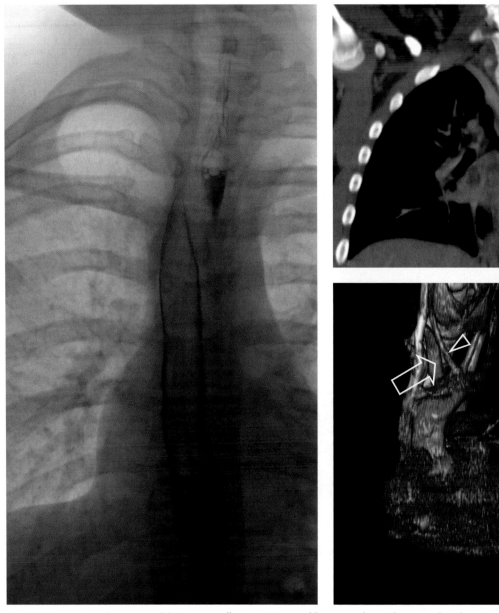

Fig. 1.225a–c Lusorian artery. (a) Barium swallow in a 17-year-old girl shows an oblique posterior impression on the esophagus. **(b)** CT angiography, coronal multiplanar reconstruction 5-mm slice thickness, shows the anomalous lusorian artery. **(c)** Shaded surface display (SSD) of the lusorian artery (arrow). Note the aberrant right carotid artery arising from the aorta (arrowhead).

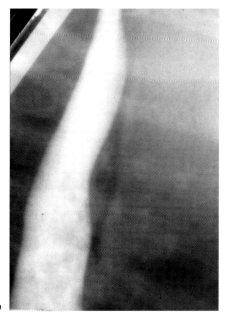
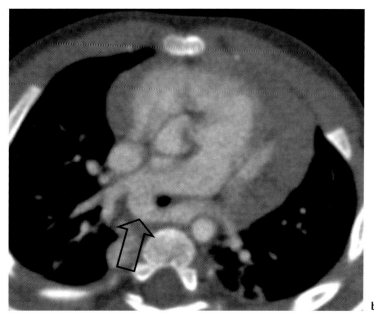

a

b

Fig. 1.226a, b   Pulmonary artery sling. (**a**) Left pulmonary sling on barium swallow. Note the posterior impression on the trachea and anterior impression on the esophagus. (**b**) Left pulmonary artery sling (arrow). (Courtesy of A. Taylor, MD, FRCP, FRCR, Cardio-respiratory Unit UCL Institute of Child Health & Great Ormond Street Hospital for Children, London, United Kingdom.)

Cardiovascular Devices

Table 1.88   Cardiovascular devices

Diagnosis	Findings	Comments
Coarctation of aorta ▷ Fig. 1.227a, b	Stent.	For adolescent patients.
Patent ductus arteriosus ▷ Fig. 1.216, p. 125	Coil; vascular clip; Amplatzer duct occluder.	

(continues on page 132)

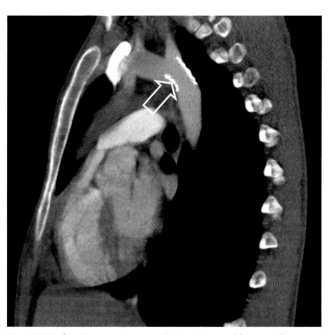
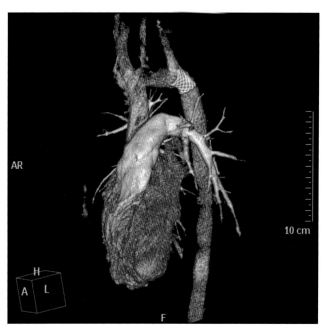

a

b

Fig. 1.227a, b   Coarctation aorta. (**a**) An 18-year-old man with coarctation aorta after endovascular stent treatment (arrow). (**b**) Three-dimensional SSD of the endovascular stent.

Table 1.88   (Cont.) Cardiovascular devices

Diagnosis	Findings	Comments
Pulmonary valve stenosis ▷ *Fig. 1.228a–c*	Melody stent.	After dysfunctioning pulmonary homograft. Beware of strut fractures.
VSD, ASD, and patent foramen ovale ▷ *Fig. 1.229*	Amplatzer occluder device.	Beware of migration.
Cardiac arrythmia: postcardiac surgery ▷ *Fig. 1.230a–c*	Pacemaker.	Beware of lead dislocation or fracture.
Valvular dysfunction ▷ *Fig. 1.231, p. 134* ▷ *Fig. 1.232, p. 134*	Valve replacement.	Projection on radiograph defines the valve replacement.

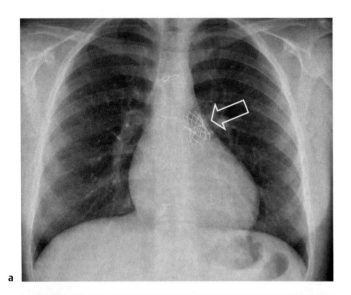

a

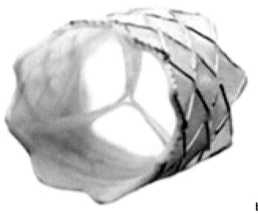

b

Fig. 1.228a–c   Melody stent. (**a**) A 14-year-old girl after Melody stent placement (arrow). (**b**) Melody stent. (**c**) Melody stent with broken strut (see inset).

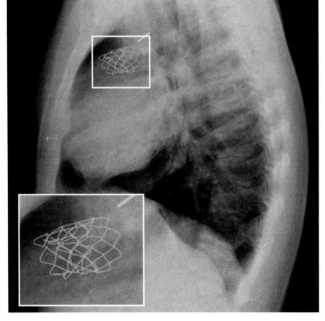

c

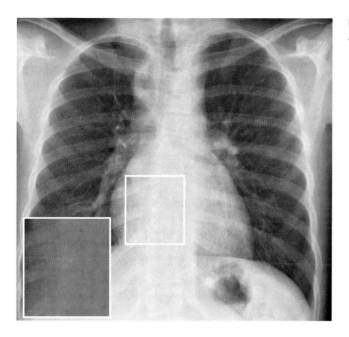

Fig. 1.229 A 16-year-old boy after endovascular treatment of ASD using an Amplatzer device (see inset).

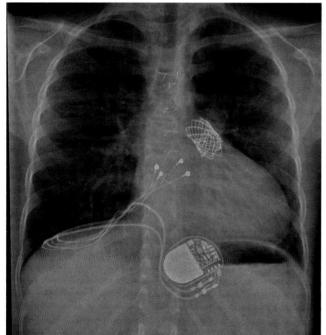

a

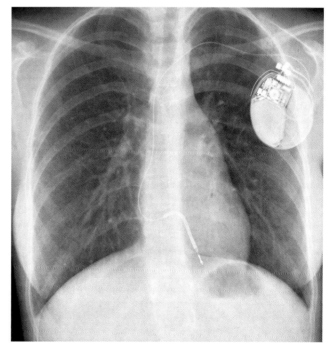

b

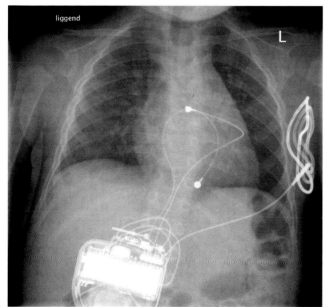

c

Fig. 1.230a–c Cardiac arrhythmia. (a) A 9-year-old girl with tetralogy of Fallot. An epicardial pacemaker has been placed. Note the presence of a Melody valve replacement. **(b)** A 15-year-old girl with an implantable cardioverter defibrillator; the lead is positioned within the right ventricle. **(c)** A 1-year-old boy with a subcutaneous implantable cardioverter defibrillator in combination with electrocardial pacing.

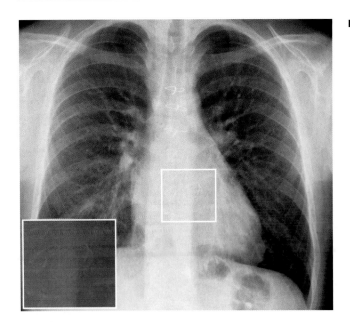

Fig. 1.231 A 17-year-old boy with a mitral valve replacement.

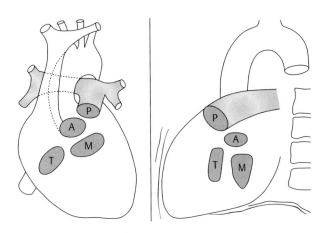

Fig. 1.232 Schematic representation of valve replacements on the anteroposterior/posteroanterior chest radiograph (left) and lateral radiograph (right).

P Pulmonary
A aortic
T tricuspid
M mitral

■ Further Reading

Ablin DS, Azouz EM, Jain KA. Large intrathoracic tumors in children: imaging findings. AJR Am J Roentgenol 1995;165:925–934

Andrén-Sandberg A, Dervenis C. Pancreatic pseudocysts in the 21st century. Part I: classification, pathophysiology, anatomic considerations and treatment. JOP 2004;5:8–24

Andronikou S, Wieselthaler N. Modern imaging of tuberculosis in children: thoracic, central nervous system and abdominal tuberculosis. Pediatr Radiol 2004;34(11):861–875

Agrons GA, Courtney SE, Stocker JT, Markowitz RI. From the archives of the AFIP: lung disease in premature neonates: radiologic-pathologic correlation. Radiographics 2005;25(4):1047–1073

Backer CL, Mavroudis C. Congenital Heart Surgery Nomenclature and Database Project: vascular rings, tracheal stenosis, pectus excavatum. Ann Thorac Surg 2000;69(4 Suppl):S308–318

Beall DP, Ly J, Bell JP, et al. Pediatric extraskeletal osteosarcoma. Pediatr Radiol 2008;38:579–582

Berdon WE. Rings, slings, and other things: vascular compression of the infant trachea updated from the midcentury to the millennium—the legacy of Robert E. Gross, MD, and Edward B. D. Neuhauser, MD. Radiology 2000;216(3):624–632

Bining HJ, Saigal G, Chankowsky J. Kingella kingae spondylodiscitis in a child. Br J Radiol 2006;79(947):e181–183

Brien EW,Mirra JM, Ippolito V, Vaughan L. Clear-cell chondrosarcoma with elevated alkaline phosphatase, mistaken for osteosarcoma on biopsy. Skeletal Radiol 1996;25:770–774

Brill PW, Winchester P, Kleinman PK. Differential diagnosis I: diseases simulating abuse. In: Kleinman PK, ed. Diagnostic imaging of child abuse. 2nd ed. St. Louis: Mosby, 1998:178–196

Calder AD, Owens CM. Computed tomography of the central and peripheral airways. In: Donoghue VP, ed. Radiological imaging of the neonatal chest. Berlin: Springer-Verlag Berlin and Heidelberg GmbH & Co, 2007:177–195

Carden KA, Boiselle PM, Waltz DA, Ernst A. Tracheomalacia and tracheobronchomalacia in children and adults: an in-depth review. Chest 2005;127(3):984–1005

Castellote A, Enriquez G, Lucaya J. Congenital malformations of the chest beyond the neonatal period. In Carty H, Brunelle F, Stringer DA, Kao SC-S, eds. Imaging children. Oxford, UK: Churchill Livingstone, 2005:1049–1074

Chao S, Mullins ME, Slanetz PJ. Posterior mediastinal pheochromocytoma. AJR Am J Roentgenol 2001;176:1408

Cheema JI, Grissom LE, Harcke HT. Radiographic characteristics of lower-extremity bowing in children. Radiographics 2003;23:871–880

Chernick V, Boat TF, Wilmott RW, Bush A. Kendig's disorders of the respiratory tract in children. Philadelphia: Elsevier Inc., 2006

Cleveland RH. A radiologic update on medical diseases of the newborn chest. Pediatr Radiol 1995;25(8):631–637

Cohen MM Jr. A comprehensive and critical assessment of overgrowth and overgrowth syndromes. Adv Hum Genet 1989;18:181–303, 373–376

Dahnert W. Radiology review manual. Philadelphia: Lippicott Williams and Wilkins, 2007

Diren HB, Kutluk MT, Karabent A, Göçmen A, Adalioğlu G, Kenanoğlu A. Primary hypertrophic osteoarthropathy. Pediatr Radiol 1986; 16:231–234

Dodd GD 3rd, Ledesma-Medina J, Baron RL, Fuhrman CR. Posttransplant lymphoproliferative disorder: intrathoracic manifestations. Radiology 1992;184(1):65–69

Donnelly LF. Practical issues concerning imaging of pulmonary infection in children. J Thorac Imaging 2001;16(4):238–250

Donnelly LF, Frush DP. Langerhans cell histiocytosis showing low-attenuation mediastinal mass and cystic lung sisease. AJR 2000; 174:877–878

Donnelly LF, Klosterman LA. The yield of CT of children who have complicated pneumonia and noncontributory chest radiography. AJR Am J Roentgenol 1998;170(6):1627–1631

Donoghue VP. Hyaline membrane disease and its complications. In: Donoghue VP, ed. Radiological imaging of the neonatal chest. Berlin: Springer-Verlag Berlin and Heidelberg GmbH & Co, 2007:67–79

Donoghue VP. Transient tachypneoa of the newborn. In: Donoghue VP, ed. Radiological imaging of the neonatal chest. Berlin: Springer-Verlag Berlin and Heidelberg GmbH & Co, 2007:81–83

Ebel KD, Blickman H, Willich E, Richter E, eds. The mediastinum. In: Differential diagnosis in pediatric radiology. Stuttgart: Thieme, 1999:155–200

Edwards DK 3rd, Berry CC, Hilton SW. Trisomy 21 in newborn infants: chest radiographic diagnosis. Radiology 1988;167:317–318

Effmann EL, Merten DF, Kirks DR, Pratt PC, Spock A. Adult respiratory distress syndrome in children. Radiology 1985;157(1):69–74

Effman EL. Chest wall. In Kuhn JP, Slovis TL, Haller JO, Caffey J, eds. Caffey's pediatric diagnostic imaging. Philadelphia: Elsevier Inc., 2004:817–856

Effman EL, Kuhn JP. Lungs and airways. In Kuhn JP, Slovis TL, Haller JO, Caffey J, eds. Caffey's pediatric diagnostic imaging. Philadelphia: Elsevier Inc., 2004:891–1072

Elliott M, Roebuck D, Noctor C, et al. The management of congenital tracheal stenosis. Int J Pediatr Otorhinolaryngol 2003;67 Suppl 1:S183–192

Feigin RD. Textbook of pediatric infectious diseases. 5th ed. Philadelphia: Saunders, 2004

Garcés-Iñigo EF, Leung R, Sebire NJ, McHugh K. Extrarenal rhabdoid tumours outside the central nervous system in infancy. Pediatr Radiol 2009;39:817–822

Gardner DJ, Azouz EM. Solitary lucent epiphyseal lesions in children. Skeletal Radiol 1988;17:497–504

Gartner L, Pearce CJ, Saifuddin A. The role of the plain radiograph in the characterisation of soft tissue tumours. Skeletal Radiol 2009;38:549–558

Geier A, Lammert F, Gartung C, Nguyen HN, Wildberger JE, Matern S. Magnetic resonance imaging and magnetic resonance cholangiopancreaticography for diagnosis and pre-interventional evaluation of a fluid thoracic mass. Eur J Gastroenterol Hepatol 2003; 15:429–431

Gilsanz V, Perez FJ, Campbell PP, Dorey FJ, Lee DC, Wren TA. Quantitative CT reference values for vertebral trabecular bone density in. Radiology 2009;250:222–227

Giron J, Fajadet P, Sans N, et al. Diagnostic approach to mediastinal masses. Eur J Radiol 1998;27(1):21–42

Gladish GW, Sabloff BM, Munden RF, Truong MT, Erasmus JJ, Chasen MH. Primary thoracic sarcomas. Radiographics 2002;22:621–637

Glass RB, Norton KI, Mitre SA, Kang E. Pediatric ribs: a spectrum of abnormalities. Radiographics 2002;22:87–104

Goldfarb CA, Manske PR, Busa R, Mills J, Carter P, Ezaki M. Upper-extremity phocomelia reexamined: a longitudinal dysplasia. J Bone Joint Surg Am 2005;87:2639–2648

Goldman AB, Kaye JJ. Macrodystrophia lipomatosa: radiographic diagnosis. AJR Am J Roentgenol 1977;128:101–105

Grayev AM, Boal DK, Wallach DM, Segal LS. Metaphyseal fractures mimicking abuse during treatment for clubfoot. Pediatr Radiol 2001;31:559–563

Green DM, Breslow NE, Beckwith JB, Norkool P. Screening of children with hemihypertrophy, aniridia, and Beckwith-Wiedemann syndrome in patients with Wilms tumor: a report from the National Wilms Tumor Study. Med Pediatr Oncol 1993;21:188–192

Greenspan A, Jundt G, Remagen W. Differential diagnosis in orthopaedic oncology. 2nd ed. Philadelphia: Lippincott Williams & Wilkins, 2007

Heller GD, Haller JO, Berdon WE, Sane S, Kleinman PK. Punctate thymic calcification in infants with untreated Langerhans' cell histiocytosis: report of four new cases. Pediatr Radiol 1999;29(11):813–815

Hernanz-Schulman M. Vascular rings: a practical approach to imaging diagnosis. Pediatr Radiol 2005;35(10):961–979

Houser JR, Kan JH. Langerhans cell histiocytosis of the epiphysis. Pediatr Radiol 2008;38:351

Howling SJ, Northway WH Jr, Hansell DM, Moss RB, Ward S, Muller NL. Pulmonary sequelae of bronchopulmonary dysplasia survivors: high-resolution CT findings. AJR Am J Roentgenol 2000;174(5):1323–1326

Hussmann J, Russell RC, Kucan JO, Khardori R, Steinau HU. Soft-tissue calcifications: differential diagnosis and therapeutic approaches. Ann Plast Surg 1995;34:138–147

Jaggers J, Balsara K. Mediastinal masses in children. Semin Thorac Cardiovasc Surg 2004;16(3):201–208

Jaramillo D, Shapiro F, Hoffer FA, et al. Posttraumatic growth-plate abnormalities: MR imaging of bony-bridge formation in rabbits. Radiology 1990;175:767–773

Jeanes AC, Owens CM. Chest imaging in the immunocompromised child. Paediatr Respir Rev 2002;3(1):59–69

Jeung MY, Gangi A, Gasser B, et al. Imaging of chest wall disorders. Radiographics 1999;19:617–637

Jeung MY, Gasser B, Gangi A, et al. Imaging of cystic masses of the mediastinum. Radiographics 2002;22:S79–93

John SD, Ramanathan J, Swischuk LE. Spectrum of clinical and radiographic findings in pediatric mycoplasma pneumonia. Radiographics 2001;21(1):121–131

Jolles H, Henry DA, Robertson JR, Cole TJ, Spratt JA. Mediastinitis following median sternotomy: CT findings. Radiology 1996; 201:463–466

Keller KA, Barnes PD. Rickets vs. abuse: a national and international epidemic. Pediatr Radiol 2008;38:1210–1216

Khanna G, Sato TS, Ferguson P. Imaging of chronic recurrent multifocal osteomyelitis. Radiographics 2009;29:1159–1177

Kilic D, Tercan F, Sahin E, Blien A, Hatipoglu A. Unusual radiological manifestations of the echinococcus infection in the thorax. J Thorac Imaging 2006;21(1):32–36

Kimonis VE, Mehta SG, Digiovanna JJ, Bale SJ, Pastakia B. Radiological features in 82 patients with nevoid basal cell carcinoma (NBCC or Gorlin) syndrome. Genet Med 2004;6:495–502

Klein DM, Barbera C, Gray ST, Spero CR, Perrier G, Teicher JL. Sensitivity of objective parameters in the diagnosis of pediatric septic hips. Clin Orthop Relat Res 1997;338:153–159

Kleinman PK. Diagnostic imaging of child abuse. 2nd ed. St. Louis: Mosby, 1989

Kleinman PK. Problems in the diagnosis of metaphyseal fractures. Pediatr Radiol 2008;38 Suppl 3:S388–394

Kleinman PK. Skeletal trauma: general considerations. In: Kleinman PK, ed. Diagnostic imaging of child abuse. 2nd ed. St. Louis: Mosby, 1998:168–177

Ko SF, Hsieh MJ, Ng SH, et al. Imaging spectrum of Castleman's disease. AJR Am J Roentgenol 2004;182:769–775

Koh DM, Hansell DM. Computed tomography of diffuse interstitial lung disease in children. Clin Radiol 2000;55(9):659–667

Kothari NA, Kramer SS. Bronchial diseases and lung aeration in children. J Thorac Imaging 2001;16(4):207–223

Kozlowski K, Sutcliffe J, Barylak A, et al. Hypophosphatasia. Review of 24 cases. Pediatr Radiol 1976;5:103–117

Kuhn JP. Diaphragm. In Kuhn JP, Slovis TL, Haller JO, Caffey J, eds. Caffey's pediatric diagnostic imaging. Philadelphia: Elsevier Inc., 2004:857–866

Kuhn JP. Mediastinum. In Kuhn JP, Slovis TL, Haller JO, Caffey J, eds. Caffey's pediatric diagnostic imaging. Philadelphia: Elsevier Inc., 2004:1160–1224

Kuhn JP. Pleura. In Kuhn JP, Slovis TL, Haller JO, Caffey J, eds. Caffey's pediatric diagnostic imaging. Philadelphia: Elsevier Inc., 2004:867–890

Kumar R, Madewell JE, Swischuk LE, Lindell MM, David R. The clavicle: normal and abnormal. Radiographics 1989;9:677–706

Lachman R. Taybi and Lachman's radiology of syndromes, metabolic disorders and skeletal dysplasias. 5th ed. St. Louis: Mosby, 2006

Laor T, Jaramillo D. MR imaging insights into skeletal maturation: what is normal? Radiology 2009;250:28–38

Le Goff C, Cormier-Daire V. Genetic and molecular aspects of acromelic dysplasia. Pediatr Endocrinol Rev 2009;6:418–423

Levesque M, Legmann P, Le Cloirec A, Deybach JC, Nordmann Y. Radiological features in congenital erythropoietic porphyria (Gunther's disease). Report of 3 cases. Pediatr Radiol 1988;18:62–66

Levine MS, Borden S 4th, Gill FM. Sternal cupping: a new finding in childhood sickle cell anemia. Radiology 1982;142:367–370

Makley JT, Dunn MJ. Prostaglandin synthesis by osteoid osteoma. Lancet 1982;2:42

Mar WA, Taljanovic MS, Bagatell R, et al. Update on imaging and treatment of Ewing sarcoma family tumors: what the radiologist needs to know. J Comput Assist Tomogr 2008;32:108–118

McCahon E. Lung tumours in children. Paediatr Respir Rev 2006; 7(3):191–196

McCarville MB, Kaste SC, Pappo AS. Soft-tissue malignancies in infancy. AJR Am J Roentgenol 1999;173:973–977

McHugh K. Mediastinal and chest tumours. In Carty H, Brunelle F, Stringer DA, Kao SC-S, eds. Imaging children. Oxford, UK: Churchill Livingstone, 2005:1147–1172

McPhillips M. Infection. In Carty H, Brunelle F, Stringer DA, Kao SC-S, eds. Imaging children. Oxford, UK: Churchill Livingstone, 2005:1075–1118

McQueen FM. Magnetic resonance imaging in early inflammatory arthritis: what is its role? Rheumatology (Oxford) 2000;39:700–706

Mehta AV, Chidambaram B, Suchedina AA, Garrett AR. Radiologic abnormalities of the sternum in Turner's syndrome. Chest 1993; 104:1795–1799

Merten DF. Diagnostic imaging of mediastinal masses in children. AJR Am J Roentgenol 1992;158(4):825–832

Moppett J, Oakhill A, Duncan AW. Second malignancies in children: the usual suspects? Eur J Radiol 2001;38:235–248

Mora S, Gilsanz V. Establishment of peak bone mass. Endocrinol Metab Clin North Am 2003;32:39–63

Muecke EC, Currarino G. Congenital widening of the pubic symphysis: associated clinical disorders and roentgen anatomy of affected bony pelves. Am J Roentgenol Radium Ther Nucl Med 1968; 103:179–185

Newman B. Congenital bronchopulmonary foregut malformations: concepts and controversies. Pediatr Radiol 2006;36(8):773–791

Nguyen ML, Jones NF. Undergrowth: brachydactyly. Hand Clin 2009; 25:247–255

O'Connor JF, Cohen J. Dating fractures. In: Kleinman PK, ed. Diagnostic imaging of child abuse. 2nd ed. St. Louis: Mosby, 1998:168–177

Oestreich AE. The lateral clavicle hook-an acquired as well as a congenital anomaly. Pediatr Radiol 1981;11:147–150

Offiah A, van Rijn RR, Perez-Rossello JM, Kleinman PK. Skeletal imaging of child abuse (non-accidental injury). Pediatr Radiol 2009; 39:461–470

OMIM—Online Mendelian Inheritance in Man. Available at http:// www.ncbi.nlm.nih.gov/omim

Olsen OE, Owens CM. Diffuse interstitial lung disease. In Carty H, Brunelle F, Stringer DA, Kao SC-S, eds. Imaging children. Oxford, UK: Churchill Livingstone, 2005:1119–1132

Oner Y, Uzun M, Tokgöz N, Tali ET. Isolated true anterior thoracic meningocele. AJNR Am J Neuroradiol 2004;25(10):1828–1830

Owens CM. Radiology of diffuse interstitial pulmonary disease in children. Eur Radiol 2004;14 Suppl 4:L2–12

Owens CM. Meconium aspiration. In: Donoghue VP, ed. Radiological imaging of the neonatal chest. Berlin: Springer-Verlag Berlin and Heidelberg GmbH & Co, 2007:85–97

Paajanen H, Hermunen H, Karonen J. Pubic magnetic resonance imaging findings in surgically and conservatively treated athletes with osteitis pubis compared to asymptomatic athletes during heavy training. Am J Sports Med 2008;36:117–121

Patel MD, Filly RA. Homozygous achondroplasia: US distinction between homozygous, heterozygous, and unaffected fetuses in the second trimester. Radiology 1995;196:541–545

Pilling DW, Pilling P. The neonatal chest. In Carty H, Brunelle F, Stringer DA, Kao SC-S, eds. Imaging children. Oxford, UK: Churchill Livingstone, 2005:1023–1048

Poznanski AK, Fernbach SK, Berry TE. Bone changes from prostaglandin therapy. Skeletal Radiol 1985;14:20–25

Prosser I, Maguire S, Harrison SK, Mann M, Sibert JR, Kemp AM. How old is this fracture? Radiologic dating of fractures in children: a systematic review. AJR Am J Roentgenol 2005;184:1282–1286

Resnick D, Greenway G. Distal femoral cortical defects, irregularities, and excavations. Radiology 1982;143:345–354

Restrepo CS, Martinez S, Lemos DF, et al. Imaging appearances of the sternum and sternoclavicular joints. Radiographics 2009;29:839–859

Rossi UG, Owens CM. The radiology of chronic lung disease in children. Arch Dis Child 2005;90(6):601–607

Ryan S. Postnatal imaging of chest malformations. In: Donoghue VP, ed. Radiological imaging of the neonatal chest. Berlin: Springer-Verlag Berlin and Heidelberg GmbH & Co, 2007:139–162

Shabshin N, Schweitzer ME, Morrison WB, Carrino JA, Keller MS, Grissom LE. High-signal T2 changes of the bone marrow of the foot and ankle in children: red marrow or traumatic changes? Pediatr Radiol 2006;36:670–676

Simmons BP, Southmayd WW, Riseborough EJ. Congenital radioulnar synostosis. J Hand Surg Am 1983;8:829–838

Slovis TL, Chapman S. Evaluating the data concerning vitamin D insufficiency/deficiency and child abuse. Pediatr Radiol 2008;38:1221–1224

Spranger J. Radiologic nosology of bone dysplasias. Am J Med Genet 1989;34:96–104

Steinberg ME, Steinberg DR. Classification systems for osteonecrosis: an overview. Orthop Clin North Am 2004;35:273–283, vii–viii

Subbarao K. Periosteal reactions in pediatrics. Indian J Pediatr 1987; 54:45–52

Temtamy SA, Aglan MS. Brachydactyly. Orphanet J Rare Dis 2008; 3:15

Ulkü R, Eren N, Cakir O, Balci A, Onat S. Extrapulmonary intrathoracic hydatid cysts. Can J Surg 2004;47(2):95–98

Van Rijn RR, Wilde JC, Bras J, Oldenburger F, McHugh KM, Merks JH. Imaging findings in noncraniofacial childhood rhabdomyosarcoma. Pediatr Radiol 2008;38:617–634

Varich LJ, Laor T, Jaramillo D. Normal maturation of the distal femoral epiphyseal cartilage: age-related changes at MR imaging. Radiology 2000;214:705–709

Wahlgren H, Mortensson W, Eriksson M, Finkel Y, Forsgren M, Leinonen M. Radiological findings in children with acute pneumonia: age more important than infectious agent. Acta Radiol 2005;46(4):431–436

Waters PM, Smith GR, Jaramillo D. Glenohumeral deformity secondary to brachial plexus birth palsy. J Bone Joint Surg Am 1998;80:668–677

Wetherell RG, Amis AA, Heatley FW. Measurement of acetabular erosion. The effect of pelvic rotation on common landmarks. J Bone Joint Surg Br 1989;71:447–451

Whitten CR, Khan S, Munneke GJ, Grubnic S. A diagnostic approach to mediastinal abnormalities. Radiographics 2007;27(3):657–671

Williams HJ, Alton HM. Imaging of paediatric mediastinal abnormalities. Pediatr Respir Rev 2003;4(1):55–66

Wong KS, Chiu CH, Huang YC, Lin TY. Childhood and adolescent tuberculosis in northern Taiwan: an institutional experience during 1994–1999. Acta Paediatr 2001;90:943–947

Worthy SA, Flint JD, Muller NL. Pulmonary complications after bone marrow transplantation: high-resolution CT and pathologic findings. Radiographics 1997;17(6):1359–1371

Yekeler E, Tunaci M, Tunaci A, Dursun M, Acunas G. Frequency of sternal variations and anomalies evaluated by MDCT. AJR Am J Roentgenol 2006;186:956–960

Zook PD, Winter TC 3rd, Nyberg DA. Iliac angle as a marker for Down syndrome in second-trimester fetuses: CT measurements. Radiology 1999;211:447–451

Zubler V, Mengiardi B, Pfirrmann CW, et al. Bone marrow changes on STIR MR images of asymptomatic feet and ankles. Eur Radiol 2007;17:3066–3072

2 The Abdomen and Gastrointestinal Tract

The Gastrointestinal Tract

Esophagus

Stomach

Small Bowel

Duodenum

Ileocecal Area

→

Colon

Peritoneum and Peritoneal Cavity

Abdominal Masses

The Acute Abdomen

The Acute Abdomen in the Neonatal Period

Liver

Differential Diagnosis of Hepatic Diseases

■ Diffuse Parenchymal Disease

Table 2.1 Nonhomogeneous liver parenchyma

Diagnosis	Findings	Comments
Cirrhosis: Regenerative changes in biliary atresia, chronic active hepatitis, cystic fibrosis, hepatic fibrosis, Budd-Chiari syndrome, Alagille syndrome, chronic biliary obstruction—biliary cirrhosis, glycogen storage disease type IV, alpha$_1$-antitrypsin deficiency, Wilson disease, galactosemia, tyrosinemia, etc. ▷ Fig. 2.1 ▷ Fig. 2.2	Cirrhotic liver shows a small right lobe. The caudate lobe and lateral segment of the left lobe are enlarged. The margins of the liver are irregular. Hepatic parenchyma is heterogeneous because of fatty infiltration, fibrosis, and regenerative nodules. The hepatic vessels may be difficult to see because of compression by fibrosis. Findings of portal hypertension are often seen.	Differentiation of regenerative nodules from hepatocellular carcinoma may be difficult by imaging techniques.
Storage diseases	Other viscera are also involved.	Glycogen storage disease, Gaucher disease, mucopolysaccharidoses, tyrosinosis, alpha$_1$-antitrypsin deficiency, Niemann–Pick disease
Malignant diseases: multifocal or diffuse hepatocellular carcinoma, diffuse metastatic disease (neuroblastoma stage 4 and 4S). ▷ Fig. 2.3	Diffuse involvement of the liver in neuroblastoma stage 4 and 4S: "salt and pepper" pattern (good prognosis).	Compression and distortion of normal vascular anatomy.
Acute hepatitis	Nonhomogeneous echo pattern; hepatomegaly; periportal edema with increased periportal echogenicity.	Thickening of gallbladder wall; portal lymphadenopathy.
Chronic granulomatous disease	Multiple, poorly defined hepatic abscesses. Lesions may resolve or calcify with treatment.	Recurrent infections of the lung, bones, lymph nodes, or liver.
Diffuse hemangioma	Near-total replacement of hepatic parenchyma by the tumor. Below the celiac axis, the aorta has a marked decrease in caliber as a result of increased hepatic arterial flow.	In diffuse hemangiomas, cardiac failure secondary to high volume shunting, hypothyroidism, fulminant hepatic failure, abdominal compartment syndrome, and even death may occur.
Irradiated liver	In the chronic stage (after 6 wks), the liver is typically small, contracted, and fibrotic.	
Liver transplantation	A periportal area of low echogenicity (dilatation of lymphatic channels) is often seen after transplantation. On computed tomography (CT) periportal edema is seen as a central or peripheral low-attenuation area and has been called the "periportal collar" sign.	
Chronic congestion in cardiac disease	Ultrasound (US): echogenic liver parenchyma.	The hepatic veins adjacent to the vena cava are often enlarged.
Chemotherapy	US: enlarged liver, echogenic in comparison to the normal renal parenchyma due to steatosis. Differential diagnosis (DD): veno-occlusive disease, excluded by Doppler.	Toxic effect of chemotherapy.

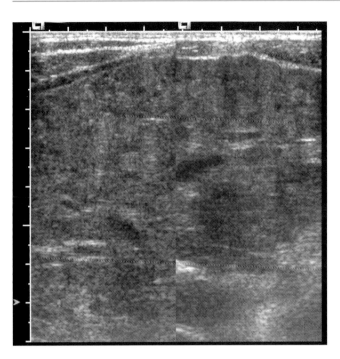

Fig. 2.1 Liver cirrhosis. High-resolution transverse US of the left hepatic lobe. A heterogeneous liver parenchyma with ill-defined hyperechoic nodules is seen in this 13-year-old boy with Wilson disease and portal hypertension.

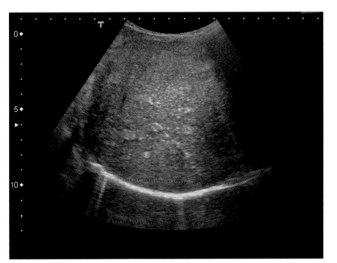

Fig. 2.2 Biliary atresia. Transverse US of the right hepatic lobe. Hepatic parenchyma is heterogeneous with hyperechoic areas related to portal spaces.

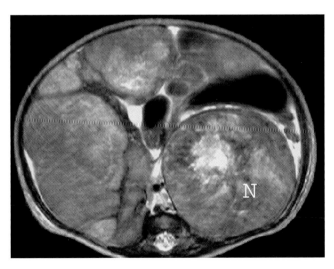

Fig. 2.3 Neuroblastoma metastases (stage 4S). T2-weighted MRI shows confined left primary adrenal neuroblastoma (N) and hepatomegaly with practically complete liver infiltration by metastases.

Table 2.2 Homogeneous liver parenchyma

Diagnosis	Findings	Comments
Diffuse fatty infiltration	US: Increased parenchymal echogenicity. Appreciation and evaluation of the hepatic echotexture is often difficult and operator-dependent. The degree of acoustic attenuation is easier evaluated when comparing the liver to the healthy kidney. An enlarged liver suggests fatty change. Further work-up: magnetic resonance imaging (MRI) in obese patients and biopsy.	Fatty liver in obesity, hyperalimentation with high fat content, hepatitis, long-term steroid therapy, Cushing disease, diabetes mellitus, severe malabsorption, protein-deficiency malnutrition, toxic and drug reactions, hyperlipidemia, familial hyperlipoproteinemia, cystic fibrosis, Reye syndrome, Wilson disease, glycogen storage disease.
Starry sky liver ▷ *Fig. 2.4a, b*	Hyperechoic portal spaces related to diffuse hypoechogenicity.	Related to fasting and/or vomiting; reverses after meals.
Edema in acute hepatitis	Hepatomegaly and lymphatic periportal edema. Progressive gallbladder wall thickening or small amounts of clear fluid in the perihepatic space and in the gallbladder fossa. Frequently enlarged lymph nodes in the hepatic ilium.	
Acute congestion in cardiac disease	US: hypoechoic liver parenchyma.	Dilated hepatic veins.
Iron deposition in the liver	MRI is the best imaging modality. Marked decrease in signal intensity on T2- and T1-weighted images.	Either in the hepatocytes (primary hemochromatosis, cirrhosis) or in the reticuloendothelial cells (hemosiderosis).

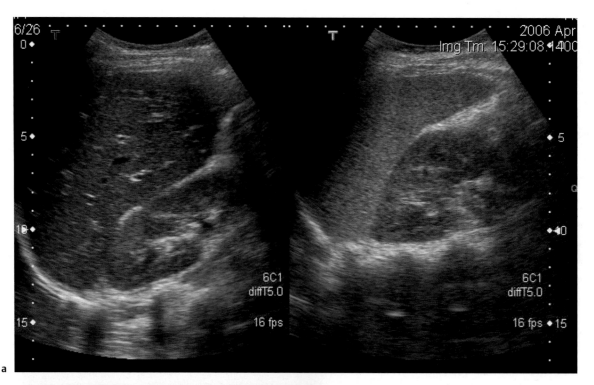

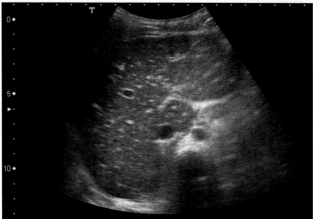

Fig. 2.4a, b Starry-sky liver. (a) US of liver (right) and spleen (left) showing a homogeneous hypoechoic parenchyma with relatively hyperechoic portal spaces. The hypoechogenicity of liver has been related with prolonged fasting and/or vomiting. **(b)** Transverse image of liver.

■ Focal Parenchymal Abnormalities

Table 2.3 Solid heterogeneous lesions

Diagnosis	Findings	Comments
Hepatoblastoma ▷ *Fig. 2.5a–d*	Large, solid mass with cystic areas (hemorrhage). Manganese-enhanced MRI may be used for increasing detection of small satellite lesions and elucidating tumoral or nontumoral thrombus.	Mean age is 0–3 y. Most common primary malignant hepatic tumor (50%). Possible venous involvement (intravascular solid material, venous encasement). Calcifications (40%).
Hepatocellular carcinoma	US: Sometimes thin hypoechoic halo (tumor capsule) and hypoechoic areas secondary to necrosis. Rare calcifications (frequent in fibrolamellar scar). CT or MRI: central scar on fibrolamellar subtype.	Mean age is 12–14 y. Underlying liver disease (50%): tyrosinemia, biliary atresia, familial cholestasis, Alagille syndrome, glycogen storage disease type 1, chronic hepatitis. Growth patterns: solitary, multifocal, or diffuse.

(continues on page 146)

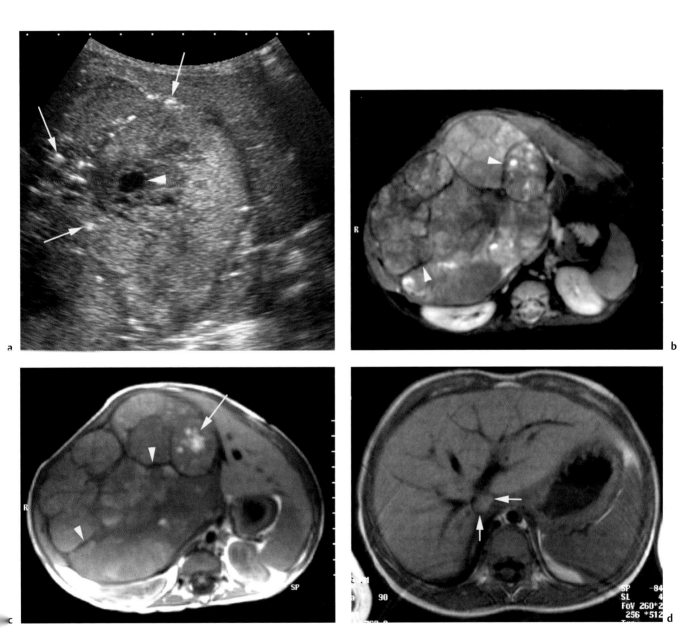

Fig. 2.5a–d Mixed hepatoblastoma. (a) Transverse US shows that calcifications (arrows) and cystic necrotic areas (arrowhead) are dominant features. Axial T2-weighted MRI **(b)** and T1-weighted MRI **(c)** show right lobe and segment 4 mass. Note areas of increased signal intensity: hemorrhage (arrow) and hypointense bands (fibrous septations; arrowheads). **(d)** T1-weighted manganese-enhanced MRI. A 4-year-old boy with resected segment 6 hepatoblastoma. A postoperative inferior vena cava (IVC) thrombus was detected (arrows). Manganese enhancement of the thrombus (equal to liver) confirms its tumoral nature.

Table 2.3 (Cont.) Solid heterogeneous lesions

Diagnosis	Findings	Comments
Undifferentiated embryonal carcinoma ▷ *Fig. 2.6a–c*	Well delineated by a fibrotic pseudocapsule. Multi-septated cystic or inhomogeneous solid appearance. Discordance between US imaging (heterogeneous solid mass) and CT or MRI (cystic appearance due to myxomatous tissue).	Mean age is 8–12 y. Most frequent pediatric hepatic sarcoma, though uncommon (5%).
Angiosarcoma ▷ *Fig. 2.7a, b*	Prominent vascularization. Peripheral or heterogeneous enhancement. Splenic or pulmonary metastases.	Very rare in children (only cases reported).
Lymphoproliferative disorders ▷ *Fig. 2.8a, b* ▷ *Fig. 2.9, p. 148*	Growth patterns: solitary, multifocal, diffuse, perihepatic, or periportal infiltration (rare but characteristic). Hepatomegaly (not necessarily due to lymphomatous infiltration).	Mean age is 2–16 y. Twelve percent of lymphomas affect the liver. Burkitt lymphoma most frequent. Posttransplantation lymphoproliferative disease: Epstein-Barr-virus–related.
Hepatic metastases ▷ *Fig. 2.3, p. 143*	Imaging: depends on some degree on the nature of the primary tumor. Typically multiple and well circumscribed masses.	Mostly Wilms tumor and neuroblastoma (neuroblastoma stage 4 and 4S).

(continues on page 148)

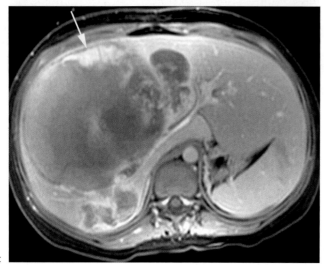
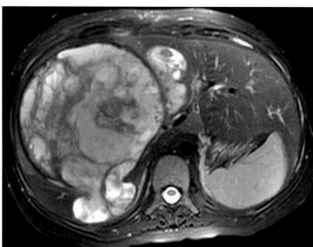
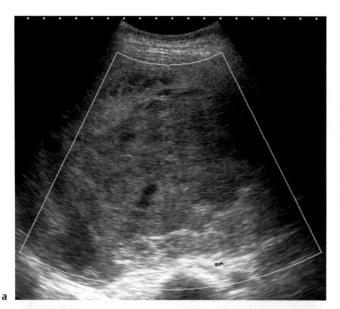

Fig. 2.6a–c Undifferentiated embryonal sarcoma in a 12-year-old boy. (**a**) Doppler US shows avascular, heterogeneous, apparently solid mass. (**b**) T2-weighted MRI shows septated, heterogeneous, but predominately cystic sarcoma. (**c**) Gadolinium-enhanced T1-weighted MRI shows enhancing parietal nodules corresponded to solid portions (arrow).

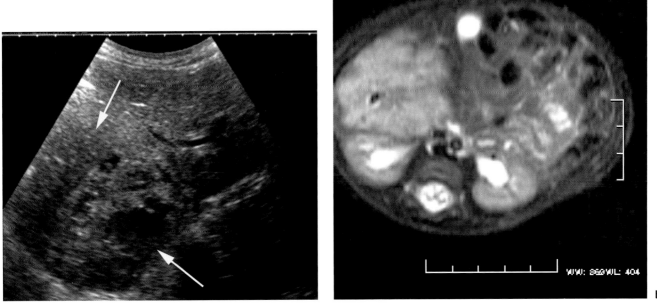

a   b

Fig. 2.7a, b   Angiosarcoma in a 9-year-old boy. (**a**) Transverse US shows poorly defined heterogeneous but mainly hyperechoic lesion (arrows). (**b**) T2-weighted MRI.

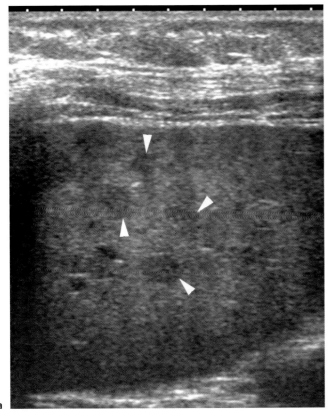

a

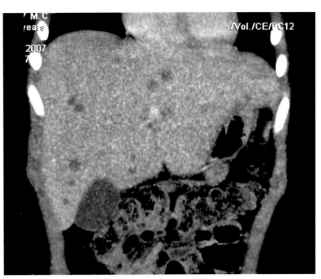

b

Fig. 2.8a, b   Multicentric Burkitt lymphoma in a 10-year-old boy with abdominal pain due to ileocolic intussusception. (**a**) US and (**b**) coronal contrast-enhanced CT show multiple, homogeneous, low echogenicity/attenuation nodules (arrowheads). The presence of hepatic nodules and the patient's age serve to rule out lymphoma.

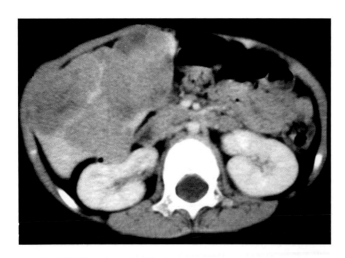

Fig. 2.9 Posttransplantation lymphoproliferative disease. Contrast-enhanced CT shows multinodular, partially enhanced hepatic lymphoma 2 years after liver transplantation in an 8-year-old girl.

Table 2.3 (Cont.) Solid heterogeneous lesions

Diagnosis	Findings	Comments
Hemangioma ▷*Fig. 2.10a–c*	Focal: Hepatic form of the cutaneous rapidly involuting congenital hemangioma (RICH). Fast spontaneous involution. Multiple hepatic lesions (multifocal) or near-total replacement of hepatic parenchyma (diffuse).	Neonates and infants, some diagnosed prenatally. Most common benign pediatric liver tumor (50%). In diffuse hemangiomas, cardiac failure, hypothyroidism, and fulminant hepatic failure may occur. Twenty to forty percent have skin hemangiomas. glucose transporter (GLUT)-1 positive in diffuse forms and GLUT-1 negative in focal forms.
Nodular regenerative hyperplasia	US: multiple nodules of variable size (frequently hyperechoic). MRI: manganese enhancement (regenerative hepatocytes uptake manganese). Absence of fibrous septa.	Associations: portal low flow conditions (Abernethy malformation, Budd-Chiari syndrome, postchemotherapy, collagen vascular diseases, hematologic disorders).
Focal nodular hyperplasia ▷*Fig. 2.11a, b*	US: mass with echogenicity similar to the liver. Central scar in 33% of the cases. T2 with ferumoxide: lesion decreased signal except scar, manganese-enhancement.	Unusual, 5% of all benign hepatic tumors. Associations: type I and type VI glycogen storage disease, Hurler syndrome, galactosemia.
Hepatic adenoma	Imaging depends on the attenuation of the surrounding liver. Low attenuation (fat, old hemorrhage) or high attenuation (recent hemorrhage, glycogen, surrounding fatty liver). No uptake of superparamagnetic iron oxide particles.	Associations: intake of androgens, type I glycogen storage disease, human immunodeficiency virus infection, and oral contraceptives.
Pyogenic abscess ▷*Fig. 2.12a, b, p. 150*	Complex mass with internal debris, air-fluid, or debris-fluid levels. Increased peripheric vascularization.	*Staphylococcus aureus*. Presentation: abdominal pain, fever, septicemia.
Amebic abscess	Chocolate-like content with leukocytes or amebae (may only be seen in abscess wall). Peripherally located (near or in contact to Glisson capsule). Peripheral "halo." Doppler: no prominent peripheral vascularization (differential finding compared to pyogenic abscess).	In 3%–7% of patients with *Entamoeba histolytica* infection. More frequent in patients younger than 3 y.
Hepatosplenic candidiasis ▷*Fig. 2.13, p. 150*	US: "wheel-within-a-wheel," "bull's eye," or hypoechoic multiple nodules.	*Candida albicans* is the most frequent pathogen. In immunocompromised patients (prolonged neutropenia).
Liver infarct	In acute phase, solid, hypoechoic lesions, mainly in the periphery of the liver.	Posttraumatic, after partial resection, or in liver transplant after an acute ischemic episode (hepatic artery stenosis or thrombosis).
Cat-scratch disease	Granulomas either resolve or calcify.	Hepatic and splenic granulomas.
Lipomatous lesions: focal fatty liver, lipoma, angiomyolipoma ▷*Fig. 2.14, p. 150* ▷*Fig. 2.15, p. 151*	Imaging: hyperechoic on US, homogenous low-attenuation lesion (less than −20 Hounsfield units [HU]) on CT, and high signal intensity on in-phase, drop in signal intensity on out-phase T1-weighted and iso- or hyperintense on T2-weighted MRI.	Rare in children.

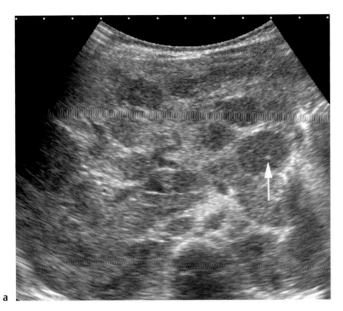

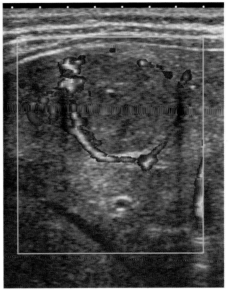

Fig. 2.10a–c   Multiple hemangiomas. (a) Transverse US shows multiple hypoechoic lesions, with central echoes, corresponding to vessels (arrow). **(b)** Doppler US shows vascular rim along the edges of the tumor, with little flow within the tumor itself. **(c)** Early postcontrast CT: peripheral enhancement of multiple diffusely distributed nodules.

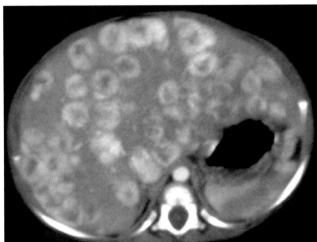

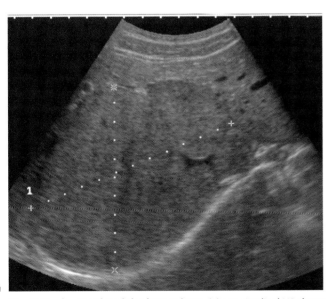

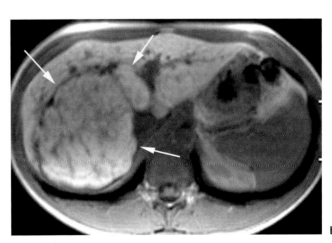

Fig. 2.11a, b   Focal nodular hyperplasia. (a) Longitudinal US shows well-defined, practically isoechoic in the right lobe of the liver (cursors). **(b)** Manganese-enhanced T1-weighted MRI shows lesion (arrows) enhancement (similar to the liver parenchyma) demonstrating hepatocellular origin.

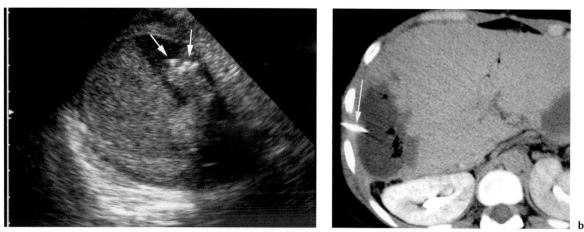

a   b

Fig. 2.12a, b   Pyogenic abscess in a 6-year-old with liver transplantation. (**a**) US: heterogeneous, encapsulated fluid collection containing gas (arrows). (**b**) Contrast-enhanced CT obtained during percutaneous drainage (arrow) confirmed collection was an abscess.

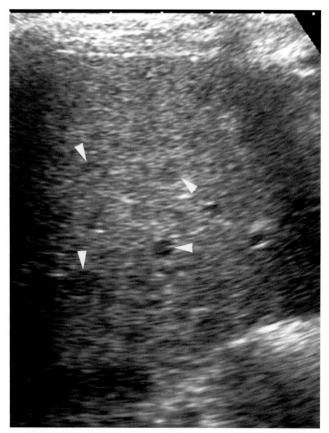

Fig. 2.13   Hepatosplenic candidiasis in a 3-year-old with acute lymphoblastic leukemia and neutropenia. US scan shows multiple hypoechoic hepatic nodules (arrowheads; most frequent US pattern).

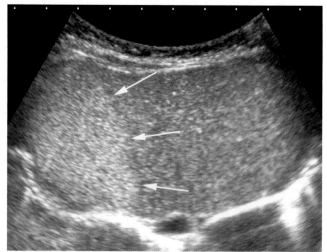

Fig. 2.14   Focal fatty liver. Transverse US shows well-marginated hyperechogenicity of liver parenchyma that affects lateral right hepatic segments (arrows), with the rest of the liver preserved.

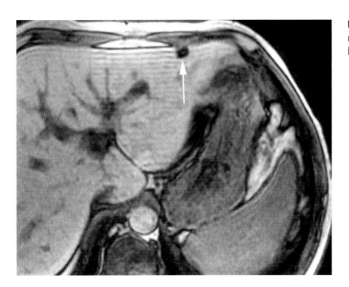

Fig. 2.15 Angiomyolipoma in a 17-year-old girl with tuberous sclerosis. T1-weighted in-phase MRI shows small hyperintense lesion in the left lateral segment (arrow).

Table 2.4 Cystic lesions

Diagnosis	Findings	Comments
Normal variants: loops of small bowel in the porta hepatis, caudate lobe, Riedel lobe	If a loop of bowel is suspected in the porta hepatis, US must be performed. In case of doubt, CT after oral contrast administration may be necessary.	
Echinococcal cysts ▷ *Fig. 2.16a, b, p. 152*	Unilocular or multilocular well-defined cystic lesions. Calcification in cyst wall or complete calcium replacement. Internal debris (hydatid sand), daughter cysts, undulating membrane (water-lily sign).	Liver is the most commonly involved organ (75%–80%) in echinococcosis. Possible superinfection and anaphylaxis secondary to rupture.
Ciliated hepatic foregut cysts ▷ *Fig. 2.17a–c, p. 152*	Well-delineated small cyst anechoic or with fine echoes (due to mucoid content) on US and hypoattenuating or isoattenuating relative to surrounding liver parenchyma on CT. MRI: hyperintense on T2-weighted, variable on T1-weighted (due to variable content).	Solitary cyst. Congenital (embryonic foregut remnant in the liver). Often < 3 cm and located in segment 4. Rarely, malignant transformation through squamous metaplasia.
Benign cystic tumors (multiple cysts): mesenchymal hamartoma	Multiseptated cystic mass, although a single dominant cyst may be seen. Echogenic material within the cyst fluid secondary to blood. Doppler: avascular. On MRI, signal intensity may vary depending on stromal, protein, or hemorrhage contents.	Patients under 2 y. Hamartoma is the second most common benign hepatic tumor (22%). Predominantly located in the right hepatic lobe.
Posttraumatic hematomas or bilomas	Intrahepatic bilomas usually present on US or CT as intrahepatic peripheral cystic lesions that communicate with the bile duct.	Image-guided aspiration of a fluid collection can be necessary to determine composition.
Mucocele	On US, mucoceles appear as cystic masses near the porta hepatis. These abnormalities are readily seen as cystic structures on MR cholangiography.	Cystic duct remnant mucocele is an uncommon complication of liver transplant that occurs when the donor cystic duct remnant becomes distended with mucus.
Post-Kasai procedure (hepatojejunostomy)	The jejunal loop is anastomosed with the bile ducts in the porta hepatis. The anastomosis may appear cystic.	
Choledochal cysts	Hepatobiliary. US and radionuclide studies usually suggest the correct diagnosis, which can be confirmed by MR cholangiography. Frequently, the intrahepatic ducts are normal. Sludge or stones may be identified within the dilated ducts.	The most common form (80%–90% of cases) is Todani type I (dilatation of the common bile duct). A characteristic triad of abdominal pain, obstructive jaundice, and fever is only seen in a minority of patients.
Caroli disease	Recognition of the connection of the ectatic ducts with one another and with the rest of the ductal system is critical in distinguishing Caroli disease from polycystic liver disease. Central dot sign.	Represents segmental or diffuse nonobstructive dilatation of the intrahepatic ducts.
Polycystic liver disease	Hepatobiliary cysts may be intrahepatic or peribiliary. Occasionally, echogenic debris can be seen if hemorrhage has occurred.	
Posttraumatic cysts and posthepatic infarct cysts (liver transplant)	In late phase posthepatic infarct, cystic image is similar to posttraumatic or echinococcal cysts, mainly in the periphery of the liver. Usually after hepatic artery stenosis or thrombosis in transplanted liver.	In posttraumatic cysts, the clinical history of trauma is the diagnostic key.

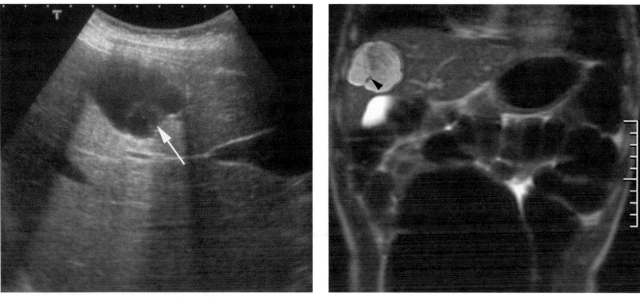

Fig. 2.16a, b   Echinococcosis. (**a**) Longitudinal oblique US: single lobular cystic lesion with thin wall, through transmission, and internal daughter cysts (type II) (arrow). (**b**) Coronal T2-weighted MRI: hyperintense cysts with internal septa (arrowhead).

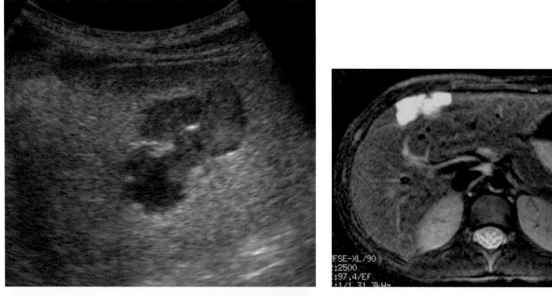

Fig. 2.17a–c   Ciliated foregut cyst in a 7-year-old girl. (**a**) Transverse US shows irregular, lobulated lesions, with fine internal echoes that increased through transmission. (**b**) T2-weighted MRI shows hyperintense lobular lesions in segment 4. (**c**) T1-weighted MRI demonstrates high signal intensity content within the lesion (asterisks), corresponding to mucoid material.

Table 2.5   Liver calcifications

Diagnosis	Findings	Comments
Metastases after chemotherapy		Neuroblastoma lesions may have calcifications, especially postchemotherapy.
Hepatic tumors: hepatoblastoma, hepatocellular carcinoma, hemangiomas, focal nodular hyperplasia		Hepatoblastoma: more evident in mixed type after chemotherapy. Hepatocellular carcinoma: calcifications frequent in fibrolamellar scar. Hemangiomas: calcifications with involution. Nodular regenerative hyperplasia: calcification is seen in only 1% of patients.
Granulomas	After acute disease, abscesses finally resolve into a calcified granuloma.	In infectious diseases.
Echinococcal cysts	Calcification in cyst wall or complete calcium replacement.	
Postinfarct calcifications		After partial hepatic resection or in liver transplant after an ischemic episode (hepatic artery thrombosis or stenosis). The larger areas of infarction may occasionally calcify.
Portal venous system or umbilical veins		In preterm infants.
Calcified hematoma (sequela of biopsy or trauma)		Calcification in the site of biopsy.

Portal Venous System and Hepatic Veins

Table 2.6   Abnormal porta hepatis

Diagnosis	Findings	Comments
Pseudotumor caused by bowel loops	US: multiple attempts at visualization and peristalsis usually suffice.	Repeat examination after fluid administration is useful. CT with oral contrast is rarely necessary.
Periportal lymphadenopathy	Multiple solid nodes of different sizes, sometimes with central vascularization.	Burkitt lymphoma is the most frequent cause.
Cavernous transformation of the portal vein ▷ Fig. 2.18, p. 154	Best demonstrated by color Doppler US and MR angiography. US shows a mass of tubular structures, within or around a previously thrombosed portal vein. Doppler US: the porta is replaced by a tangle of venous collaterals at the hepatic hilum whose purpose is to link the extrahepatic portal circulation and the intrahepatic portal branches.	
Extrahepatic and intrahepatic portal vein thrombosis	US: Direct visualization of the thrombus is rare in children. The portal vein usually appears normal or the portal lumen is absent. Doppler is essential as it demonstrates absence of blood flow. Occasionally, there can be total absence of flow in the hepatic hilum, with reversed portal flow in peripheral intrahepatic branches (spontaneous arterioportal shunts). Chronic thrombosis leads to cavernomatous transformation of the portal vein.	Causes: portal vein thrombosis (perinatal omphalitis or umbilical venous catheterization, sepsis, appendicitis, acute dehydration, coagulopathies, splenectomy, hepatic transplantation, cirrhosis related to biliary atresia, congenital hepatic fibrosis). Portal vein thrombosis leads to portal hypertension, manifested by the presence of collateral circulation, possible recanalization of the periumbilical veins, less omental thickening, or splenomegaly.

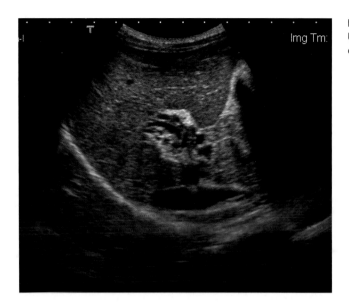

Fig. 2.18 Cavernous transformation of the portal vein. Oblique US through the hepatic hilum shows multiple tubular structures without evidence of normal portal vein.

Table 2.7 Abnormal periportal spaces

Diagnosis	Findings	Comments
Posttraumatic		A harbinger of other injury in the peritoneal cavity.
Post liver transplant		Due to lymphatic stasis.
Leukemia and lymphoma	US: Markedly enlarged and echogenic liver. Widened periportal areas, predominantly hypoechoic.	Periportal tumoral infiltration.
Cirrhosis	Bandlike echogenic, periportal areas. A rare finding in cirrhosis.	
Fatty liver	Echogenic changes in the periportal regions seen in marked obesity.	
Periportal fibrosis		Sequela of previous disease, including cytomegalovirus hepatitis, alpha$_1$-antitrypsin deficiency, post liver transplant, vascular abnormalities.
Niemann-Pick disease		Histological diagnosis: deposition of sphingomyelin.

■ Bile Ducts and Gallbladder

Ultrasound (US) is the imaging modality of choice for screening the gallbladder and biliary tract in children. The study should consist of a systematic examination of the liver, bile ducts, gallbladder, pancreas, and spleen. A complete duplex and color Doppler examination of the hepatic vessels should be performed. US guidance is very useful to guide invasive diagnostic or therapeutic procedures.

Magnetic resonance cholangiopancreatography (MRCP) is also a noninvasive, nonradiating technique; in young children, MRCP needs to be performed under sedation. MRCP uses the signal from the bile within the ducts to allow visualization of the biliary system. Fasting is necessary. The basic principle is to use a heavily T2-weighted sequence with fat suppression to show the high signal intensity of the static fluids. MRCP has the potential to replace diagnostic endoscopic retrograde pancreatography (ERCP) and percutaneous transhepatic cholangiography. A normal study obviates the need for more invasive studies.

Computed tomography (CT) has very few indications because of the use of radiation and, frequently, intravenous contrast. CT is useful in differentiating aerobilia from calculus. Multidetector equipment allows fast scans and three-dimensional (3D) reconstruction of very good quality even in non–breath-holding children.

ERCP is invasive and technically difficult. It requires general anesthesia in children and has the potential for significant associated morbidity. However, it is a useful diagnostic and therapeutic tool in selected cases.

Hepatobiliary scintigraphy is an isotopic study that uses technetium (99mTc)-labeled iminodiacetic acid that is extracted and secreted by the liver. Scintigraphic visualization of tracer in the gastrointestinal (GI) tract indicates patency of the extra hepatic biliary ducts. It is useful to demonstrate bile leakage after surgery and for diagnosing of biliary atresia.

Bile Ducts

Table 2.8 Dilated bile ducts

Diagnosis	Findings	Comments
Caroli disease ▷ *Fig. 2.19*	US findings: dilated, ectatic bile ducts, "intraluminal portal vein" or "central dot" sign with flow on Doppler, biliary sludge and calculi, enlarged gallbladder and common bile duct, abscesses, and associated renal anomalies. Recognition of the connection of the ectatic ducts with one another and with the rest of the ductal system is critical (DD between Caroli disease and polycystic disease).	Segmental nonobstructive dilatation of the intrahepatic bile ducts. Ductal plate malformation spectrum. It is associated with hepatic fibrosis, choledochal cyst, medullary sponge kidney, infantile polycystic renal disease, or nephronophthisis.
Ascending cholangitis		Associated with biliary obstruction whether congenital or acquired. Appropriate therapy has to be directed to the underlying cause.
Sclerosing cholangitis	Strictures in multiple segments of the bile ducts with intervening dilated segments. Amputation of some segmental bile ducts is common. MRCP is the first imaging modality (demonstrates the typical abnormalities with high specificity).	Inflammatory obliterative fibrosis affecting the intra- and extrahepatic biliary tree. Poor prognosis with progressive evolution to biliary cirrhosis.
Choledochal cyst ▷ *Fig. 2.20, p. 156*	US: Cystic dilatation of the common bile duct often associated with hepatic bile duct dilatation. (This affects the main left and right hepatic ducts but not the smaller ducts.) MRCP provides the anatomic map of the pancreaticobiliary ductal union and also of the biliary tree, which are critical for surgery.	Congenital. Most frequent cause of extrahepatic cholestasis in childhood.
Bile plug syndrome		Sludge in the bile ducts and gallbladder forms plugs and may cause transient gallbladder and duct dilatation in the neonatal period.
Choledocholithiasis ▷ *Fig. 2.21a, b, p. 156* ▷ *Fig. 2.22a, b, p. 156*	US: echogenic material within the dilated duct with associated acoustic shadowing.	Most frequent cause of biliary obstruction.
Biliary obstruction without calculi	DD with cavenous transformation of the portal vein by Doppler US.	Caused by biliary tumors (rhabdomyosarcoma of the biliary tree), inspissated bile, pancreatitis, congenital biliary stenosis.
Biliary obstruction in liver transplantation	US: dilated intrahepatic ducts with dilatation of the proximal common bile duct to the level of the surgical anastomosis MR cholangiography can be used to delineate the anatomy and morphology of bile ducts and to search for biliary strictures.	Children with reduced-size transplantation have a higher risk. Most anastomotic strictures are secondary to scar tissue causing retraction and narrowing of the common bile duct at the suture site, although ischemia may also be a factor. Segmental saccular dilatations in transplanted livers are mostly secondary to arterial thrombosis or stenosis.

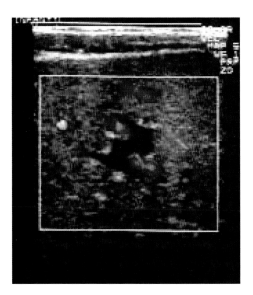

Fig. 2.19 Caroli disease. Doppler US of the liver shows an avascular cysticlike structure with surrounding portal vessels that correspond to an intrahepatic biliary duct.

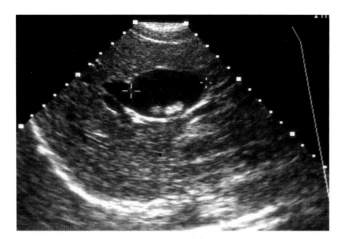

Fig. 2.20 Choledochal cyst. Transverse US image depicts a cystic dilatation of the common biliary duct at the hepatic hilum (between calipers) with lithiasis inside the lumen.

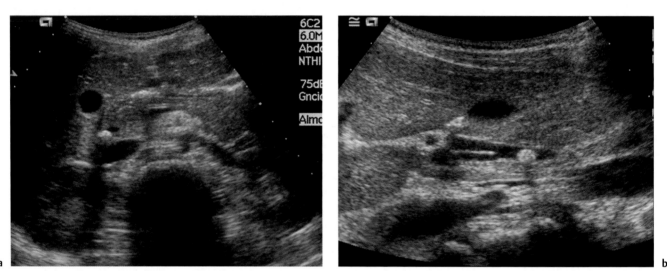

a   b

Fig. 2.21a, b Choledocholithiasis. (a) Transverse and **(b)** longitudinal US scans showing a hyperechoic biliary stone with posterior shadowing located in the common bile duct. The cystic duct is also dilated in the longitudinal image.

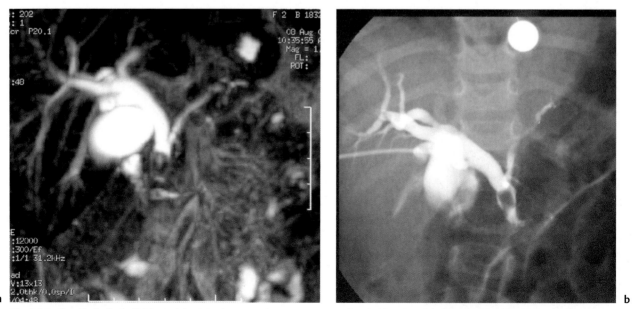

a   b

Fig. 2.22a, b Choledocholithiasis. (a) MRCP shows an obstructing material in the distal common bile duct and the biliary and pancreatic ducts dilatation. **(b)** Percutaneous cholecystography also demonstrates the stone producing the bile duct dilatation.

Table 2.9   Abnormal nondilated bile ducts

Diagnosis	Findings	Comments
Aerobilia	DD: portal venous air in necrotizing enterocolitis. Abdominal radiographs and Doppler US are the best imaging modalities for diagnosing aerobilia.	After biliary tract surgery or manipulation, as well with incompetent ampulla of Vater; in biliary atresia, after Kasai procedure; in reduced-size liver transplant (choledochojejunostomy).
Sclerosing cholangitis	Irregular segmentary narrowing of the bile ducts with cholestasis. Secondary pancreatitis may occur. Diagnosis is made on liver biopsy.	Associated with ulcerative colitis, Crohn disease, autoimmune hepatitis, or idiopathic causes.
Bile duct tumors		Papilloma and adenoma.

Gallbladder

Table 2.10   The enlarged gallbladder

Diagnosis	Findings	Comments
Gallbladder hydrops	US: transducer compression over the distended gallbladder causes pain. Marked dilatation of the gallbladder (sonographic Murphy sign) with usually normal wall thickness and a biconvex appearance on longitudinal scans. Sludge is seen in some cases. Spontaneous regression is common.	Acute gallbladder distension without any mechanical cystic duct obstruction. Causes: long-term bowel rest or parenteral hyperalimentation, sepsis, cholecystitis, hepatitis, Wilson disease, Kawasaki syndrome, familial Mediterranean fever, scarlet fever, leptospirosis, ascaris, typhoid fever.
Cystic duct obstruction	Visualization of cause is the clue to diagnosis.	Due to calculi, biliary sludge, large lymph nodes, choledochal cyst, sclerosing cholangitis, parasites in the common bile duct.
Kawasaki syndrome (mucocutaneous lymph node syndrome)		Classic: hydropic gallbladder, fever, coronary aneurysms, mucosal changes, lymphadenopathy.
Cystic gallbladder		Congenital. The gallbladder appears to contain numerous septa.
Bile plug syndrome		Rare cause of perinatal jaundice in which sludge in the bile ducts and gallbladder forms plugs and may cause transient gallbladder hydrops and duct dilatation.
Post abdominal trauma		Transitory.
Acalculous or calculous acute cholecystitis		(see **Table 2.12**)

Table 2.11   The small gallbladder

Diagnosis	Findings	Comments
Normal finding		Postprandial.
Extrahepatic biliary atresia	US: absent gallbladder or < 2 cm in longitudinal diameter. Hepatobiliary scintigraphy is usually required to differentiate between neonatal hepatitis and biliary atresia.	In most patients, the gallbladder cannot be visualized. In about one-fifth of cases, however, it may appear smaller than expected in a fasting infant. There is no postprandial contraction. Surgery: Kasai procedure.
Cystic fibrosis		Gallbladder hypoplastic because of tenacious, inspissated bile.
Intrahepatic biliary atresia with normal extrahepatic bile ducts	DD with extrahepatic biliary atresia by MR cholangiography. In extrahepatic atresia, there is no common bile duct.	
Cirrhosis		The gallbladder may be small, not seen, or have stones, depending on the primary disease leading to the cirrhosis.

Table 2.12 Generalized thickened gallbladder wall

Diagnosis	Findings	Comments
Acute cholecystitis ▷ *Fig. 2.23*	US findings: distended gallbladder. Gallbladder thickened wall < 3 mm with hypoechoic halo due to edema. Localized tenderness (sonographic Murphy sign) and pericholecystic fluid. Gallbladder wall thickened. In acute calculous cholecystitis, the calculi are present in the gallbladder. Irregularity of the gallbladder wall may suggest gangrenous changes.	Acalculous or calculous. Conditions predisposing to acalculous cholecystitis: recent surgery, sepsis, burns, and debilitation.
Chronic cholecystitis	US: may be normal or show sludge, gallstones, or a thickened gallbladder wall.	Usually results from chronic irritation of the gallbladder secondary to gallstones or cystic fibrosis and rarely by recurrent attacks of acute cholecystitis.
Gallbladder empyema	US: irregular thickening of the gallbladder wall, which may contain small air collections. Multiple intraluminal echoes within the gallbladder.	
Conditions unrelated to gallbladder disease	DD at US: In all these conditions, there is wall thickening but a sonolucent rim or halo around the gallbladder has been reported only in acute cholecystitis. DD by Doppler US: in acute cholecystitis there is an increase in blood vessels of the gallbladder wall not seen in noninflammatory diseases.	Ascites, viral hepatitis, portal hypertension, severe hypoalbuminemia, congestive heart failure, partial emptying of the gallbladder.

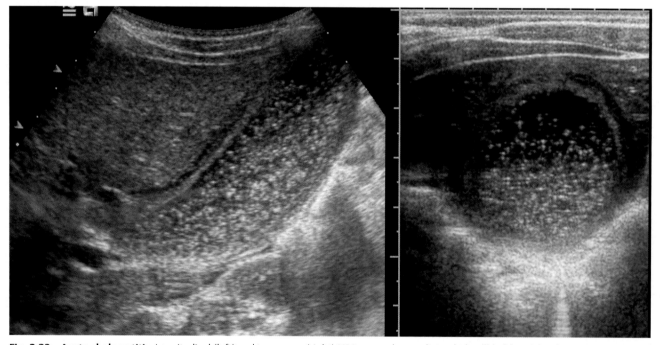

Fig. 2.23 Acute cholecystitis. Longitudinal (left) and transverse (right) US images show a distended gallbladder with echogenic content and thickened wall.

Table 2.13   Localized thickened gallbladder wall

Diagnosis	Findings	Comments
Adenomyomatosis	US: diffuse or segmental thickening of the gallbladder wall and intramural diverticula. Diverticula that contain bile appear anechoic, and diverticula that are small or contain sludge appear echogenic.	Represents proliferation of the gallbladder epithelium surface with glandular formation and Rokitansky-Aschoff sinuses.
Cholesterolosis	US: single or multiple adherent nonshadowing echogenic masses, protruding into the gallbladder lumen. DD: adenomas, papillomas, inflammatory polyps, mucus retention cysts, heterotopic pancreatic and gastric tissue, and carcinomas.	Abnormal accumulations of triglycerides and cholesterol esters in the lamina propria of the gallbladder wall.
Polyp, heterotopic pancreatic of gastric tissue, gallbladder neoplasia	A fixed lesion on multiple projections.	

Table 2.14   Solid-content gallbladder

Diagnosis	Findings	Comments
Cholelithiasis ▷ Fig. 2.24	The diagnosis is made by US: mobile, echogenic foci with acoustic shadowing inside the gallbladder.	Usually asymptomatic. Pain in the right upper quadrant (RUQ) and jaundice indicate migration into the common bile duct.
Bile sludge	US: Nonshadowing low-to-medium level echoes that layer in the dependent part of the gallbladder lumen. Because of its viscous nature, the fluid-fluid level produced by the sludge moves slowly with changes in patient position.	Presence of calcium bilirubinate granules within the bile. Secondary to bile stasis (obstruction at the gallbladder neck) or following a prolonged fast or after hyperalimentation.
Limey bile	Bile debris in the gallbladder that is dense enough to cause attenuation of X-ray. It is usually seen as a high attenuation fluid in the gallbladder on CT.	Due to bile stasis.
Porcelain gallbladder	The gallbladder wall calcifies and is seen on abdominal radiograph as an opacity to the RUQ.	Due to chronic, low-grade inflammation.

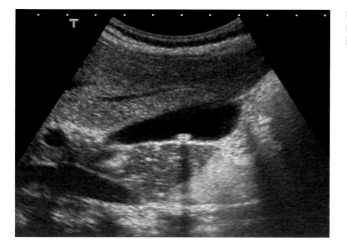

Fig. 2.24   Cholelithiasis. Longitudinal US image depicts a mobile hyperechoic gallstone with posterior acoustic shadowing in the gallbladder lumen.

Pancreas

Differential Diagnosis of Pancreatic Diseases

Sonography is the modality of choice for the initial evaluation of suspected pancreatic disease in children because ionizing radiation is not involved and sedation is not required. Pancreatic magnetic resonance imaging (MRI) is indicated after suboptimal or equivocal US findings and a high clinical suspicion of pancreatic pathology. Although not recommended as the initial routine imaging study for the pancreas, CT is useful when sonographic findings are not diagnostic, the MRI is not available, and, also, for guidance of diagnostic and therapeutic procedures (aspiration biopsy, drainage, etc.).

■ Diffuse Pancreatic Involvement

Table 2.15 Normal-sized pancreas

Diagnosis	Findings	Comments
Preterm or term healthy newborn	The echogenicity of the pancreas in most cases is similar to that of the liver, although it can be less or more echogenic in premature and term newborns during the first 4 wk of life.	
Cystic fibrosis		In first stages, when complete pancreatic replacement by fat without fibrosis is visualized.
Shwachman-Diamond syndrome ▷ Fig. 2.25	On US, the pancreas is hyperechoic (echogenicity similar to that of the retroperitoneal fat) but unchanged in size.	Exocrine pancreatic insufficiency that leads to malabsorption, with normal results on the sweat test, short stature, and bone marrow dysfunction. The characteristic pathologic finding is fatty infiltration of the pancreas
Johanson-Blizzard syndrome	The pancreas can show complete fatty replacement similar to Shwachman-Diamond syndrome.	Associated anomalies: nasal alar hypoplasia, hypothyroidism, congenital deafness, absent permanent teeth, midline ectodermal scalp defects, mental retardation, and urogenital anomalies.
Acute pancreatitis		A normal pancreas does not exclude pancreatitis.
Fatty infiltration: obesity, Cushing disease, long-term treatment with corticosteroids, cytostatics, parenteral nutrition	US: hyperechoic pancreas with normal size. CT: low-attenuation tissue interposed between normal pancreatic parenchyma. On MRI, the fatty infiltrated pancreas has a signal intensity higher than the normal pancreas on in-phase T1-weighted images and loss of signal intensity on opposed-phase T1-weighted images.	The pancreatic body and tail are the dominant areas of fatty replacement.
Other storage diseases (hemosiderosis)	Similar to fatty infiltration. MRI: loss of signal intensity related to normal pancreas on gradient-echo T2-weighted sequences.	Structural change due to hemosiderin deposition.

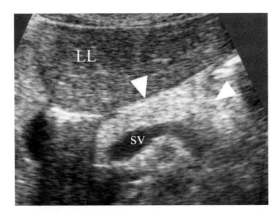

Fig. 2.25 Shwachman-Diamond syndrome. Transverse sonogram shows a pancreas of normal size with increased echogenicity similar to that of the retroperitoneal fat (arrowheads).
LL Left lobe of the liver
sv Splenic vein

Table 2.16   Enlarged pancreas

Diagnosis	Findings	Comments
Normal variant		Can be focal or diffuse.
Acute pancreatitis ▷ *Fig. 2.26*	The most common US finding is diffuse/focal glandular enlargement and decreased echogenicity with poorly defined borders. CT shows diffuse pancreatic enlargement, heterogeneous attenuation (there is a striking decrease or total lack of enhancement, related to the development of pancreatic zones of ischemia and necrosis), a poorly defined pancreatic contour, and peripancreatic fluid, that are most commonly found in the anterior pararenal space and lesser sac. More than a third of patients with acute pancreatitis have an initially normal CT.	Clinical entity caused by a wide variety of etiological agents: viral infections, drugs, and hereditary abnormalities. Trauma is the most common cause in children.
Infiltration in malignant diseases (Burkitt lymphoma, leukemia) ▷ *Fig. 2.27*	Diffuse pancreatic enlargement is the second pattern in frequency (15%–44% of cases). Pancreatic contour may be smooth or lobulated. The next most frequent US pattern is diffuse in almost all cases, other abdominal organ involvement is present: lymphadenopathies, bowel wall mass, and/or visceral tumoral infiltration (kidneys, liver, etc.).	Non-Hodgkin lymphoma is the most frequent tumoral pancreatic disease in children, involving the pancreas secondarily in approximately 30% of patients with widespread disease.
Metabolic diseases		Hyperlipidemia, hyperparathyroidism.

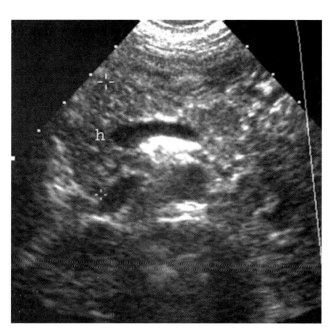

Fig. 2.26   Acute pancreatitis. Focal acute pancreatitis in a 3-year-old girl with acute abdominal trauma. Sonogram shows a pancreatic head (h, between calipers) of increased size and normal hypoechogenicity.

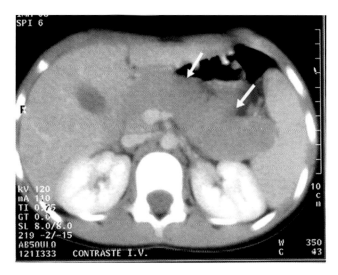

Fig. 2.27   Burkitt lymphoma. A diffuse pancreatic involvement in Burkitt lymphoma. CT image shows homogeneously increased size of the pancreas (arrows).

Table 2.17   Reduced-size pancreas

Diagnosis	Findings	Comments
Cystic fibrosis ▷ *Fig. 2.28*	The classic sonographic findings are an increase in the echogenicity and a decrease in pancreatic size with the typical fine-lobular (cobblestone-like) normal echo pattern of the pancreas no longer detectable. Complete pancreatic atrophy without any fatty replacement can also be found. In those cases, the pancreas shows a decreased size with normal echogenicity. On MRI: soft-tissue attenuation without scattered areas of fat attenuation or high signal intensity. Calcifications and multiple cysts within the pancreas can also be found.	The most significant autosomal recessive pancreatic disorder in the Caucasian white population.
Chronic pancreatitis ▷ *Fig. 2.29* ▷ *Fig. 2.30a, b*	US: parenchymal atrophy with increased echogenicity, calcifications, ductal dilatation, irregular pancreatic outline, and pseudocysts. CT: intraductal calcifications that may be scattered or clustered, focal or diffuse, have parenchymal atrophy, and have both main pancreatic and biliary ductal dilatation. MR: decreased signal intensity on T1-weighted images, decreased heterogeneous enhancement on postgadolinium images, atrophy of the gland, and irregular dilatation of the pancreatic duct.	Chronic inflammatory process with irreversible exocrine and endocrine dysfunction. Hereditary pancreatitis is the most frequent cause of chronic pancreatitis in children.
Familial hereditary pancreatitis		Autosomal dominant disorder with variable penetrance. Usually by 11 y of age. There is a long-term risk present for pancreatic cancer (20%).

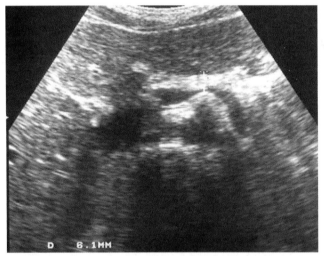

Fig. 2.28   Cystic fibrosis. Sonogram shows an echogenic pancreas of reduced thickness.

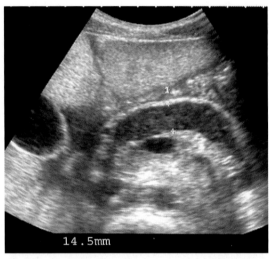

Fig. 2.29   Chronic pancreatitis. Transverse sonogram through the pancreas demonstrates a small, hyperechoic pancreas and dilatation of the main pancreatic duct (between calipers: 1 = 14.5 mm).

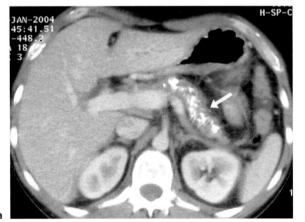
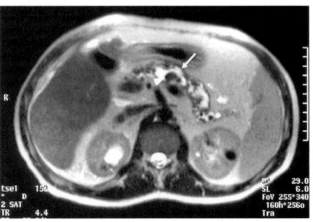

Fig. 2.30a, b   Chronic pancreatitis. (a) CT shows multiple calcifications in the pancreatic body and tail (arrow). **(b)** Axial T2-weighted half-Fourier acquisition single-shot turbo spin echo (HASTE) MRI shows a dilated main pancreatic duct and side branches (arrows) and a calculus in the pancreatic duct (arrowhead).

■ Focal Pancreatic Involvement

Table 2.18   Cystic lesions

Diagnosis	Findings	Comments
Congenital cyst ▷ *Fig. 2.31*	Rounded uni- or multilocular fluid-filled collections, generally located in pancreatic tail.	A true pancreatic cyst is lined by epithelium, as opposed to a pseudocyst, which has only a fibrous wall. May be single or multiple. May appear isolated or in association with systemic diseases (von Hippel-Lindau syndrome, autosomal dominant polycystic kidney disease).
Pseudocysts ▷ *Fig. 2.32* ▷ *Fig. 2.33a, b, p. 164*	On US, appear as anechoic structures with well-defined borders and posterior reinforcement. On CT, they are round or oval and have a thin capsule and fluid content of < 15 HU; the capsule can later calcify. Higher attenuation values > 40 to 50 HU are indicative of intracystic hemorrhage. MRI: usually homogeneous, and of water-signal intensity on T1-weighted and T2-weighted images.	The most usual type of pancreatic cysts. The most common complication of the acute pancreatitis. May be intrapancreatic or extrapancreatic (usually in the lesser sac). Diagnosis requires at least 4 wk waiting following an episode of acute pancreatitis.
Pseudoaneurysm of the splenic artery	US: rounded cystic lesion. Doppler US: confirms vascular origin of mass.	Suspected pseudoaneurysm after pancreatitis may be noted on Doppler US.
Pancreatic cystosis (cystic fibrosis) ▷ *Fig. 2.34a, b, p. 164*	Rarely in cystic fibrosis, aggregates of cysts up to several centimeters replace the pancreas. This condition has been called pancreatic cystosis. US, CT, and MRI: complete replacement of the pancreas by uni- or multiloculated cystic masses.	Cyst formation probably occurs secondary to duct obstruction by inspissated secretions.

(continues on page 164)

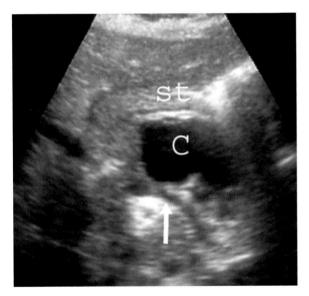

Fig. 2.31   Congenital cyst. Transverse sonogram of a newborn that shows a well-defined, thin-walled anechoic mass in the tail of the pancreas (C). The splenic vein is noted (arrow).
st Stomach

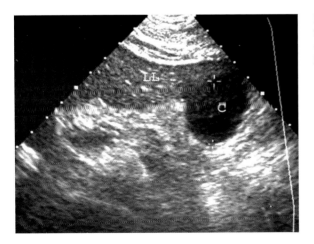

Fig. 2.32   Pseudocyst. Sonogram shows an anechoic structure (c) anterior to the pancreatic tail. Note that the cyst wall has no layering, in contrast to duplication cysts.
LL Left lobe of the liver

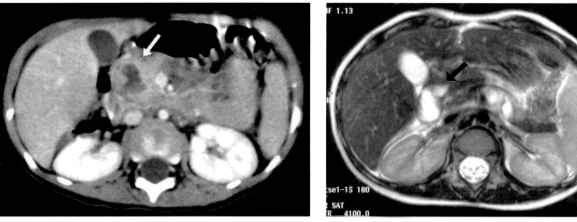

a
b

Fig. 2.33a, b Pseudocyst. (a) Pseudocyst in a 12-year-old boy with history of recurrent acute pancreatitis. CT shows fully encapsulated pancreatic fluid content of < 15 HU, (arrow). **(b)** Same patient: axial T2-weighted HASTE MRI reveals a multiloculated high signal intensity pseudocyst in the pancreatic head and body (arrow).

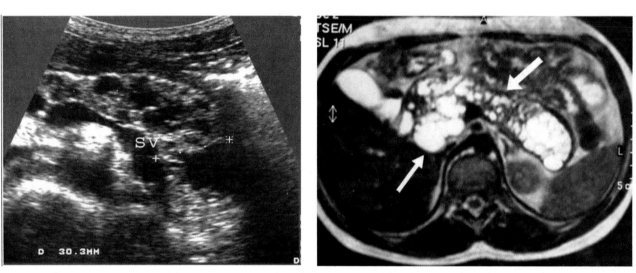

a
b

Fig. 2.34a, b Pancreatic cystosis. (a) Transverse US scan through the pancreatic body and tail demonstrates numerous sonolucent (cystic) lesions distributed throughout the gland. A small amount of echogenic pancreatic tissue is observed among the cysts. **(b)** Axial T2-weighted turbo spin echo MRI of the same patient at the same level shows an enlarged pancreas presenting numerous, different sized cysts with high signal intensity (arrows).
sv Splenic vein

Table 2.18 (Cont.) Cystic lesions

Diagnosis	Findings	Comments
Von Hippel-Lindau syndrome ▷ *Fig. 2.35*	Pancreatic lesions include single or multiple cysts, cyst replacement of the pancreas, microcystic adenomas, and islet cell tumors. Cysts can be associated with focal calcifications.	Autosomal-dominant disease; comprises the triad: retinal angiomatosis, cerebellar hemangioblastoma, and cysts of various organs.
Autosomal dominant polycystic renal disease	Renal disease is the diagnostic clue.	Hepatic cysts occur in approximately one-third of adults with the disease, but there is usually no periportal fibrosis. Cysts may also be found in the pancreas, lungs, spleen, ovaries, seminal vesicles, and testes.
Mucinous cystadenoma or macrocystic adenoma	Large uni- or multilocular cyst with internal echoes (mucinous material or hemorrhagic fluid). Capsular or septal calcifications in approximately 10% of lesions.	The majority (70%–90%) occur in the body and pancreatic tail.
Microcystic adenoma (serous cystadenoma)	Generally composed of numerous small cysts, separated by fibrous septae that radiate from the center. These fibrous bands form a central stellate scar that can calcify.	Increased frequency in patients with Von Hippel-Lindau disease. Benign and usually located in the pancreatic head.
Macrocystic lymphangioma	US: septated, cystic mass. CT: The soft-tissue septations may enhance following intravenous contrast. The cystic components have near-water attenuation and do not enhance.	Benign tumor arising from lymphatic vessels.

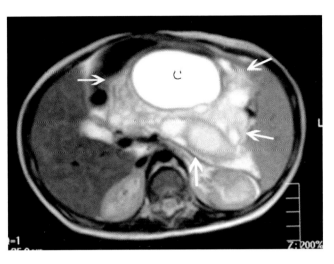

Fig. 2.35   Von Hippel-Lindau syndrome in a 10-year-old boy. Axial T2-weighted HASTE MRI shows multiple pancreatic cysts of different sizes with high signal intensity (arrows). The biggest one (C) is located in the pancreas body, measuring approximately 33 × 42 mm. Hepatic and renal cysts were not present.

Table 2.19   Solid lesions

Diagnosis	Findings	Comments
Acute focal pancreatitis	Localized involvement with mild duct dilatation. Fluid collections due to focal edema.	
Metastases: lymphoma and leukemia ▷ *Fig. 2.36*	Solid nodular, hypoechoic, solitary or multiple lesions.	Metastases are more frequent than primary neoplasms. Burkitt lymphoma is the most frequent cause of pancreatic metastasis. The mean age at presentation is 11 y. Often accompanied by concurrent extrapancreatic metastases.
Functioning islet-cell tumors (insulinoma, glucagonoma, gastrinoma, VIPoma, somatostatinoma) ▷ *Fig. 2.37, p. 166*	US: Round or oval, well defined, and hypoechoic to the normal parenchyma. Tend to be small (< 2 cm in diameter). CT and MRI: arterial-phase imaging with either CT or MRI detect and characterize these lesions by demonstrating a hypervascular tumor involving the pancreas.	The most common is insulinoma.
Nonfunctioning islet-cell tumors	Usually large (3–20 cm in diameter) and sometimes contain calcifications. They may develop a cystic appearance secondary to degeneration and necrosis.	
Epithelial pancreatic tumors of nonendocrine origin (pancreatoblastoma, carcinoma, etc.)	US: solid, heterogeneous mass in the body or pancreatic tail. CT: heterogenous enhancement with or without foci of calcification.	There is an association between pancreatoblastoma and the Beckwith-Wiedeman syndrome. These solid tumors tend to be large (7–18 cm), solitary masses that can occur in any region of the pancreas.
Solid pseudopapillary neoplasm		Mainly in adolescent girls.

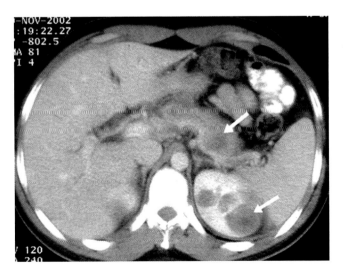

Fig. 2.36   Metastases of Burkitt lymphoma. A 17-year-old boy with mediastinal non-Hodgkin lymphoma. CT shows hypodense masses when compared with the normal parenchyma (arrows) corresponding to pancreatic and renal focal involvement.

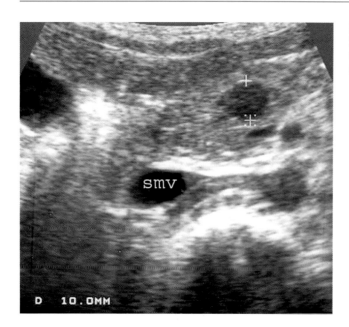

Fig. 2.37 Insulinoma. An 8-year-old boy with sustained hypoglycemia. Sonogram shows a small, hypoechoic, well-defined, solid lesion (between calipers) in the pancreatic body, measuring 10 mm.
smv Superior mesenteric vein

Table 2.20 Mixed solid-cystic lesions

Diagnosis	Findings	Comments
Pancreatic abscess ▷ *Fig. 2.38*	May have thin walls or ill-defined borders. The content is fluid-filled occasionally with gas. Pancreatic abscesses can have imaging features similar to pseudocysts.	After severe acute pancreatitis. Immunocompromised children. The diagnosis is commonly made by percutaneous aspiration under imaging guidance.
Necrotizing pancreatitis	CT: Area of nonenhancing parenchyma that is > 3 cm in diameter or involves 30% or more of the pancreas. Gas bubbles may be noted when there is infected pancreatic necrosis.	It is the most severe form of the disease and is produced by rapid escape of lytic enzymes into the pancreatic parenchyma.

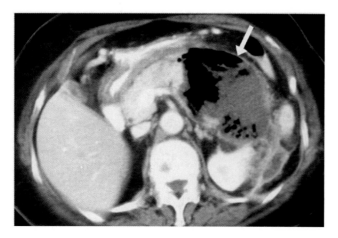

Fig. 2.38 Pancreatic abscess. CT shows a complex, gas-containing fluid collection in the pancreatic tail (arrow).

Table 2.21 Partial absence of pancreas

Diagnosis	Findings	Comments
Congenital short pancreas	US: rounded, enlarged pancreatic head with normal echogenicity. Only a globular pancreatic head can be identified on CT.	This anomaly has been described in patients with the polysplenia syndrome.
Nesidioblastosis after 90% pancreatectomy	A remnant of pancreatic tissue (0.5–1 cm), mainly the head, is left to protect the common bile duct.	Near-total pancreatectomy (95% pancreatectomy) is recommended to avoid repeated operations associated with smaller resections.
Partial agenesis	Incidental finding at cross-sectional imaging with deficient pancreatic body and tail.	Associations: Shwachman-Diamond syndrome, Johanson-Blizzard syndrome, and leprechaunism. Polysplenia can be an associated finding.

The Spleen

The spleen is a wedge-shaped organ that is convex supero-laterally and concave inferomedially with a vascular hilum. It can be affected either by primary pathologic process or by multiorgan or systemic disease. Its histology varies with age, with little white pulp in the neonate, which increases with age.

Table 2.22 Normal imaging

Diagnosis	Findings	Comments
US	Homogeneous, slightly hyperechoic than normal kidney.	With high-frequency transducers, a granular pattern can be seen in children aged 1 to 5 y.
CT	Unenhanced CT: Homogeneous. With contrast, irregular, bizarre patterns of enhancement that disappear in portal phase (> 70 s).	
MR	Neonate: Hypointense on T2 and hyperintense (to liver) on T1. From 1 year of age, adult pattern: hyperintense on T2 and hypointense on T1. Irregular pattern of enhancement.	
Nuclear medicine (NM)	99mTc-labeled heat-damaged red cells are only taken up by the spleen.	Useful if a normal spleen is not detected by other imaging methods.

Table 2.23 Changes in position and shape

Diagnosis	Findings	Comments
Notches, clefts, and lobulations	Lobules are located near the hilum or extending anterior to the upper pole of the kidney. Clefts are sharp, located in the superior border, and sometimes 2–3 cm deep.	Normal in fetal period, usually disappear, but may be present into adult life.
Positional anomalies ▷ *Fig. 2.39*	Situs inversus. Wandering spleen: migration from its original position to a more caudal location because of laxity or lack of ligament fixation.	Wandering spleen is more common in females. It usually presents as an abdominal mass or as an acute abdomen due to torsion of the vascular pedicle with possible infarction.

(continues on page 168)

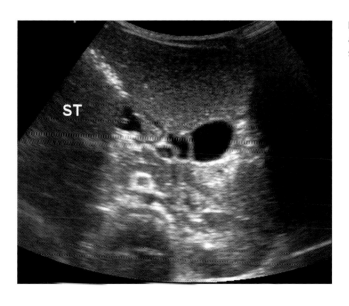

Fig. 2.39 Situs inversus. Transverse US through epigastrium shows a left-located liver and gallbladder and a right-sided air-distended stomach (ST).

Table 2.23 (Cont.) Changes in position and shape

Diagnosis	Findings	Comments
Accessory spleen(s) ▷ *Fig. 2.40*	Common anomaly (> 30%). Usually < 15 mm and located near the hilum, but can be multiple and in other locations. Same pattern that normal spleen.	Clinically insignificant. Increase in size after splenectomy.
Polysplenia syndrome (levoisomerism)	Multiple discrete spleens, right- or left-sided (at the same side of the stomach). Cardiac anomalies. Liver centrally located. No intrahepatic IVC, with azygous continuation. Mirror location of GI organs.	Wide range of abdominal anomalies. Most patients have severe cardiac anomalies, but 5%–10% reach adulthood without symptoms. More frequent in females.
Asplenia syndrome (dextro-isomerism) ▷ *Fig. 2.41*	Absence of spleen. Severe congenital heart disease. Liver and gallbladder in midline. IVC and aorta lie on the same side of column. Short pancreas. Midgut malrotation.	Most die in the first year. Male predominance.
Vascular shunts	Splenogonadal, splenorenal, splenohepatic.	

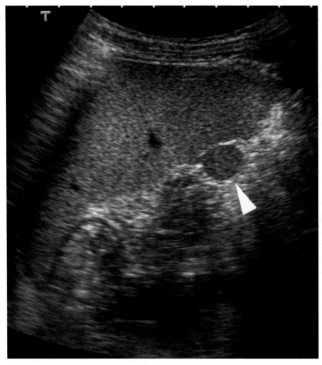

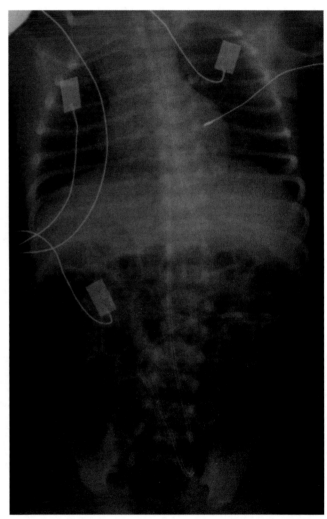

Fig. 2.40 Accessory spleen. Longitudinal US shows an isoechoic splenic parenchyma nodule (arrowhead) near the splenic hilum, representing accessory tissue.

Fig. 2.41 Asplenia syndrome. Plain film in a neonate showing the central position of liver.

Table 2.24   Splenomegaly

Diagnosis	Findings	Comments
Infection, sepsis	Usually homogeneous splenomegaly.	Many causative organisms: Bacterial, viral, protozoal, fungal. Some of them produce isolated spleno-megaly: Ebstein-Barr virus, malaria, histoplasma, mycobacterium.
Portal hypertension	Often due to extrahepatic portal vein thrombosis: Doppler US with absent or reversed flow or with cavernomatous transformation. Splenomegaly with heterogeneous hepatomegaly with lobulated margins.	Common causes: liver disease, umbilical vein catheterization, tumor, dehydration, omphalitis, hypercoagulability states.
Malignant diseases: leukemia, lymphoma, Langerhans cell histiocytosis, metastases	Either homogeneous splenomegaly or single or multiple masses can be present.	Look for other manifestations of disease.
Metabolic disease: Gaucher, Niemann-Pick, mucopolysac-charidosis, tyrosinosis	Homogeneous splenomegaly. Usually correlates with severity of disease.	Abnormal products of metabolism are stored in spleen parenchyma.
Hemolytic anemia		Due to sequestration of abnormal red cells.
Extracorporeal membrane oxygenation		Due to increased number of damaged red cells.
Right heart failure		Due to congestion.

Table 2.25   The small spleen

Diagnosis	Findings	Comments
Normal variant		Congenital hypoplasia.
Infarction (late phase)	Small spleen, sometimes with capsular calcification.	Secondary to emboli, torsion, portal hypertension, Gaucher disease.
Autosplenectomy		In sickle cell disease, thalassemia.
Celiac disease		In late phases of disease.

Table 2.26   Focal anomalies, solitary

Diagnosis	Findings	Comments
Cyst: serous, epidermoid, dermoid, echinococcal, pseudocyst (trauma, infarct) ▷ Fig. 2.42a, b, p. 170	Usually unilocular, with clear and homogeneous fluid. Echinococcal and pseudocyst may calcify	Echogenicity (US), density (CT), and signal intensity (MR) may vary due to composition of fluid.
Hemangioma	Septate, subcapsular cystic lesions. No contrast enhancement.	Solitary or multiple.
Lymphangioma	May appear cystic, solid, or a combination.	May cause Kasabach-Merritt syndrome if large.
Hamartoma	Solid and avascular lesions, heterogeneous.	Most common primary neoplasm.
Solitary focus of a typically multifocal disease (see Table 2.27)		

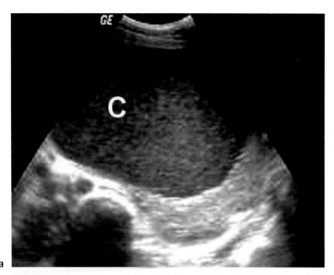
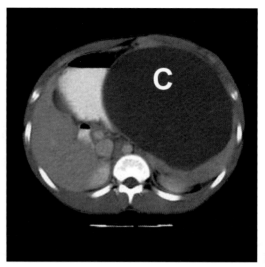

a
b

Fig. 2.42a, b   Epidermoid cyst. (a) Longitudinal US depicts a splenic cystic mass (C) with low-level echoes. **(b)** Contrast-enhanced CT of the same cyst.

Table 2.27   Focal anomalies, multiple

Diagnosis	Findings	Comments
Abscess ▷ *Fig. 2.43* ▷ *Fig. 2.44* ▷ *Fig. 2.45*	Centrally located, rounded, or irregular in shape with central fluid/necrosis. Avascular. Fungal abscess are small lesions (few millimeters).	Seen in immunosuppressed population (on chemotherapy, acquired immunodeficiency syndrome [AIDS])
Trauma	Lacerations, rupture, intrasplenic and subcapsular hematomas.	Sometimes, minor trauma can affect spleen.
Lymphoproliferative disorders, Langerhans cell histiocytosis, metastases ▷ *Fig. 2.46* ▷ *Fig. 2.47*	Multiple focal masses. Lymphoma can invade the capsule. Lymphadenopathy in hilum and retroperitoneum can be seen.	Look for other manifestations of disease.
Gaucher, Niemann-Pick disorders	Multiple nodules. On MRI, T1 signal is lower than for normal spleen.	

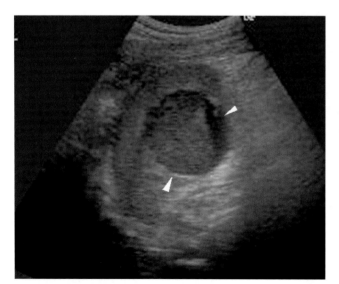
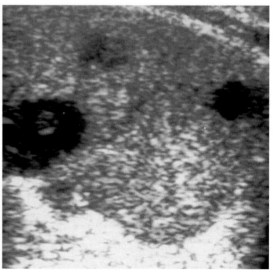

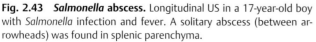

Fig. 2.43   *Salmonella* abscess. Longitudinal US in a 17-year-old boy with *Salmonella* infection and fever. A solitary abscess (between arrowheads) was found in splenic parenchyma.

Fig. 2.44   *Candida* abscess. In a neutropenic 5-year-old girl treated for neuroblastoma, transverse US shows multiple fungal abscess cavities.

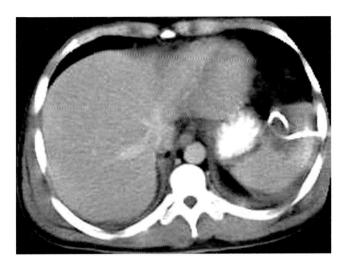

Fig. 2.45   Pyogenic abscess. Contrast-enhanced CT in a 15-year-old boy with a pyogenic abscess treated with percutaneous drainage.

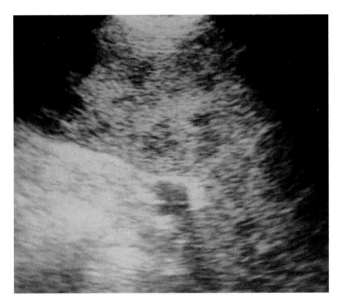

Fig. 2.46   Non-Hodgkin lymphoma. Longitudinal US shows multiple heterogeneous solid nodules.

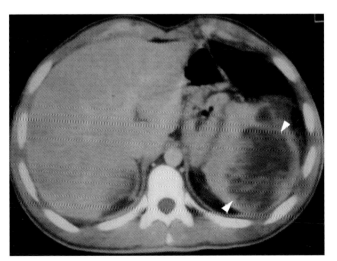

Fig. 2.47   Metastasis. Contrast-enhanced CT shows a discrete splenic mass (between arrowheads) representing metastasis from renal sarcoma.

Table 2.28 Diffuse anomalies

Diagnosis	Findings	Comments
Lymphoproliferative disorders, Langerhans cell histiocytosis, metastases		Depending on underlying disease.
Infarction (early phase)	Hypoattenuating (CT) spleen, with only capsular enhancement.	Patients with sickle cell disease are prone to infarction.
Iron deposition disease	MRI: low signal on T1 and T2.	
Hemangioma, hemangioendothelioma		May affect the entire spleen.

Table 2.29 Splenic calcifications

Diagnosis	Findings	Comments
Granulomatous diseases	Multiple tiny foci of calcium.	Histoplasma, cat-scratch, chronic granulomatous disease.
Infarction	Isolated peripheral, associated with scarring.	
Cysts, hematoma, abscesses	Peripheral calcification.	
AIDS	Arterial splenic calcifications.	

The Gastrointestinal Tract

Esophagus

■ Displacement and Compression

Esophageal displacement can be demonstrated by means of an
upper GI (UGI) study, MRI, or CT.

Table 2.30 Esophageal displacement

Diagnosis	Findings	Comments
Neurogenic tumors (neuroblastoma, neurofibroma)	Solid homogeneous masses in the posterior mediastinum. Anterolateral displacement of the esophagus. May calcify.	May produce osseous involvement. Additional investigation: MRI, (123)I-metaiodobenzylguanidine [(123)I-MIBG] scintigraphy, biopsy.
Anterior intrathoracic meningocele	Fluid-filled soft-tissue density tumor in the posterior mediastinum. Dysraphic changes are common.	Often associated with neurofibromatosis. Additional imaging: CT, MRI.
Esophageal duplication ▷ Fig. 2.58a, b, p. 180 ▷ Fig. 2.59a, b, p. 180	(see Table 2.34)	May be associated with dysraphic vertebral bodies (neurenteric cyst) and other bowel duplications.
Abscess	Displacement by a spindle-shaped fluid collection on both sides of the vertebral bodies.	Descended retropharyngeal abscesses or secondary to spondylitis and discitis
Paraesophageal hernia	Lateral/anterior displacement of the distal esophagus.	Commonly filled with air. Either congenital or posthiatal hernia repair.
Cardiomegaly	Posterior displacement of the esophagus.	See Chapter 1
Aberrant vessels		See Chapter 1
Enlarged lymph nodes	Multiple solid homogeneous masses often in anterior and/or middle mediastinum.	Most often due to lymphoma.
Bronchogenic cysts	Cystic homogeneous lesion frequently in the middle mediastinum compressing the esophagus according to the size.	Arise from disruption in fetal separation of the esophagus and trachea. Work-up: CT, MRI.
Teratoma	Solid or cystic usually anterior mediastinal masses. May contain bony elements and calcifications.	Work-up: CT, MRI.
Enlarged thymus	Posterior proximal esophageal displacement.	Rarely associated with swallowing or breathing difficulties.
Cystic lymphangioma	Cystic multiseptated mass with anterior mediastinum widening and causing posterior esophageal displacement.	The mass may extend from the cervical area through the thoracic inlet to the anterior mediastinum.
Pulmonary volume loss	Lateral displacement of the esophagus and the entire mediastinum to the side of the volume loss. Compensatory emphysema of the normal side.	Pulmonary aplasia, pulmonary volume loss/atelectasis, total lung atelectasis (foreign body), status postpulmonary resection.
Increased hemithorax volume	Lateral mediastinal displacement toward the uninvolved side.	Congenital lobar emphysema, congenital pulmonary cysts, cystic adenomatoid malformation, tension pneumothorax, diaphragmatic hernia.

Table 2.31 The esophagus: Dilatation and stricture

Diagnosis	Findings	Comments
Physiologic	Distention of esophagus during deglutition.	Due to swallowing of air or belching. In contrast to adults, gas in the esophagus is a frequent finding in children.
Hypotonia ▷ *Fig. 2.48*	Generalized esophagus distention.	Secondary to inflammation and gastroesophageal reflux (GER).
GER (incompetent lower esophageal sphincter) ▷ *Fig. 2.49* ▷ *Fig. 2.50*	US or contrast examination show passage of gastric content to the esophagus.	Physiologic up to 18 mo of age. Endoscopic Ph-measure is the gold standard for diagnosis. Imaging is essential to rule out GER secondary to gastric outlet obstruction. Is the most frequent cause of aspiration pneumonia. Roviralta syndrome: hiatal hernia secondary to hypertrophic pyloric stenosis (HPS).
Hiatal hernia ▷ *Fig. 2.51*	Anteroposterior X-ray: basal lucency within the outline of the cardiac silhouette. Confirmation with contrast examination. to demonstrate GER and its sequelae (esophagitis and reflux stricture).	Mostly congenital. Sliding hernias varying in size. DD: small epiphrenic ampulla.
Reflux esophagitis ▷ *Fig. 2.52*	Contrast examination: irregular and gross mucosal folds in distal esophagus with ulcerations.	The most important cause is hiatal hernia. Endoscopy for diagnosis.
Caustic injury	The mucosa is initially edematous and thickened. Later, atonic dilatation occurs, as well as irregular mucosal pattern due to necrosis.	Nonionic contrast medium for diagnosis at early stage due to perforation risk. Late sequelae: long stenosis. Most often with alkalis.
Other esophagitis (mycotic, viral, bacterial)	Spasm, pseudodiverticula ulcerations, edema, cobblestone pattern, stenosis.	Can affect the esophagus at any level. Usually diffuse. Immunocompromised patients.

(continues on page 176)

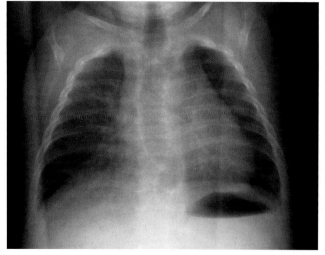

Fig. 2.48 Hypotonia. Plain anteroposterior chest radiograph shows a dilated hypotonic esophagus in a patient with GER.

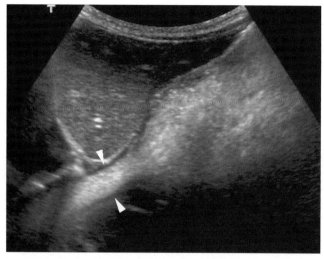

Fig. 2.49 Gastroesophageal reflux. US sagittal view of an infant with GER: the lower esophageal sphincter is open and a large amount of gastric content is seen passing into the distal esophagus (arrowheads).

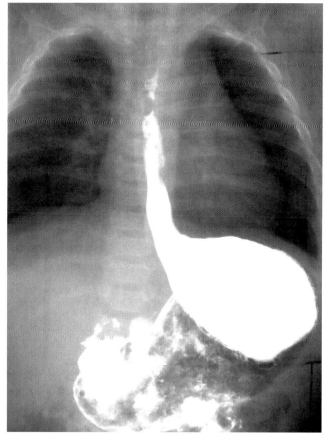

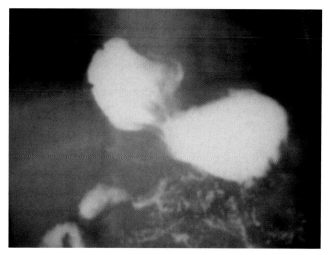

Fig. 2.50 Gastroesophageal reflux. Upper gastrointestinal (UGI) series in supine position: barium is seen refluxing into the esophageal hiatus to the lower esophagus.

Fig. 2.51   Hiatal hernia. UGI series in an infant: the barium-filled stomach is partially herniated and has an hourglass configuration.

Fig. 2.52   Peptic acid esophagitis. UGI series of an infant with esophageal stricture with some tiny lineal ulcerations caused by prolonged GER and peptic acid esophagitis.

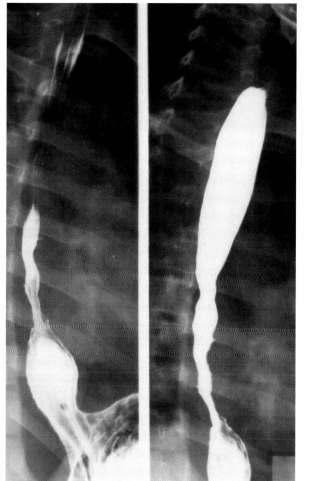

Table 2.31 (Cont.) The esophagus: Dilatation and stricture

Diagnosis	Findings	Comments
Foreign bodies ▷ *Fig. 2.53*	Contrast examination: filling defects. Foreign body impaction often at stenotic areas.	Barium or nonionic contrast medium in cases of perforation suspicion. Endoscopic extraction.
Achalasia	Atonic esophagus dilatation (megaesophagus). Heterogeneous air-fluid level due to air and retained food. The stomach bubble is small or absent. Contrast examination: characteristic beak deformity at the distal esophagus.	Rare in infants. Unknown cause. Clinically: swallowing difficulty and retrosternal pain. DD: distal esophageal strictures.
Congenital esophageal stricture	Membranous-, hour-glass–, or tubular-shaped.	Associated with tracheoesophageal fistula or isolated as a cartilaginous ring in bronchial remnant syndromes.
Secondary esophageal stricture ▷ *Fig. 2.52, p. 175*	Narrowed lumen with possible prestenotic dilatation. The contracture and scarring are more often in the middle and lower esophagus.	Causes: Most often due to reflux esophagitis. After operative repair for esophageal atresia, at the level of the anastomosis, after caustic esophagitis (alkalis, acids), with epidermolysis bullosa; postirradiation; with vascular anomalies.
Radiation damage	Mural scar formation and distortion with loss of motility. The lumen is narrowed.	Extent of the damage depends on the size of the radiation field.
Leukemic infiltration	Narrowing of the lumen, mostly in the distal esophagus.	Other tumors are rare.
Epidermolysis bullosa dystrophica	Circumferential constriction can occur, as well as long segment strictures.	Hereditary. Presents in infancy. Minimal trauma can result in blister production.
Scleroderma, dermatomyositis, lupus erythematosus	Dilatation. Absent peristalsis.	Hiatus hernia and reflux esophagitis may develop distal stenosis.

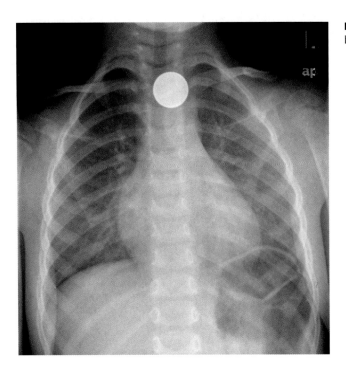

Fig. 2.53 Foreign body. Plain chest film shows a radiopaque foreign body (coin) impacted in the upper third of the esophagus.

■ Mucosal Changes and Filling Defects

Table 2.32   The esophagus: Mucosal changes and filling defects

Diagnosis	Findings	Comments
Inflammation		
Caustic burns	Superficial ulcerations. Thickened, weeping, edematous mucosa and local spasm. Scarring. Contrast examination after the acute phase to exclude stricture or fistulas.	Inflammation due to alkalis or acids (mostly affects the stomach). DD: thermal esophagitis (heals without scarring).
Reflux esophagitis ▷ *Fig. 2.52, p. 175*	Mucosal swelling or ulceration in the distal atonic esophagus.	
Radiation esophagitis	Irregularity of the wall contours, cobblestone mucosal pattern with possible ulceration. Narrowed lumen.	Damage can occur after low doses of radiation when combined with systemic chemotherapy.
Infectious esophagitis	Alteration of mucosal pattern with erosions, ulcerations, and irregular outline. Reduced tone and peristalsis. Late fibrosis and stricture formation.	Candidiasis (immunocompromised patients). Herpes simplex infection (generalized primary infection in nonimmunized infants).
Granulomatous infections (tuberculosis, syphilis, actinomycosis, lymphogranulomatosis)	Superficial ulcers. Submucosal granulomata may resemble tumors.	Endoscopy and biopsy are necessary to make the diagnosis.
Epidermolysis bullosa	Well-defined narrowing in the upper third of the esophagus.	Autosomal recessive (AR). Minimal trauma causes blistering and scarring of mucosa and skin.
Crohn disease	Concentric narrowing distally.	Rare.
Neoplasms		
Leukemia	(see **Table 2.31**)	
Hemangiomatosis	Long, superficial, well-defined raised lesions in the dilated and atonic distal esophagus.	In mucocutaneous hemangiomatosis.
Sarcoma		Rare. Biopsy is necessary for diagnosis.
Other Causes		
Varices in portal hypertension	Thick, serpiginous mucosal folds, varying in size in barium exam.	
Scleroderma	Diminished peristalsis. The esophagus becomes a rigid tube.	GI tract involvement occurs later than bone and skin changes.

Table 2.33   Esophageal atresia: Classification according to Vogt (Fig. 2.54)

Diagnosis	Findings
Type I ▷ *Fig. 2.55, p. 178*	Esophageal atresia (very rare). No air in the esophagus and stomach.
Type II	Atresia without a fistula, relatively distended and large blind-ending pouch. No air in the GI tract.
Type IIIa	Atresia with a proximal fistula, nondistended blind-ending pouch. No air in the GI tract.
Type IIIb ▷ *Fig. 2.56, p. 178*	The most common type. Atresia with a proximal blind-ending pouch and fistulous connection between the trachea and distal esophageal segment. Air in the GI tract.
Type IIIc	Atresia with a fistulous connection between the proximal and distal segments of the trachea (approximately 2%–3%). Small caliber proximal blind-ending pouch. Air in the GI tract. GI-tract anomalies are associated with congenital cardiac anomalies.
H-Fistula ▷ *Fig. 2.57, p. 179*	Tracheoesophageal fistula without atresia. DD: fistula secondary to foreign bodies.

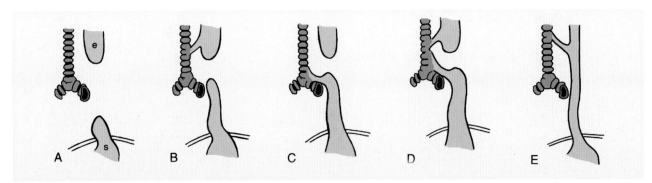

Fig. 2.54a–e The classification of esophageal atresias and tracheoesophageal fistulas. (**a**) Type II. (**b**) Type IIIa. (**c**) Type IIIb. (**d**) Type IIIc. (**e**) H-type (see **Table 2.33** for descriptions).

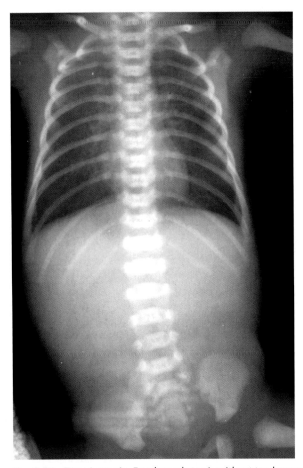

Fig. 2.55 Type I atresia. Esophageal atresia without tracheoesophageal fistula. Plain chest and abdominal film of a day-old newborn with a gasless GI tract.

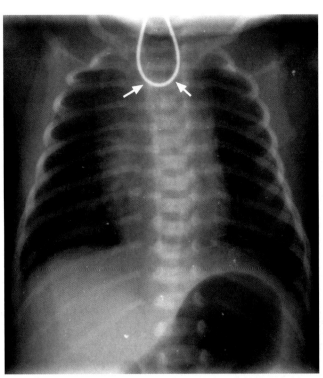

Fig. 2.56 Type IIIb atresia. Esophageal atresia with distal tracheoesophageal fistula in a newborn with a nasogastric tube in a blind proximal esophageal pouch. There is gas in stomach, proving the presence of the fistula.

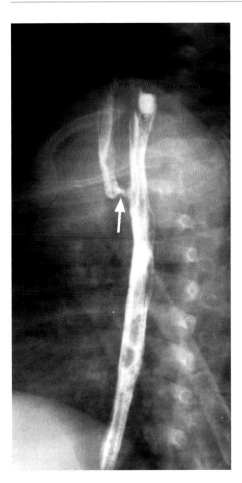

Fig. 2.57   H-type atresia. Tracheoesophageal fistula without atresia. Barium is seen passing from the esophagus to the trachea through a fistula (arrow).

■ Diverticula and Duplications

Table 2.34   The esophagus: Diverticula and duplications

Diagnosis	Findings	Comments
Diverticulum	Well-defined saccular-like projections of contrast beyond the esophageal lumen.	Thought to be incomplete neuroenteric duplications. Pulsion or traction mechanism (related to inflamed nodes, e.g., tuberculosis).
Pseudodiverticulum		Due to multiple outpouching of the esophagus in tertiary contractions or due to iatrogenic sinus tract.
Duplication ▷ *Fig. 2.58a, b, p. 180* ▷ *Fig. 2.59a, b p. 180*	Chest radiographs: posterior mediastinal mass. Esophagogram: esophagus displaced to the side opposite the mass or an intramural extramucosal mass. CT: mass sharply marginated, with homogeneous near-water density and not enhanced after intravenous contrast administration. MRI: low signal intensity on T1-weighted images and very high signal intensity on T2 weighted images.	DD: neoplasms arising from the sympathetic chain, bronchogenic or neurenteric cysts, pulmonary sequestration, anterior meningocele, and hemangioma.

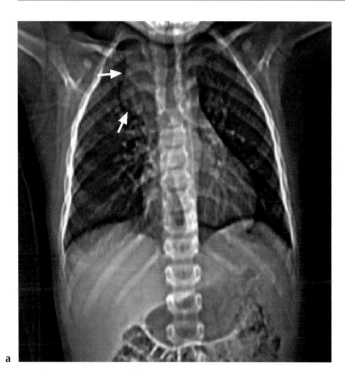

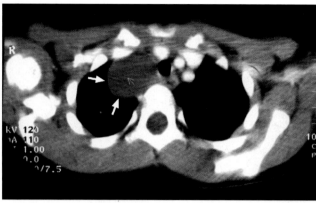

Fig. 2.58a, b   Duplication cyst. (a) Chest radiograph shows a widening of the right superior mediastinum produced by a mediastinal mass (arrows). **(b)** Same patient: contrast-enhanced CT image demonstrates a fluid-filled, thin-walled, near-water density mass adjacent to the trachea and esophagus (arrows).

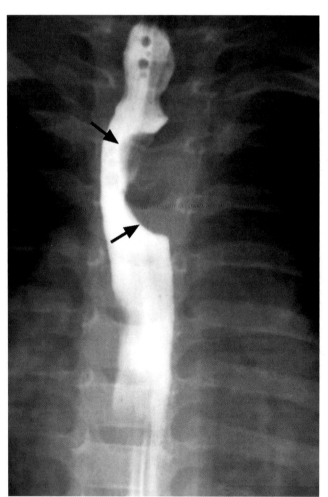

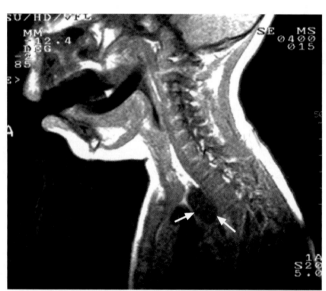

Fig. 2.59a, b   Duplication cyst in a 2-year-old girl with recurrent episodes of vomiting. **(a)** Esophagogram shows extrinsic compression on the left wall of the esophagus (arrows). **(b)** On sagittal T1-weighted MRI, a sharply defined low signal intensity mass (arrows) is seen adjacent to the left side of the esophagus. The mass had very high signal intensity on T2-weighted MRI (not shown).

■ Disturbances of Motility and Function

Table 2.35   The esophagus: Disturbances of motility and function

Diagnosis	Findings	Comments
Immaturity	Swallowing views (fluoroscopic): poorly coordinated contraction and relaxation of the esophagus.	Dysphagia. Nonpathologic in the first few months of life, mostly in premature infants.
Atony	Absent peristalsis. Linear mucosal folds. Hold-up of contrast in the esophagus in the absence of abnormality of the cardia.	Causes: sepsis, pneumonia, peritonitis, brain injury in infancy. Dermatomyositis, scleroderma. DD: esophagitis, achalasia, etc.
Spasm	Rapid esophageal contraction obliterates stripping wave. Mucosal changes depend on the underlying cause.	Reflex spasm in the lower esophagus: with foreign body impaction, caustic, mechanical or thermal injury, esophagitis, and ulceration.

Stomach

■ Dilatation

Table 2.36   Gastric dilatation

Diagnosis	Findings	Comments
Aerophagia	Marked gastric distention due to swallowed air	Caused by crying. May be exacerbated during feeding in the supine position.
Mask breathing	Progressive gastric distention, frequently accompanied by small-bowel dilatation.	Air forced to pass through esophagus and stomach due to increased airway resistance (e.g., in respiratory distress syndrome [RDS]).
Tube malposition ▷ Fig. 2.60, p. 182	The endotracheal tube may be malpositioned in the esophagus with resultant overdistention of the stomach.	
Hypotonia, paralysis	Increased gastric content sometimes accompanied by decreased bowel air due to impaired gastric emptying.	Causes: perinatal brain damage, RDS, sepsis, metabolic imbalance, surgery, acute pancreatitis, etc.
Hypertrophic pyloric stenosis (HPS) ▷ Fig. 2.61, p. 182 ▷ Fig. 2.62, p. 182	US: best imaging screen method. US findings: elongation of the pyloric channel ($\geq$ 16 mm). Persistent thickening of the pyloric muscle ($>$ 3 mm) in the elongated portion of the canal. Hypoechoic "doughnut" (thickened muscle) on axial projection. Vigorous peristalsis.	Gastric outlet obstruction leads to emaciation. "Projectile" vomiting. DD: congenital pyloric stenosis, "prostaglandin E induced stenosis outlet": the stenosis is produced by central foveolar hyperplasia. Mucosal changes are different from the muscular thickening observed in HPS. Roviralta syndrome: HPS and hiatal hernia.
Pylorospasm	US: Persistent spasm of the pyloric canal with little fluid passing into duodenum. Borderline measurements. No evidence of hyperperistalsis.	Typically intermittent. Serial US useful to differentiate from hypertrophic pyloric stenosis (HPS).
Antral ulcer	Located in the antrum.	
Congenital intrinsic obstruction: antral membrane (web), pyloric atresia ▷ Fig. 2.63, p. 183 ▷ Fig. 2.64, p. 183	Plain X-ray: "single bubble" image: distention of the stomach proximal to the obstruction and absence of gas in the small bowel and colon.	Usually produced by a membranous diaphragm, sometimes incomplete. Predominant symptom: free of bile vomiting.
Volvulus	(see **Table 2.39**)	

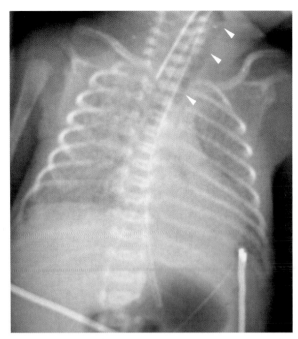 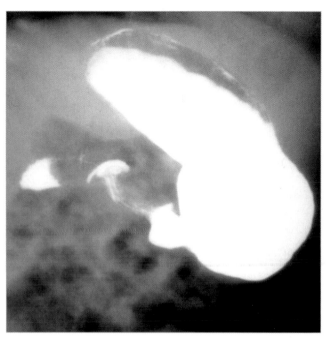

Fig. 2.60   Tracheal tube malposition. Chest X-ray in a newborn with neonatal respiratory distress. The endotracheal tube is malpositioned inside the esophageal lumen. Note that the tracheal lumen (arrowheads) is located anterior to the nasogastric and tracheal tubes.

Fig. 2.61   Hypertrophic pyloric stenosis. UGI series of a newborn with persistent vomiting shows gastric distension with emptying difficulty throughout an elongated pyloric channel with "double channel" image.

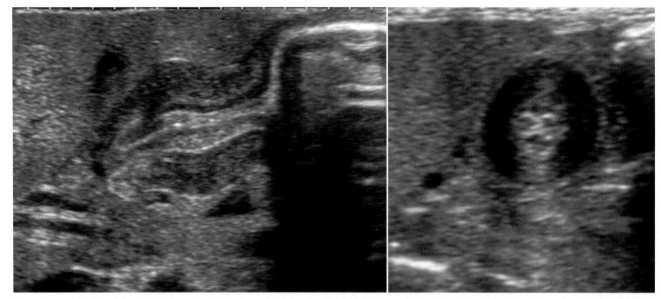

Fig. 2.62   Hypertrophic pyloric stenosis. US images of pylorus in a 21-day-old boy with persistent vomiting. In the longitudinal image (left), the pyloric channel is elongated and the muscular layer is hypoechoic and thickened. Axial scan (right) shows a doughnut image in the subhepatic region with a double pyloric channel image produced by folding of the hyperechoic mucosal surface. No passage of gastric content is observed during the exploration period.

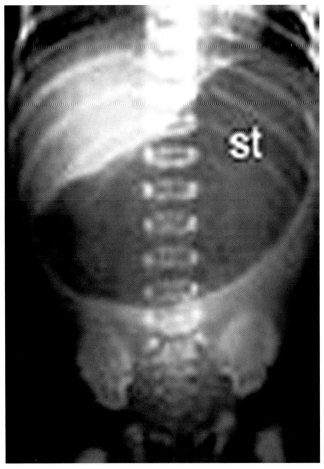

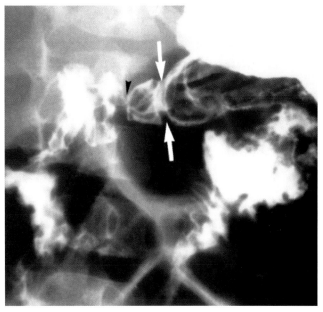

Fig. 2.63 Pyloric atresia. Anteroposterior plain abdominal radiograph in a newborn with pyloric atresia that shows distention of the stomach (st) and absence of air in the small bowel and colon, resulting in the characteristic "single bubble" image.

Fig. 2.64 Antral web. UGI series shows an incomplete antral web. In this oblique view, a concentric radiolucent band (arrows) is seen, resulting in discrete antral lumen reduction. The arrowhead indicates where the pylorus is located.

■ Mucosal Changes

Table 2.37   The stomach: Mucosal changes and filling defects

Diagnosis	Findings	Comments
Inflammatory Changes		
Infectious gastritis	*Helicobacter pylori*: enlarged gastric folds in the body and antropyloric regions of the stomach. Cytomegalovirus (CMV): often causes deep ulcerations, submucosal masses resulting from edema, or local microabscesses.	*Helicobacter pylori* has been related to gastritis and peptic ulcer. Associated with AIDS, CMV, *Toxoplasma gondii*, *Cryptosporidium*, or human immunodeficiency virus direct damage.
Caustic injury (chemical gastritis)	Plain radiographs: always, to assess perforation. Double-contrast exam: in absence of perforation (if perforation exists, water-soluble contrast materials are mandatory). Severe mucosal edema and spasm and narrowing of the stomach are the most common findings.	Alkali is the most common substance. Despite it usually causing esophagitis, antral and pyloric channel gastritis is found in up to 20% of cases.

(continues on page 184)

Table 2.37 (Cont.) The stomach: Mucosal changes and filling defects

Diagnosis	Findings	Comments
Ménétrier disease ▷ *Fig. 2.65*	UGI exam: marked enlargement of the fundal rugae, commonly along the greater curvature. US: Thickening of the gastric mucosal folds if examination is performed with an empty stomach. In a fully filled stomach, hypertrophied rugae collapse. Thickening occurs on the submucosal layer of the stomach.	Uncommon self-limited disease. Cause unknown (hypersensitivity response and viral infection have been reported). Nausea and vomiting in association to protein-loss enteropathy. Pleural effusion, ascites, and peripheral edema.
Ulcer disease	Ulcer crater usually associated with thickening mucosal folds (superficial in stress ulcer and drug erosive gastritis).	Peptic ulcer, steroid ulcer, stress ulcer.
Chronic granulomatous disease of childhood ▷ *Fig. 2.66*	US: thickening of antropyloric wall that sometimes might simulate HPS but beyond infancy. Barium exam: Narrowing of antropyloric lumen secondary to inflammation and fibrosis. Duodenum is often affected.	Recurrent infection, usually bacterial or fungal. Pathophysiology: phagocytosis disorders.
Crohn disease	Barium exam: double-contrast technique is mandatory to detect mucosal detail (aphtha, small mucosal ulcers).	Stomach affected in 2%–20%.
Benign Tumors		DD: ectopic pancreatic tissue.
Polypoid gastric tumors, solitary or multiple	Filling defect on a stalk.	Peutz–Jeghers syndrome (hamartomas). Occult bleeding and perioral pigmentosus. Cowden disease.
Mesenchymal tumors ▷ *Fig. 2.67*	Polypoid filling defect that may have a central dimple.	Leiomyoma, lipoma. DD: neuroma, teratoma.
Malignant Tumors		Extremely rare. Lymphoma, usually the non-Hodgkin variety, is the most common malignancy.
Non-Hodgkin lymphoma ▷ *Fig. 2.68* ▷ *Fig. 2.69*	Barium exam: marked enlargement and thickening of folds of the body and pyloric region. CT: very rarely seen, but sometimes might present as bull's-eye lesions.	Mostly associated with disseminated disease.
Metastases	Rounded areas of infiltration, may ulcerate.	From sarcomas.

(continues on page 186)

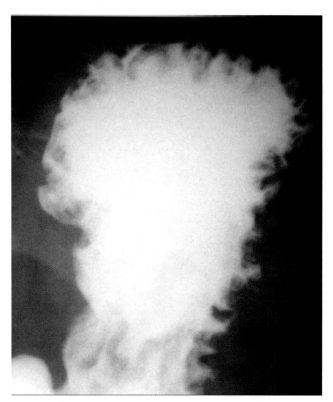

Fig. 2.65 Ménétrier disease. UGI series shows rugal hypertrophy in a 5-year-old boy with hypoproteinemia and Ménétrier disease

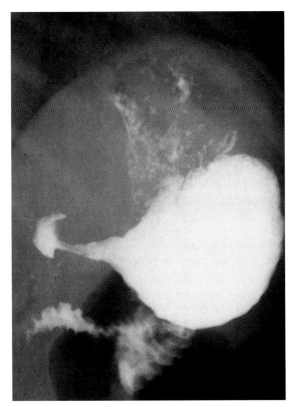

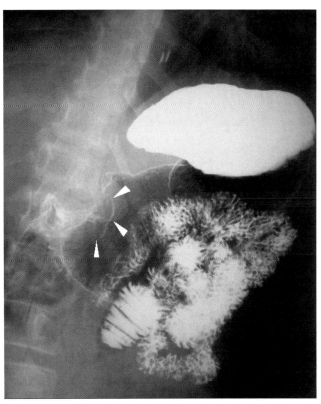

Fig. 2.66 Chronic granulomatous disease. UGI series depicts a tapered antral stenosis with benign appearance in a 9-year-old boy with chronic granulomatous disease. Contrast retention in the stomach is also noted.

Fig. 2.67 Leiomyoblastoma. UGI series depicts a filling defect in the antral region (arrowheads) produced by a submucosal tumor (leiomyoblastoma).

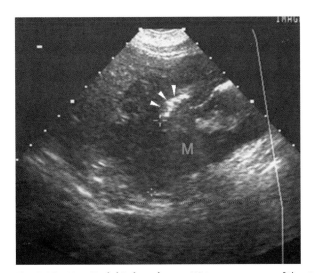

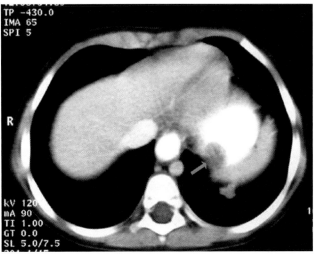

Fig. 2.68 Non-Hodgkin lymphoma. US transverse scan of the stomach in a 5-year-old girl shows a narrow hyperechoic mucosal lumen (arrowheads) and a thickened, tumoral infiltrated wall, depicted as a rounded hypoechoic mass (M).

Fig. 2.69 Burkitt lymphoma and gastric involvement. CT scan of a 7-year-old boy: note the existence of a small homogeneous, polypoid, rounded mass located in the posterior fundic wall (arrow).

Table 2.37 (Cont.) The stomach: Mucosal changes and filling defects

Diagnosis	Findings	Comments
Gastrointestinal stromal tumors ▷ *Fig. 2.70a, b*	Barium examination, US, CT, and MRI: Intramural masses in all sort of sizes. Occasionally might be multilobar and show an exophytic growing.	Less well-differentiated stromal tumors of the GI tract.
Carcinoma	Varied appearances. CT: very useful to demonstrate the extragastric component of the tumor.	
Anomalies		
Microgastria	The shape of the stomach is tubular or saccular, small in size, usually nonrotated, and in some cases located partially in the intrathoracic space. Almost all cases are associated with severe GER and a dilated lower esophagus.	Extremely rare abnormality. Associations: asplenia (most common), intestinal malrotation, duodenal atresia, upper limb anomalies, micrognathia, and spinal deformities.
Antral web, pyloric atresia		(see **Table 2.36**)
Ectopic pancreatic tissue ▷ *Fig. 2.71*	Barium examination: Small (1–3 cm) broad-based submucosal mass on the larger curvature. At times, central umbilication (rudimentary pancreatic duct). Can easily be misinterpreted as a gastric submucosal tumor.	Pancreatic tissue that lacks anatomic and vascular continuity with the main body of the pancreas. Most common location: gastric antrum. May prolapse into the pylorus, producing intermittent obstruction.
Miscellaneous		
Bezoars (trichobezoars, phytobezoars, lactobezoars) ▷ *Fig. 2.72*	Plain X-ray: intragastric mass with solid or bizarre appearance, frequently rounded by air. Barium exams: contrast may either soak or superficially coat the mass. US: hyperechoic line with progressive sound attenuation.	Trichobezoars: swallowed hair. In adolescence. Phytobezoars: vegetal matter (coconut, raw oranges). Lactobezoars: incorrectly prepared powdered milk formula (highly concentrated).
Prolapsed gastric mucosa	Filling defects in duodenal bulb.	
Gastric (fundal) varices	GI series: serpiginous filling defects in antrum and lesser curvature.	Associated with esophageal varices in patients with portal hypertension. More common in splenic vein thrombosis.
Hematoma/hemorrhage	Thickened mucosal folds.	Trauma, child abuse, hemophilia.

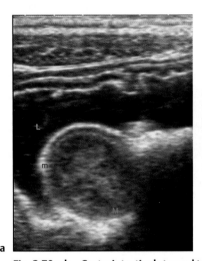
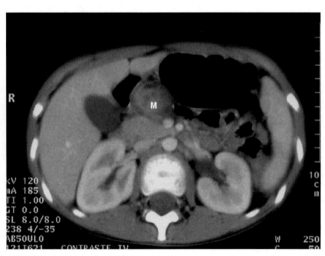

a   b

Fig. 2.70a, b Gastrointestinal stromal tumor. (a) US performed with the stomach lumen fully filled with water (L). A solid, mostly hypoechoic, submucosal mass (M) is depicted. Note that the mucosal layer (m) is patent and unaffected. **(b)** Axial CT with intravenous contrast in the same patient. Note that the mass (M) is not enhancing despite the intravenous contrast administration.

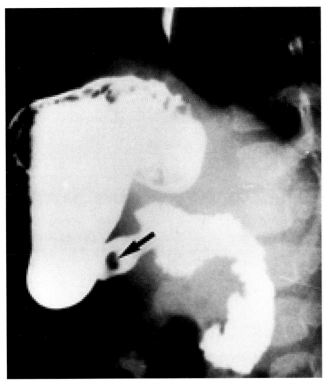

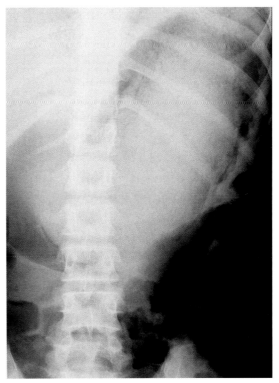

Fig. 2.71 Ectopic pancreas. A left-posterior oblique view of a UGI series performed in a 7-year-old boy: The ectopic pancreatic tissue measures less than 2 cm in size and is classically located within 6 cm from the pylorus in the gastric antrum (arrow). The presence of ulceration could not be assessed in this study despite the clinical diagnosis of microcitic anemia.

Fig. 2.72 Large gastric trichobezoar. A 13-year-old girl with abdominal pain: plain abdominal film shows a distended air-filled stomach with a large intraluminal mass outlined by air.

Table 2.38 The stomach: Diverticula and duplications

Diagnosis	Findings	Comments
Diverticulum	Barium exam: round or oval pouch with a small neck that typically changes in shape and size.	Uncommon in any age group. Represent communicating duplications. Usually in the cardiofundal and antropyloric regions.
Duplication ▷ *Fig. 2.73a–d, p. 188*	US: well-defined cystic mass lying close to the greater curvature of the stomach. The presence of an echogenic inner rim and hypoechoic outer muscle layers is highly suggestive. CT: sharply marginated, with a homogeneous near-water density, not enhancing after intravenous contrast material injection. MRI: low signal intensity on T1-weighted images and high signal intensity on T2-weighted images.	Seven percent of GI tract duplications.

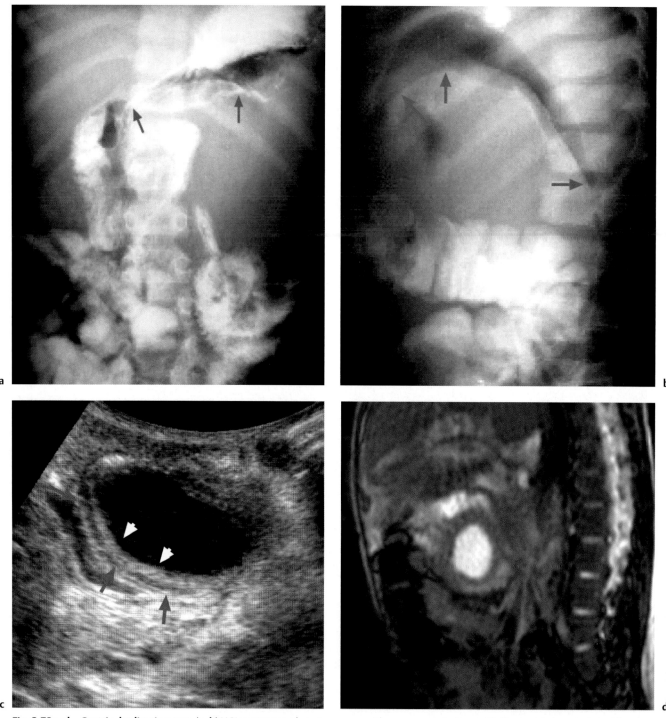

Fig. 2.73a–d   Gastric duplication cyst. (a, b) UGI contrast study outlines an intra-abdominal mass displacing the stomach and bowel up and to the right. **(c)** US scan through the gastric body shows a cystic mass with no communication with the gastric lumen and with a double-layered wall (landmark of duplication). **(d)** Sagittal T2-weighted MRI shows a cystic mass compressing the stomach wall.

Table 2.39   Alteration in gastric shape and position

Diagnosis	Findings	Comments
Cascade stomach	Fundus folded posteriorly that empties into the antrum (horizontal stomach).	Caused by overdistention of transverse colon, splenomegaly, tumors, etc.
Gastric volvulus ▷ *Fig. 2.74*	Dilated stomach. Mesenteroaxial volvulus: the cardia is inferiorly displaced and the pylorus is in a higher subdiaphragmatic position. Organoaxial volvulus: greater curvature to the right of the lesser one.	Mesenteroaxial volvulus: Associated with left hemidiaphragm elevation. Associated with big hiatal hernias, particularly paraesophageal. Organoaxial volvulus asymptomatic in neonates.

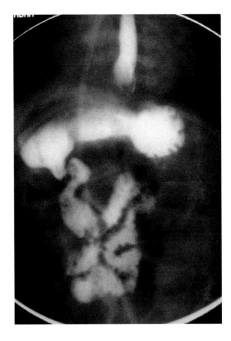

Fig. 2.74 Organoaxial volvulus. A 3-month-old boy with persistent vomiting: UGI series shows the greater curvature located to the right and superior to the lesser curvature. The twisting is only of 180 degrees, thus permitting the passing of oral contrast.

Small Bowel

The diagnosis of small-bowel diseases is a challenge to the clinician because of the overlapping of nonspecific symptoms.

Disorders affecting the small bowel are a significant cause of morbidity in infants and children, frequently requiring multiple imaging modalities for diagnosis. By enteroscopy, only 50% of small-bowel loops can be visualized. The radiologist, therefore, has come to play an important role in the evaluation of a variety of small-bowel conditions.

The plain radiograph examination is often the first radiologic investigation, particularly when obstruction or pneumoperitoneum is suspected in neonates. In young children, the differences of density are hardly pronounced, and loops are densely packed in a polygonal appearance. Air usually reaches the rectum by 24 hours after birth. Plain film with horizontal beam (supine, lateral decubitus, erect) may be essential to demonstrate free air and air-fluid levels. Neonatal obstructions are classified as high or low. Obstructions that occur proximal to the middle ileum are called high or upper intestinal obstructions. Obstructions that involve the distal ileum or colon are called low intestinal obstructions. The distinction is critical because children with high obstructions usually need little or no radiologic evaluation after plain radiographs, and the specific diagnosis is made in the operating room. Newborns with low obstructions need a contrast enema, which usually provides a specific diagnosis and may be therapeutic. In older children, some authors prefer to start the abdominal investigation with US, because abdominal X-ray has less accuracy for usual pathologies (appendicitis, intussusception [IT], obstruction)

and inherent radiation risk. Because abdominal symptoms are occasionally referred from lower lobe chest pathology, the diaphragmatic area should be adequately depicted on plain films.

Contrast examination, usually with barium, is a primary technique and widely used (despite its low index accuracy/cost benefits) because of the limitations of endoscopy in depicting the small bowel pathologies and the current decreased availability of MR enterography exams. The goal of barium examination is to establish the presence or absence and the nature of the disease with a minimal radiation dose. The transit time takes a mean of 70 minutes. Rarely used today, an enteroclysis examination can depict the entire small bowel, including mucosal detail and smaller luminal defects. The use of MRI to do the same is currently being investigated.

On cross-sectional techniques, the small-bowel wall is thin, usually less than 3 to 4 mm.

By US, the bowel wall appears mostly as a hypoechoic band limited by two hyperechoic surfaces and divided by a hyperechoic line, which is the submucosa. Sonography may visualize five concentric layers of alternating echogenic/hypoechoic layers from the lumen outward (**Fig. 2.75**).

MRI and CT are indicated to determine the extent of a lesion for masses and trauma, provide important 3D information about the extraluminal component of bowel disease, the relationships to adjacent organs, as well as vascular information. Accurate imaging of the small bowel requires the administration of both intravenous and oral contrast medium, sometimes by enteroclysis.

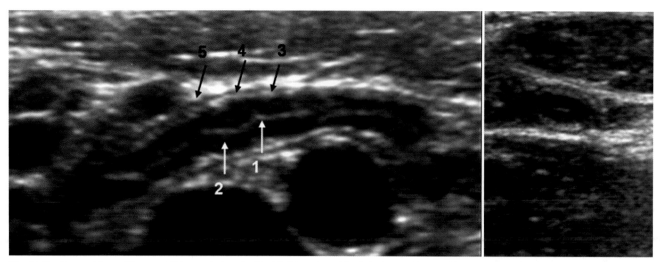

Fig. 2.75 Normal bowel layers. US image in longitudinal (left) and axial (right) planes of normal bowel (appendix) shows the normal layered appearance that can be seen in any location in a GI tube.
1 hyperechoic mucosal surface
2 hypoechoic mucosa
3 hyperechoic submucosa
4 hypoechoic muscular
5 hyperechoic serosa

Table 2.40	Normal bowel wall layers seen by US
First echogenic layer	*Mucosal surface*: Interface between the lumen contents and mucosa.
Second hypoechoic layer	*Mucosa*: Deeper mucosa and muscularis mucosae.
Third echogenic layer	*Submucosa*: Submucosa and inner muscularis propria.
Fourth hypoechoic layer	*Muscular*: Middle to deep muscularis propria.
Fifth echogenic layer	*Serosa*: Interface between serosa and adjacent tissue.

Duodenum

Table 2.41	The duodenum mucosal wall changes and filling defects	
Diagnosis	**Findings**	**Comments**
Duodenitis ▷ *Fig. 2.76*	Coarse and transverse thickening of the folds.	Involvement of the stomach is frequent. Crohn disease.
Duodenal ulcer ▷ *Fig. 2.77*	Area of localized swelling with central crater, converging folds where there is scarring.	Clinical symptoms unreliable. Multiple ulcers are frequent. Endoscopy.
Benign polyps	Filling defects of variable size, single or multiple. Mostly at the region of the duodenal bulb or at the inferior portion of the duodenal loop.	Differentiation is only possible histologically. Ectopic pancreas may be present. Malignant tumors have not been described in children.
Foreign bodies	UGI: may delineate a nonopaque foreign body.	Hair clips, peanuts, hot dogs, etc. Danger of perforation.
Erosive duodenitis	Filling defects with punctuate depressions.	Colicky abdominal pain.
Gastric, bulbar, and duodenal varices	Round, oval impressions in the bulb and/or duodenum; alteration with change in position on the contrast examination.	Portal hypertension.

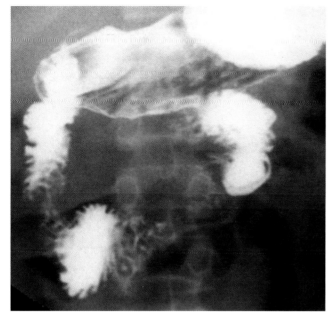

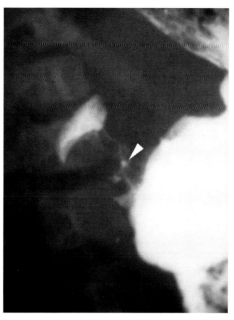

Fig. 2.76 Duodenal ulcer. Two small ulcers (aphtha) with a central barium-filled hole and rounded peripheral edema are seen in the third duodenal portion in a patient with Crohn disease.

Fig. 2.77 Duodenal ulcer. An additional image (arrowhead) is seen in the pyloric channel, with peripheral edema.

Table 2.42 Duodenal atresia and stenosis

Diagnosis	Findings	Comments
Duodenal atresia	X-ray: "double bubble" sign. Rarely require further radiologic investigation and most patients are taken directly to surgery.	Most frequent cause of complete duodenal obstruction. Sixty percent are premature. Thirty percent have Down syndrome. DD: annular pancreas, midgut volvulus, duodenal web, Ladd band, preduodenal portal vein.
Congenital duodenal stenosis ▷ *Fig. 2.78, p. 192*	X-ray: dilatation of the stomach and duodenum with a normal or diminished amount of air in the small bowel. UGI series: necessary to differentiate between midgut volvulus and partial duodenal obstruction caused by a web or stenosis, etc. US: to rule out midgut volvulus ("whirlpool" sign) and extraluminal causes (duplication cyst, etc.).	Causes of partial duodenal obstruction: duodenal web, Ladd bands, annular pancreas, midgut volvulus, preduodenal portal vein, duplication cyst, and superior mesenteric artery compression.
Traumatic duodenal hematoma	Intramural lesion narrowing the duodenal lumen.	Due to fall, for example, onto bicycle handlebars.
Postoperative changes	Narrowed caliber with proximal dilatation. Paucity of small-bowel air.	Disparity of bowel caliper after removing stenotic or atretic segment may remain after surgical repair.
Superior mesenteric artery compression	Lineal abrupt intermittent obstruction of the third duodenal portion depending on patient position.	Small angle between aorta and the mesentery artery in a thin patient (body cast). May be familial.

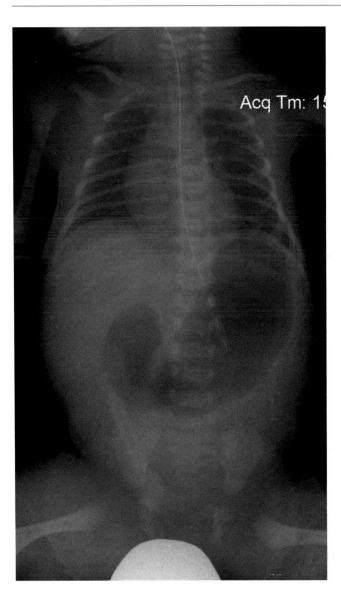

Fig. 2.78   Duodenal web. The classic "double-bubble" image is depicted, with distention of the stomach and the duodenum proximal to the stenotic area, located in the fourth portion. No distal air is seen in this film, which was taken 6 hours after birth.

Table 2.43   The duodenum: Diverticula and duplications

Diagnosis	Findings	Comments
Duplication ▷ *Fig. 2.79a–c*	Contrast examinations: the duodenum compressed by intramural mass in the duodenal c-loop ("beak" sign). US: cystic image with echogenic inner rim and outer hypoechoic muscle layers ("double-halo" sign) is highly suggestive.	Usually noncommunicating and located along the first and second portion of the duodenum on the mesenteric side. Clinically: Symptoms of obstruction. They may cause biliary obstruction and pancreatitis.
Congenital diverticulum ▷ *Fig. 2.80*	In antimesenteric side.	May be multiple.

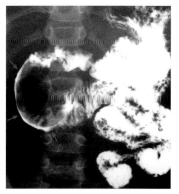
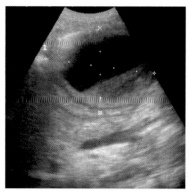
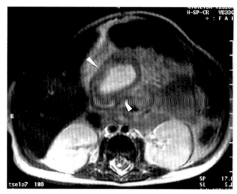

a   b   c

Fig. 2.79   Duodenal duplication. (a) UGI series: The C-shaped duodenum is widened by a rounded mass. The lumen is compressed, but contrast passage is not blocked. **(b)** US shows the cystic mass. The clue to the diagnosis is the layered appearance of the wall ("double-wall" sign). The content has a fluid-fluid level. **(c)** T2-weighted MRI shows the cystic mass with wall identical to the rest of the bowel (arrowheads).

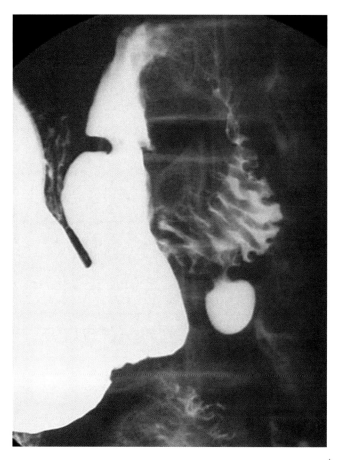

Fig. 2.80   Duodenal diverticulum. UGI series shows a diverticulum of the third portion.

■ Small Bowel

Table 2.44   Displacement or separation of loops of small bowel

Diagnosis	Findings	Comments
Inflammatory, vascular, and development diseases	Thickened bowel wall.	Crohn disease, Henoch-Schönlein purpura, lymphangiectasia.
Morbid obesity		
Ascites	Supine abdominal radiograph: generalized high density, central position of bowel loops, and separated bowel luminogram (differentiate from thickened bowel wall or increased content).	
Masses and tumors	Usually focal displacement depending on tumor origin.	Due to generalized lymphadenopathy (leukemia, Hodgkin disease), mesenteric cysts, inflammatory masses in Crohn disease, ovarian tumors, small bowel exophytic tumors, etc.

Table 2.45 Diminished or absent air in the small bowel

Diagnosis	Findings	Comments
Proximal Mechanical Obstruction ▷ *Fig. 2.55, p. 178*	Distal absent bowel air. DD with distal obstructions with bowel loops filled. Upright X-ray can show air-fluid levels.	Congenital: esophageal atresia types I, II, and IIIa (no fistulous connection with the dilated esophagus), duodenal atresia, agastria, pyloric atresia. Scaphoid abdomen.
Proximal Functional Obstruction		
Neonates and infants	Absent or diminished air/content in the small and large bowel. Normal GI tract may be patent insufflating air through a nasogastric tube.	Poor sucking and swallowing. Prematurity, perinatal brain anoxia, severe RDS, parenteral hyperalimentation, maternal medication (e.g., sedation during delivery).
All age groups		Frequent vomiting of any etiology, poor swallowing (consumption).

Table 2.46 Small-bowel distention: Neonates

Diagnosis	Findings	Comments
High small-bowel obstruction (SBO) ▷ *Fig. 2.81*	Abdominal X-ray: three or four air bubbles (more than in duodenal atresia and fewer than in ileal atresia). An upper GI series is clearly not indicated. In cases of doubt, aspiration and insufflation of air through a nasogastric tube. US: to differentiate multiple dilated loops filled with fluid from ascites in patients with lack of air on the plain radiograph.	Causes: atresia or stenosis of the jejunum or proximal ileum. Clinically: bilious vomiting (frequently delayed until after the first feeding), and abdominal distension. Normal barium enema.
Ileal atresia ▷ *Fig. 2.82a, b*	Plain X-ray: numerous dilated loops of bowel occupying the entire abdominal cavity. Meconium may be noted in the distal ileal loops. Contrast enema is mandatory: the colon is normally placed but has an abnormally small caliber (functional microcolon) (DD with colonic atresia).	Fifty percent of small bowel atresias. Intraperitoneal calcifications, indicative of meconium peritonitis, are not uncommon in ileal atresia. Pneumoperitoneum contraindicates colon examination.
Congenital short gut	Shortened narrow caliper bowel.	Anomalous mesenteric position, possibly associated with malrotation. Failure to thrive.
Meconium ileus ▷ *Fig. 2.83*	US: hyperechoic intestinal content (DD with ileal atresia). Contrast enema: microcolon with multiple small filling defects (meconium pellets). Therapeutic enema (high osmolar, nonionic water-soluble agents are the best choice) to help the passage of the sticky meconium relieving obstruction and avoiding surgery.	Low intestinal obstruction produced by impaction of abnormal meconium in the distal ileum. Almost always in cystic fibrosis. The diagnosis may be confirmed by finding an increased concentration of sodium chloride in sweat.

(continues on page 196)

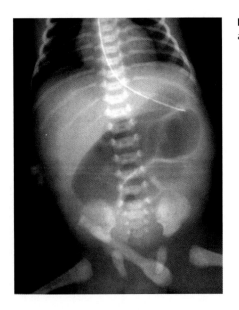

Fig. 2.81 Jejunal atresia. Supine radiograph shows a few dilated air-filled intestinal loops, about four "bubbles," which indicates a high obstruction. No distal air is seen.

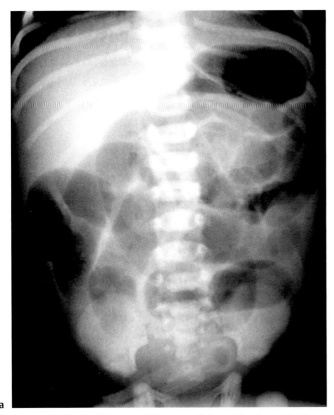

a

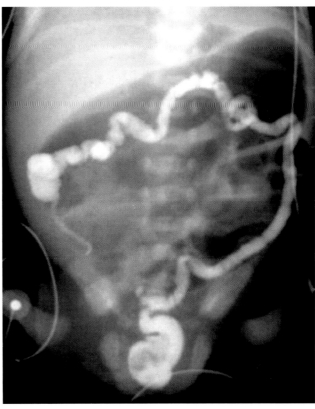

b

Fig. 2.82a, b   Ileal atresia. (a) Supine abdominal radiograph shows multiple dilated air-filled bowel loops occupying the entire abdominal cavity. With any degree of distention, it is impossible to differentiate the small bowel from the colon. **(b)** Contrast enema outlines the small size of the colon corresponding to an unused colon.

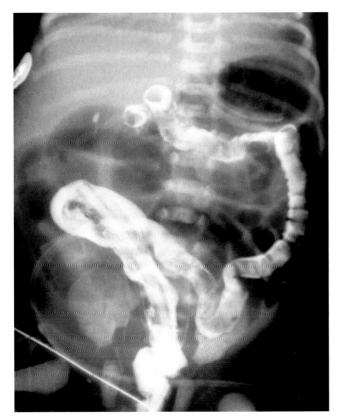

Fig. 2.83   Meconium ileus. Water-soluble contrast enema shows a microcolon with scattered filling defects that correspond to inspissated meconium.

Table 2.46   (Cont.) Small-bowel distention

Diagnosis	Findings	Comments
Meconium peritonitis with bowel obstruction ▷ *Fig. 2.84* ▷ *Fig. 2.85*	Abdominal X-ray: linear or punctate calcifications over the serosal surfaces of the abdominal viscera. Distended loops of the bowel with air-fluid levels may be present due to the underlying intestinal obstruction. Ascites may be present.	In utero perforation of fetal GI tract during the last 6 months of pregnancy. If perforation is patent at birth, free air will be seen in the peritoneal cavity or trapped in a walled-off loculus or pseudocyst.
Functional immaturity of the colon: meconium plug syndrome and small left colon syndrome	Low bowel obstruction. Contrast enema: narrow (micro) descending colon. Diagnose and treat with contrast enemas. Typically, there is clinical improvement after the enema.	Premature infants. Both entities are associated with dysmotility of the colon. Causes: diabetic mothers, septicemia, hypothyroidism, and hypoglycemia. DD: meconium ileus and Hirschsprung disease.
Functional ileus of prematurity	Bowel distention usually is less severe than in organic obstruction. Few air-fluid levels.	Temporary poor intestinal function during the first days of life (immaturity of the neural plexus).
Necrotizing enterocolitis (NEC)	Abdominal X-ray: gaseous distention and thickened bowel walls. *Pneumatosis intestinalis* (submucosal or subserosal air). May be linear (submucosal) or cystic collections (subserosal). Portal vein gas: finely branching radiolucencies from the porta hepatis to the periphery of the liver.	Premature infants, within the first 2 weeks of life. See **Figs. 2.112** to **2.116** and **Table 2.54**.

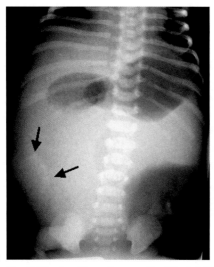 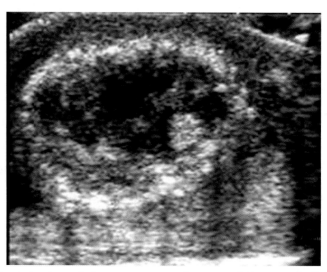

a   b

Fig. 2.84a, b   Meconium peritonitis. (a) Abdominal radiograph demonstrates a small amount of air in a markedly distended abdomen. A calcified mass within the peritoneal cavity is observed (arrows). There is no pneumoperitoneum. **(b)** Sonography of the same patient shows a pseudocyst containing debris with peripheral calcification.

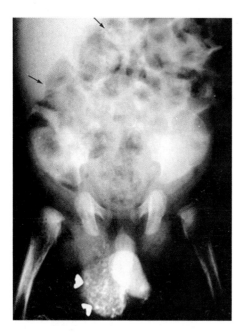

Fig. 2.85   Meconium peritonitis with calcified meconium in the scrotum. Plain radiograph at birth shows scattered areas of calcification in the scrotum (arrowheads). Small flakes of intra-abdominal calcifications are also observed (arrows).

Table 2.47   Small-bowel distention: Infants, toddlers, and older children

Diagnosis	Findings	Comments
Prominent intestinal air	Slightly dilated bowel loops.	Caused by long bouts of crying in young children. Distended stomach predominance.
Mechanical obstruction (SBO)	Disparity in size between obstructed proximal and distal bowel loops. Hyperactive peristalsis/aperistalsis ("fatigued" small bowel). Supine X-ray: progressive increase in luminal fluid/gas relation leads to sequential features: "stretch sign," "stepladder appearance," and "string of beads." In cases of fluid-filled intestine without air, SBO may be overlooked in supine X-ray films.	All age groups. Complete SBO: colon empties in 12–24 h. Supine X-ray has sensitivity of less than 50% in SBO.
Mechanical obstruction (SBO): Extrinsic bowel lesions		
Hernia ▷ *Fig. 2.86a, b*	Soft-tissue density or abnormal gas over the herniary orifice.	Usually inguinal, umbilical, spigelian, etc.
Adhesions and congenital bands	Angulated and fixed bowel segment. US and CT: "beak sign" at the point of obstruction.	Commonly in ileum.
Large masses		Duplication cyst, neoplasm, abscess. Meckel diverticulum.
Midgut volvulus ▷ *Fig. 2.87a–d, p. 198* ▷ *Fig. 2.88a–c, p. 199*	"Whirlpool" sign: twisting of the gut and mesentery around the superior mesenteric arterial axis.	Malrotation. Arrest of rotation and fixation of intestine. Fatal strangulation: 3.5 mesenteric turns
Mechanical obstruction (SBO): Luminal occlusion		
Small bowel intussusception (IT) ▷ *Fig. 2.89, p. 199*	Coiled-spring appearance on contrast exams. Cross-sectional methods: "crescent-in-doughnut" sign (axial images) and "sandwich" sign (longitudinal). Ileocecal valve not involved.	Usually transient, asymptomatic, mobile, and smaller (< 3 × 2 cm) than ileocolic intussesception. Frequent in sprue and enteritis. Consider surgery in cases with peritoneal trapped fluid, lead point (polyp, lymphoma, Meckel), obstruction, or when longer than 3.5 cm.

(continues on page 200)

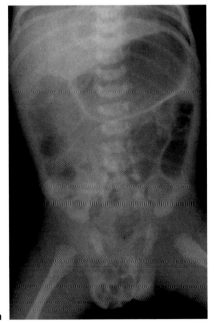
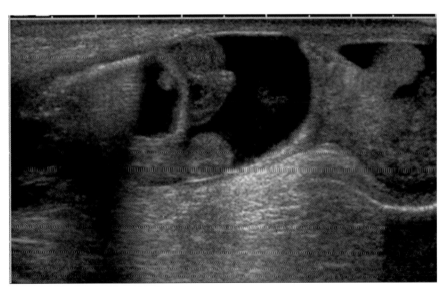

a

b

Fig. 2.86a, b   Inguinal hernia. (a) Plain abdominal film shows bowel loops inside the right scrotum; a mild proximal bowel dilatation is seen. **(b)** Scrotal longitudinal US shows the scrotal hernia with ascitis and bowel loops inside the iguinal channel superior to the scrotal content.

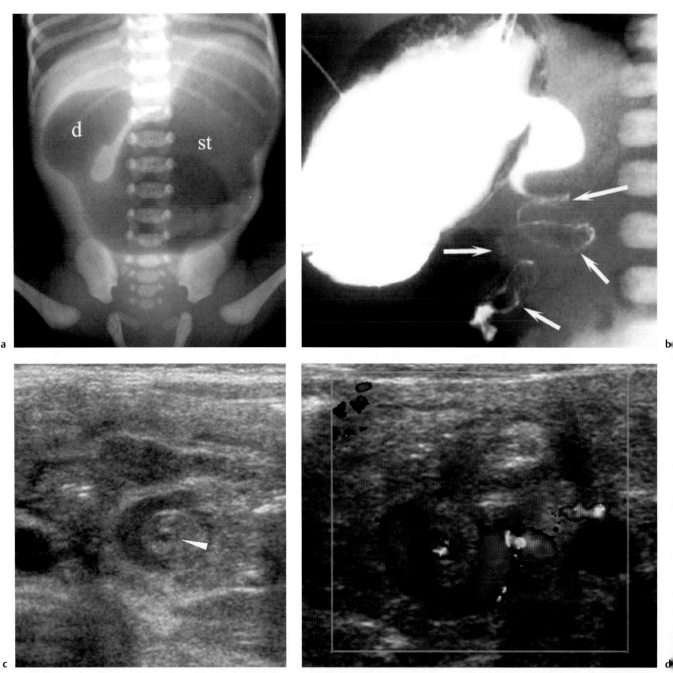

Fig. 2.87a–d Midgut volvulus. A 12-day-old girl with bilious vomiting. (**a**) Plain abdominal film with "double bubble" sign in a neonate with a complete duodenal obstruction. Note the dilated stomach and duodenum. (**b**) UGI series that shows the pathognomonic "corkscrew appearance" (arrows). (**c**) Transverse B-mode sonography of the upper abdomen shows the twisting of bowel, mesentery, and superior mesenteric vein around the axis of superior mesenteric artery (arrowhead). (**d**) Color Doppler image demonstrates a circle of vascularity that represents the superior mesenteric vein twisting around the superior mesenteric artery, producing the characteristic "whirlpool" sign.

d duodenum
st stomach

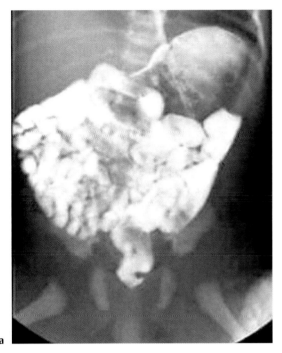

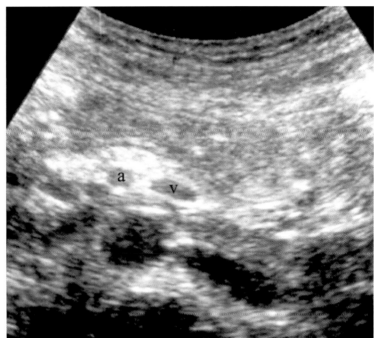

a

b

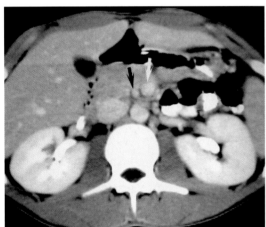

c

Fig. 2.88a–c Intestinal malrotation. (**a**) UGI series demonstrates the small intestine located in the right hemiabdomen and the colon in the left, corresponding to a nonrotation. (**b**) Transverse sonogram that shows the superior mesenteric vein lying to the left of the superior mesenteric artery. (**c**) Contrast-enhanced CT scan shows the same findings as an US. Note the superior mesenteric artery (black arrow) and superior mesenteric vein (white arrow).

a superior mesenteric artery
v superior mesenteric vein

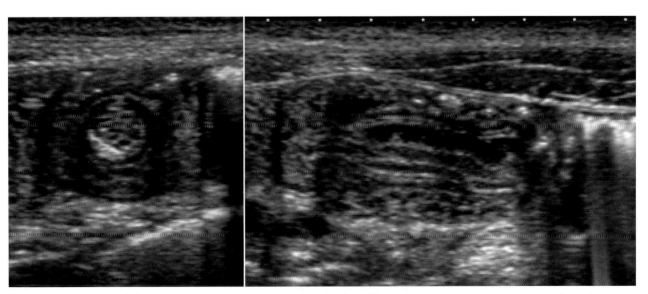

Fig. 2.89 Transient small bowel intussesception. US images: As an incidental finding in an asymptomatic patient, a transient intussesception is found. A small crescent-in-doughnut image (less than 2 cm) is seen in the transverse image (left). In the longitudinal scan (right), the intussesception is short with no lymphadenopathies inside. During the scan, peristalsis is seen inside the intussesception.

Table 2.47   (Cont.) Small-bowel distention: Infants, toddlers, and older children

Diagnosis	Findings	Comments
Foreign bodies		
Bezoars	Inhomogeneous filling defect.	Lactobezoar (inspissated milk: highly concentrated prepared milk formula), fitobezoar, trichobezoar.
Bolus of Ascaris lumbricoides ▷ *Fig. 2.90*	Elongated densities in the intestinal lumen.	Contrast ingested by the worms will outline their digestive tract.
Tumor (rare)		Mostly polyps.
Meconium ileus equivalent	Large amount of stools. Inspissated feces.	In teenagers with cystic fibrosis particularly caused by postfebrile dehydration. Stercoral ulcers predispose to perforation.
Mechanical obstruction (SBO): Intrinsic lesion of the bowel wall		
Inflammatory stricture	Smooth edges. Multiple stenotic lesions in Crohn disease.	Crohn disease, tuberculosis (TB) enteritis, NEC, irradiation.
Congenital stricture	Microcolon distal to stenosis.	
Hemorrhage	(see **Table 2.48**)	Blunt trauma, Henoch-Schönlein purpura.
Neoplastic stricture	Irregular abrupt edges.	Lymphoma rarely produce stricture. Carcinoma and Gastrointestinal stromal tumors are uncommon.
Complicated mechanical obstruction (SBO): Strangulated obstruction	Edema and hemorrhage of the bowel wall with peritoneal fluid. If necrosis develops, gas may be present in the bowel wall, portal venous system, and in the peritoneal cavity (patent perforation). Supine X-ray: "coffee-bean" sign (gas-filled loop excluded) and "pseudotumor" sign (fluid-filled loop). "Whirl" sign (twisting of bowel and mesentery) on cross-sectional imaging.	Mechanical obstruction with interruption of arterial blood supply. Closed-loop obstruction: bowel obstruction at two points. Caused by: volvulus, incarcerated hernia, adherences, etc.
Adynamic-paralytic ileus	Generalized dilatation (including stomach and rectum) with normal folds and air-fluid levels. "Sentinel loop" if ileus is localized.	No need for surgery.
Intra-abdominal inflammation/ infection ▷ *Fig. 2.91*		Appendicitis, peritonitis, pancreatitis. Gastroenteritis (hyperperistalsis often detected on US). Perforation.
Extra-abdominal disease		Pneumonia, pleuritis, discitis.
Systemic disease		Sepsis, urticaria, diabetes, hypothyroidism, porphyria, neuromuscular disorders.
Drug and electrolyte imbalance	Delayed small bowel transit < 6 h.	Anticholinergic: atropine, morphine derivatives, glucagon, chemotherapy. Hypokalemia.
Postoperative	Pneumoperitoneum may be associated.	Previous history. Usually resolves by fourth day.
Malabsorption syndromes: Celiac disease (sprue) and lactase deficiency	Fluid distended loops of the small bowel (hypotonic) with normal fold thickness and some air-fluid levels due to secretions. See **Table 2.48**.	Sprue: Malabsorption due to gluten intolerance. Atrophy of folds. Intestinal biopsy confirmatory. Lactase deficiency: Addition to lactose to the barium contrast reproduces symptoms and malabsorptive findings.
Visceral pain		Ureteral stone, ovarian torsion, trauma.
Vascular compromise or disease	Dilatation and regular thickened mucosal folds.	Vascular insufficiency: venous or arterial occlusion, low cardiac output. Acute radiation enteritis. Henoch-Schönlein purpura.
Pseudoobstruction		Transient (electrolyte imbalance, renal or heart failure) or chronic idiopathic (females).

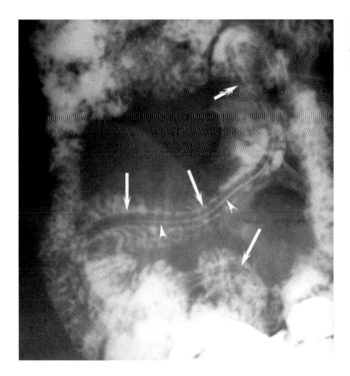

Fig. 2.90   Ascariasis. Barium examination shows the ascaris worms as elongated tubular filling defects (arrows). The intestines of the worm are seen as stringlike white densities outlined by ingested barium (arrowheads).

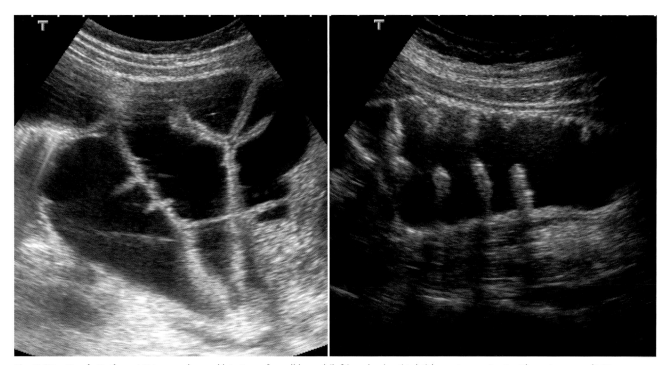

Fig. 2.91   Paralytic ileus. US image shows dilatation of small-bowel (left) and colon (right) loops in a patient with acute appendicitis.

Table 2.48   The small bowel: Diffuse parietal involvement

Diagnosis	Findings	Comments
Edema ▷ *Fig. 2.92*	Regular thickening of the bowel wall with smooth folds.	Hypoproteinemia (cirrhosis, nephrotic syndrome, GI protein loss). Dilated bowel if albumin < 2.7 g/dL. Increased capillary permeability (gastroenteritis). Portal venous hypertension.
Hemorrhage ▷ *Fig. 2.93* ▷ *Fig. 2.94a, b*	Usually thickened smooth folds, but occasionally irregular folds, scalloping, and thumbprinting may be seen. Henoch-Schönlein purpura (nephritis, abdominal and joint pain) causes effacement small bowel wall layers (on US) and anechoic ascites. Often transient small-bowel IT and lymphadenopathy may be seen. Rarely affects the colon (DD hemolytic-uremic syndrome).	Ischemia, trauma. Vasculitis (connective tissue diseases, Henoch-Schönlein purpura, irradiation). Hypocoagulability (drugs, hemophilia, idiopathic thrombocytopenic purpura, neoplastic bleeding diathesis). Graft versus host disease.
Infection ▷ *Fig. 2.95a, b*	Hyperperistaltic intestine. Transient intussesception. Late stage: Thickened bowel wall with regular/irregular folds, depending of the infectious agent and the evolution stage. Rarely ascites.	Generalized or jejunal predominance: Nonspecific viruses. Rotavirus, Giardiasis (protozoan). AIDS-related infection (cryptosporidium, *Mycobacterium avium* complex). Terminal ileitis: *Yersinia enterocolitica*, *Salmonella*, TB.
Inflammation: Crohn disease ▷ *Fig. 2.96a–d, p. 204* ▷ *Fig. 2.97a–c, p. 205*	Granular and linear ulcerations (cobblestone pattern), thickening of bowel wall with submucosal enlargement followed by loss of the stratification in fibrous rigid narrow segments. Fistulas, abscesses, fibrofatty proliferation of the mesentery, and lymphadenopathies separating the bowel loops.	Chronic idiopathic disease related to immunologic disorder in predisposed genetic patients, post GI infection in some cases. May affect any part of the GI tract, particularly the terminal ileum. Discontinuity (skip lesions), transmural and mesenteric involvement, ulceration, and fistula are characteristic.
Neoplasia	Variable patterns: Dilatation, thickened smooth/irregular folds. Masses. Strictures. Pseudoaneurysmal loop.	Lymphoma, pseudolymphoma.
Malabsorptive syndromes	Increased intraluminal fluid with dilution and flocculation of oral contrast agent.	
Celiac disease ▷ *Fig. 2.98a, b, p. 205*	Dilatation and hypomotility. Excessive fluid in dilated small bowel with no fold thickening, (except at the duodenojejunal area) with normal fold pattern in the ileum ("jejunization of the ileum"): reversal of the jejunoileal fold pattern. Transient intussesceptions.	Sprue: Malabsorption due to gluten intolerance. Atrophy of the intestinal villi and folds. Small bowel flaccid and poorly contracting. Some air-fluid levels. Intestinal biopsy confirmatory. Complication: diffuse intestinal lymphoma.

(continues on page 206)

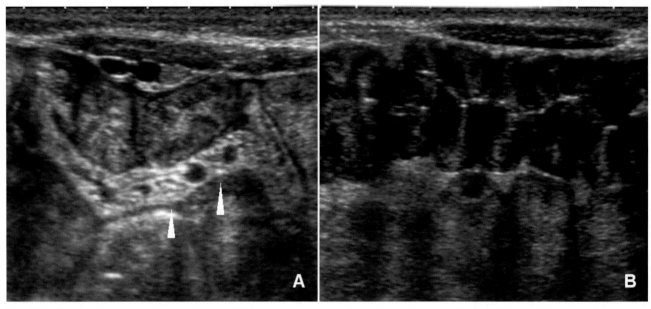

Fig. 2.92   Bowel edema in portal hypertension. US image shows edema of small bowel (**a**) and colon (**b**). Note in (**a**) that mesenteric edema is also present (arrowheads).

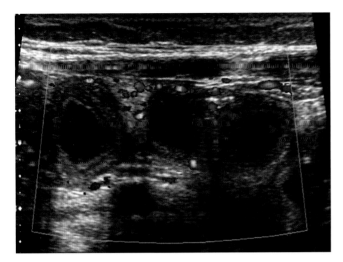

Fig. 2.93 Bowel hemorrhage in a patient with Henoch-Schönlein purpura. Doppler US shows vascularized, fluid-filled small-bowel loops with parietal thickening.

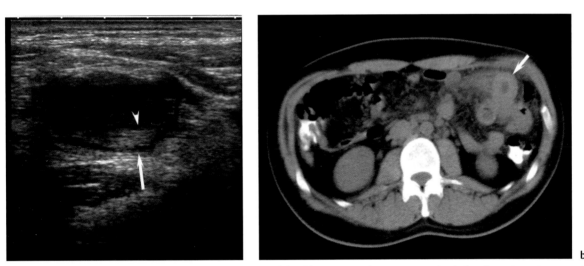

a b

Fig. 2.94a, b Intramural hematoma in a boy with hemophilia. (**a**) Sonogram (transverse section) of an ileum loop shows marked bowel wall thickening (arrow and arrowhead) with poorly defined wall stratification. (**b**) Unenhanced CT scan shows circumferential thickening in cross-section of ileal wall (arrow) with adjacent stranding of mesentery.

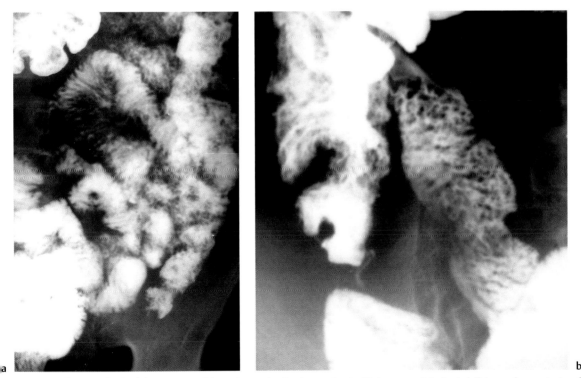

a b

Fig. 2.95a, b Giardiasis. (**a**) Barium small-bowel examination in a patient with immunoglobulin A deficiency demonstrates dilution of barium and an apparent fold thickening. (**b**) The same patient shows a fine nodular pattern at the terminal ileum.

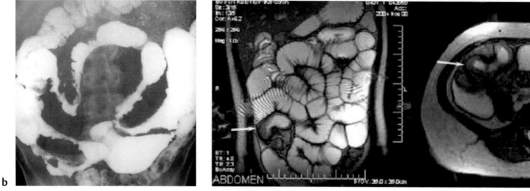

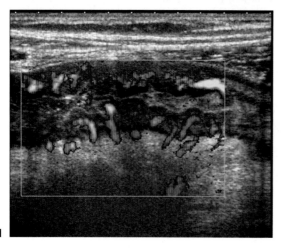

Fig. 2.96a–d   Crohn disease. (a) Barium small-bowel examinations. (**1**) Aphtha (arrows) in the proximal jejunum with more advanced disease is found distally (not shown). (**2**) Transversely oriented linear ulcers (fissures) are a frequent finding in Crohn disease. (**3**) Many linear and transverse ulcerations separating islands of protruding mucosa are present and give rise to a cobblestone appearance. (**b**) Barium small-bowel examination shows extensive ulcerated Crohn disease with ulcers, thickened folds, strictured segments, pseudodiverticula, and mesenteric involvement. (**c**) True fast imaging with steady state precession MRI (coronal: left; axial: right) demonstrates bowel wall thickening at the distal ileum (arrows) and a slight distortion of the bowel folds. (**d**) Doppler sonogram demonstrates an increased flow in the affected intestinal segment.

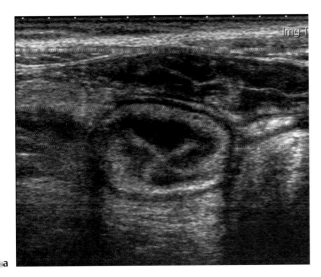

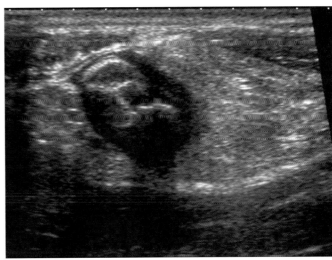

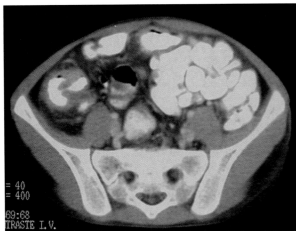

Fig. 2.97a–c Crohn disease of the terminal ileum. (**a**) US axial image shows transmural regular thickening with conspicuous submucosal layer. (**b**) In another area, with more advanced stage, the wall thickening is asymmetric with irregular mucosal surface due to ulcerations. The mesentery is also affected. (**c**) CT shows the ileocecal region with the valve rigid and open and parietal thickening both the caecum and the terminal ilium.

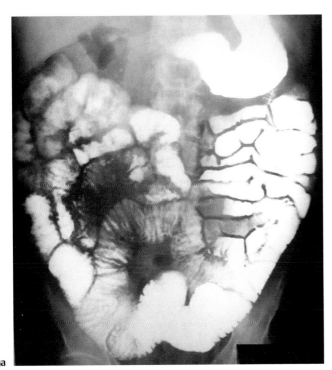

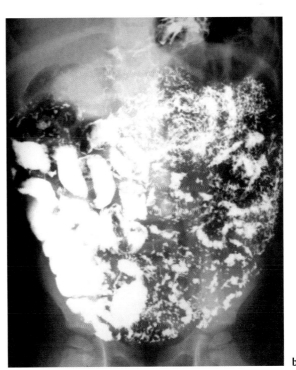

Fig. 2.98a, b Celiac disease. (**a**) Barium small-bowel examination shows dilatation with hypersecretion and flocculation. There is an increase of normal fold pattern in the ileum ("jejunization of the ileum") and their reduction in the jejunum ("moulage" sign). Hypomotility was demonstrated fluoroscopically. (**b**) Barium examination shows severe flocculation and segmentation of the barium as a consequence of a very slow transit.

Table 2.48   (Cont.) The small bowel: Diffuse parietal involvement

Diagnosis	Findings	Comments
Lactase deficiency	Addition to lactose to the barium contrast reproduces symptoms and malabsorptive findings.	Hydrogen breath test.
Connective tissue diseases (rare)	Hypomotility and "hidebound" sign of the folds (close together) due to the wall atrophy.	Symptoms depend on the type of autoimmune disease.
Food allergy or food intolerance	Bowel loops separated by edema of the wall and mesentery. Hypersecretion.	Allergic (food intolerance type IV) or immunologic etiology. Eosinophilia. GI symptoms related to ingestion of specific foods. Self-limiting nature. Steroid therapy response.
Eosinophilic enteritis	Usually thickened irregular mucosal folds with jejunum predominance and concomitant gastric involvement. Rigidity, separation of the bowel loops, and hyperplastic lymph nodes may simulate Crohn disease.	
Lymphangiectasia	Edematous regular thickening of small bowel mucosal folds (due to lymphatic dilatation and protein loss) with no evidence of liver, kidney, or heart disease is suggestive.	Primary or secondary (inflammatory or neoplastic lymph nodes) block lymphatic outflow.
Whipple disease	Duodenal and jejunal thickened irregular distorted folds. Large hypoechoic/hypodense bulky lymphadenopathy in the mesentery and retroperitoneum is very characteristic.	Arthritis, fever, and lymphadenopathy may precede diarrhea. Macrophages and glycoprotein granules are positive for periodic acid–Schiff in the lamina propria. It is caused by *Tropheryma whippleii*, a Gram-positive bacilli. Revert to postantibiotic therapy.
Cystic fibrosis ▷ *Fig. 2.99*	Thickened mucosal folds in proximal jejunum associated with duodenal findings (thickened coarse fold pattern: nodular, poor defined folds, kinking, and distortion of duodenum).	Associate changes in the liver, bile ducts, and pancreas (see **Tables 2.15** and **2.17**). Adherent collections of viscous mucus, hyperplastic appearance of the colon mucosa. Residual thick secretions.
Lymphoma ▷ *Fig. 2.100* ▷ *Fig. 2.101a, b*	Localized in a segment (75%) usually ileum, multifocal (polyp/stenosis) or diffuse (thick or obliterated folds). Exophytic and mesenteric masses. Aneurysmal dilatation (slough of the necrotic core of a large mass).	Primary or secondary. Possible enlargement of mesenteric and retroperitoneal lymph nodes.
Alpha-beta-lipoproteinemia	Dilatation and moderate regular thickness of the small bowel.	Rare inherited malabsorption of fat, neurologic deterioration and retinitis pigmentosa.
Xanthomatosis	Regular thickness of the small bowel.	Multicentric proliferation of lipid-laden cells is initially a cutaneous disorder.
Giardiasis ▷ *Fig. 2.90, p. 201*	Irregular thickness of the small bowel due to the infiltration of inflammatory cells most apparent in the duodenum and jejunum. Hypermotility, secretions.	Acute gastroenteritis (GE), malabsorption syndrome associated with GI immunodeficiency syndrome. Characteristic cyst in the mucus (smear/bowel biopsies).
Other		Radiation injury. Mastocytosis. Mucositis.

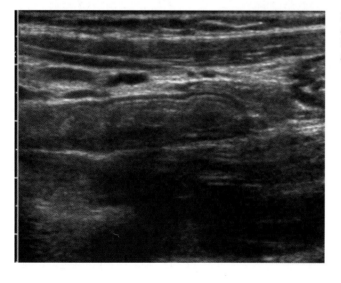

Fig. 2.99   Cystic fibrosis. Longitudinal US of the appendix shows dilatation of lumen due to inspissated mucus and feces. The incidentally increased diameter of the appendix (> 6 mm) must not be interpreted as a sign of acute appendicitis.

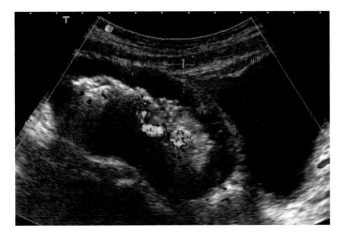

Fig. 2.100   Small bowel Burkitt lymphoma. Longitudinal Doppler US scan shows a pseudokidney image cranial to the bladder.

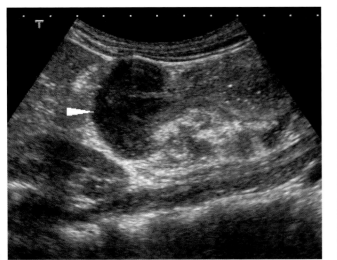

a

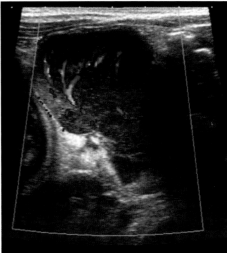

b

Fig. 2.101a, b   Small bowel non-Hodgkin lymphoma with intussusception. (a) Longitudinal image in the right flank shows an ileocolic intussesception with a hypoechoic mass at the apex (arrowhead), located in the subhepatic area. (b) Hypervascular lymph nodes are seen in the mesogastric area in the Doppler US image.

Table 2.49 The small bowel: Focal parietal involvement and filling defects (solitary)

Diagnosis	Findings	Comments
Duplication cyst	Smooth margins	(see **Table 2.48**)
Benign Tumors (rare)		
Mesenchymal tumors	Luminal smooth defect. Variable echogenicity, density, and homogenicity depending on cellularity (fat) and ulceration/necrosis (if large).	Fibroma, leiomyofibroma, fibromyoma, GIST, etc. Gross pathologic diagnosis. Intraluminal, parietal, or extrinsic masses.
Adenomyoma		Duodenum, jejunum.
Polypoid lesions	Polyplike appearance.	Often cause small-bowel intussesception.
Malignant Tumors		
Non-Hodgkin lymphoma (see Table 2.45)	Multiple coarse, nodular outline of the lumen; wall infiltration with long segment narrowing of the lumen; polypoid form has a tendency to intussesception, endoenteric and exoenteric types with crater and fistula formation; tumor infiltration in the mesentery with a spruelike appearance.	Depicted accurately on cross-sectional imaging techniques.
Carcinoid	Parietal ileal small lesion with desmoplastic response (kinking and rigidity of the bowel, mesentery, and vessels).	Elevated 5-indolacetic acid. Scintigraphy with (123) I-MIBG is diagnostic.

Table 2.50 The small bowel: Multifocal parietal involvement and filling defects (multiple)

Diagnosis	Findings	Comments
Polyposis syndromes	(see **Table 2.54**)	Peutz–Jeghers syndrome (hamartomatous): Hereditary. Oral and perioral pigmentosus. Intussusception. Anemia. Most frequent in the jejunum. Juvenile polyposis: predominantly colonic. Multiple simple adenomatous polyps. Gardner syndrome: diagnosis based on histology.
Hemangiomatosis		In Rendu-Osler syndrome.
Lymphangioma		US and MRI are diagnostic.
Malignant tumors		Lymphoma. Metastatic Wilms tumor (rare, filling defects impinges on the bowel lumen); intussesception.

Table 2.51 The small bowel: Diverticula and duplications

Diagnosis	Findings	Comments
Meckel diverticulum	Contrast demonstration of the diverticulum is rarely accomplished. May produce intussesception, obstruction, diverticulitis, and enterolith formation.	Remnant of the omphalomesenteric duct in the antimesenteric side. Ectopic gastric mucosa present in 30% of cases may cause hemorrhage (positive scintigraphy).
Duplications (enteric cysts, neurenteric cysts)	Barium examination: compression may produce a "beak" sign. On the mesenteric side US: a cystic image with echogenic inner rim and outer hypoechoic muscle layers ("double halo" sign) is highly suggestive of duplication. DD: choledochal cyst, pancreatic pseudocyst, and mesenteric cysts.	Most common location is the ileum, followed by the duodenum. May be cystic or tubular, the second being more frequent in the rectum. A cyst located in the ileum at the ileocecal junction can manifest as an intussesception.
Diverticulum	On the antimesenteric side.	Complication: infection, ulceration, and perforation.

Ileocecal Area

A large number of GI diseases can manifest as right lower quadrant (RLQ) acute pain, and some of them are potentially surgical. Knowledge of ileocecal region pathology is crucial in order to achieve an adequate differential diagnosis.

Table 2.52   Diseases of distal ileum, cecum, and appendix

Diagnosis	Findings	Comments
Acute appendicitis	(see **Table 2.68**)	
Ileocolic IT	(see **Table 2.68**)	Represents more than 95% of intussesception.
Enteritis		
Nonspecific enteritis: nodular lymphoid hyperplasia ▷ *Fig. 2.102* ▷ *Fig. 2.103*	Symmetric, fairly sharply demarcated, small mucosal follicles with central umbilication.	Mostly considered as a variant related to the immunization process.

(continues on page 210)

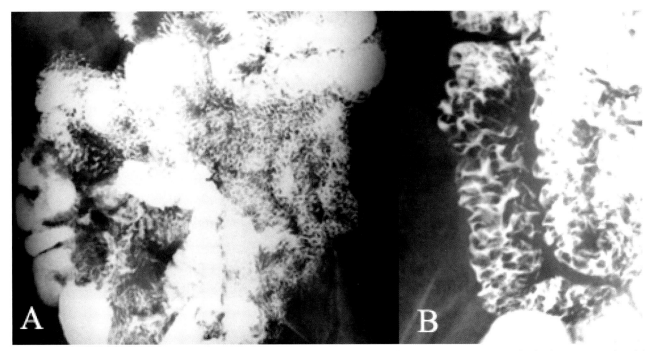

Fig. 2.102   Nodular lymphoid hyperplasia in a patient with hyperimmunoglobulin E syndrome. (a) Multiple discrete, round nodules throughout the small bowel are seen. **(b)** Irregular mucosal fold thickening with an added pattern of fine nodulation is noted.

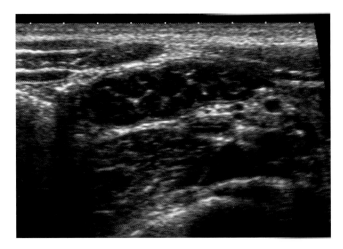

Fig. 2.103   Nodular lymphoid hyperplasia of ileum. Longitudinal US scan of terminal ileum is depicted between the abdominal wall muscles and psoas. The wall is slightly thickened with hypoechoic mucosal predominance. The serrated lumen is delineated by the hyperechoic mucosal surface.

Table 2.52 (Cont.) Diseases of distal ileum, cecum, and appendix

Diagnosis	Findings	Comments
Acute enteritis: acute terminal ileitis, ileocaequitis, nonsclerosing ileitis ▷ Fig. 2.104a, b ▷ Fig. 2.105	Symmetrical thickness due to mucosal lymphoid hyperplasia of the terminal ileum (Peyer patches). Cobblestone appearance or adenitis. Colonic involvement associated.	Clinically simulates appendicitis and radiologically simulates nonstenotic Crohn disease. Caused by *Yersinia enterocolitica* or *Campylobacter jejuni* (Gram-negative rod), *Salmonella typhosa* infection (typhoid fever) with splenomegaly, anisakiasis.
Chronic nonspecific enteritis: inflammatory disease (Crohn disease, ulcerative colitis)		
Chronic specific enteritis: bowel TB, amebiasis ▷ Fig. 2.106a, b		Mimics Crohn disease: more localized in the ileocecal region. Commonly, ileitis extends to the colon (coned cecum).
Acute agranulocytic cecal enteritis: typhlitis	Dilatation. Marked thickening of the bowel wall with submucosal (edema and hemorrhage) predominance can be observed. Thumbprinting. Risk of perforation.	Commonly in immunosuppressed leukemic therapy (second week). Necrotizing enteritis of the right colon and ileocecal region. Nonsurgical appendicitis.
Non-Hodgkin lymphoma (Burkitt)	(see **Table 2.45**)	Frequently secondary intussesception.
Complications postappendectomy	(see **Table 2.54**)	Appendiceal abscess. Stump.
Meckel diverticulum	(see **Table 2.48**)	

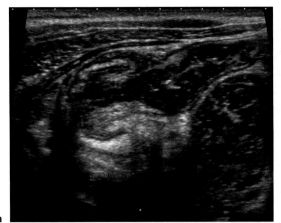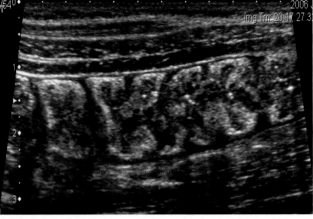

a   b

Fig. 2.104a, b Ileocecitis due to *Yersinia*. (a) Ileocecal area. **(b)** Ascending colon: US shows parietal thickening of the ileum, cecum, and ileocecal valve. The ileum predominates the hypoechoic follicular mucosal hyperplasia, although in the cecum the hyperechoic submucosal layer is dominant. In the ascending colon, an accordion appearance is seen.

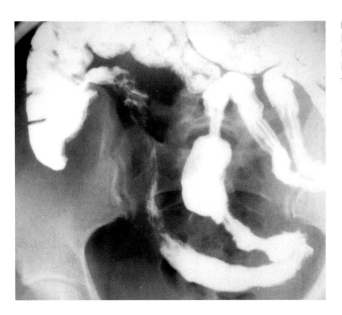

Fig. 2.105 Yersiniosis. Compression spot radiograph of a small-bowel examination in a patient with a self-limited diarrheal illness and RLQ pain shows fold thickening with nodulation and ulcers in the distal ileum. Differentiation from Crohn disease is impossible. Resolution of the disease with antibiotic treatment provided a definitive diagnosis.

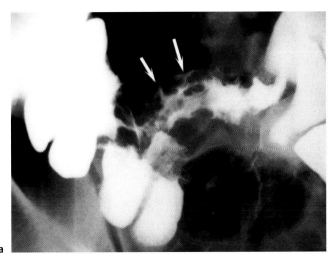
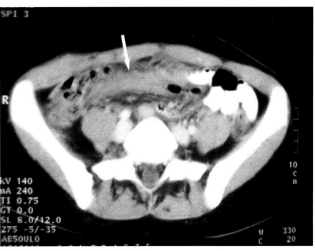

Fig. 2.106a, b Tuberculosis. (a) Compression spot radiograph of a small-bowel examination. Note the nodular and edematous appearance of the distal ileum. Ulceration (arrows) and medial cecal affec-

tation are present. **(b)** Contrast-enhanced CT scan shows bowel wall thickening in the distal ileum (arrow) with diffuse infiltration in the regional mesentery.

Colon

Endoscopy with biopsy and/or microbiological investigation is a definitive tool for the diagnosis of colonic diseases, whether inflammatory or tumoral. However, imaging techniques remain essential in the evaluation of some entities like:

- Anorectal anomalies: atresia with or without fistulas (contrast examinations, US, and MR to determine its level and the presence of fistulas). Radiograph neither useful nor diagnostic.

- Hirschsprung disease: a well-done low-pressure enema may detect the transition zone between the distal aganglionic segment and the proximal dilated colon, otherwise it is difficult to assess even with biopsy
- Appendicitis: US has high accuracy without radiation risks.

Table 2.53 Increased colonic air with distention

Diagnosis	Findings	Comments
Neonates and Infants		
Congenital megacolon (aganglionic megacolon, Hirschsprung disease) ▷ *Fig. 2.107a, b, p. 212*	Plain X-ray: similar to other forms of low SBO. Barium enema *(lateral view)*: transition zone between the normal or relatively narrow aganglionic segment and the dilated bowel proximal to it.	Low intestinal obstruction caused by the absence of normal myenteric ganglion cells in a segment of the colon. Abdominal distention, failure to pass meconium in the first 24 h of life, constipation, and bilious vomiting are the predominant symptoms.
Neonatal small left colon syndrome		(see **Table 2.69**)
Colonic atresia ▷ *Fig. 2.108, p. 212*	Proximal dilatation with obstruction to the flow of contrast in contrast enema at the site of the atresia; distal microcolon (DD with ileal atresia).	Less common than ileal atresia.
Post-neonatal period, infants, toddlers, and older children		
Organic or neurogenic megacolon	Marked air-filled colon with stools.	Organic: congenital stenosis, fibrotic strictures, post-NEC, etc. Neurogenic causes: spinal cord infarcts, cord transection, and cerebral palsy. DD: Hirschsprung disease by clinical findings and (rarely) radiographic examination. Suction biopsy.
Chronic constipation ▷ *Fig. 2.109, p. 212* ▷ *Fig. 2.110, p. 213*	Large amounts of air mixed with stools throughout the entire large bowel. Acquired fecal retention, especially in the sigmoid colon and rectum.	Most common cause of colonic dilatation in infancy and school-age children. Causes: difficult toilet training, neuropsychogenetic abnormalities, hypothyroidism, malnutrition, etc.
Toxic megacolon	Marked dilatation of the transverse colon in particular. Nodular thickening and rigidity of the colonic wall. Increased perforation risk: air-fluid levels and ascites.	Infrequent complication of ulcerative colitis and other colitis. Enema is contraindicated.
IT (see Table 2.68)	Predominant small bowel dilatation. A normal X-ray does not exclude intussesception(s). US is diagnostic.	Less than 5% of intussesception(s) are colocolic.

(continues on page 213)

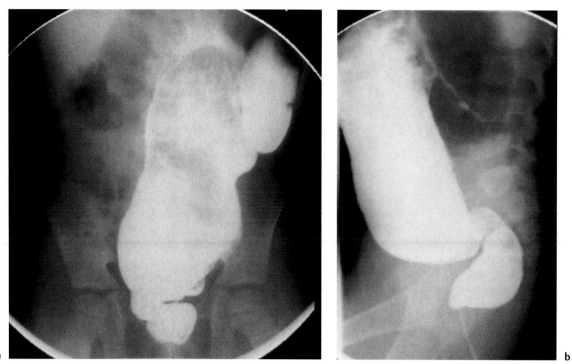

a b

Fig. 2.107a, b Hirschsprung disease. Anteroposterior (**a**) and lateral (**b**) views of a contrast enema show the significant dilatation of the sigmoid and proximal rectum. The distal rectum is not dilated, representing the aganglionic segment.

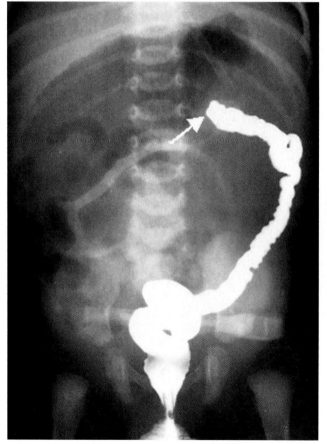

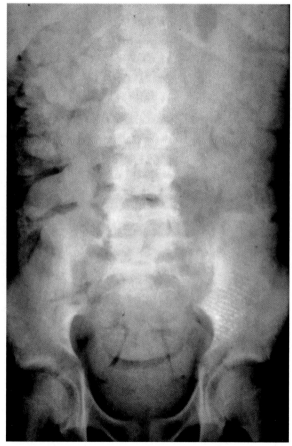

Fig. 2.108 Colon atresia. Contrast enema shows abnormally small colon (microcolon) with complete obstruction to retrograde flow of contrast material proximal to the middle transverse portion of colon (arrow). There is gaseous distention of proximal bowel.

Fig. 2.109 Chronic constipation. Plain abdominal film shows colonic distention by feces that occupies all the segments.

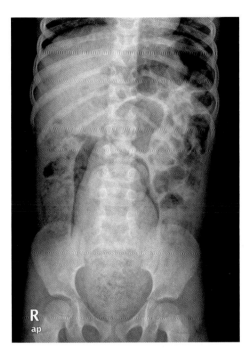

Fig. 2.110   Fecaloma. Plain abdominal film shows fecaloma in rectum outlined by gas in a girl with abdominal pain and with no evacuation in the last 10 days.

Table 2.53   (Cont.) Increased colonic air with distention

Diagnosis	Findings	Comments
Chilaiditi syndrome ▷ *Fig. 2.111*	Distended colon interposed between the liver and the anterior abdominal wall.	Common in neurologically impaired children. Abdominal wall muscle weakness promotes intestinal content accumulation. DD: subphrenic abscess.
Sigmoid volvulus	"Coffee-bean" sign. Low obstruction	Unusual but possible.
Neuronal degeneration	Radiographically resembles Hirschsprung disease.	
Anal rhabdomyosarcoma	Circumferential narrowing without mucosal destruction.	Constipation. Palpable tumor.
Other distal colonic obstructions		Huge distended bladder, hematoma, pelvic masses (abscess, tumors), hernia (diaphragmatic: transverse, inguinal: sigma).

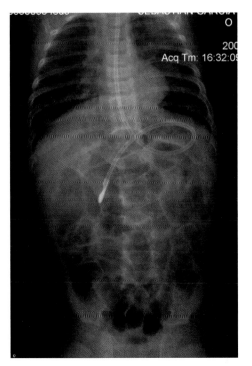

Fig. 2.111   Chilaiditi syndrome. Plain abdominal films shows transverse colon interposition between the liver and the anterior abdominal wall. Nasoduodenal tube is seen.

Table 2.54 The colon parietal changes

Diagnosis	Findings	Comments
NEC ▷ *Fig. 2.112* ▷ *Fig. 2.113* ▷ *Fig. 2.114a, b* ▷ *Fig. 2.115* ▷ *Fig. 2.116a, b, p. 216*	Abdominal X-ray: linear or cystic pneumatosis intestinalis (submucosal or subserosal air). Portal vein gas: finely branching radiolucencies extending from the porta hepatis to the periphery of the liver. US: bright, shifting echogenic foci within the portal vein.	In premature infants weighing < 1500 g. Factors: ischemia, decreased mucus production, diminished immune response of the premature infants, Hirschsprung. Complications: perforation, strictures.
Infectious colitis ▷ *Fig. 2.117, p. 216*	Nonspecific moderate continuous and mostly generalized thickening of the colon wall.	Often due to *Salmonella* infection. Not a primary radiographic diagnosis.
Chronic nonspecific enteritis: Crohn disease, ulcerative colitis (rare) ▷ *Fig. 2.118, p. 216*	Crohn: Asymmetric changes in the wall. Skip lesions and fistulas.	Crohn: more frequent in the ileocecal region. DD: TB and amebic dysentery. Ulcerative colitis begins in the rectum and ascends. Fistulas are very rare.

(continues on page 217)

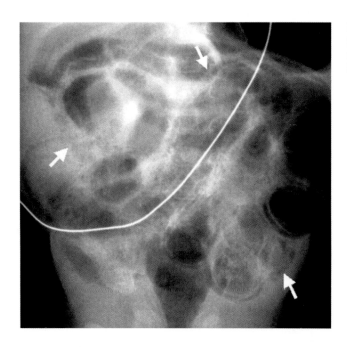

Fig. 2.112 Pneumatosis intestinalis in a 1-week-old infant. Anteroposterior plain radiograph shows small and large bowel loops sharply outlined by collections of air in bowel wall (arrows). Most of these collections of air are linear, suggesting a submucosal location.

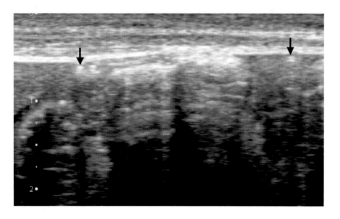

Fig. 2.113 Necrotizing enterocolitis. Longitudinal US scan at the transverse colon shows air bubbles (arrows) within the colonic wall corresponding to pneumatosis intestinalis.

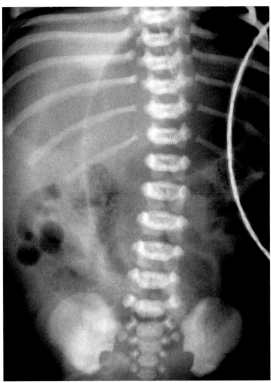

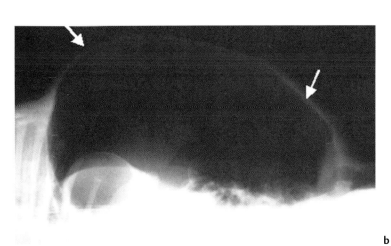

a

b

Fig. 2.114a, b   Pneumoperitoneum complicating necrotizing enterocolitis. (**a**) Supine radiograph in a 1-month-old premature infant shows intramural air in the small bowel and free intraperitoneal air secondary to bowel perforation. The central lucency and the falciform ligament are seen ("football" sign). (**b**) Horizontal beam decubitus radiograph in another patient that shows pneumoperitoneum (arrows) due to bowel perforation in a premature infant.

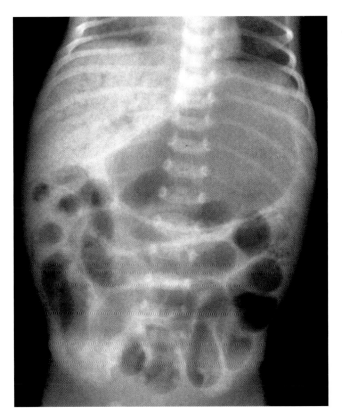

Fig. 2.115   Portal vein air. Plain radiographs: air is observed within the portal vein branches, complicating pneumatosis intestinalis in a 3-week-old premature infant.

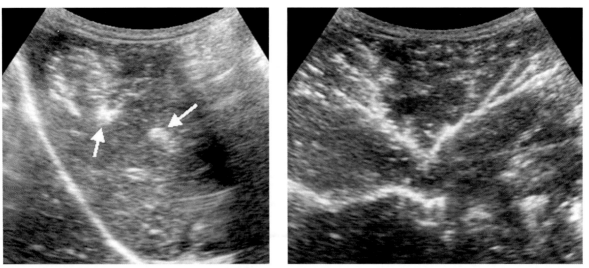

a   b

Fig. 2.116a, b   Portal vein air. (a) Transverse sonogram of the liver shows multiple echogenic areas (arrows) corresponding to air within the portal vein branches. **(b)** Air is also observed within the hepatic veins.

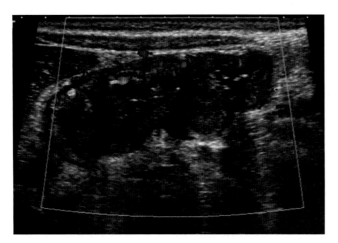

Fig. 2.117   Salmonellosis. Axial Doppler US through the transverse colon depicts a hypervascularized thickened colonic wall with a patent hyperemic submucosal layer.

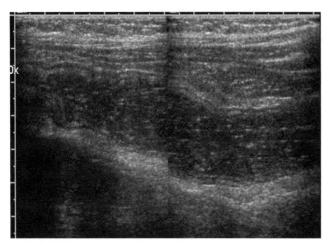

Fig. 2.118   Ulcerative colitis. Longitudinal US ultrasound through the left colon: The normal folds are lost and the lumen is filled with fluid. This is the US counterpart of the "lead-pipe" appearance on a contrast enema.

Table 2.54 (Cont.) The colon parietal changes

Diagnosis	Findings	Comments
Pseudomembranous enterocolitis	Marked thickening of the colon wall. Mucosal irregularity and ulcerations. Pseudomembranes on contrast studies.	Complication of oral antibiotic therapy. Caused by *Clostridium difficile*.
Hemolytic uremic syndrome	Thickening of the colon with irregular narrowing of the lumen and "thumbprinting" pattern due to intramural hemorrhage. Lost of bowel wall layering.	Hemolytic anemia, renal failure, and thrombocytopenia. DD: Henoch-Schönlein purpura predominates in the small bowel and shows flow on Doppler US. US examination of the kidneys.
Acute appendicitis	(see **Table 2.68**)	Nonfilling of the appendix occurs in 30% of normal contrast studies.
Appendiceal abscess ▷ *Fig. 2.119*	Deformed cecum or rectum and adjacent bowel loops.	DD: gynecological pathology.
Complications postappendectomy ▷ *Fig. 2.120, p. 218*	Cecal filling defect due to an inflamed appendiceal stump. Cecal fistulas.	Particularly significant when they appear soon after surgery.
Benign Tumors		
Lymphoid hyperplasia	Small (2–3 mm) mucosal follicles with central umbilication.	Considered normal variant.
Juvenile polyp	Often pedunculated solitary filling defect.	Benign hyperplastic polyp; autoamputation is frequent.
Juvenile colonic polyposis	Multiple round filling defects.	Malignant degeneration has not been described.
Generalized juvenile gastrointestinal polyposis	Changes throughout the GI tract.	Histology.
Hereditary adenomatous colonic polyposis	Multiple polyps of various sizes.	Premalignant; autosomal dominant (AD); histology.
Adenomatous polyps of the colon (Gardner and Turcot syndromes)	Sessile or pedunculated.	Malignant degeneration is described.
Cavernous hemangioma ▷ *Fig. 2.121a, b, p. 218*	Nodular or polypoid wall thickening with flow detected on Doppler US; phleboliths.	Prone to hemorrhage; may involve any segment of GI tract.
Malignant Tumors		
Non-Hodgkin lymphoma ▷ *Fig. 2.122a, b, p. 218*	Several patterns; homogenously hypoechoic high vascularized lesions.	Predominate in the ileocecal region; intussesception.
Carcinoma of the colon ▷ *Fig. 2.123, p. 219*	Irregular polypoid filling defect, mural rigidity, erosions crater, stenosis.	Secondary to inflammatory intestinal disease, adenomatous polyposis, sporadic.

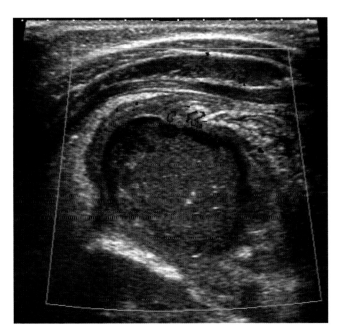

Fig. 2.119 Retrocecal appendical abscess. Axial Doppler US: A fluid collection with high-level echoes and with hypoechoic thick wall is seen in the retrocecal area (between the abdominal muscular wall and the right kidney posteriorly). Doppler signal is depicted in the abscess wall.

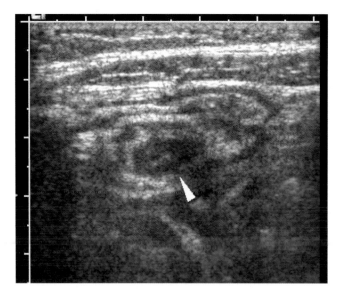

Fig. 2.120 Inflamed appendiceal stump. Axial US image through cecal area shows a multilayered image (arrowhead; bowel inside bowel) due to the remaining inflamed submucosa in the invaginated appendiceal stump (tobacco bag).

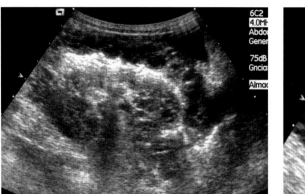

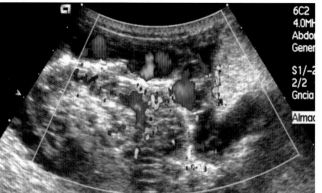

a   b

Fig. 2.121a, b Sigmoid hemangiomatosis. B-mode (**a**) and Doppler (**b**) US through the left iliac fossa show a sigmoid colon with parietal thickening and hypoechoic areas with prominent flow.

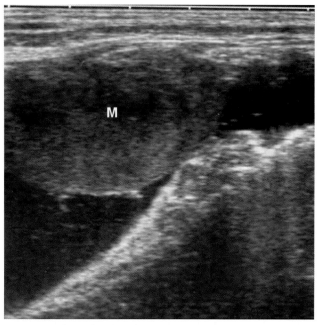

a

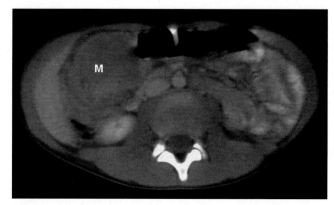

Fig. 2.122a, b Colon lymphoma. A 6-year-old boy diagnosed with intussesception with a pathologic lead-point by US. A saline enema was performed, achieving full reduction. (**a**) The postreduction US image shows a hypoechoic homogenous mass in the anterior wall of the ascending colon. The mass was biopsied and diagnosed as Burkitt lymphoma. (**b**) The CT image depicts a hypoattenuating mass with no lymphadenopathies or other findings present. This procedure avoided the necessity to perform a partial colectomy.
M Mass

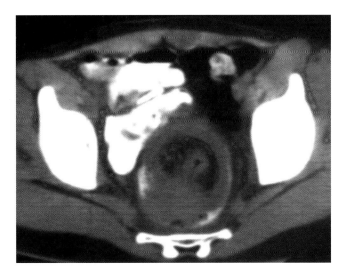

Fig. 2.123 Intussuscepted sigmoid carcinoma. A 12-year-old boy with constipation and rectal mass at examination. CT examination with rectal contrast depicts a parietal colonic mass with mucosal irregularity and outlined with contrast. This mass is the lead-point of a sigmoid-rectal intussesception: the crescent-shaped intussuscepted mesentery is depicted.

Table 2.55 Anorectal anomalies in neonates

Diagnosis	Findings	Comments
High anomaly without fistula	Blind-ending pouch above the I-point (lowest point of the pubis or below the tip of the ischium). Voiding cystourethrogram (VCUG).	MRI may be of help.
Intermediate anomaly without fistula ▷ *Fig. 2.124a, b* ▷ *Fig. 2.125, p. 220*	Blind-ending pouch at the level of the I-point.	MRI.
Rectourethral fistula, rectovaginal/vestibular	Demonstration of fistula with VCUG in boys or contrast filling from the anus in girls.	May present with air in bladder or meconium in urine.
Perineal and vulvar fistulas	Retrograde contrast evaluation.	Always low anomalies.
Transscrotal fistulas	Retrograde contrast evaluation.	Intermediate anomaly.

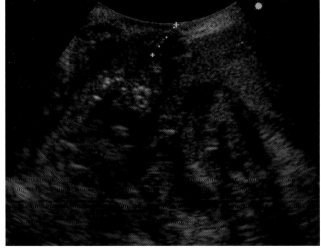

a

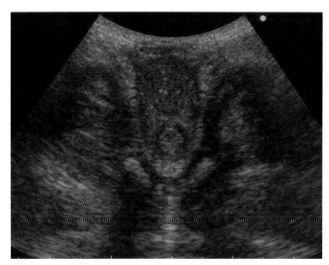

b

Fig. 2.124a, b Anal atresia. (a) Sagittal US in transperineal approach shows the blind-ended rectum filled with meconium (hyperechoic dots). The calipers measure the distance between rectum and perineal surface.

(b) Axial US from the posterior shows the normal muscular pelvic anatomy, which is encircling the rectal pouch.

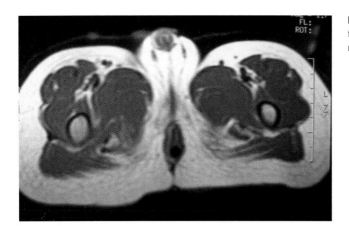

Fig. 2.125   Anal atresia, postoperative. Axial T1 MRI with a rectal tube inserted, which helps to evaluate the proper position of descended rectum. In this case, the rectum is slightly lateralized to the left.

Table 2.56   The colon: Diverticula and duplications

Diagnosis	Findings	Comments
Diverticulum	Isolated colonic diverticulum.	Rare.
Duplications ▷ *Fig. 2.126a, b*	The cecum accounts for about 40% of cystic colonic duplications, and its imaging features are similar to those of small bowel duplications. US: a cystic image with echogenic inner rim and outer hypoechoic muscle layers ("double-halo" sign) is highly suggestive.	Colonic duplications can be cystic or tubular, the second being more frequent in the rectum. If the cyst contains ectopic gastric mucosa or pancreatic tissue and communicates with the rectum, rectal bleeding may occur.

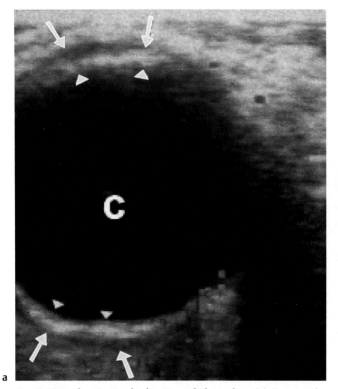

a

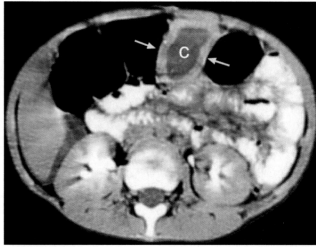

b

Fig. 2.126a, b   Cystic duplication of the colon. (a) Sonography shows a round, fluid-filled image (C). Note the inner echogenic layer (arrowheads) and the outer hypoechoic rim (arrows). (b) CT scan of the same patient demonstrates a water-density cystic mass (C) surrounded by transverse colon gas (arrows).

Table 2.57   Intramural air in the gastrointestinal tract

Diagnosis	Findings	Comments
Pneumatosis intestinalis (small and large bowel; see Table 2.54)	Abdominal X-ray: linear or cystic (submucosal or subserosal) air in intestinal wall.	In NEC (perforation risk). May also occur in obstruction, Hirschsprung disease, cystic fibrosis, immunosuppression, etc.
Gastric pneumatosis	Linear or cystic lucencies in the gastric wall.	Tube malposition, after endoscopy, volvulus, ulcer disease, and from chemical damage.

Table 2.58   Calcifications and foreign bodies within the gastrointestinal tract

Diagnosis	Findings	Comments
Appendicolith and foreign body ▷ *Fig. 2.127* ▷ *Fig. 2.128*	Often single round or oval calcification in the RLQ. Specific finding (just seen in the 10% of appendicitis).	Delayed surgery is indicated even if asymptomatic due to the increased risk of perforated appendicitis.
Foreign bodies	Abdominal radiograph.	Coins, stones, marbles, metallic toys, ingested soil (geophagia).
Calcified meconium ▷ *Fig. 2.116a, b, p. 216*	Small flecks of calcification in the lumen with meconium ileus and other congenital forms of obstruction.	Neonates.
Enterolith		Due to chronic fecal retention with anorectal anomalies. Begins as a soft-tissue density and later increased in density due to peripheral apposition of calcium salts.
Enterolith in a Meckel diverticulum		Rare.

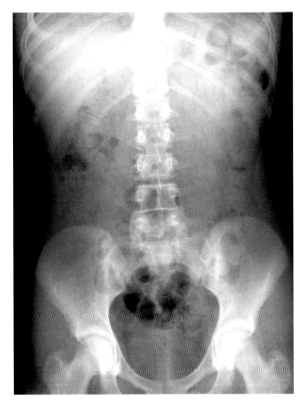

Fig. 2.127   Appendicolith. An appendicolith is seen in this abdominal plain film adjacent to right L4 transverse process.

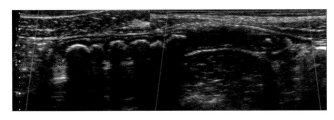

Fig. 2.128   Appendicolith. Doppler US longitudinal scan shows several hyperechoic stones with acoustic shadowing inside the lumen of a dilated, inflamed appendix.

Peritoneum and Peritoneal Cavity

Table 2.59 Clear peritoneal fluid (ascites)

Diagnosis	Findings	Comments
Normal finding	Small pouches of fluid between bowel loops or in Douglas pouch.	Visible in up to 22% of normal children. Also in patients in peritoneal dialysis, with ventriculoperitoneal shunts, in postovulation period.
Pitfalls		Fluid-filled bowel loops. Fluid-filled rectum.
Fetal hydrops	Also pleural and pericardial effusion, subcutaneous edema.	Clinically evident.
Urinary ascites	Uni-/bilateral dilatation of excretory system.	Caused by lower obstruction and upper rupture: urethral valves, neurogenic bladder, extrinsic mass.
Cardiac disease	Dilatation of hepatic veins with mono- or biphasic flow on Doppler US.	In latter phase, hepatic veins are narrowed.
Portal hypertension ▷ *Fig. 2.129*	Intrahepatic portal obstruction: neonatal hepatitis with portal cirrhosis, biliary atresia. Extrahepatic obstruction: atresia, compression.	Look for other findings: heterogeneous hepatomegaly, splenomegaly, portosystemic shunts.
Trauma	Small amounts of fluid are normal after blunt trauma.	If amount of fluid is larger, look for organ injuries: liver, spleen, kidney, mesentery, bowel, bladder.
Hemorrhage	Subacute and chronic hemorrhage, after cloth formation and sedimentation may resemble clear fluid.	Usually after trauma, ruptured ovarian cyst, or hydrometrocolpos.
Peritoneal carcinomatosis	Ascites with peritoneal or mesenteric nodules. The primary tumor is usually depicted.	In peritoneal seeding of gastric, pancreatic, or ovarian tumors. Also lymphoma.

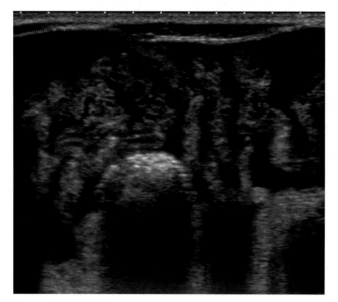

Fig. 2.129 Ascites. Free anechoic peritoneal fluid is seen in a neonate with biliary cirrhosis and portal hypertension.

Table 2.60　Dense peritoneal fluid (ascites)

Diagnosis	Findings	Comments
Hemorrhage	In acute phase, blood is echogenic (US) and hyperattenuating (CT).	After blunt trauma with solid organ injury, cystic mass rupture, etc.
Biliary ascites		After perinatal trauma or surgery.
Chylous ascites	Low-level echoes (US) and hypoattenuating (CT).	Postprandial, after birth, trauma, or surgery. In filariasis, lymphangiectasia.
Secondary peritonitis ▷ Fig. 2.130 ▷ Fig. 2.131	In late cases, the origin of peritonitis may be not clearly depicted.	In appendicitis, pancreatitis, pelvic inflammatory disease, perforation of hollow viscus.
Primary peritonitis ▷ Fig. 2.132a, b	Ascites with peritoneal engorgement that enhances with contrast (CT). Loculations can be seen.	Bacterial, TB, viral.
Meconium peritonitis ▷ Fig. 2.133a, b, p. 224	Proximal bowel obstruction. Dense fluid. Calcifications.	

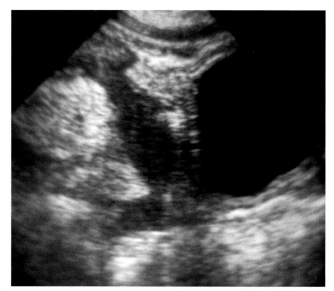

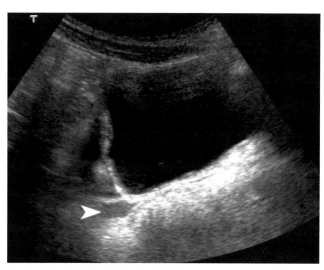

Fig. 2.130　Peritonitis secondary to free perforation of acute appendicitis. Sagittal US image of pelvis in a 3-year-old boy shows echogenic fluid surrounding the hyperechoic omentum and intestinal loops over the distended bladder. The appendix was not identified, even at surgery.

Fig. 2.131　Douglas fluid. Sagittal US image shows a small amount of hyperechoic free fluid in the pouch of Douglas (arrowhead) in a patient with suspected acute appendicitis. This finding suggests this diagnosis, particularly if seen after 48 hours of evolution, even if the appendix itself is not depicted. In this case, surgery confirmed the diagnosis of acute appendicitis.

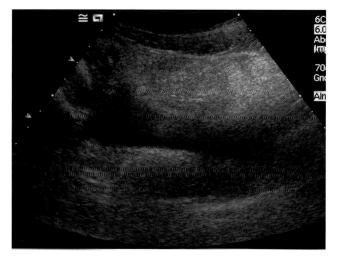

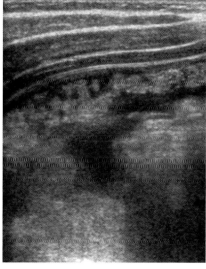

Fig. 2.132a, b　Tuberculous peritonitis. US abdominal scans at mesogastrium (a) and RLQ (b) show the thickened hyperechoic omentum located in contact with the whole anterior abdominal wall. In (a), the omentum is seen homogeneously hyperechoic, whereas in

(b) it is more heterogeneous. Slightly echogenic ascites is present. Note that in appendicular peritonitis, the omentum is in contact with the appendicular area, not the abdominal wall.

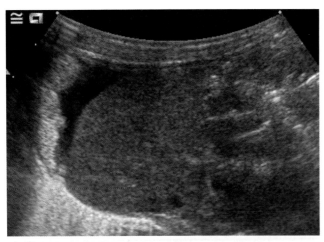 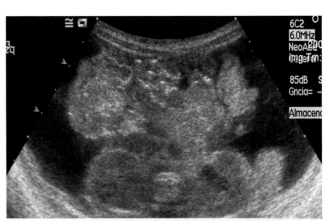

a

Fig. 2.133a, b Meconium peritonitis. Transverse abdominal US through the right upper quadrant (RUQ) (**a**) and in mesogastrium (**b**). Ascites is present. In (**a**), the meconium deposits are seen in subdiaphragmatic area. In (**b**), meconium is seen beside the left kidney. Also in (**b**), the bowel loops are outlined by a thin hyperechoic meconium rim.

Table 2.61 Localized fluid collections

See **Tables 2.64** and **2.66** (abdominal cystic masses) and free peritoneal air (pneumoperitoneum) in neonate.

Diagnosis	Findings	Comments
NEC	Air dissecting colonic wall with free air in late stages.	Seen in premature infants.
Gastric perforation	Large amount of peritoneal air.	Spontaneous idiopathic perforation in premature infants.
GI tract obstruction	Obstruction is evident.	Usually in low tract obstruction: imperforate anus, Hirschsprung disease, meconium ileus.
Extra-abdominal air dissection	From pneumomediastinum.	
Iatrogenic		After laparotomy, thermometer injury in rectum, traumatic tube placement in stomach or bladder.

Table 2.62 Free peritoneal air (pneumoperitoneum) in neonates

Diagnosis	Findings	Comments
GI tract perforation	Location of air depends on location of perforation.	After gastric or duodenal ulcer, appendicitis, inflamed Meckel diverticulum.
Extra-abdominal air dissection	From pneumomediastinum.	
Iatrogenic	After surgery.	
Fistulas		To abdominal wall, GI tract, vagina.
Air-producing intra-abdominal infections	Gas may be contained or disseminate to peritoneum.	In emphysematous infections: appendicitis, pancreatitis, other origin abscesses, etc.

Table 2.63 Peritoneal calcifications

Diagnosis	Findings	Comments
Tumors		
Neuroblastoma	Over 30% of tumors show coarse or stippled calcifications. Most common locations: paravertebral and suprarenal.	Up to 70% of tumors have calcifications on CT exam.
Teratoma	Coarse calcifications, but also frequently well-defined structures, like teeth.	Also fat density can be depicted in radiograph.
Wilms tumor	Mass effect in the renal fossa, with curvilinear or phlebolithic calcifications in 15%.	Calcifications are not stippled.
Hepatoblastoma	Heterogeneous, coarse, ill-defined calcifications in 12%–30%. In some cases, osseous matrix.	Also, hemangioendothelioma may show fine granular calcifications. Hepatoma has no calcium on radiograph.
Mesenteric cysts	Rim calcification.	

(continues on page 225)

Table 2.63   (Cont.) Peritoneal calcifications

Diagnosis	Findings	Comments
Inflammatory—trauma		
Calcified abscesses	Frequent in paravertebral tuberculous abscesses, less frequent in bacterial.	Secondary to spondylodiscitis.
Tuberculous peritonitis	Small foci of calcifications in multiple locations.	Usually other signs of TB (in most cases pulmonary) are not seen.
Calcified hematoma		Usually posttrauma.
Hydatid cysts	Eggshell-like calcification, most of them located in the liver, but also splenic, peritoneal.	Caused by calcification of external (adventitial) layer. In endemic areas.
Meconium peritonitis	Small flecks of calcification scattered throughout abdomen. Lineal calcifications along inferior surface of liver.	In neonates, with obstructive signs following birth. Pathologic obstetric US. Also accompanied with meconium pseudocysts.
Peritoneal dialysis	Lineal calcifications of peritoneum.	Deposit of calcium-binding protein after several years of dialysis.
Lymph nodes	Single or multiple, usually in central or lower abdomen, rounded or irregular.	After a wide variety of infections: TB, salmonella, other bacteria.
Other		
Phlebolith	Small, rounded calcifications with central radiolucent dot.	Frequent in pelvis.
Renoureteral calculi	Irregular or rounded calcifications of variable sizes, located superimposed to the kidneys and to the ureteral trajectory.	Uric acid stones only show calcification with CT.
Biliary calculi	Rounded calcification, usually multiple and sometimes with central low-density area.	
Foreign bodies ▷ *Fig. 2.134*	Located anywhere in the GI tract, but more frequent in physiological low-caliper areas: antrum, ileocecal.	Wide variety of sizes and shapes. Ingestion has sometimes been noted.
Enterolith	In chronic constipation, usually with anorectal anomalies.	Formed by deposition of calcium over inspissated feces.
Appendicolith	Usually laminated and located in RLQ, but may be present also in right flank, pelvis, etc.	Present in 7%–15% of appendicitis (usually complicated).
Lithiasis in Meckel diverticulum	Similar to appendicolith, but usually centrally located.	Difficult DD with appendicolith (much more frequent).

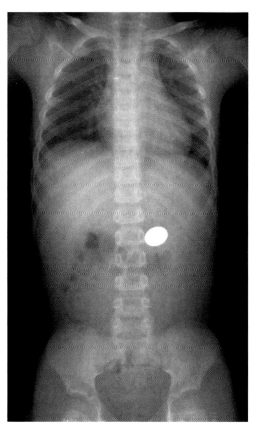

Fig. 2.134   GI foreign body. An ingested coin is depicted on plain abdominal film superimposed over the stomach.

Abdominal Masses

Imaging is essential in management of suspected abdominal masses. Data to be obtained are the composition of the mass (solid, cystic, or mixed), its limits, its location and organ dependence, its vascularization, and the presence of additional findings (lymphadenopathy, ascites, etc.). Afterward, an approximation about the nature of the mass (benign/malignant) and a possible differential diagnosis can be inferred. US is almost always the first imaging modality used, and can provide essential information. CT, MR, NM, and PET are useful to complete the diagnosis.

Table 2.64   Neonatal cystic masses

Diagnosis	Findings	Comments
Hydronephrosis	Depending if uni-/bilateral and on level of obstruction.	Most common mass in neonate. Usually diagnosed in utero.
Multicystic dysplastic kidney	Cluster of cysts in renal fossa	In rare occasions may be focal.
Multilocular cystic nephroma	Noncommunicating cysts with thick septa.	
Hydrometrocolpos ▷ Fig. 2.135a, b	Fluid-filled dilated vagina and uterus. In midline.	May be associated with other congenital anomalies.
Ovarian cyst	Lateral mass, usually unilocular.	May appear rather abdominal than pelvic.
GI duplication	Layered wall, with muscle.	May produce obstruction.
Mesenteric-omental cyst	Thin walled. Uni- or multilocular.	
Meconium pseudocyst	Formed by twisted and fused loops of bowel.	
Adrenal hemorrhage	Anechoic if subacute.	Decreases in size in serial controls.
Cystic neuroblastoma	Usually echogenic.	Equal or increasing in size.
Hepatic or splenic cyst	Unilocular. May be multiple.	
Mesenchymal hamartoma of liver	Multiple rounded cystic areas, hypovascular.	
Choledochal cyst	Usually located in or near the hepatic hilum	NM can confirm the diagnosis.
Gallbladder hydrops	Usually biliary sludge and/or echogenic bilis is depicted on US examination.	
Cystic hygroma/lymphangioma ▷ Fig. 2.136	Multilocular, thin wall, grows among other structures without displacing.	
Sacrococcygeal teratoma	Mixed cystic-solid pattern.	

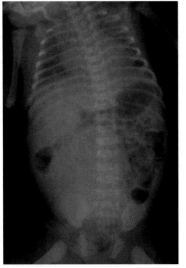
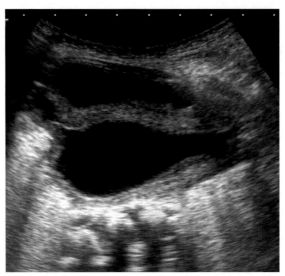

a   b

Fig. 2.135a, b   Hydrometrocolpos. A newborn with abdominal distension. (**a**) Plain film depicts a pelvic mass with intestinal loop displacement. (**b**) Sagittal pelvic US obtained after partial drainage shows a fluid-filled vagina and a uterus with mildly distended endometrial lumen, located behind the bladder.

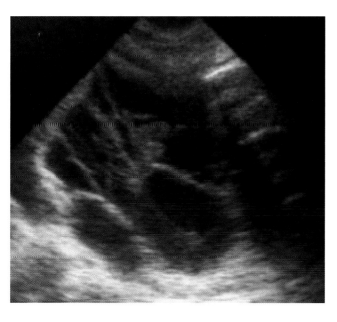

Fig. 2.136   Peritoneal lymphangioma. Transverse US image in mesogastrium depicts a characteristic polylobulated cystic mass with thin septa.

Table 2.65   Neonatal solid masses

Diagnosis	Findings	Comments
Polycystic kidney disease	Bilateral enlarged distorted kidneys.	In autosomal recessive form.
Mesoblastic nephroma	Large ill-defined mass.	May be cystic.
Renal ectopia	Empty renal fossa.	Usually pelvic kidney or crossed-fused ectopia.
Renal vein thrombosis	Unilateral enlarged kidney with absent flow (acute phase), subsequent atrophy.	Secondary to dehydration, sepsis, umbilical vein catheterization.
Nephroblastomatosis-Wilms tumor	Large tumors uni- or multifocal and uni- or bilateral.	Most common solid renal mass in children.
Neuroblastoma	Large, heterogeneous, irregular mass. Adrenal, retroperitoneum, or other locations.	Good prognosis.
Hemangioendothelioma—hemangioma of liver	Diffuse mass affecting entire liver.	Benign tumor. Tendency to involute.
Hepatoblastoma	Large heterogeneous mass	Elevated alpha fetoprotein.

Table 2.66   Older children cystic masses

Diagnosis	Findings	Comments
Hydronephrosis		
Renal cyst	Usually unilocular.	May be multiple.
Renal cystic disease	Usually bilateral and symmetric.	In autosomal dominant form.
Rhabdoid renal tumor	Mostly cystic.	Bad prognosis.
Perirenal hematoma		Post trauma or biopsy.
Teratoma ▷ Fig. 2.137a, b, p. 228	Mixed solid-cystic pattern.	
Appendiceal abscess	Thick irregular wall.	May contain appendicolith.
Mesenteric-omental cyst	Uni- or multilocular.	
Hepatic parasitic cyst	Well defined.	Echinococcal cyst.
Cerebrospinal fluid pseudocyst	Cyst related with the tip of a catheter.	In patients with ventriculoperitoneal shunt.
Hepatic/renal/splenic cyst	Thin wall. Single or multiple.	
Hepatic/renal/splenic abscess	Thick wall, irregular.	
Hematometrocolpos	Midline, echogenic.	Girls in puberal age.
Urachal cyst/abscess	Midline, related to bladder dome and umbilicus.	

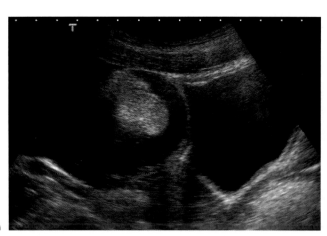

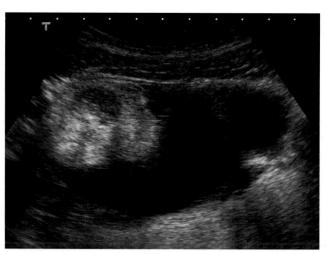

a

b

Fig. 2.137a, b **Mature teratoma** in a 13-year-old girl. Sagittal (**a**) and transverse (**b**) US images show a complex cystic mass cranial to the uterus and positioned over the bladder with solid hyperechoic components representing fat and hairs, which was confirmed at pathologic examination.

Table 2.67 Older children solid masses

Diagnosis	Findings	Comments
Wilms tumor	Large tumor, hypervascular, heterogeneous. May invade IVC and cross midline.	
Neuroblastoma	Adrenal, retroperitoneal, or in other locations. Irregular margins, heterogeneous, crosses midline, with retroperitoneal lymph nodes. Stippled calcifications.	Worst prognosis than in neonate. Two-thirds of patients > 2 y have disseminated disease.
Rhabdomyosarcoma	Lobulated solid soft-tissue masses, with local invasion, and nodal and distant metastases.	Usually genitourinary (bladder, prostate, vagina, cervix, paratesticular) or biliary.
Burkitt lymphoma	Rapidly growing infiltrative mass originated in ileal lymphoid follicles that extends to adjacent bowel mesentery.	Usually in boys between the ages of 5 and 10 y. May present as a small bowel obstruction or intussesception.
Hepatocellular carcinoma	Well-circumscribed mass with central scar and calcifications.	In older children. Fibrolamellar subtype.
Hepatic adenoma	Well-defined mass without arterial-phase enhancement.	Predisposed in children with von Gierke disease.
Hepatic metastasis	Multiple and solid nodules. Some cases: diffuse heterogeneous hepatomegaly.	From neuroblastoma or Wilms tumor.
Wandering spleen	Not really a tumor, but an unexpected abdominal mass.	May become infarcted if pedicle torsion occurs.

The Acute Abdomen

Table 2.68   The acute abdomen in infants, toddlers, and older children

Diagnosis	Findings	Comments
Appendicitis ▷ *Fig. 2.138a, b* ▷ *Fig.2.139* ▷ *Fig.2.140* ▷ *Fig.2.141, p. 230*	US: Dilated or collapsed blind-ending structure ≥ 6 mm, with thickened or vanished submucosal layer; prominent hyperechoic periappendicular fat, echogenic fluid. Appendicolith (25%). Sonographic Blumberg (+). Hyperemia in Doppler images.	Mechanical or paralytic ileus may associate. DD: bacterial ileocecitis, inflammatory intestinal disease (IID), adenitis, right-sided omental infarction, Henoch-Schönlein purpura, primary peritonitis, ovarian pathology. US: diagnostic modality of choice. CT/MRI in equivocal cases.

(continues on page 230)

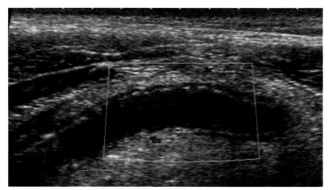
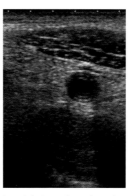

b

Fig. 2.138a, b   Acute appendicitis. RLQ US, longitudinal (**a**) and axial (**b**) views, shows a dilated obstructed appendix with a thin-rings pattern: the normal bowel wall layers are patent, unless their thickness is decreased and the lumen is occupied by purulent anechoic content.

In axial view, there is an increased sound transmission pointing to the fluid nature of the content. The hyperechoic mesenteric fat is enlarged. The Doppler signal (longitudinal view) is increased in appendix wall.

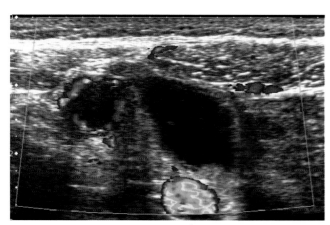
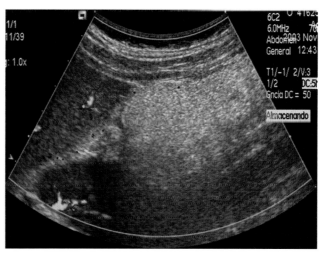

Fig. 2.139   Acute appendicitis. Transverse Doppler US image of RLQ: An inflamed hypervascularized appendix is depicted. Note the difference in size and vascularization with the adjacent fluid-filled ileum.

Fig. 2.140   Omental segmental infarction. Sagittal Doppler US scan in mesogastric area: A hyperechoic avascular thickened omentum is seen beside the liver and kidney. The inflamed fat-containing omentum progressively attenuates the US beam.

Table 2.68 (Cont.) The acute abdomen in infants, toddlers, and older children

Diagnosis	Findings	Comments
Intussusception ▷ *Fig. 2.142* ▷ *Fig. 2.143* ▷ *Fig. 2.144* ▷ *Fig. 2.145* ▷ *Fig. 2.146a, b* ▷ *Fig. 2.147*	US: "crescent-in-doughnut" sign: mesenteric fat encircling entering intussusceptum. Sandwich sign. Can produce obstruction signs.	Mean age is 6 mo to 2 y. More than 95% ileocolic. Successfully enema reduction in more than 80% of cases. Less of 5% nonidiopathic: Meckel diverticulum, lymphoma (thick hypoechoic apex), etc.
Mechanical obstruction (see Table 2.44)	Proximal dilatation. Air-fluid levels.	AAIIMM (appendicitis, adhesions, IT, incarcerated hernia, Meckel diverticula, miscellanea).
Postoperative, postinfection adhesions	Dilated bowel loops proximal to the obstruction. Decreased or absent distal intestinal content.	May be present as early as 48 h. After 4% of surgeries.

(continues on page 232)

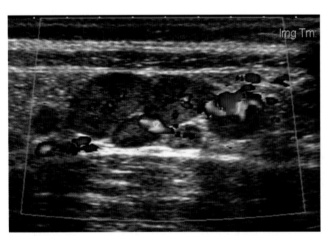

Fig. 2.141 Mesenteric adenitis. Transverse Doppler US image in mesogastric area: There are several slightly increased in size (> 6 mm) mesenteric lymph nodes with patent vascularization. This is a nonspecific finding, and other causes of acute abdomen must be ruled out. In this case, the appendix (not shown) was normal.

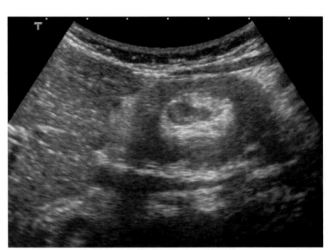

Fig. 2.142 Intussusception. US axial image of an intussesception depicted at the subhepatic region. There is a thick hypoechoic outer "doughnut" with a crescent-shaped hyperechoic mesentery inside, eccentrically surrounding a hypoechoic central limb of the intussusceptum. This is the "crescent-in-doughnut" sign.

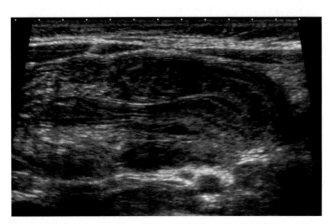

Fig. 2.143 Intussusception. US longitudinal image of an intussesception. There are several alternating bands that represent the hypoechoic intussesception and the hyperechoic mesentery. This is the "sandwich" sign.

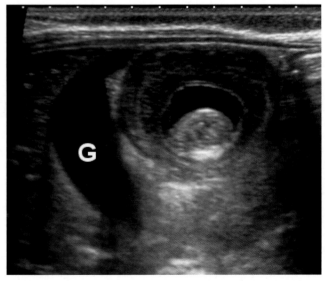

Fig. 2.144 Intussusception. US axial image of an intussesception in the subhepatic region shows the double "crescent-in-doughnut" sign. There is an additional anechoic crescent inside the doughnut formed by trapped ascites located opposite to the mesenteric hyperechoic crescent. The presence of ascites is related with bowel ischemia and low reducibility rates.
G Gallbladder

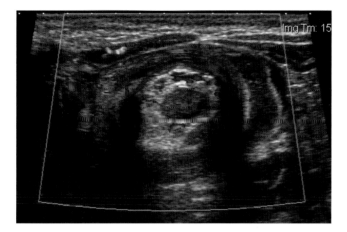

Fig. 2.145   Intussusception. Doppler US axial image of an intussesception showing blood flow in the peripheral doughnut and in the central mesentery. The presence of blood flow is a good prognostic sign of reducibility.

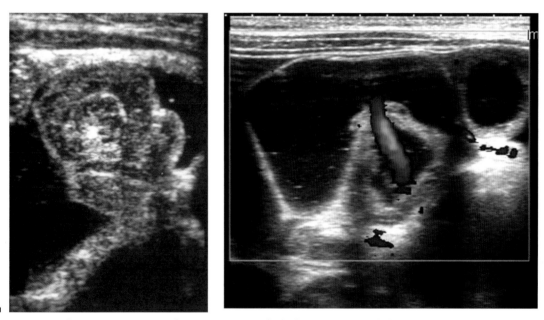

a   b

Fig. 2.146a, b   Intussusception reduction. (**a**) During the hydrostatic echo-guided enema, the intussesception is seen partially reduced at the level of the ileocecal valve. (**b**) After intussesception reduction, the valve is seen open and with fluid passage through terminal ileum (blue color in the Doppler image).

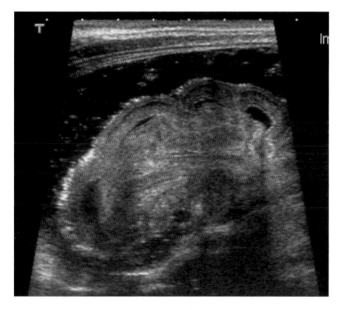

Fig. 2.147   Ileoileocolic intussusception. Longitudinal US during hydrostatic echo-guided enema shows a complex polylobulated ileo-ileo-colic intussesception with fluid trapped inside attempting to pass through the valve. In this case, the reduction was not possible.

Table 2.68 (Cont.) The acute abdomen in infants, toddlers, and older children

Diagnosis	Findings	Comments
Incarcerated hernia	Gas can be depicted beyond the abdominal cavity.	Obstruction complicated with strangulation: worse prognosis.
Volvulus ▷ *Fig. 2.148a, b*	Of stomach, duodenum, small bowel, sigmoid colon.	
Midgut volvulus **(see Table 2.44)**	"Whirlpool" sign.	Rare but severe. Prerequisite: malrotation.
Adynamic (paralytic) Ileus ***(see Table 2.44)***		
Inflammatory causes	Generalized or focal (sentinel loop) distended bowel loops with distal gas.	Gastroenteritis, appendicitis, enteritis, ovarian pathology.
Postoperative		
Posttraumatic		After blunt abdominal trauma, including child abuse.
Extra-abdominal causes		Pneumonia, discitis, sepsis, metabolic, medication.
Toxic megacolon		
Traumatic acute abdomen (AA): blunt abdominal trauma	Pneumoperitoneum, intraperitoneal or retroperitoneal hemorrhage/laceration of viscera.	Multidetector CT in polytrauma patients can be necessary.
Nontraumatic hemorrhagic AA: GI bleeding from other causes ▷ *Fig. 2.88a–c, p. 199* ▷ *Fig. 2.89, p. 199*	Angio-CT or MRI, angiography, endoscopy.	Massive bleed from a Meckel diverticulum: uptake of 99mTc pertechnetate if ectopic gastric mucosa is present. Hemolytic-uremic syndrome, ulceration, IID, tumors, angiodysplasia, intussesception.

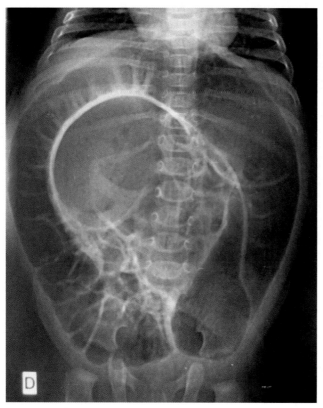
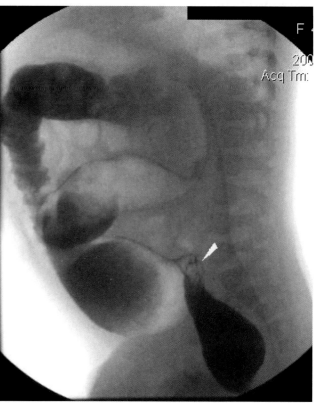

Fig. 2.148a, b Sigmoid volvulus. (a) Plain abdominal film shows a distal colonic obstruction with the "coffee-bean sign," which is formed by twisted sigmoid colon and distended proximal colonic loops. **(b)** Contrast enema delineates the areas of sigmoid narrowing after devolvulation (arrowhead).

The Acute Abdomen in the Neonatal Period

Table 2.69   Acute abdomen in the neonatal period

Diagnosis	Findings	Comments
Gastric outlet obstruction	Plain X-ray: "single-bubble" image. When a single bubble is observed, most patients are taken directly to surgery.	Causes: antral or pyloric atresia, congenital peritoneal bands, annular pancreas Cardinal symptom: free of bile vomiting.
Pyloric hypertrophy in the neonatal period ▷ *Fig. 2.149, p. 234*	US: mucosal thickening often with polypoid or lobular appearance (DD with the muscular thickening observed in hypertrophic pyloric stenosis).	After administration of prostaglandin E to infants with ductus-dependent congenital heart disease. The stenosis is produced by central foveolar hyperplasia.
Complete duodenal obstruction	More frequent than gastric obstruction. Plain radiograph: "double-bubble" image. Rarely require further radiologic investigation.	Causes: duodenal atresia, annular pancreas, and midgut volvulus. Less frequently secondary to duodenal web, Ladd band, or preduodenal portal vein.
Incomplete duodenal obstruction	Plain X-ray: distention of the stomach and duodenum with a diminished air in the small bowel. DD with HPS by US. UGI series: to differentiate midgut volvulus from a web or stenosis. US: to rule out extraluminal causes (duplication cyst).	Causes: duodenal stenosis, duodenal web, Ladd bands, midgut volvulus, annular pancreas, preduodenal portal vein, and duplication cyst.
High small bowel obstruction (SBO)	Abdominal X-ray: three or four air bubbles (more than in duodenal atresia and fewer than in ileal atresia). A UGI series is clearly not indicated. In cases of doubt, aspiration and insufflation of air through a nasogastric tube. US to differentiate multiple dilated loops filled with fluid from ascites in patients with lack of air on the plain radiograph.	Causes: atresia or stenosis of the jejunum or proximal ileum. Clinically: bilious vomiting (frequently delayed until after the first feeding) and abdominal distention.
Low intestinal obstruction	Plain X-ray: multiple dilated air-filled bowel loops occupying the entire abdomen. Contrast enema: the critical DD finding on the contrast enema of a neonate with low obstruction is the presence or absence of a microcolon.	Occurring in the distal ileum or colon. Symptoms: vomiting, abdominal distention, and failure to pass meconium. Causes: ileal atresia, meconium ileus, colonic atresia, Hirschsprung disease, and functional immaturity of the colon.
Meconium peritonitis	Plain X-ray: linear or punctate calcifications over the serosal surfaces of the abdominal viscera. Decubitus X-ray to determine the presence of free air with a persistent perforation is essential. US: especially indicated in the presence of a relatively airless abdomen.	In-utero perforation of the fetal GI tract during the last 6 mo of pregnancy. May occur with meconium ileus but may occur with any type of obstruction and in utero perforation.

(continues on page 234)

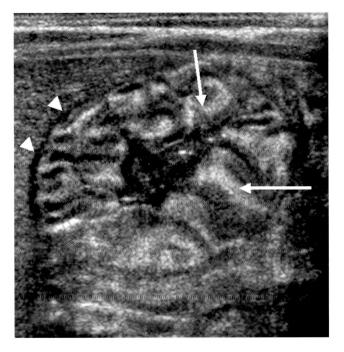

Fig. 2.149   Pyloric hyperthropy. A neonate with ductus-dependent congenital heart disease treated with prostaglandin E to keep the ductus open. Axial US scan through the gastric antrum reveals markedly hypertrophic mucosal folds (arrows) with an undulating appearance. The thickness of the muscular layer is normal (arrowheads).

Table 2.69   (Cont.) Acute abdomen in the neonatal period

Diagnosis	Findings	Comments
Anorectal malformations		Anorectal malformations are almost always evident on physical examination.
Pneumoperitoneum of GI origin	Left lateral decubitus radiograph most reliable.	It is usually the result of a hollow viscus perforation. In healthy neonates, is usually iatrogenic. Other causes: necrotizing enterocolitis, atresias, meconium ileus, congenital megacolon.
Pneumoperitoneum of pulmonary origin		Air passes to the abdomen through the normal diaphragmatic foramina. There is no perforation of the GI tract in these cases.
Necrotizing enterocolitis	Abdominal X-ray: linear or cystic pneumatosis intestinalis (submucosal or subserosal air). Portal vein gas: finely branching radiolucencies extending from the porta hepatis to the periphery of the liver. On US: bright, shifting echogenic foci within the portal vein.	Pathophysiology: ischemia, decreased mucus production, diminished immune response of the premature infants.
Massive ascites	US, abdominal radiograph to exclude complications, free air, or calcifications.	In congenital hydrops, urinary tract perforation (e.g., urethral valves), or GI perforation.

■ Further Reading

Baltazhar EJ. Complications of acute pancreatitis: clinical and CT evaluation. Radiol Clin North Am 2002;40:1211–1229

Benya EC. Pancreas and biliary system: imaging of developmental anomalies and diseases unique to children. Radiol Clin North Am 2002;40:1355–1362

Berrocal T, del Pozo G. Imaging in pediatric gastrointestinal emergencies. In: Devos AS, Blickman H, ed. Radiological imaging of the digestive tract in infants and children. Berlin: Springer Verlag, 2008:1–78

Berrocal T, Lamas M, Gutieérrez J, et al. Congenital anomalies of the small intestine, colon and rectum. Radiographics 1999;19:1219–1236

Berrocal T, Parrón M, Alvarez-Luque A, Prieto C, Santamaría ML. Pediatric liver transplantation: a pictorial essay of early and late complications. Radiographics 2006;26:1187–1209

Berrocal T, Torres I, Gutiérrez J, Prieto C, del Hoyo ML, Lamas M. Congenital anomalies of the upper gastrointestinal tract. Radiographics 1999;19:855–872

Boudiaf M, Jaff A, Soyer P, Bouhnik Y, Hamzi L, Rymer R. Small bowel diseases: prospective evaluation of multi-detector row helical CT enteroclysis in 107 consecutive patients. Radiology 2004;233:338–344

Callahan MJ, Rodriguez DP, Taylor GA. CT of appendicitis in children. Radiology 2002;224(2):325–332

Carty HM. Paediatric emergencies: non-traumatic abdominal emergencies. Eur Radiol 2002;12(12):2835–2848

Cazier PR, Sponaugle DW. "Starry sky" liver with fasting: variation in glycogen stores? J Ultrasound Med 1996;15:405–407

Christison-Lagay ER, Burrows PE, Alomari A, et al. Hepatic hemangiomas: subtype classification and development of a clinical practice algorithm and registry. J Pediatr Surg 2007;42:62–68

Daneman A, Navarro O. Intussusception. Part 2: an update on the evolution of management. Pediatr Radiol 2004;34:97–108

del-Pozo G, Albillos JC, Tejedor D. Intussusception: US findings with pathologic correlation—the crescent-in-doughnut sign. Radiology 1996;199:688–692

del-Pozo G, Albillos JC, Tejedor D, et al. Intussusception in children: current concepts in diagnosis and enema reduction. Radiographics 1999;19:299–319

del-Pozo G, González-Spinola J, Gómez-Ansón B, et al. Intussusception: trapped peritoneal fluid detected with US-relationship to reducibility and ischemia. Radiology 1996;201:379–386

del-Pozo G, Miralles M, Sánchez L, et al. Apendicitis aguda en la infancia. Hallazgos ecográficos frecuentes e infrecuentes. Radiología 1994;36:411–424

Furukawa A, Saotome T, Yamasaki M, et al. Cross-sectional imaging in Crohn disease. Radiographics 2004;24:689–702

Gonzalez-Spinola J, del Pozo G, Tejedor D, et al. Intussusception: the accuracy of ultrasound-guided saline enema and the usefulness of a delayed attempt at reduction. J Pediatr Surg 1999;34: 1016–1020

Grazioli L, Federle MP, Brancatelli G, Ichikawa T, Olivetti L, Blachar A. Hepatic adenomas: imaging and pathologic findings. Radiographics 2001;21:877–892

Ha A, Levine M, Rubesin S, Laufer I, Herlinger H. Radiographic examination of the small bowel: survive of practice patterns in the United States. Radiology 2004;231:407–412.

Hammond N, Miller FH, Sica GT, Gore RM. Imaging of cystic diseases of the pancreas. Radiol Clin North Am 2002;40:1243–1263

Helmberger TK, Ros PR, Mergo PJ, Tomczak R, Reiser MR. Pediatric liver neoplasms: a radiologic-pathologic correlation. Eur Radiol 1999;9:1339–1347

Hilmes MA, Strouse PJ. The pediatric spleen. Semin Ultrasound CT MR 2007;28(1):3–11

Jamieson D, Shipman P, Israel D, Jacobson K. Comparison of multidetector CT and barium studies of the small bowel: inflammatory bowel disease in children. AJR Am J Roentgenol 2003;180:1211–1216

Jamieson D, Stringer DA. Small bowel. In: Stringer DA, Babin PS, ed. Pediatric gastrointestinal imaging and interventional. Hamilton, Ontario, Canada: BC Decker, 2000:396–400

Kaiser S, Frenckner B, Jorulf HK. Suspected appendicitis in children: US and CT—a prospective randomized study. Radiology 2002;223(3): 633–638

Kehagias D, Moulopoulos L, Antoniou A, et al. Focal nodular hyperplasia: imaging findings. Eur Radiol 2001;11:202–212

Keyzer C, Tack D, de Maertelaer V, Bohy P, Gevenois PA, Van Gansbeke D. Acute appendicitis: comparison of low-dose and standard-dose unenhanced multi-detector row CT. Radiology 2004;232(1): 164–172

Kimmey MB, Martin RW, Haggitt RC, Wang KY, Franklin DW, Silverstein FE. Histologic correlates of gastrointestinal ultrasound images. Gastroenterology 1989;96:433–441

King LF, Scurr ED, Natajaran M, Williams SGF, Westaby D, Healy JC. Hepatobiliary and pancreatic manifestations of cystic fibrosis: MR imaging appearances. Radiographics 2000;20:767–777

Kuhn JP, Slovis TL, Haller JO, ed. Caffey's pediatric diagnostic imaging. Philadelphia, PA: Elsevier Inc., 2004

Ly JN, Miller FH. MR imaging of the pancreas: a practical approach. Radiol Clin North Am 2002;40:1289–1307

Marincek B. Nontraumatic abdominal emergencies: acute abdominal pain: diagnostic strategies. Eur Radiol 2002;12:2136–2150

Metreweli C, So NM, Chu WC, Lam WW. Magnetic resonance cholangiography in children. Br J Radiol 2004;77:1059–1064

Norton KI, Glass RB, Kogan D, Lee JS, Emre S, Shneider BL. MR cholangiography in the evaluation of neonatal cholestasis: initial results. Radiology 2002;222:687–691

Pariente D. The liver, biliary tract and spleen. In: Carty H, Brunelle F, Shaw D, Kendall B, ed. Imaging children. London, England: Churchill Livingstone, 1994:485–560

Park NH, Park SI, Park CS, et al. Ultrasonographic findings of small bowel intussusception, focusing on differentiation from ileocolic intussusception. Br J Radiol 2007;30:798–802

Paterson A, Frush DP, Donnelly LF, Foss JN, O'Hara SM, Bisset GS 3rd. A pattern-oriented approach to splenic imaging in infants and children. Radiographics 1999;19(6):1465–1485

Puylaert JB. Right-sided segmental infarction of the omentum: clinical, US, and CT findings. Radiology 1992;185:169–172

Puylaert JB. Ultrasonography of the acute abdomen: gastrointestinal conditions. Radiol Clin North Am 2003;41(6):1227–1242

Puylaert JB, Vermeijden RJ, Van der Werf SDJ, Doornbos L, Koumans RK. Incidence and sonographic diagnosis of bacterial ileocaecitis masquerading as appendicitis. Lancet 1989;2:84–86

Remer EM, Baker ME. Imaging of chronic pancreatitis. Radiol Clin North Am 2002;40:1229–1243

Robertson F, Leander P, Ekberg O. Radiology of the spleen. Eur Radiol 2001;11(1):80–95

Roebuck DJ, Olsen Ø, Pariente D. Radiological staging in children with hepatoblastoma. Pediatr Radiol 2006;36:176–182

Rubesin S. Simplified approach to differential diagnosis of small bowel abnormalities. Radiol Clin North Am 2003;41:343–364

Scatarige JC, Horton KM, Sheth S, Fishman EK. Pancreatic parenchymal metastases: observations on helical CT. AJR Am J Roentgenol 2001;176:695–699

Strouse P. Disorders of intestinal rotation and fixation ("malrotation"). Pediatr Radiol 2004;34:837–851

Taylor GA. Suspected appendicitis in children: in search of the single best diagnostic test. Radiology 2004;231(2):293–295

Valls C, Iannacconne R, Alba E, et al. Fat in the liver: diagnosis and characterization. Eur Radiol 2006;16:2292–2308

Ziegler MM. The diagnosis of appendicitis: an evolving paradigm. Pediatrics 2004;113:130–132

3 Urogenital Tract

The Kidneys

Anomalous Renal Size

Abnormal Renal Contour

Agenesis, Dysplasia, and Ectopia

Positional Anomalies of the Kidneys

Pelvicaliceal System

Ureters, Urinary Bladder, and Urethra

→

The Scrotum and Testes

The Adrenal Glands

Adrenal Masses

Adrenal Calcification

The Kidneys

Abnormalities can affect part or all of a kidney and may be unilateral or bilateral. There can be associated involvement of the collecting system and bladder, and, especially in females, ipsilateral genital anomalies. Although ultrasound (US) remains the mainstay of renal imaging, there has been a decline in the use of excretory urography and a rise in the use of computed tomography (CT) and magnetic resonance imaging (MRI). MRI is particularly useful as it provides functional and anatomic information in one study, but availability and the need for sedation or anesthesia limit its use in many centers.

Anomalous Renal Size

■ Unilateral Small Kidneys

A kidney is small if it is > 2 standard deviations (SDs) below normal size for age. Causes may be congenital, secondary to abnormal development, or acquired due to parenchymal loss from a multitude of factors. The remaining normal renal tissue can undergo compensatory hypertrophy. Postnatally, this can be seen 12 to 18 months later (**Tables 3.1** and **3.2**).

Table 3.1 Unilateral small kidneys without pelvicaliceal (PC) dilatation

Diagnosis	Findings	Comments
Congenital hypoplasia (rare)	US: normal echogenicity and corticomedullary differentiation. Voiding cystourethrogram (VCUG): normal. Excretory urography (EU): often decreased number of calyces. Nuclear medicine (NM): Decreased function. Scars suggest segmental hypoplasia/infection.	Small kidney, normal calyces, but often fewer in number. Normal histology. No familial link Segmental hypoplasia (Ask-Upmark kidney): Can lead to severe hypertension. May actually be secondary to infection.
Dysplasia ▷ *Fig. 3.1, p. 240* ▷ *Fig. 3.2, p. 240*	Can involve all or part of a kidney and can be bilateral. US: Increased echogenicity, loss of corticomedullary differentiation. Multiple cortical cysts (small to large). Doppler: increased resistive index (RI) in affected segment. EU: May show ectopic insertion of ureter. May have dilated PC system and ureter from vesicoureteral reflux (VUR) or obstruction. NM: Non- or poorly functioning kidney depending on the extent of dysplasia.	Can be associated with ureteral agenesis or atresia; ureteropelvic junction obstruction; ectopic ureteric insertion (with distance from normal insertion proportional to dysplasia). Can be secondary to obstruction in the first half of pregnancy. Often associated with VUR.
Renal artery stenosis ▷ *Fig. 3.3, p. 240* ▷ *Fig. 3.4, p. 240*	US: Decrease in size of all or part of kidney. Doppler: Increased velocity (> 180 cm/s) immediately distal to the stenosis. Tardus et parvus waveform on intrarenal arteries. Decreased diastolic flow. NM: Delayed perfusion and decreased maximal peak. Increased sensitivity with captopril. Angiography/MRI/CT: narrowing of renal artery.	Associated with fibromuscular hyperplasia, neurofibromatosis, radiation arteritis, and Takayasu disease. Multiple renal arteries may be present and not all affected.
Atrophy secondary to renal artery occlusion	Doppler: absent blood flow with capsular collaterals. Contrast-enhanced CT (CECT): Nonenhancement. Absent or small renal artery.	Causes: thrombotic/thromboembolic, umbilical artery catheter, postsurgery.
Atrophy secondary to radiation	Smooth renal outline with cortex and medulla affected.	Radiation > 30 Gy will result in renal damage.
Atrophy secondary to renal vein thrombosis	US/CT/MRI: Secondary calcification of small intrarenal veins (dystrophic calcification around pyramids). Collateral veins at renal hilum. Renal vein may recanalize.	Can be bilateral.

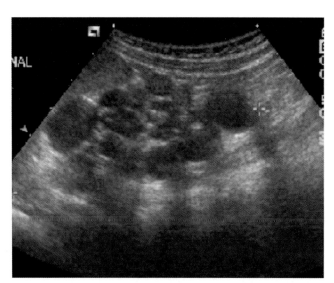

Fig. 3.1   MCDK. US image of a MCDK showing multiple cysts of varying sizes with no discernible intervening renal parenchyma.

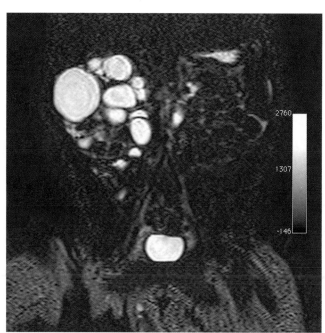

Fig. 3.2   MCDK. Coronal T2-weighted image of the abdomen shows multiple cysts of varying sizes in the right kidney. A nonfunctioning kidney was noted on nuclear scan.

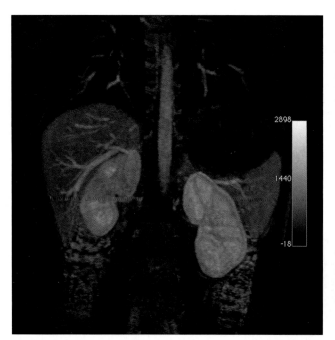

Fig. 3.3   Renal artery stenosis. MRI coronal image: smaller hypoperfused right kidney.

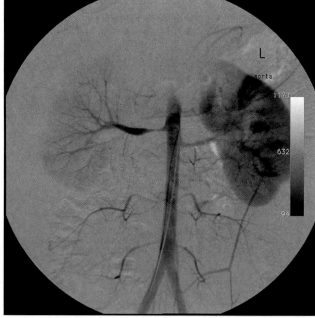

Fig. 3.4   Severe right renal artery stenosis is seen on digital subtraction angiography. Note the delay in the arterial phase of opacification between the two kidneys.

Table 3.2   Unilateral small kidney with PC dilatation

Diagnosis	Findings	Comments
Dysplastic kidneys	(see unilateral dysplastic kidneys in **Table 3.1**)	Renal dysplasia associated with in utero ureteric obstruction or reflux
Postobstructive atrophy	US: Dilated PC system. Thinned cortex with increased echogenicity. CT/MRI: can show level of obstruction.	Can be associated with dysplasia especially if prenatal obstruction.
Decreased size due to pyelonephritis ▷ *Fig. 3.5*	US: small kidney, asymmetric scarring/cortical thinning over calyces. NM (dimercaptosuccinic acid [DMSA]): focal scarring with photopenic areas and decreased function. MRI: dynamic postcontrast imaging can show scarring as areas of cortical thinning and decreased contrast uptake. Can also assess PC system, ureters, split renal function, and glomerular filtration rate (GFR).	Also known as "reflux nephropathy." VCUG may show reflux in approximately 80%. Intravenous urogram (IVU) is no longer indicated.

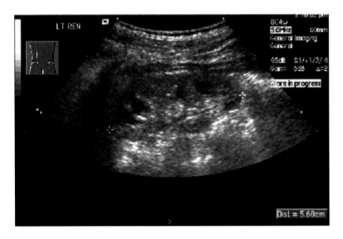

Fig. 3.5   Chronic pyelonephritis. US image shows a small irregular kidney in a child with recurrent renal tract infections.

■ Bilateral Small Kidneys

Similarly to unilateral small kidneys, bilateral small kidneys may be due to congenital or acquired causes; as such, any unilateral cause can also result in bilateral small kidneys. In their end stage, almost all causes of renal disease have similar imaging findings.

Table 3.3   Bilateral small kidneys

Diagnosis	Findings	Comments
Hypoplasia ▷ *Fig. 3.6a, b, p. 242*	(see unilateral hypoplasia)	
Dysplasia ▷ *Fig. 3.7, p. 242*	(see unilateral dysplasia in **Table 3.1**)	Severe renal failure in the neonatal period. May have associated chromosomal abnormalities
Postpyelonephritis shrunken kidneys	(see **Table 3.2**)	Due to recurrent infections and bilateral reflux.
Chronic glomerulonephritis	US: small diffusely hyperechogenic kidneys with loss of corticomedullary differentiation.	Imaging findings are nonspecific and similar to any end-stage renal failure. Renal biopsy establishes diagnosis.
Papillary necrosis ▷ *Fig. 3.8a, b, p. 242*	US: No loss of renal substance. Normal or enlarged calyces. May get calcification of necrosed calyces in chronic cases. IVU: Calcification if chronic. Tracks and horns from calyces. Egg-in-cup appearance. Clubbed, blunt calyces. Filling defects/obstruction from sloughed papillae.	Causes: sickle cell anemia, hemodynamic shock, diabetes, analgesics.
Oligomeganephronia	EU: decreased excretion with decreased number of calyces, sometimes single.	Decreased number of nephrons but markedly hypertrophied.

(continues on page 243)

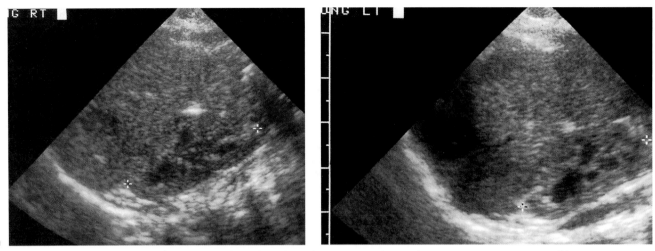

Fig. 3.6a, b   Hypoplasia. US: both kidneys are hypoplastic but otherwise normal. Length: R 3.4 cm; L 3.2 cm. Normal function in a 3-year-old. These lengths might be normal if this were a neonate.

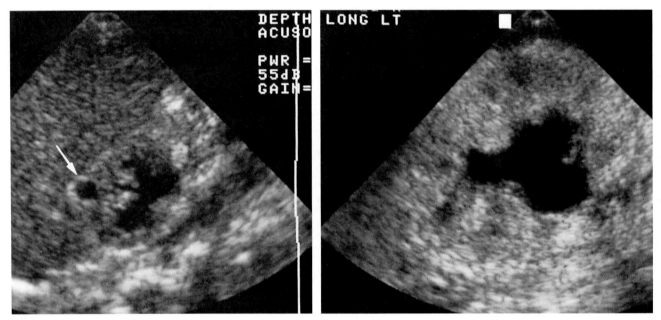

Fig. 3.7   Dysplasia. Urethral valves and bilateral renal hypoplasia and dysplasia. Subcapsular (cortical) cysts on the right (arrow).

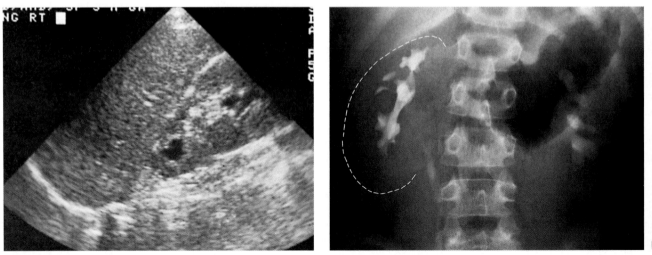

Fig. 3.8a, b   Papillary necrosis. (a) US: postobstructive atrophy and papillary necrosis, significant parenchymal loss in the right kidney and absent medullary pyramids. (b) EU: multiple deformed calyces, parenchymal loss, and abnormal rotation of the right kidney.

Table 3.3   (Cont.) Bilateral small kidneys

Diagnosis	Findings	Comments
Juvenile nephronophthisis (medullary cystic disease complex or hereditary tubulointerstitial nephritis)	US: loss of corticomedullary differentiation initially, then increased cortical echogenicity, decreased size, and small cysts at the corticomedullary junction. CT/MRI: also demonstrate cysts.	Most common genetic cause of end-stage renal disease in children. Usually autosomal recessive with early onset. Autosomal dominant is late onset. May be associated with retinal, oculomotor abnormalities and hepatic fibrosis. Chronic sclerosing tubulointerstitial nephritis on biopsy.
Alport syndrome	US: Hyperechogenic, no corticomedullary differentiation. Progressive decrease in size.	Hereditary nephritis (often X-linked). Hematuria, proteinuria, renal failure. Bilateral hearing loss and ocular defects.
Amyloidosis	Kidneys are initially large then progressively shrink.	

■ Unilateral Renal Enlargement

Large kidneys (> 2 SD above the mean for age) can occur with normal, increased, or decreased renal parenchyma depending on the degree of PC dilatation and the presence of cysts or masses. Unilateral enlargement can be a physiologic response to absence of or loss or decreased function in the contralateral kidney.

Table 3.4   Unilateral renal enlargement without PC dilatation

Diagnosis	Findings	Comments
Duplex kidney ▷ *Fig. 3.9* ▷ *Fig. 3.10*	US: Large kidney with subtle duplication of renal collecting systems and echogenic central sinus complexes. May show ureterocele in bladder. EU: Two renal pelves and ureters. The ureters may fuse distally.	Frequency is approximately 1%. May be complete (major) duplex or partial (minor) duplex. Complete duplex systems may show upper pole obstruction and lower pole reflux. Upper pole tends to insert ectopically in the bladder and be associated with an ureterocele (Weigert-Meyer rule).
Compensatory hypertrophy (solitary kidney)	Large but normal kidney with abnormal or absent kidney on the other side.	Secondary to decreased renal function in the opposing kidney.
Nephromegaly	Large, normal appearance. No duplication of collecting system.	Associated with hemihypertrophy, Beckwith-Wiedemann syndrome, Perlman syndrome.

(continues on page 244)

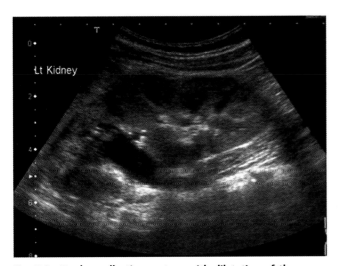

Fig. 3.9   Duplex collecting system with dilatation of the upper moiety.

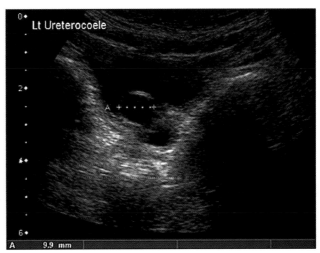

Fig. 3.10   Ureterocele. US image of the urinary bladder shows the presence of an ureterocele in the same patient as in **Fig. 3.9**.

Table 3.4 (Cont.) Unilateral renal enlargement without PC dilatation

Diagnosis	Findings	Comments
Crossed renal ectopia ▷ *Fig. 3.11a, b*	(see agenesis, dysplasia, and ectopia in **Table 3.10**)	
Renal contusion/laceration ▷ *Fig. 3.12a, b*	CECT: Wedge-shaped areas of decreased attenuation. Will show extent of hemorrhage, renal perfusion, and acute ongoing hemorrhage. Delayed CT will show damage to pelvis/ureters and continuity of ureters.	Secondary to blunt abdominal trauma. CT is the modality of choice and allows assessment of other areas.
Acute pyelonephritis ▷ *Fig. 3.13*	US: May be normal. Renal swelling, loss of corticomedullary differentiation, focal areas of abnormal echogenicity. Thickening of walls of pelvis/ureter and renal sinus hypoechogenicity. Doppler: wedge-shaped areas of hypoperfusion. DMSA: focal/diffuse decrease in tracer uptake.	Most commonly upper pole. Imaging has limited role but may show structural abnormality that predisposes to infection or complications such as abscess.
Acute obstructive nephropathy	US: variable dilatation of collecting system. CT: may show calculus. CECT/EU: persistent nephrogram and swollen parenchyma. MRI: persistent nephrogram and delayed renal transit. MAG3: delayed renal transit time.	Causes: calculus, acute obstruction of partially obstructed system.
Nephroblastomatosis ▷ *Fig. 3.14*	US: enlarged kidney with hypoechoic nodules and loss of corticomedullary differentiation. CECT/MRI: Low attenuation nodules with poor enhancement. Predominantly subcapsular. Can be diffuse.	Usually bilateral. Neonate to 2 y. Increased risk of Wilms tumor, especially with Beckwith-Wiedemann syndrome. Requires follow-up but can spontaneously regress.
Mesoblastic nephroma ▷ *Fig. 3.15a, b*	US: predominantly solid hypoechoic/mixed echogenicity lesion. Doppler: may show anechoic vascular ring around tumor. CT: enhances postcontrast but less than normal renal parenchyma.	Cysts, hemorrhage, and necrosis rarely found. Most common neonatal solid tumor. Ninety percent of patients are aged < 1 y. Although benign, can rarely metastasize to lungs, brain, and bone.

(continues on page 246)

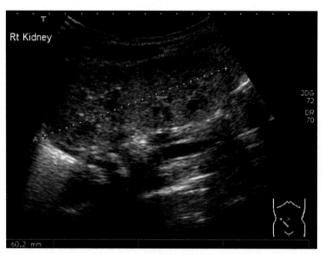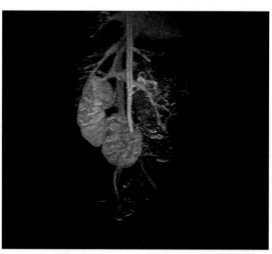

Fig. 3.11a, b Enlarged right kidney. (a) US image showing enlarged right kidney with altered axis; the left renal bed was empty. **(b)** MRI coronal postgadolinium image shows crossed fused renal ectopia of the left kidney.

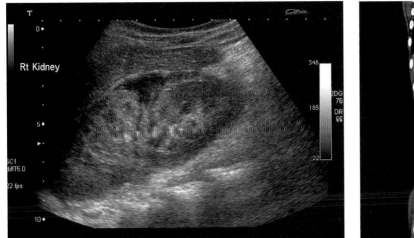
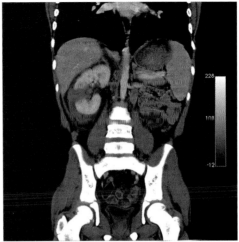

Fig. 3.12a, b   Focal contour defect. (a) US image of a focal contour defect in the right kidney from laceration caused by blunt abdominal trauma. **(b)** CECT image in the same patient defines the extent of laceration along with perinephric hematoma well.

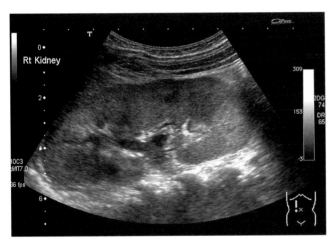
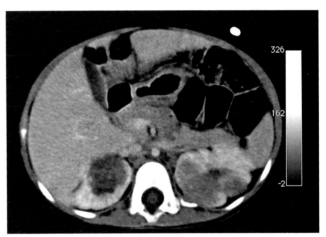

Fig. 3.13   Enlarged kidney. US image of the right kidney in a child presenting with fever and urinary sepsis shows enlarged kidney with heterogeneously altered echotexture of the kidney. The normal corticomedullary distinction is somewhat lost.

Fig. 3.14   Nephroblastomatosis. CECT axial image in a child with nephroblastomatosis. Multiple hypoechoic nodules in both kidneys. The right kidney shows transformation of one of the rests into Wilms tumor.

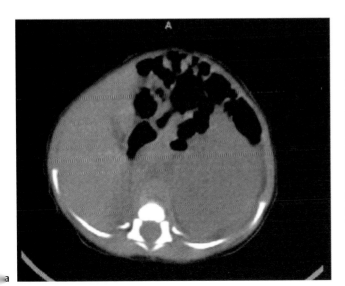
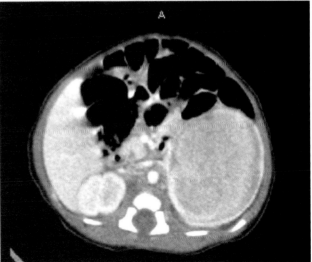

Fig. 3.15a, b   Mesoblastic nephroma. (a) Pre- and **(b)** postcontrast axial CT images show a mesoblastic nephroma in a neonate. The mass is hypodense and enhances heterogeneously with contrast.

Table 3.4   (Cont.) Unilateral renal enlargement without PC dilatation

Diagnosis	Findings	Comments
Wilms tumor	US/CT/MRI: heterogeneous mass. Inferior vena cava and renal vein may show thrombus. Does not encase vessels. Nodal metastases. Low signal on T1-weighted and high on T2-weighted MRI. MRI most sensitive for caval patency.	Eighty percent occur before 5 y of age. Four to thirteen percent are bilateral; 1% are familial. Five to ten percent have calcifications. Associated with cryptorchidism, hemihypertrophy, hypospadias, sporadic aniridia.
Multilocular cystic renal tumor	US/CT/MRI: Well-demarcated cystic intrarenal mass. Septae enhanced. Cysts may show evidence of hemorrhage or protein on MRI.	Two age peaks: 3 mo to 4 y (boys > girls). Adults (mainly women). Benign.
Autosomal dominant polycystic kidney disease (ADPKD) ▷ *Fig. 3.16a, b*	See **Table 3.6**	May be unilateral initially in young patients.
Renal transplant rejection	US: Increased echogenicity. Loss of corticomedullary differentiation. Doppler: decreased blood flow and increased resistive indices.	Acute tubular necrosis has a similar appearance.
Medullary sponge kidney ▷ *Fig. 3.17*	(see bilateral medullary sponge kidneys, **Table 3.6**)	
Xanthogranulomatous pyelonephritis ▷ *Fig. 3.18a, b*	US/CT: Calcified nodule in otherwise normal kidney seen in localized form. Diffuse form shows large lesion replacing entire kidney with loss of corticomedullary differentiation, cystic/necrotic areas, calcification/stones around renal pelvis.	Severe atypical, chronic renal parenchymal infection. Multiple causes: 70% stones. Difficult to differentiate from tumor.
Acute renal vein thrombosis ▷ *Fig. 3.19*	US: Enlarged, hypoechoic kidney with hyperechoic streaks. Loss of corticomedullary differentiation. Thrombus not always visible. Doppler: Lack of flow in renal vein. Absent/reversed end-diastolic flow in intrarenal arteries. MRI: most sensitive if US equivocal.	May be bilateral. On the left, may be associated with adrenal hemorrhage. Causes: asphyxia, shock, dehydration, infant of diabetic mother.

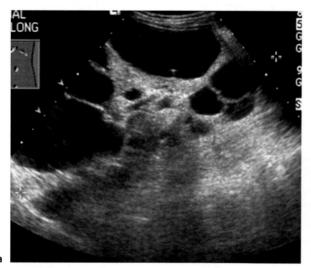
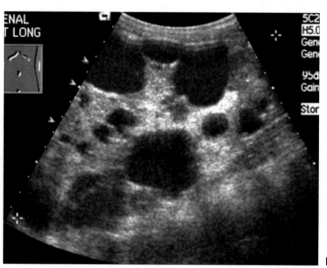

a   b

Fig. 3.16a, b   ADPKD. US images of bilaterally enlarged kidneys with multiple cysts in a child with ADPKD.

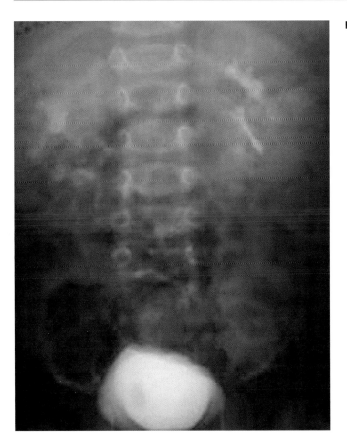

Fig. 3.17   **Bilateral renal calcifications** with dilated tubules on the EU.

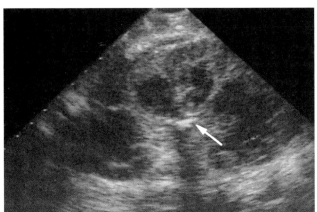
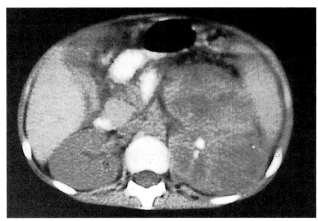

a   b

Fig. 3.18a, b   **Xanthogranulomatous pyelonephritis. (a)** US: markedly enlarged right kidney, focal alterations in echogenicity, calculi (arrow). **(b)** Precontrast CT: marked hydronephrosis on the left and intrarenal calcification.

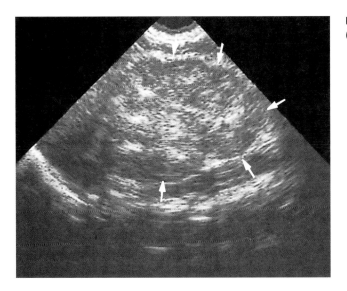

Fig. 3.19   **Acute renal vein thrombosis.** Markedly enlarged kidney (arrows) with areas of echogenic hemorrhage.

Unilateral Renal Enlargement with Pelvicaliceal Dilatation

Hydronephrosis can be obstructive, nonobstructive, or secondary to reflux. The degree of dilatation depends predominantly on duration of reflux or obstruction and less on severity and can be assessed well on US. The presence of a dilated ureter helps determine cause. However, US is unable to assess severity of obstruction and function. Technetium-99m (99mTc) mercaptoacetyltriglycine scintigraphy with Lasix washout is able to assess the degree of obstruction and remaining renal function, but if function is reduced in both kidneys, then erroneously "normal" results can be obtained. MRI is increasingly being used and is able to assess level and cause of hydronephrosis as well as function of kidneys, including GFR.

Table 3.5   Unilateral renal enlargement with PC dilatation

Diagnosis	Findings	Comments
Ureteropelvic junction (UPJ) obstruction ▷ *Fig. 3.20a–c*	US: Dilatation of renal pelvis and calyces with varying parenchymal loss. Anteroposterior renal pelvis diameter > 10 m. MAG3: Test of choice. Delayed excretion and retention of counts in pelvis. Activity curves allow quantitation of obstruction. Also allows indirect VCUG for reflux. MRI: With gadolinium-diethylene triamine pentaacetic acid. Allows activity curves similar to NM as well as split renal function, GFR, and anatomic detail.	Associated with VUR (14%, which can be shown by VCUG), horseshoe kidney, lithiasis. Ten to thirty percent are bilateral. Usually obstruction is partial. Often diagnosed on prenatal US.
Hydronephrosis due to VUR	Dilated collecting system (see bilateral renal enlargement with PC dilatation, **Table 3.7**)	
Nonobstructive hydronephrosis or status postsurgically repaired urethral obstruction	US: hydronephrosis. MAG3: normal washout of tracer with diuretic.	

(continues on page 249)

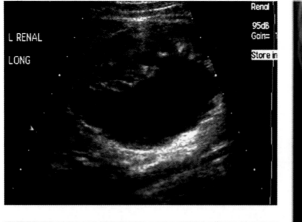

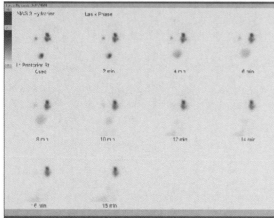

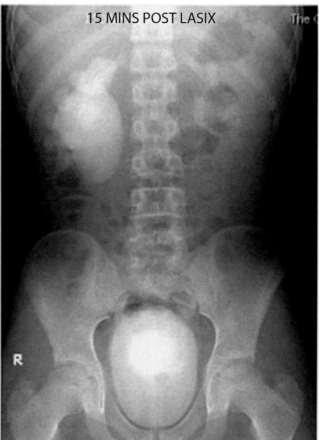

Fig. 3.20a–c   UPJ obstruction. (a) US image of dilated renal pelvis and hydronephrosis. **(b)** IVU shows persistent hydronephrosis after intravenous Lasix. **(c)** MAG3 scan postintravenous Lasix shows tracer retention in the renal PC system with delayed clearance in keeping with UPJ obstruction.

Table 3.5 (Cont.) Unilateral renal enlargement with PC dilatation

Diagnosis	Findings	Comments
Megacalycosis/polycalycosis	EU: Polygonal multifaceted appearance of 15+ calyces. Cortical thinning. MAG3: no evidence of obstruction.	May be associated with primary megaureter. At risk for lithiasis, infection. Thought to be secondary to underdevelopment of renal pyramids.
Multicystic dysplastic kidneys (MCDK) ▷ Fig. 3.1, p. 240 ▷ Fig. 3.2, p. 240	US: Multiple large and some small noncommunicating cysts. Echogenic dysplastic tissue between cysts. No normal renal parenchyma. NM: no renal excretion of isotope.	Associated with abnormal or atretic ipsilateral ureter. Ipsilateral genital abnormalities in 50% (e.g., cystic dysplasia of the rete testis). Thirty percent of contralateral kidneys/ureter abnormal.
Distal ureteral stenosis	Variable dilatation of ureters and collecting system. Often with minimal renal enlargement.	Associated with renal dysplasia.

Bilateral Renal Enlargement Without Pelvicaliceal Dilatation

Table 3.6 Bilateral renal enlargement without PC dilatation

Diagnosis	Findings	Comments
Tamm-Horsfall nephropathy (stasis nephropathy)	US: hyperechoic medulla and normal cortex. CT: prolonged nephrogram.	Usually seen in first 5 d of life. Reversible.
Nephromegaly in infants of diabetic mothers	US: large but otherwise normal kidneys.	Renal vein thrombosis is also more common in infants of diabetic mothers. Caused by transient hyperinsulinism.
Bilateral duplex kidneys	(see duplex kidney, Table 3.4)	
Autosomal recessive polycystic kidney disease (ARPKD) ▷ Fig. 3.21, p. 250 ▷ Fig. 3.22a, b, p. 250	US: large homogenous echogenic kidneys with barely discernible subcapsular cysts measuring up to 3 mm. EU: radial streaks and tubular stasis ("brush" pattern).	Live births: 1:40,000. Associated with hepatic fibrosis. If severe may have hypoplastic lungs and Potter phenotype.
ADPKD ▷ Fig. 3.16a, b, p. 246	US: Often normal in early childhood. At least two cysts in one kidney and family history is diagnostic. Can be asymmetric/unilateral in childhood. CT/MRI: Sensitive for showing size and number of cysts. Can show evidence of infection or hemorrhage.	Occurrence: 1:1000. Associated with intracranial aneurysms, colonic diverticula, mitral valve regurgitation. Cysts occur in other organs, especially liver in adults. Usually manifests after three decades of life. Increasing volume of cysts corresponds with increasing renal failure.
Acute lymphoblastic leukemia (ALL)/lymphoma ▷ Fig. 3.23, p. 250	US: Diffuse (or nodular in lymphoma) enlargement of kidneys. Loss of corticomedullary differentiation. Hypoechoic. CT/MRI: Similar findings. Deposits enhance poorly.	Lymphoma is usually bilateral and associated with other sites of disease. Older children than Wilms tumor.
Medullary sponge kidneys ▷ Fig. 3.17, p. 247	US: large kidneys with nephrocalcinosis around papillae. EU/CT: Nephrocalcinosis. Radial patchy contrast in pyramids in excretory phase of scan.	Rare in pediatrics. Manifests in adults. Can be segmental or affect whole kidney. Causes by cystic dilatation of collecting tubules.
Nephroblastomatosis Fig. 3.14, p. 245	(see unilateral renal enlargement without PC dilatation, Table 3.4)	

(continues on page 251)

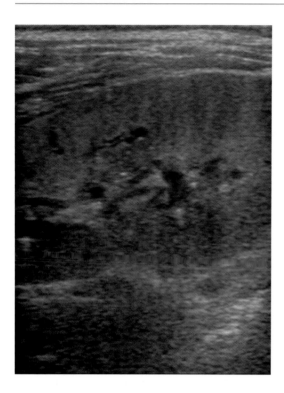

Fig. 3.21 ARPKD. US image of a kidney in a neonate with ARPKD. The parenchyma is echogenic with poor corticomedullary differentiation. Note the small juxtamedullary cysts.

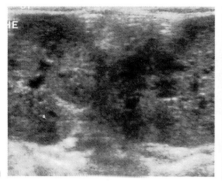

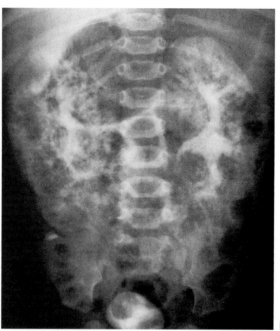

Fig. 3.22a, b ARPKD. (a) Transverse section US at the level of the umbilicus: markedly echogenic kidneys (5-day-old neonate). **(b)** EU: classic appearance with markedly enlarged kidneys and delayed nephrogram (2 hours post injection; 9-day-old neonate).

b

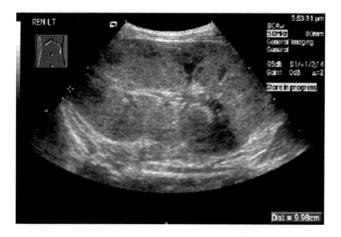

Fig. 3.23 Leukemic infiltration. Diffusely enlarged kidneys in a child with ALL representing leukemic infiltration. Note that the kidneys retain their reniform shape despite the parenchymal infiltration.

Table 3.6   (Cont.) Bilateral renal enlargement without PC dilatation

Diagnosis	Findings	Comments
Acute tubular necrosis (shock kidneys) ▷ Fig 3.24a, b	US: large swollen echogenic kidneys with loss of corticomedullary differentiation. Doppler: Nonspecific increase in RI. EU/CT: persisting dense nephrogram that may develop slowly	Causes: Prerenal failure, drugs, anoxic injury in neonates. Acute sequelae of renal transplant. Kidney returns to normal following treatment.
Acute/subacute glomerulonephritis	US: Renal enlargement with increased cortical echogenicity. Doppler: may show halo sign on power Doppler with peripherally reduced renal flow.	Increased risk of renal vein thrombosis.
Nephrotic syndrome with minimal change nephritis	US: Renal enlargement with increased echogenicity of the cortex. Pleural effusions and ascites common.	Sonographic changes correspond with clinical course.
Acute pyelonephritis ▷ Fig. 3.13, p. 245	(see unilateral renal enlargement without PC dilatation, **Table 3.4**)	Rarely bilateral.
Kawasaki syndrome	US: Large, echogenic kidneys. Hydropic gallbladder. Doppler: arteritis may lead to renal artery stenosis/aneurysms.	Medium vessel arteritis. Coronary arteries often involved. Nephrotic syndrome.
Human immunodeficiency virus nephropathy	US: large echogenic kidneys.	
Sickle cell anemia	US: increased echogenicity of renal pyramids but no hypercalciuria. Doppler: increased RI/infracts. EU: Papillary necrosis. Vertebral body changes.	Renal failure in 5% to 18% at median age of 23 y. Scarred shrunken kidneys in the late stage. At risk of renal medullary carcinoma.
Glycogen storage disease	US: Large kidneys with nonspecific changes in echogenicity. Hepatomegaly.	Type 1 most associated with renal involvement.
Cystinosis	US: Large kidneys with increased echogenicity. May get severe nephrocalcinosis.	Autosomal recessive. Chromosome 17p13. Causes tubular dysfunction.
Amyloidosis	US: diffusely increased echogenicity and enlarged kidneys.	Causes: cystic fibrosis, bronchiectasis, familial Mediterranean fever, chronic osteomyelitis.

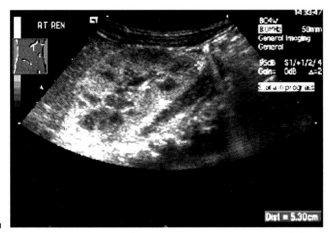 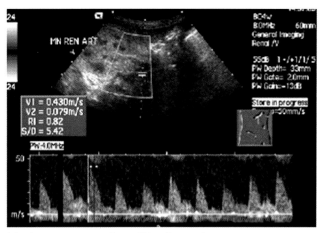

b

Fig. 3.24a, b   Acute tubular necrosis. (a) On US, echogenic kidneys with high-resistance waveforms (**b**) in the renal arteries are seen.

Bilateral Renal Enlargement with Pelvicaliceal Dilatation

Table 3.7 Bilateral renal enlargement with PC dilatation

Diagnosis	Findings	Comments
Duplex kidneys ▷ *Fig. 3.10, p. 243*	(see duplex kidney, **Table 3.5**)	
UPJ obstruction ▷ *Fig. 3.20a–c, p. 248*	(see UPJ obstruction, **Table 3.5**)	
UVJ obstruction	(see distal ureteral obstruction, **Table 3.5**)	
VUR ▷ *Fig. 3.25a, b* ▷ *Fig. 3.26* ▷ *Fig. 3.27*	US: may show dilated renal pelvis and calyces. VCUG: Definitive examination. Reflux from bladder into ureters and kidney. MAG3: Indirect radionuclide cystography in continent children. Increased counts in the renal pelvis following micturition.	Graded 1 to 5 on VCUG, based on level of reflux and amount of dilatation of ureter and PC system. May be associated with duplex kidneys (usually lower pole) and posterior urethral valves. Obstruction may coexist.
Megacalycosis/ polycalycosis	(see unilateral renal enlargement with PC dilatation, **Table 3.5**)	

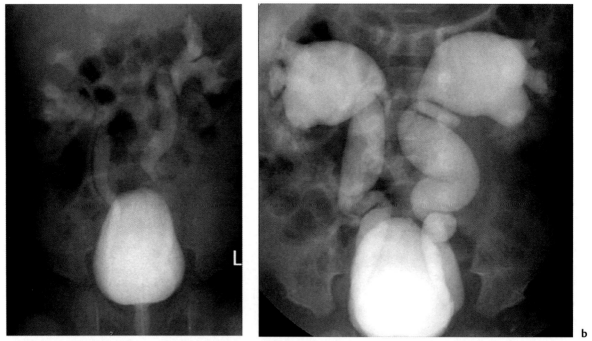

Fig. 3.25a, b   Bilateral VUR on a micturating cystourethrogram. (a) Note the duplex collecting system on the right side with Grade 2 reflux in the upper moiety and Grade 3 reflux in the lower moiety. **(b)** Bilateral Grade 5 VUR with intrarenal reflux.

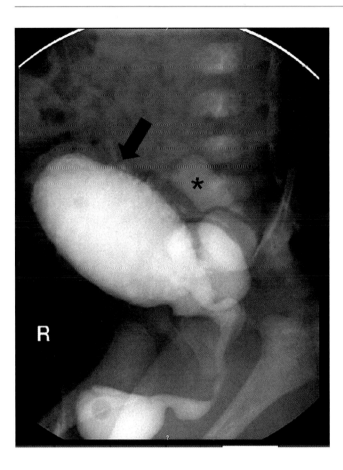

Fig. 3.26 Urethral diverticulum. VCUG image in the micturition phase in a boy with anterior urethral stricture shows posterior urethral diverticulum. Note the trabeculated contours of the bladder (arrow) and reflux (asterisk).

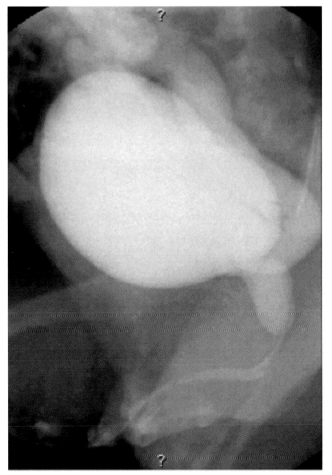

Fig. 3.27 VCUG image in the micturition phase shows posterior urethral valve causing obstruction and dilatation of the posterior urethra. Sometimes, the valve itself may be seen as a lucent filling defect at the posterior urethra on the urethrograms. Note the gross VUR on this image.

Abnormal Renal Contour

Renal function and contour change with age. In the neonatal period, the kidney has a more rounded appearance with a thinner hyperechogenic cortex and more apparent fetal lobulation (**Fig. 3.29**). The pyramids are hypoechogenic and prominent with little sinus fat. By 2 to 3 months, the cortex takes on a more adult echogenicity. With increasing age, the kidneys elongate and there is a gradual reduction in lobulation (illustrated in **Fig. 3.28**). Common normal variants in renal contour include hypertrophied column of Bertin (**Fig. 3.30**) and dromedary hump (**Fig. 3.31**). Incomplete fusion of the two renal masses that form the kidney result in an echogenic strip of nonrenal tissue toward the upper pole, called the interrenicular junction line (**Fig. 3.32**), and should not be mistaken for scarring. Persistence of fetal lobulation may also occur.

Abnormal position of the kidneys can occur, ranging from minor unilateral displacement to complete displacement of both kidneys. Kidneys may fail to ascend during development, resulting in a pelvic kidney, or cross the midline with a consequent cross-fused ectopic kidney. A horseshoe kidney where the lower poles (or upper in 10%) of the kidneys are connected across the midline by abnormal renal or fibrous tissue is the most common fusion anomaly and is associated with chromosomal disorders such as Turner syndrome.

Acquired changes include flattening from hepato- or splenomegaly, or the presence of renal cysts or masses deforming the renal contour. Loss of renal tissue such as from scarring also alters contour.

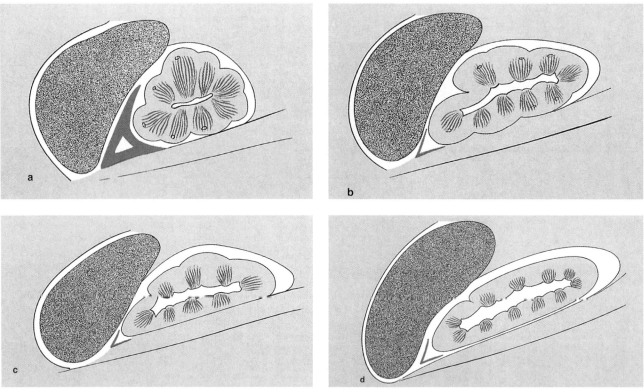

Fig. 3.28a–d   Progression of renal development. Alteration in the shape and outline of the kidney in neonate (**a**), infant (**b**), young child (**c**), and adult (**d**). Note the decreasing size of the adrenal gland.

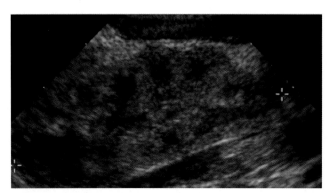

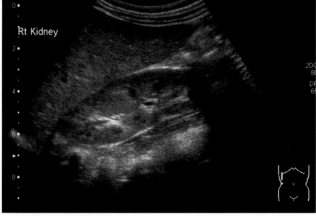

Fig. 3.29   Dromedary hump. US image of the left kidney shows a bulge on its lateral aspect owing to the adjacent spleen: the dromedary hump.

Fig. 3.30   Fetal lobulations. US image in a neonate shows the presence of fetal lobulations at the renal contours. This is a normal appearance and may be seen up to 6 months of age.

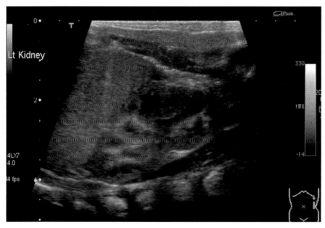

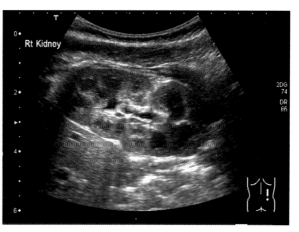

Fig. 3.31 A prominent column of Bertin may be mistaken for an isoechoic renal neoplasm.

Fig. 3.32 Junctional cortical defect or interrenicular septum may be mistaken for a focal scar.

Table 3.8 Focal areas of renal hyperplasia

Diagnosis	Findings	Comments
Dromedary hump ▷ *Fig. 3.30*	US: left kidney triangular with bulge on lateral aspect.	More common in neonates, becomes less common with age.
Pseudotumor: hypertrophied column of Bertin ▷ *Fig. 3.29*	US: extension of cortex between two calyces towards the renal pelvis. DMSA: will show increased uptake at site of column.	
Renal cyst	US: simple cyst shows clear, well-defined thin wall with anechoic fluid and posterior acoustic enhancement. CT/MRI: classic appearance. Fluid (0–20 Hounsfield units [HU] on CT).	Rare in children (0.22%). May be part of an inherited syndrome such as ADPKD if multiple.
Focal nephritis	As for glomerulonephritis/pyelonephritis but focal (see **Table 3.4**)	May result in scarring which is well demonstrated on DMSA.
Intrarenal tumor ▷ *Fig. 3.33, p. 256* ▷ *Fig. 3.14, p. 245* ▷ *Fig. 3.15a, b, p. 245*	US: usually heterogenous mildly hyperechogenic mass (but angiomyolipoma usually echo bright). CT/MRI: low attenuation precontrast with enhancement postcontrast.	Nephroblastomatosis, Wilms tumor, lymphoma, renal cell carcinoma, medullary carcinoma, rhabdoid tumor, clear cell carcinoma, etc. Benign: mesoblastic nephroma, angiomyolipoma.
Intrarenal hematoma	US: Heterogeneously hyperechoic initially, becoming hypoechoic with time. May have subcapsular hematoma flattening underlying renal cortex. CT: heterogenous, initially high attenuation.	Usually secondary to blunt trauma or biopsy.
Acute renal infarct	Focal enlargement with hypoechogenicity on US and low attenuation on CT. Doppler: decreased vascularity of affected segment.	Causes: embolus or thrombosis (secondary to vasculitis).
Renal absces ▷ *Fig. 3.34, p. 256*	US: Abscess appears as a mass with variable echogenicity depending on degree of liquefaction. Surrounding fat may show increased echogenicity due to inflammation. CT: best technique to show extent of abscess and subcapsular and perinephric spread.	Usually secondary to delayed or incorrect diagnosis of acute pyelonephritis.

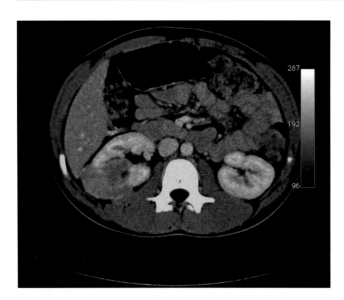

Fig. 3.33 Angiomyolipoma. CECT image shows a right renal mass in a child with tuberous sclerosis. The mass has heterogenous attenuation with areas of fat density as is often seen with an angiomyolipoma.

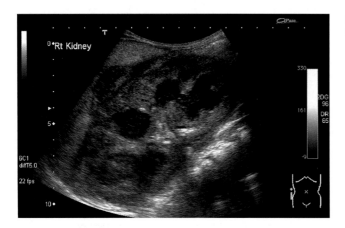

Fig. 3.34 Pyonephrotic kidney. US image of pyonephrotic kidney with concomitant renal abscess extending into the perinephric space.

Table 3.9 Focal areas of renal hypoplasia

Diagnosis	Findings	Comments
Segmental hypoplasia	US/CT/MRI: Localized cortical loss and thinning. Often associated with duplex kidneys. Doppler: hypoplastic region may be paucivascular.	Reflux nephropathy, renal artery stenosis in presence of multiple renal arteries, arteritis, Ask-Upmark kidney.
Renal scarring	US/CT/MRI: Caliceal deformity and loss of parenchyma overlying the calyx. Upper pole most common. DMSA: wedge-shaped photopenic areas.	Causes: Reflux nephropathy, pyelonephritis. Also surgery, intervention, infarction, trauma.
Localized intrarenal obstruction, caliceal diverticulum	US/CT/MRI: hydrocalyx and focal parenchymal reduction.	Causes: Obstruction by blood clot or stone. Infundibular stenosis. Obstruction due to external blood vessel (Fraley syndrome).

Agenesis, Dysplasia, and Ectopia

During development, the kidney arises from the presacral mesenchyme. As it matures, it ascends craniad and rotates to lie in the retroperitoneum lateral to the T10–L2 vertebral bodies. Problems during this phase can result in agenesis, dysplasia, and ectopia. Thus absence of a kidney in its normal location should raise the possibility of an ectopic location or severe hypoplasia as well as agenesis. US may provide the answer, as may scintigraphy if there is functioning renal tissue. MRI is becoming increasingly valuable as it is able to assess anatomy of the whole renal tract as well as function.

Table 3.10   Agenesis, dysplasia, and ectopia

Diagnosis	Findings	Comments
Renal agenesis	US/scintigraphy: Unilateral kidney with compensatory hypertrophy. No renal tissue demonstrated elsewhere	Incidence is 1:450. Ipsilateral adrenal agenesis in 10%. Associated with genital abnormalities in females
Multicystic dysplastic kidney ▷Fig. 3.1, p. 240 ▷Fig. 3.2, p. 240	(see unilateral renal enlargement with PC dilatation, Table 3.5)	
Horseshoe kidney ▷Fig. 3.35a–c	US/CT/MRI: Medial orientation of long axis. Renal pelves and ureters anterior. Joined at poles by parenchymal or fibrous band. May have reflux or UPJ obstruction.	Incidence is 1:2000. Ninety percent are in the lower pole, and 10% in the upper. Associated with Turner syndrome, trisomy 18, malformations of central nervous system, cardiovascular, anorectal, genitourinary, etc.
Crossed (fused) renal ectopia ▷Fig. 3.11a, b, p. 244	US: May see anterior or posterior notch. Two collecting systems with different orientation. Absent kidney on other side. EU: two collecting systems and ureters with one crossing the midline to insert in the bladder. MRI: multiplanar imaging allows assessment of position, rotation, ureters, fusion, and vascular supply.	Incidence is 1:5000. Left to right more common. Associated with reflux, chromosomal abnormalities. Ninety percent are fused, and 10% are unfused.
Pancake kidney	Fused kidneys lying in the lumbar or presacral region.	Normal insertion of the ureters.
Pelvic kidney	US/scintigraphy: pelvic position of kidney.	Associated with reflux, obstruction, vertebral body anomalies, and genital anomalies in females.
Thoracic kidney ▷Fig. 3.36a, b, p. 258	Kidney lies in thorax.	Ninety percent are left-sided. Associated with diaphragmatic defects.

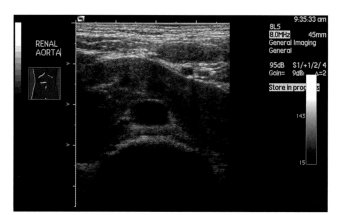

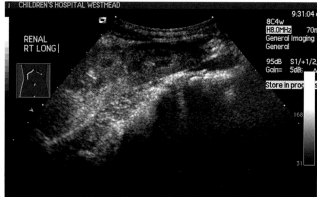

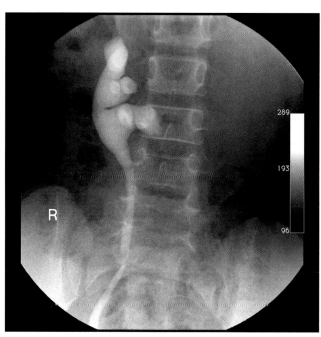

Fig. 3.35a–c   Horseshoe kidney. (**a**) US image in the axial plane shows renal cortical tissue forming an isthmus (bridge) anterior to the abdominal aorta in a horseshoe kidney. (**b**) Long axis view of the right kidney shows the inferior pole extending toward the midline to form the isthmus. (**c**) VCUG shows reflux in the right moiety in a horseshoe kidney. Note the orientation of the PC system.

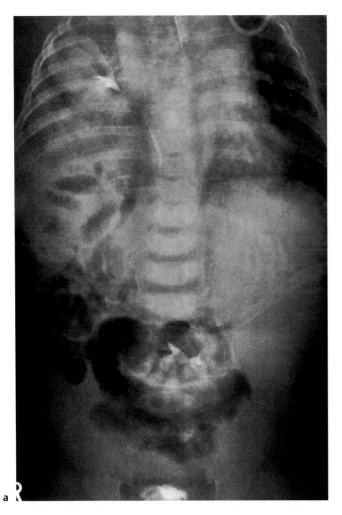

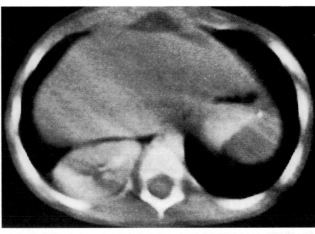

Fig. 3.36a, b Thoracic kidney. (a) Kidney of normal size and good function: right diaphragmatic hernia and left lumbosacral ectopic kidney. **(b)** CT reveals a kidney in the right costophrenic angle.

Positional Anomalies of the Kidneys

The kidney may be in an anomalous position whether due to ectopia (**Table 3.10**) or due to secondary displacement arising from surrounding structures (**Table 3.11**). The kidney itself is rarely compromised by displacement. MRI and multidetector CT offer the best imaging with both cause and effect demonstrated. US can also be helpful, but changes in position can be subtle. EU has no role to play.

Table 3.11 Secondary renal displacement

Diagnosis	Findings	Causes
Inferior renal displacement ▷ *Fig. 3.37* ▷ *Fig. 3.38a–c*	Kidney low lying and may be rotated. May have indentation of upper pole.	Adrenal tumor (neuroblastoma, adenoma, carcinoma). Adrenal hemorrhage. Adrenal cysts or phaeochromocytoma.
Lateral renal displacement	Whole kidney may be displaced, or upper/lower pole may be displaced with rotation of the kidney. Can be missed on US.	Hydronephrotic upper pole of duplex kidney. Paravertebral mass (neuroblastoma, lymphoma). Retroperitoneal hemorrhage. Psoas abscess/hemorrhage Masses arising from the vertebral column.
Anterior renal displacement	Mild elevation of the lower pole, which is difficult to appreciate on US.	Psoas muscle abscess, hemorrhage, hypertrophy. Retroperitoneal soft-tissue tumor. Perirenal subcapsular hematoma.

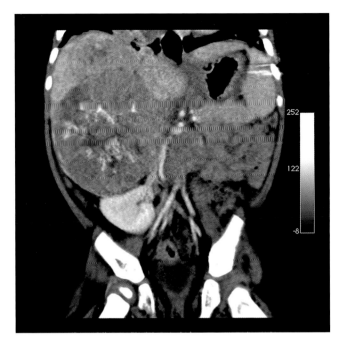

Fig. 3.37   Suprarenal neuroblastoma. CECT coronal reconstruction shows a large right suprarenal neuroblastoma with calcifications.

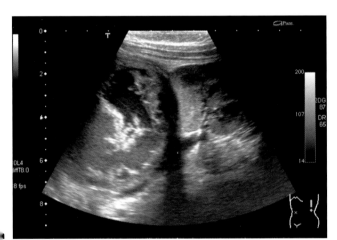

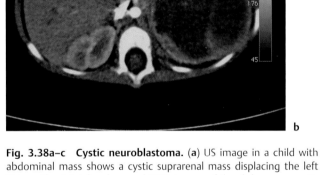

b

Fig. 3.38a–c   Cystic neuroblastoma. (a) US image in a child with abdominal mass shows a cystic suprarenal mass displacing the left kidney. **(b, c)** Axial and coronal CECT images of the abdomen: a cystic left suprarenal mass with enhancing capsule and thick septation solid components is seen. Biopsy revealed a cystic neuroblastoma.

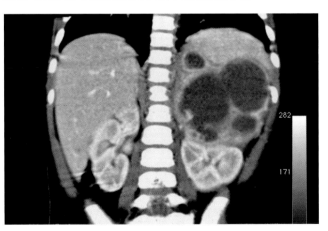

Pelvicaliceal System

Table 3.12 Dilatation of the entire PC system

Diagnosis	Findings	Comments
UPJ obstruction	(see UPJ obstruction, **Table 3.5**)	
Intrinsic ureteral obstruction	Plain X-ray: calculus (but 30% false negative). CT (noncontrast): Sensitive and specific for calculi. Periureteral/-nephric stranding suggestive of obstructing lesion. MR: contrast urography delineates function and morphology of renal tract.	Causes: calculi (most common), blood clot, fungal ball, papillary necrosis, polyp, ureteral valve, strictures, ureteroceles, and bladder masses
Extrinsic ureteral obstruction ▷ *Fig. 3.39*	Plain X-ray: Displaced loops of bowel. Calcification in mass. US: Hydronephrosis and proximal ureteric dilatation. May show extrinsic mass or vascular cause. CECT/MRI: can show mass, crossing vessels, retrocaval ureter, etc.	Medial ureteric deviation: retrocaval ureter, renal mass/hemorrhage. Lateral deviation: retroperitoneal tumors, lymphadenopathy, hematoma. Deviation/compression of lower ureter: lymphadenopathy, diverticula, surgery, pelvic mass/lipomatosis/hematoma
Megacalycosis/polycalycosis	(see megacalycosis/polycalycosis, **Table 3.5**)	
Infundibulopelvic stenosis	EU/CT/MRI: Caliceal dilatation and infundibular stenosis. Small renal pelvis. US: Nonspecific. Caliceal dilatation. No renal pelvis dilatation.	Rare form of congenital hydrocalycosis. Dilated calyces drain through stenotic infundibula into a hypoplastic/stenosed renal pelvis. Different from infundibular stenosis, which has normal pelvis.

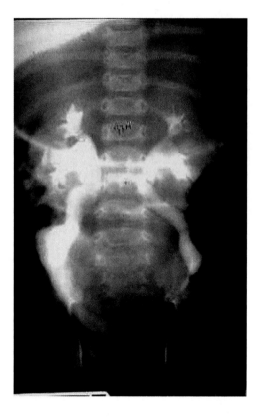

Fig. 3.39 EU in a young girl shows obstructed ureters on both sides displaced laterally by a pelvic "mass." The extrinsic mass was found to be an enlarged uterus from hydrometrocolpos.

Table 3.13   Partial dilatation of the PC system

Caliceal diverticulum	EU/CT/MRI: Delayed opacification and drainage of diverticulum. Smooth margins and caliceal communication. May arise from any part of PC system. US: cystic parenchymal lesion.	Congenital or acquired. Typically asymptomatic, but may be complicated by infection or stones.
Upper caliceal dilatation	CECT/MRI: demonstrates caliceal dilatation and cause. US: focal caliceal dilatation. Doppler: may show compressing vessel.	Extrinsic infundibular stenosis: congenital vascular compression, trauma, space occupying lesion (SOL). Intrinsic infundibular stenosis: tumor, trauma, infection (especially tuberculosis).
Dilated upper pole of a duplex kidney ▷ *Fig. 3.9, p. 243* ▷ *Fig. 3.10, p. 243*	US: dilated upper system, large kidney. EU: Drooping lily sign with nonfunctioning upper moiety. Shows ectopic ureteric insertion. CECT/MRI: can show ureteral and renal morphology.	Causes: stenosis of upper pole ureteral orifice, ectopic insertion of upper pole ureter, and ureterocele. Associated with lower moiety reflux, which can be seen on VCUG.

Table 3.14   Filling defects in the PC system and ureter

Diagnosis	Findings	Comments
Calculi ▷ *Fig. 3.40*	Noncontrast CT: perinephric and periureteral stranding with stone in renal tract. US: echogenic focus in kidney or PC system.	Plain films are only 60% sensitive.
Renal cysts	(see **Table 3.8**)	
Renal tumors	(see **Table 3.8**)	
Pyonephrosis ▷ *Fig. 3.41, p. 262* ▷ *Fig. 3.42, p. 262* ▷ *Fig. 3.34, p. 256*	US: dependent debris in dilated renal tract. CECT: Dilated renal tract with increased attenuation over urine. Urothelial thickening.	Causes: infection post obstructing calculus or in preexisting obstruction.
Intraluminal air	Abdominal X-ray: streaky, bubbly lucencies in renal tract. US: echogenic foci with dirty shadowing or ring-down artifacts. CT: air attenuation within renal tract.	Causes: iatrogenic, penetrating trauma, fistulae. Rarely infection.
Blood clot	Noncontrast CT: intraluminal density with HU consistent with blood. US: echogenic focus with no Doppler signal.	Causes: trauma, intervention, surgery, tumor, and rarely infection.
Papillary necrosis	(see bilateral small kidneys, **Table 3.3**)	
Fungal ball	US: Echogenic mass in collecting system. No Doppler signal. EU: CT irregular; castlike filling defect in the collecting system.	*Candida* is most common infection. Usually an opportunistic infection in the immunocompromised patient.
Fibroepithelial polyp	EU: irregular filling defect attached by a stalk at one end to the ureter.	

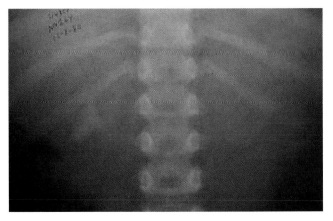

Fig. 3.40   Right renal staghorn calculus. The shape of the calculus conforms to the collecting system.

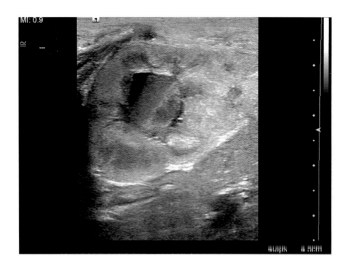

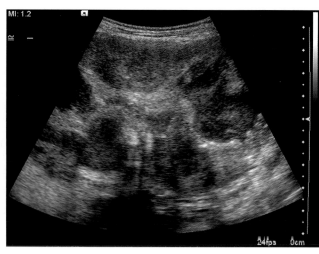

Fig. 3.41 Pyonephrosis. US image of kidney shows dilated collecting system with layering echogenic debris.

Fig. 3.42 Pyonephrosis. US image of the kidney in another child with pyonephrosis shows dilated calyces with particulate internal echoes and debris.

Ureters, Urinary Bladder, and Urethra

Table 3.15   The dilated ureter

Diagnosis	Findings	Comments
VUR ▷ *Fig. 3.25a, b, p. 252* ▷ *Fig. 3.26, p. 253* ▷ *Fig. 3.27, p. 253*	(see bilateral renal enlargement with PC dilatation, **Table 3.7**)	
Primary megaureter	EU/MRI/CT: dilated whole or part of ureter, most marked and fusiform distally with suddenly above vesicoureteral junction (VUJ). US: may show adynamic distal dilatation.	Bilateral in 20%. More common in males.
Intrinsic ureteral compression	(see **Table 3.12**)	
Extrinsic ureteral compression	(see **Table 3.12**)	
Ureterocele ▷ *Fig. 3.43* ▷ *Fig. 3.10b, p. 243*	US: thin-walled cystic structure in bladder, extending from ureter. CT/EU: cobra head appearance of orthotopic ureterocele. VCUG: filling defect in bladder on early filling films.	Ectopic ureteroceles: Associated with upper pole of duplex kidney. More common in females (6 times more common). Orthotopic ureteroceles: Rarer. Often incidental findings in older children/adults. Normal position at trigone.
Ectopic (subvesical) ureter	Dilated ureter and dysplastic upper moiety of duplex system may be shown on all modalities. EU/CT/MRI: can show ectopic insertion. VCUG: reflux in 30%.	Presentation: dribbling in girls, epididymo-orchitis in boys. Sixty-eight to 80% are associated with duplication, where the ectopic ureter inserts caudal and medial to the normal ureteric insertion (Weigert-Meyer law). May drain into lower bladder, urethra, vestibule, or vagina in girls; lower bladder, posterior urethra, seminal vesicles, or vas deferens in boys.
Functional dilatation of the ureter	US/CT/MRI: dilated ureter with no intraluminal obstruction.	May be seen with postobstructive diuresis, diabetes insipidus.
Ureteral stump	US: stump may appear as diverticulum or blind-ending ureter. CT/MRI: may show reflux into stump on delayed imaging.	Results from heminephrectomy of duplex system or nephrectomy from any cause.
Retrocaval ureter	EU/CT/MRI: Medial deviation of ureter at L3 level, passing behind ureter. Classic sigmoid or "fish-hook" appearance.	Almost always right-sided. Results from persistence of the posterior cardinal venous system.
Ureteral dysplasia	US/CT/MRI: Very dilated tortuous ureters with absent peristalsis. May show dysplastic kidneys. VCUG: gross reflux.	Histology shows poor muscularization of ureteral wall, leading to absent/poor peristalsis. Association of renal dysplasia is less than expected.

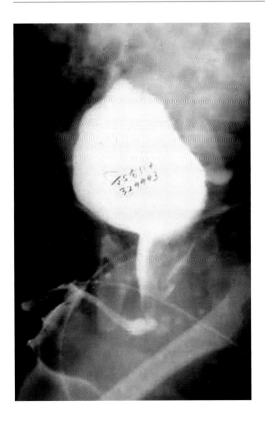

Fig. 3.43   Ureterocele. VCUG image shows a filling defect in the posterior urethra caused by prolapsed ureterocele of an ectopically inserted ureter.

Table 3.16   The enlarged bladder

Diagnosis	Findings	Comments
Functional disturbance of bladder emptying	US: Large capacity but normal appearing bladder. Large residual. VCUG: no reflux.	Causes: status postcatheterization, intervention, analgesia, infection, trauma.
Infrequent voider, lazy bladder syndrome	Large but otherwise normal bladder with large residual. US: may have prominent upper tracts. VCUG: urodynamics show hypotonic bladder, prolonged decreased voiding.	No/infrequent urge to void every 8–12 h. Incontinence. Frequent urinary tract infections. Associated with constipation. Need to exclude neuropathic bladder.
Bladder diverticulum ▷ *Fig. 3.44, p. 264* ▷ *Fig. 3.45, p. 264* ▷ *Fig. 3.26, p. 253*	US: usually paraureteral outpouching of the bladder wall with narrow or wide neck. VCUG: demonstrates size and number with drainage assessed postvoid.	Causes: primary, secondary to neurogenic bladder, posterior urethral valves, and prune belly syndrome.
Posterior urethral valve ▷ *Fig. 3.46, p. 264* ▷ *Fig. 3.27, p. 253*	US: Thick-walled, trabeculated bladder with dilated, elongated posterior urethra. Variable upper tract dilatation and renal dysplasia. VCUG: trabeculated bladder, urethral valve below verumontanum. Reflux in 50%.	Exclusively in boys and increasingly diagnosed antenatally (may get oligohydramnios). Incidence is 1:5000 to 1:8000.
Urethral stenosis, stricture ▷ *Fig. 3.47a, b, p. 264* ▷ *Fig. 3.48, p. 265*	VCUG: Bladder wall trabeculation. Stricture and dilated proximal segment of urethra noted. Ascending urethrography shows true distal extent of stricture.	Causes: usually iatrogenic (catheterization and cystoscopy), but also trauma, foreign bodies, extrinsic compression from pelvic floor tumors.
Neuropathic bladder	Abdominal X-ray: may show spinal dysraphism, sacral agenesis, spinal trauma. US/VCUG: Thick-walled, trabeculated, or large atonic bladder depending on level of lesion. Pseudodiverticula. Elongated funnel-shaped posterior urethra on voiding.	Suprasacral lesions give an elongated pine cone appearance to the bladder. Suprapontine lesions give a rounded serrated appearance. Peripheral (below S2–S4) lesions demonstrate a large atonic bladder.
Urachal diverticulum ▷ *Fig. 3.49, p. 265*	Vesicourachal diverticulum is an outpouching at the apex of the bladder resulting from incomplete closure of the proximal urachus. The majority of patients are asymptomatic because the diverticula drain well with bladder emptying.	

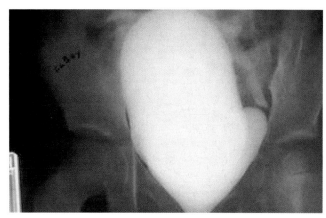

Fig. 3.44 Bladder diverticulum. Cystogram during VCUG demonstrates a smooth-walled posterior bladder diverticulum.

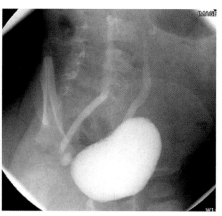

Fig. 3.45 Bilateral reflux on VCUG image. A diverticulum is present in relation to the right VUJ, which is typical of a Hutch diverticulum.

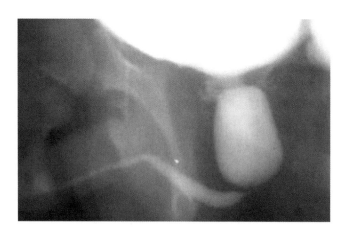

Fig. 3.46 A posterior urethral valve resulting in dilatation of the posterior urethra.

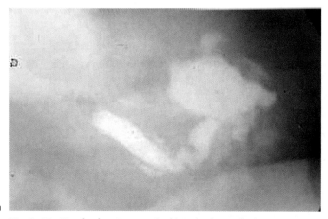

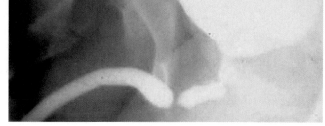

a   b

Fig. 3.47 Urethral strictures. (a, b) Multiple urethral strictures are seen on cystourethrogram causing focal narrowing and dilatation of the membranous and posterior urethra.

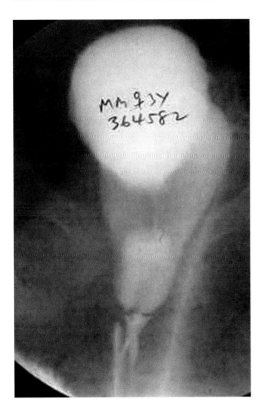

Fig. 3.48 **Urethral stenosis** causing urethral dilatation in a girl. Note the vaginal reflux, which is common during cystourethrography in the female child.

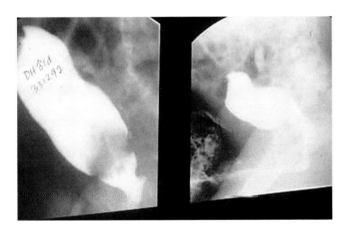

Fig. 3.49 **Urachal diverticulum.**

Table 3.17   Urethral narrowing

Diagnosis	Findings	Comments
Urethral stenosis, urethral stricture ▷ *Fig. 3.47a, b* ▷ *Fig. 3.48*	(see **Table 3.16**)	
Meatal stenosis	VCUG: Difficult to catheterize. Pinpoint meatus on voiding. Trabeculated bladder with residual.	Pinpoint appearance of meatus on visual inspection. May be congenital or secondary to surgery (circumcision/hypospadias) or trauma.
"Spinning top" urethra	VCUG: triangular appearance of the urethra in girls.	Associated with bladder instability.
Wide bladder-neck deformity		

Table 3.18   Filling defects in the urethra

Diagnosis	Findings	Comments
Posttraumatic	VCUG/retrograde urethrography: Acutely, will show contrast extravasation at site of injury; evaluate bladder. Later, will get irregular polypoid changes in the lumen. MRI: can assess urethra and distinguish type IV from type IVa injuries.	More common in males. Goldman classification from type I to V.
Ureterocele ▷*Fig. 3.50*	Can prolapse into the urethra on voiding.	Almost exclusively girls.
Urethral polyp ▷*Fig. 3.51a, b*	Polyp on stalk in proximal urethra, extending into the bladder. Obstruction is rare.	Similar to ureteral polyp. Benign fibroepithelial hyperplasia.

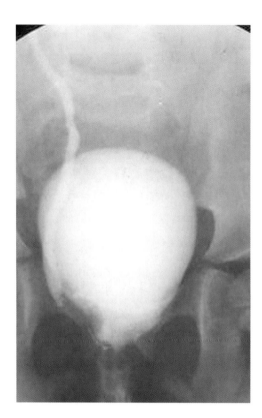

Fig. 3.50   Filling defect. Cystogram demonstrates a well-defined filling defect at the base of bladder on the right side from a prolapsed ureterocele.

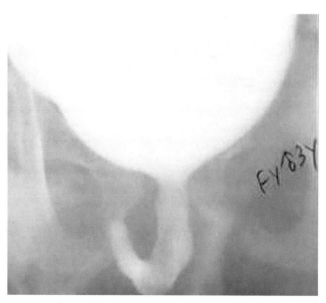
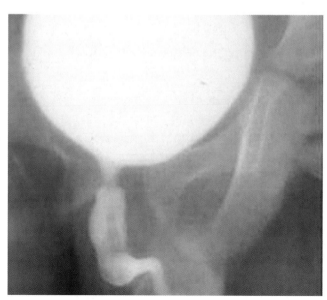

a   b

Fig. 3.51a, b   Urethral polyp. Cystourethrogram shows a lucent filling defect within the urethra caused by a urethral polyp.

Table 3.19   Calcifications in the renal fossa

Diagnosis	Findings	Comments
Nephrolithiasis	US: Echogenic foci with posterior shadowing. Doppler may show twinkle sign. CT: definitive, but radiation dose.	
Medullary sponge kidney ▷ *Fig. 3.17, p. 247*	(see **Table 3.6**)	
Nephrocalcinosis (cortical)	US: increased cortical echogenicity with shadowing. EU/CT: patchy cortical calcifications with occasional tramlines.	Causes: Ischaemia, shock, glomerulonephritis, Alport syndrome. Chronic dialysis.
Nephrocalcinosis (medullary) ▷ *Fig. 3.52a, b*	US: initially nonshadowing increased echogenicity in a rim around the pyramids (Anderson-Carr kidney), then get increasing echogenicity and shadowing. EU/CT: calcifications in a medullary distribution.	Causes: hyperparathyroidism, renal tubular acidosis.
Xanthogranulomatous pyelonephritis	(see unilateral large kidney without PC dilatation, **Table 3.4**)	
Oxalosis	US/EU/CT: widespread faint medullary calcification, with early stone formation.	Can be inherited or secondary to extensive small bowel resection. Acquire osteosclerosis.
After renal trauma	Calcification of a perirenal hematoma.	

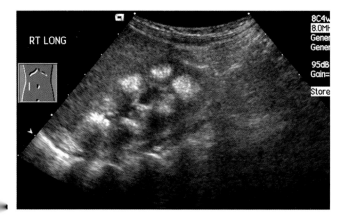

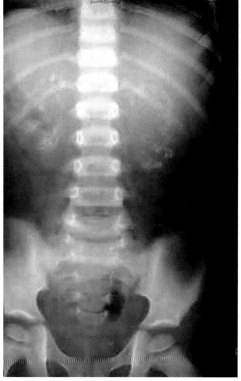

Fig. 3.52a, b   Renal pyramids. (a) US image shows hyperechoic pyramids in a child with nephrocalcinosis. **(b)** Abdominal radiograph shows calcifications in both renal areas, conforming to the renal pyramids.

Table 3.20 The small capacity bladder

Diagnosis	Findings	Comments
Detrusor hyperreflexia instability	US: Normal or small bladder with wall thickening. Normal upper renal tracts. VCUG: Small, hypertonic bladder, with intermittent widening and contraction of bladder neck. VUR may be seen.	Increased day time frequency; normal urine examination. benign and self limiting condition.
Cystitis	Plain X-ray: bladder calculi; intramural or intraluminal air in emphysematous cystitis. US: small capacity bladder with irregular thick walls (> 3.5 mm), internal echoes, postvoid residual urine. CT: may show bladder calculi, diverticula, fistula formation, or pelvic abscess with complicated cystitis. MRI: small capacity bladder with wall thickening, increases T2 signal in wall, and enhancement with gadolinium	Acute hemorrhagic cystitis, cyclophosphamide-induced and tumoral cystitis are the most important forms of pediatric cystitis. Correlation with urine examination is essential.
Neuropathic bladder	Plain X-ray: may show associated spinal anomalies, calculi. US/VCUG: thick-walled trabeculated bladder with or without upper tract dilatation (from VUR); abnormal bladder shape—Christmas tree type (elongated) or atonic type (with diverticula or pseudodiverticula).	Urodynamic studies may confirm elevated intravesical pressures, detrusor sphincter dyssynergia. MRI is usually done to evaluate associated neurologic abnormalities.
Status postbladder surgery	US: small capacity, irregular outline, with significant postvoid, postoperative collections. VCUG: extravasation or fistula formation. CT/MRI: pelvic collections or fistulae.	
Bladder rupture	US: free fluid in pelvis. CT: Pelvic fractures in case of trauma. Delayed CECT images or CT cystography shows extravasated contrast (in paracolic gutters and interloops in case of intraperitoneal rupture or perivesical space and perineum and upper thighs with extraperitoneal rupture). Combined intra- and extraperitoneal rupture may occur. Retrograde ureteral study shows associated urethral rupture.	Intraperitoneal rupture occurs at the dome, which is weakest part. Extraperitoneal rupture is close to bladder base anterolaterally.
Bladder exstrophy, status post surgery	(see status postbladder surgery) US: Small bladder capacity, wall thickening, upper tract dilatation, calculi (due to urinary stasis). Postoperative collections. Scrotal US for epididymitis as a late complication. NM: DMSA for renal cortical scarring.	Surgery includes closure of bladder exstrophy, bladder neck reconstruction, and epispadias repair in a staged manner with or without bladder augmentation. Appendicovesicostomy allows for percutaneous bladder catheterization. VUR is seen almost always postoperatively.
Bilateral ectopic ureters	US: small capacity bladder with dysplastic kidneys. VCUG: associated reflux. EU/CT or MRI urography abnormal course and ectopic insertion of ureters (see dilated ureter, **Table 3.15**)	Rare. More common in girls. Kidneys are usually dysplastic. Ectopic ureters may drain into rectum, posterior urethra, or vas deferens in boys; into rectum, urethra, uterus, or vagina in girls.

Table 3.21   Filling defects in the bladder

Diagnosis	Findings	Comments
Cystitis	(see **Table 3.20**)	
Ectopic ureterocele ▷ *Fig. 3.43, p. 263*	(see **Table 3.15**)	
Blood clot ▷ *Fig. 3.53* ▷ *Fig. 3.54a, b, p. 270*	US: irregular echogenic masses, dependent debris, no acoustic shadowing, may move with change in position. CT: irregular hyperdense areas in the bladder.	
Bladder calculus ▷ *Fig. 3.55, p. 270*	Plain X-ray: radiopaque density in pelvis. Cystogram: filling defect in the bladder. US: echogenic mass with strong shadowing. CT: can show calcified or noncalcified calculi.	Ninety percent of vesical calculi are radiopaque.
Foreign bodies	Plain X-ray: radiopaque foreign body. US: confirms foreign body in bladder; good for detection of nonradiopaque foreign body.	
Orthotopic ureterocele	(see **Table 3.15**)	
Rhabdomyosarcoma ▷ *Fig. 3.56a, b, p. 271*	US: Lobulated, polypoid mass usually from trigone > bladder neck > dome. Local spread to lymph nodes. MRI for extent.	Most common neoplasm of urinary tract. Occurs most often in bladder but can occur in prostate or vagina. Embryonal type most common. Age < 5 y. M > F. Diagnosis confirmed with biopsy.
Hemangioma	US: Discrete mass usually arising from bladder dome. Doppler imaging for assessment of vascularity. Calcifications may be present. CT: May show vascular mass enhances with contrast. MRI: better for characterization and evaluation of extent.	Most common benign bladder tumor. Coexisting cutaneous hemangioma over lower abdomen, pelvis, or thigh may be found. Venolymphatic malformations may also present as filling defects in bladder although they present commonly with hematuria. Mulitiple visceral hemangiomas, rectal varices, and genitourinary venolymphatic malformations may be seen in Klippel Trenauney syndrome.

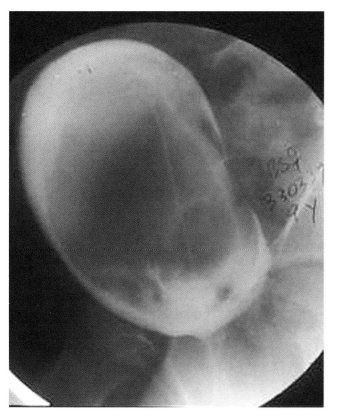

Fig. 3.53   Bladder hematoma. Cystogram shows a distended bladder opacified by contrast, with a large filling defect.

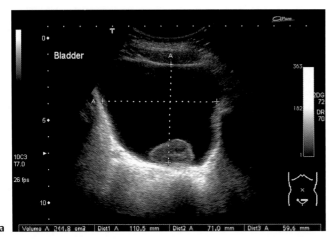

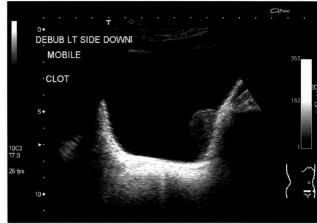

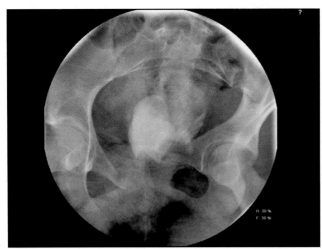

Fig. 3.54a, b   Intraperitoneal rupture of the bladder. (a) US image of the urinary bladder clot seen as mobile echogenic material within the lumen. **(b)** Cystogram in a child who sustained pelvic fractures shows contrast extravasation, confirming intraperitoneal rupture of the bladder.

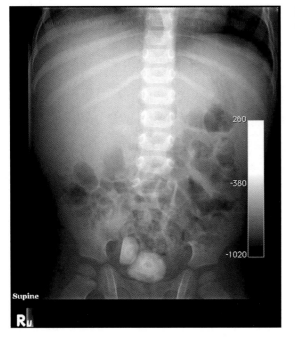

Fig. 3.55   Vesical calculi. Abdominal radiograph demonstrates two well-defined large radiopaque vesical calculi.

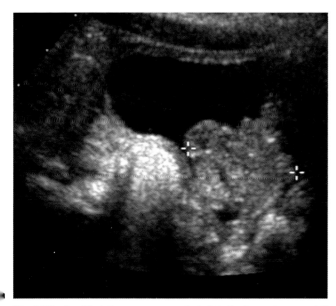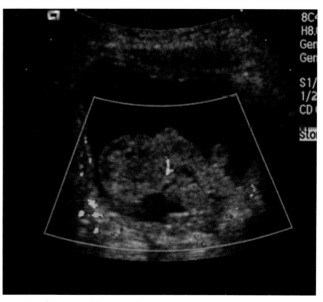

b

Fig. 3.56a, b   Rhabdomyosarcoma. Lobulated echogenic mass at the base of bladder and the prostate.

Table 3.22   Urethral dilatation

Diagnosis	Findings	Comments
Posterior urethral valve ▷ *Fig. 3.27, p. 253* ▷ *Fig. 3.46, p. 264*	(see **Table 3.16**)	
Urethral diverticulum ▷ *Fig. 3.57, p. 272* ▷ *Fig. 3.26, p. 253*	VCUG: oval contrast–filled outpouching along ventral aspect of anterior urethra. High-resolution ultrasonography: shows the diverticulum if filled and the anterior lip.	May be congenital or acquired (secondary related to trauma, catheter, etc.).
Prune belly syndrome	VCUG: large bladder ± VUR, dilated high placed posterior urethra. US: large bladder, dilated posterior urethra, hydro-nephrosis/dysplastic kidneys.	Predominantly seen in males. Triad of deficient anterior abdominal wall musculature, undescended testes, and urinary tract anomalies, particularly dysplastic kidneys and dilated posterior urethra.
Urethral duplication ▷ *Fig. 3.58a, b, p. 272*	VCUG: Demonstrates partial or complete urethral duplication. Retrograde urethrogram (RGU) can be used for diagnosis.	Partial duplication can be proximal or distal. Can be epispadiac or hypospadiac depending on the position of accessory external openings.
Megaurethra	VCUG: Marked dilatation of penile urethra with proximal and distal tapering into normal caliber urethra. There is no obstruction. US: may show deficiency/absence of corpus spongiosum and corpora cavernosa.	May be associated with prune belly syndrome or can present as an isolated anomaly. Can be of scaphoid or fusiform shape; scaphoid is more commonly seen as a ventral bulge of penile urethra during voiding. Only part of anterior urethra may be affected.
Status postepispadias repair	VCUG/RGU: Postoperative strictures and prestenotic dilatation. Urethro- or vesicocutaneous fistulas if present.	
Lacuna magna	VCUG/RGU: displays the lesion as dorsal and parallel to distal anterior urethra.	Dorsal diverticulum in the roof of fossa navicularis. Approximately 5 mm in size. Rarely symptomatic. Pain postvoid spotting or hemorrhage may be present.

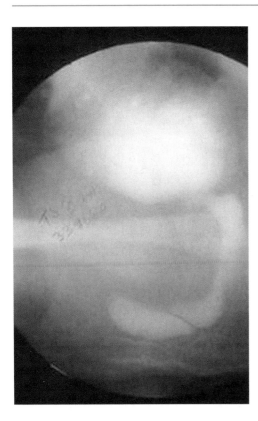

Fig. 3.57   Urethral diverticulum. Contrast-opacified outpouching from the anterior urethra resulting from urethral diverticulum.

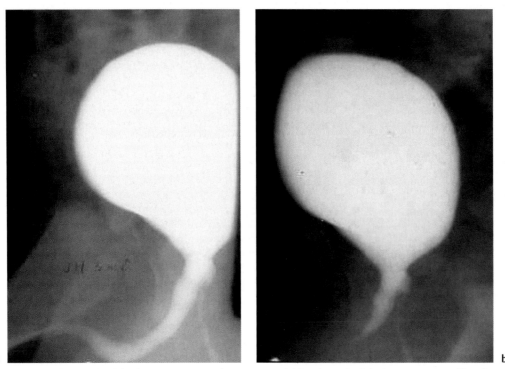

a   b

Fig. 3.58a, b   Urethral duplication. Cystourethrogram in a child with urethral duplication. Note a dilated posterior urethra and the accessory anterior urethral channel of a smaller caliber.

The Scrotum and Testes

The testes are located in the scrotum in 90% of full-term infants. When not in the scrotum, they are usually to be found within the inguinal canal. Rarely, they are intra-abdominal. Testicular size varies with age and with the onset of puberty. US is the gold standard for evaluating the testis and epididymis as it can demonstrate changes in size and texture, as well as assessing blood flow using spectral and color Doppler. NM (99mTc pertechnetate) has been used in cases of suspected torsion, but as it uses radiation it is not usually recommended. MRI can also assess the testis but is rarely indicated because of the cost.

On US, the normal testis is primarily of homogeneous echogenicity (**Fig. 3.59**). A not uncommon finding is microcalcification within the testicular parenchyma (**Fig. 3.60**) and is usually of no clinical significance.

An undescended testis, seen in 0.5% of boys prior to puberty, is the most common abnormality seen. Congenital aplasia of one testis is rare, and bilateral aplasia is very rare. US is the modality of choice to search for the testes, but if they are not within the inguinal canal they may be difficult to see within the abdomen due to bowel gas; in that case, MRI may be useful.

If there is scrotal swelling without pain or inflammation, the most common cause is a hydrocele (**Fig. 3.61**). If there is pain and/or evidence of inflammation, then testicular torsion has to be the first consideration, as this is a surgical emergency.

Testicular torsion is indicated if there is disorganization of the echo texture, usually enlarged and hypoechoic, (**Fig. 3.62**) with loss of blood flow within the testis on color Doppler; however, this is not always reliable, particularly if the torsion is intermittent. The most common radiologic diagnosis with an acutely tender testis is epididymitis (with or without orchitis). Seeing marked increase in blood flow to a swollen epididymis on color Doppler can make the diagnosis (**Fig. 3.63**). If the testis is involved with increased blood flow, then it is orchitis as well as epididymitis. Torsion of the testicular appendage is the other diagnosis to be considered and is seen as a swollen appendage separate from the epididymis. Torsion is the most common cause in infants and adolescents, and 50% of boys with torsion of the testicular appendage are between 9 and 12 years old.

Trauma can result in testicular hematomas. These can remain for an extended period of time and hence be mistaken for a more sinister lesion (**Fig. 3.64**). If there is a patent processus vaginalis, herniation of bowel loops or fluid from the peritoneal cavity can occur and extend into the scrotum. This can also happen with meconium peritonitis resulting in calcification.

Tumors are rare before puberty. The most common involvement of the testis by tumor is in leukemia.

Tables 3.23 and **3.24** tabulate the changes seen.

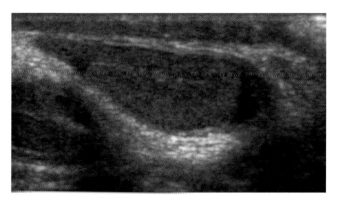

Fig. 3.59 **Normal testis.** Normal echotexture shown on US.

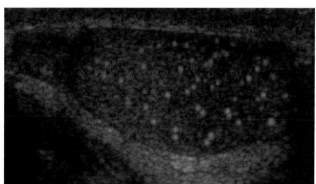

Fig. 3.60 **Testicular microlithiasis.** Microcalcification is seen sonographically as multiple echogenic foci.

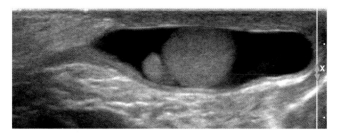

Fig. 3.61 **Hydrocele.** The fluid extent is well shown by US in a young infant boy.

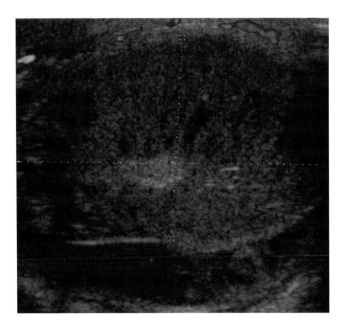

Fig. 3.62   Testicular torsion with infarction. The testis is enlarged and hypoechoic, with no flow on color Doppler study.

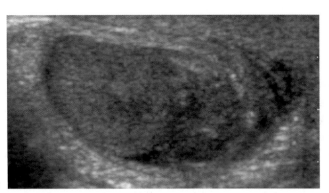

a

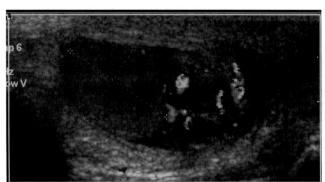

Fig. 3.63a, b   Right epididymitis. The epididymis is enlarged and of mixed echogenicity (**a**) and shows marked increase in blood flow on color Doppler study (**b**).

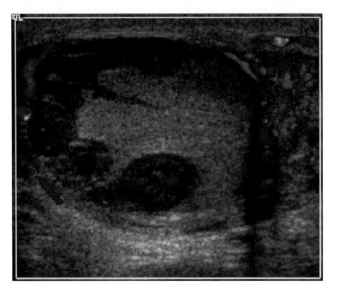

Fig 3.64   Testicular trauma. Multiple hypoechoic areas are seen in the testis, which has a mixed echotexture.

Table 3.23   Testicular enlargement

Diagnosis	Findings	Causes and comments
Hypertrophy	Homogeneously enlarged testes of normal echogenicity on US.	Atrophy or agenesis of the contralateral testis; bilateral hypertrophy is caused by hormone-secreting tumors.
Hydrocele ▷ *Fig. 3.61, p. 273*	Fluid collection in the scrotal sac around normal testes on US.	Common in infants and small children.
Testicular torsion ▷ *Fig. 3.62*	Enlarged hypoechoic testes with decreased or absent perfusion on color Doppler and scintigraphy. Not 100% reliable as torsion can be intermittent with flow returning intermittently.	Torsion of the vascular pedicle with resultant necrosis of the testis. Peak incidence in the neonatal period and in adolescence.
Testicular appendage torsion	Testis and epididymis are normal with a swollen appendage showing increased vascularity on color Doppler.	Torsion of the vascular pedicle and resultant necrosis of the appendage.
Epididymitis ▷ *Fig. 3.63a, b*	Enlarged epididymis, compared with the opposite side, fluid in the scrotal sac on US. Often shows markedly increased perfusion on scintigraphy and color Doppler.	Orchitis, postcatheterization, cystoscopy. Rarely due to ectopic insertion of the ureter into ductus deferens.
Orchitis	Testis and epididymis are enlarged with irregular echogenic parenchyma and increased vascularity on color Doppler.	Mumps, bacterial infection.
Scrotal trauma ▷ *Fig. 3.64*	Inhomogeneous testicular echogenicity and/or hemorrhage in the scrotal sac and testis	Direct perineal trauma, impaling trauma. Child abuse, sexual abuse.
Leukemia ▷ *Fig. 3.65*	Enlargement of one or both testes with abnormal echotexture on US.	Common in ALL.
Testicular tumor ▷ *Fig. 3.66*		Various histology, such as teratoma, embryonal cell carcinoma, seminoma, gonadoblastoma, rhabdomyosarcoma.
Adrenogenital syndrome	Focally decreased parenchymal echogenicity and calcification on US. The epididymis is enlarged and lobulated; microadenomas develop later.	Caused by insufficient replacement therapy.

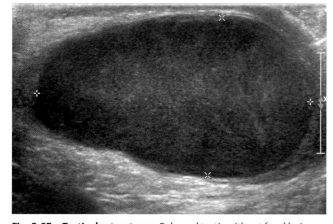

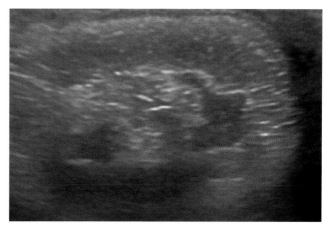

Fig. 3.65   Testicular teratoma. Enlarged testis without focal lesions.

Fig. 3.66   Testicular teratoma. There is markedly inhomogeneous and disorganized echotexture of the parenchyma.

Table 3.24   Small testes

Diagnosis	Findings	Comments
Atrophy	Diminished volume of one or both testes, echogenicity normal or decreased on US; hypertrophy of the contralateral testis.	Can occur after torsion, incomplete descent, orchitis, or orchidopexy. Also seen in cystic fibrosis and Kartagener syndrome.
Hypoplasia	Testes are small on US.	Associated with prune belly syndrome, cystic fibrosis, and chromosomal abnormalities or as late sequelae of radiation or chemotherapy.

The Adrenal Glands

The adrenal glands are Z-shaped (**Fig. 3.67a**) unless there is absence or ectopia of the adjacent kidney, in which case they are discoid (**Fig. 3.67b**). They are large in the fetus and immediately after birth (see **Fig. 3.67a, b**). On sonography, they are divided into two distinct hyperechoic and relatively hypoechoic layers: the cortex, and medulla (see **Fig. 3.67a, b**). Physiologic involution of the adrenal glands begins after the first few weeks of life, ending by the fourth month. In this time, sonography is the modality of choice and can differentiate mass lesions. After this period, CT and MRI are more useful with MRI preferred, as it has no ionizing radiation.

Adrenal Masses

Masses can be cystic (**Table 3.25**) or solid (**Table 3.26**). An adrenal mass in a fetus is usually a neuroblastoma, but after birth adrenal hemorrhage becomes more common (**Figs. 3.68** and **3.69**). Initially, the postnatal appearance can be similar, but adrenal hemorrhage changes faster than a neuroblastoma; as most neonatal neuroblastomas involute spontaneously, follow-up US will help distinguish. In long-standing cases, the adrenal hemorrhage becomes calcified, and occult adrenal hemorrhage is probably the major cause of so-called idiopathic adrenal calcification (**Fig. 3.70**). In cases where there is still concern of neuroblastoma, especially in older children, US, CT, MRI, or NM may be very useful (**Figs. 3.72, 3.73, 3.74,** and **3.75**). A rare differential diagnosis is an intra-abdominal sequestration.

Other tumors can occur in older children, the most common being pheochromocytoma, which is often predominately cystic and benign (**Fig. 3.71a–c**). CT and MRI are the most common modalities used to investigate these, although NM and positron emission tomography can be useful.

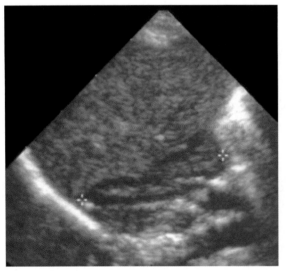
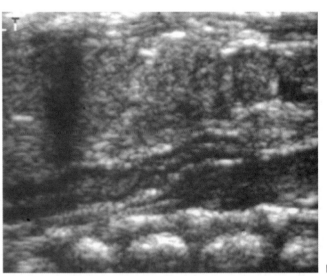

a   b

Fig. 3.67a, b   **Normal adrenal gland in neonates.** Excellent differentiation is seen between the cortex and medulla in an adrenal gland with a Z configuration (**a**) and in an adrenal gland with an elongated configuration in a neonate with an absent kidney (**b**).

Table 3.25 Predominantly cystic adrenal masses

Diagnosis	Findings	Comments
Adrenal hemorrhage ▷ *Fig. 3.68* ▷ *Fig. 3.69*	On US, echogenic, often hypoechoic, mass, with cystic change as resorption occurs over many weeks. Calcification frequently occurs later. CT may demonstrate increased attenuation but this does aid differentiation from neuroblastoma.	Nearly all related to perinatal asphyxia. The hemorrhage can affect all or part of the gland and is bilateral in 10%. Rare in older children and is associated with severe blunt injury.
Adrenal cysts	These rare cysts can be confused with the upper pole of the kidney and should not be confused with an upper pole renal cyst, hydrocalyx, or hydronephrotic upper pole of a duplex kidney.	Caused most commonly by prenatal or postnatal hemorrhage. Microcysts are associated with Beckwith-Wiedemann syndrome.
Pheochromocytoma ▷ *Fig. 3.71a–c, p. 278*	Hypoechoic, partly solid, mass with small cysts on US. CT and MRI show cystic and solid mass, with significant contrast enhancement. Iodine-123-metaiodobenzylguanidine (^{123}I-MIBG) scintigram: positive in 80% of cases.	Tumors originate from the medulla (70%) or sympathetic ganglia. Catecholamines are elevated and there may be associated endocrinopathies. In children, usually are benign. Bilateral in 24%.

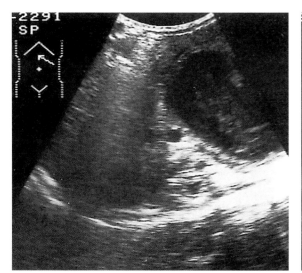 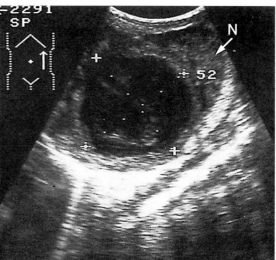

Fig. 3.68   Adrenal hemorrhage. The adrenal hemorrhage is cystic on US.

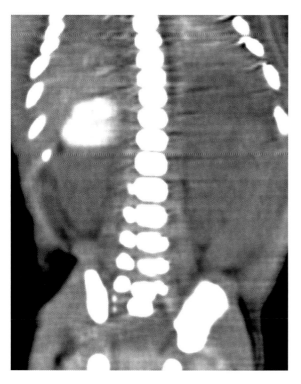

Fig. 3.69   Adrenal hemorrhage. Postmortem CT of 30-week fetus following fetal death in utero: incidental right adrenal hemorrhage. (Image kindly provided by Dr. Michelle Fink, Director of Medical Imaging, Royal Melbourne Children's Hospital, Australia.)

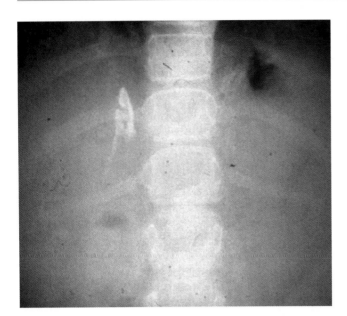

Fig. 3.70 Idiopathic adrenal calcification. Unilateral right adrenal calcification is clearly seen in this plain film.

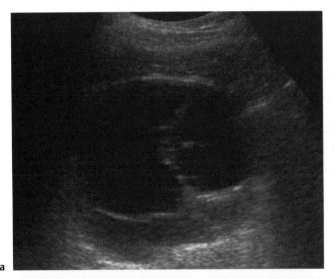

a

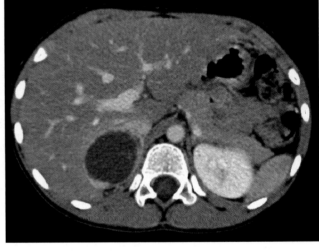

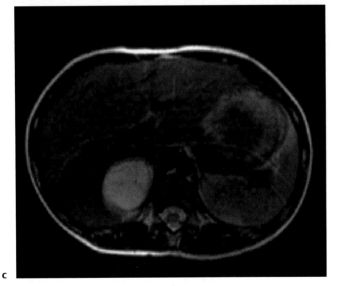

c

Fig. 3.71a–c Right pheochromocytoma. There is a cystic lesion replacing most of the right adrenal gland shown on US (**a**), CT (**b**), and MRI (**c**).

Table 3.26   Predominantly solid adrenal masses

Diagnosis	Findings	Comments
Neuroblastoma ▷ *Fig. 3.72* ▷ *Fig. 3.73a, b* ▷ *Fig. 3.74, p. 280* ▷ *Fig. 3.75, p. 280*	Usually hyperechoic on US with calcification common. Lymph node metastases are common. Radiography, CT, and MRI show enhancing mass ± calcification. The primary tumor and metastases show uptake of ^{123}I-MIBG scintigraphy	Urinary catecholamine levels are elevated. Seventy-five percent are intra-abdominal with majority in the adrenal. Usually present < 5 y old with peak in third year and up to 60% present with metastases. Paraneoplastic syndromes, such as opsoclonus-myoclonus encephalopathy and intractable diarrhea, occur secondary to hormone release.
Intra-abdominal sequestration	US shows an echogenic mass adjacent to the adrenal gland.	Rare intra-abdominal mass may be mistaken for a neuroblastoma or adrenal hemorrhage but does not show any change over time unlike neuroblastoma and adrenal hemorrhage.
Ganglioneuroma	On cross-sectional imaging, these large solid tumors are usually homogeneous (except for calcification) and may show pressure on adjacent structures such as the ribs.	These slow growing benign tumors are more common and present later than neuroblastoma.
Adrenal hemorrhage ▷ *Fig. 3.68, p. 277*	On US, acute hemorrhage is echogenic, becoming hypoechoic over a period of days to weeks and can persist for months.	(see **Table 3.25**)
Adrenal cortical tumors	Rare tumors appear as solid masses on cross-sectional imaging.	Adenoma, adenocarcinoma that presents with Cushing syndrome (rare < 7 y), or endocrine malfunction, virilization.

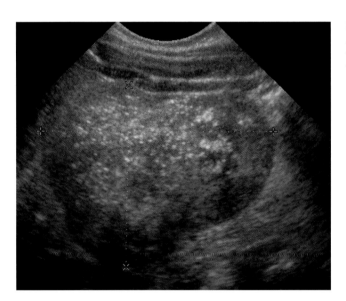

Fig. 3.72   Neuroblastoma. US in a 1-year-old girl with right-sided abdominal mass shows a solid mass in the right side of the abdomen with fine speckled hyperechoic calcifications, which were confirmed to be a neuroblastoma.

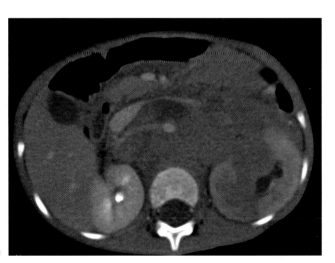 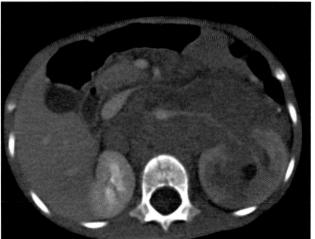

b

Fig. 3.73a, b   Neuroblastoma. There is a large mass anterior to and infiltrating the hilum of the kidney on CECT. Note the characteristic surrounding of the aorta by the mass. The right (**a**) and left (**b**) renal arteries are also encased by tumor.

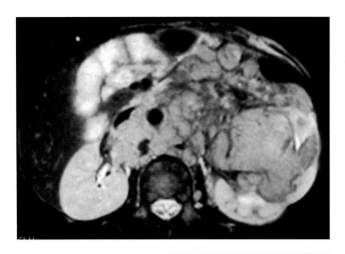

Fig. 3.74   Neuroblastoma. There is a large mass of moderately high signal intensity arising from the left but crossing the midline and surrounding the aorta on T2-weighted MRI in a different patient from **Fig. 3.73**.

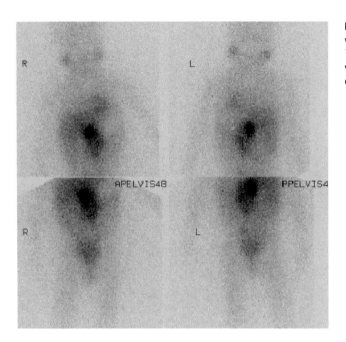

Fig. 3.75   Neuroblastoma. ^{123}I-MIBG scintigram: an 8-year-old boy with an upper abdominal mass on CT scan, and avid tumor uptake on ^{123}I-MIBG, that was proven to be adrenal at biopsy. (Image kindly provided by Dr. Arvind Kumar Sinha, Consultant Radiologist, Department of Diagnostic Imaging, National University Hospital, Singapore.)

Adrenal Calcification

Calcification in the adrenal glands is unusual without other abnormalities such as previous adrenal hemorrhage, tumor (especially neuroblastoma), or Wolman disease (**Table 3.27**).

Table 3.27   Adrenal calcification not considered in Tables 3.1 and 3.2

Disease	Type of calcification	Side	Primary disease
Idiopathic adrenal calcification ▷ *Fig. 3.70, p. 278*	Triangular	Seventy percent are right-sided, and 10% are bilateral.	Probably due to previous occult adrenal hemorrhage.
Wolman disease	Dense, triangular	Always bilateral.	Rare severe inherited lysosomal acid lipase deficiency, lethal in infancy.
Tuberculosis	Triangular		

Gynecologic Disorders in Children

US remains the gold standard for the evaluation of pediatric gynecologic abnormalities. For more complex abnormalities, genitography and MRI are useful, particularly in complex embryologic and congenital malformations.

Normal Findings

The uterus is bulky at birth because of maternal hormones; over a few months, it reduces to prepubertal dimensions with a uterus–cervical ratio of 1:1 (**Fig. 3.76a**). Postpuberty, the uterus changes with the uterine muscle, which will be more bulky; the uterine ratio becomes 2:1 (**Fig. 3.76b**). Ovarian cysts up to 0.9 cm are not uncommon in both prepubertal (approximately 5%) and postpubertal (approximately 15%) patients and are normal findings. Ovarian cysts are occasionally very large in neonates due to maternal hormones (**Fig. 3.77**). If they can be decompressed or watched conservatively, they will usually resolve.

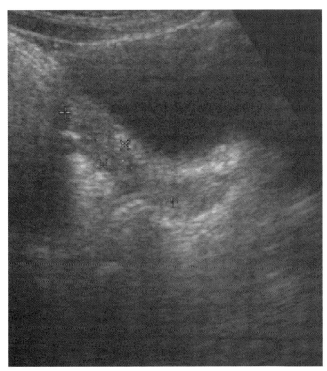 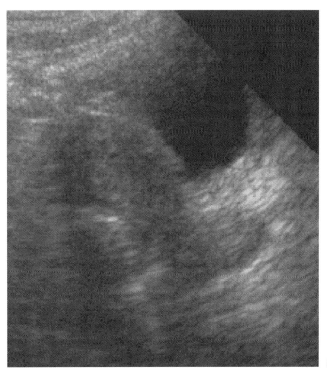

b

Fig. 3.76a, b Normal uterus. On sagittal pelvic US, the normal prepubertal uterus is bulky at birth due to maternal hormones; over a few months, it reduces to prepubertal dimensions with a small uterus compared to the cervix. The uterocervical length ratio is 1:1. Postpuberty, the uterine muscle is bulkier (**a**), and the uterocervical length ratio becomes 2:1 (**b**).

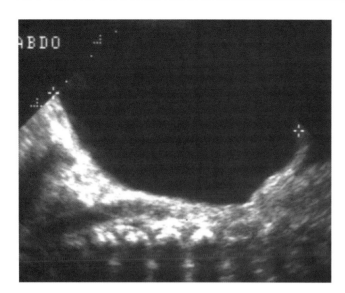

Fig. 3.77   Large ovarian cyst in a neonate. Longitudinal abdominal US shows a large ovarian cyst in a neonate filling the abdomen anterior to the lumbar vertebral bodies and aorta.

Congenital Malformation

A variety of congenital anomalies can occur, including uterine septation, which is most extreme in uterus didelphys (**Fig. 3.78a, b**) or even complete duplication of the genital tract (**Fig. 3.79a–d**). The uterus or vagina can be obstructed. An intact hymen, or more rarely a septum or atresia, will present with hydrocolpos before puberty or hematocolpos after puberty (**Fig. 3.80**). This can extend to affect the uterus, and then is hydrometrocolpos or hematometrocolpos (**Fig. 3.81**).

Cloacal, urogenital, and Müllerian duct anomalies can occur. These usually require genitography (**Fig. 3.82**) and MRI. Cloacal anomalies arise from incomplete division of the urorectal septum, leading to a single perineal orifice. In urogenital sinus anomalies (**Fig. 3.82**), the rectum and anus are usually normal but there is a single perineal orifice for the urethra and vagina. Müllerian duct anomalies are variable and may be asymptomatic and affect only the genital tract.

Intersex and ambiguous genitalia are complex embryologic, anatomic, and physiologic anomalies requiring extensive investigation. Congenital adrenal hyperplasia is the most common cause of ambiguous genitalia in females (**Fig. 3.83**). It is an autosomal recessive inborn error of metabolism. This leads to marked enlargement of the adrenal glands, which is well shown on US (see section on adrenal glands).

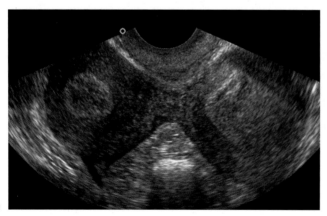
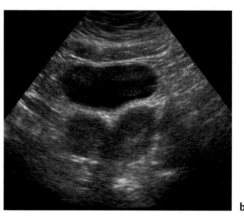

a   b

Fig. 3.78a, b   Uterus didelphys. Transverse US of the pelvis shows a duplicated uterus (**a**) and cervix (**b**).

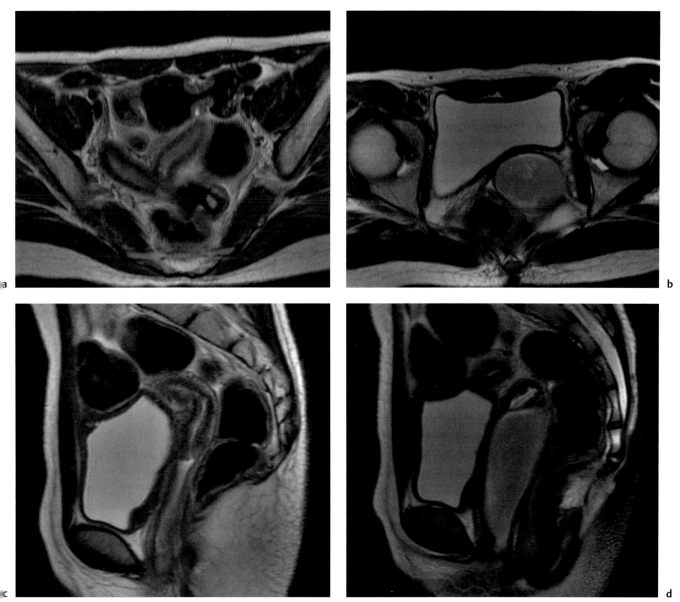

Fig. 3.79a–d   Duplication of the uterus and vagina. T2-weighted MRI demonstrates duplication of the uterus and vagina. The duplication is best seen on the transverse views (**a, b**), and the extent of the obstruction is best seen on the sagittal images (**c, d**). There is a left hematocolpos (**b, d**).

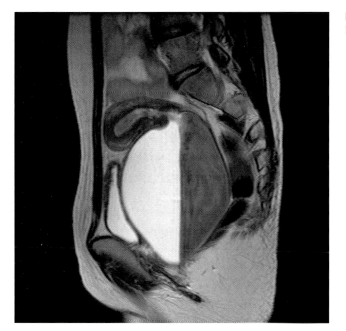

Fig. 3.80   Vaginal atresia. T2-weighted MRI demonstrates a large hematocolpos with posterior layering of blood products.

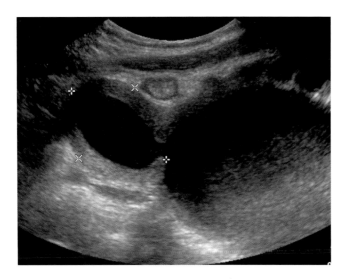

Fig. 3.81   Hydrometrocolpos. Longitudinal abdominal US demonstrates a large hydrometrocolpos with a normal uterus on transverse view.

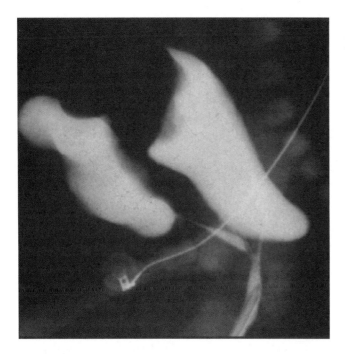

Fig. 3.82   Urogenital sinus anomaly. Genitogram shows a common channel of the distal urethra and vagina. The proximal vagina is distended and outlines the indentation of the cervix.

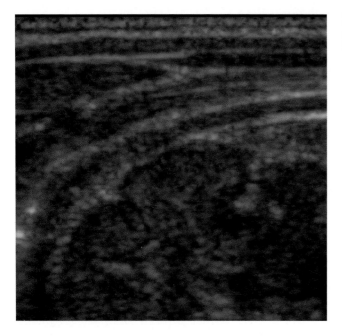

Fig. 3.83   Congenital adrenal hyperplasia. There is marked enlargement of the adrenal gland which has a "cerebriform" pattern, mimicking sulci and gyri.

Acquired Abnormalities

Ovarian torsion, usually associated with ovarian cysts, can occur at any age but most commonly in older children. Pelvic inflammatory disease, endometriosis, and ectopic pregnancy also occur in older children.

Benign and malignant tumors occur occasionally and 30% are malignant. Approximately 70% are germ cell tumors (**Fig. 3.84a, b**).

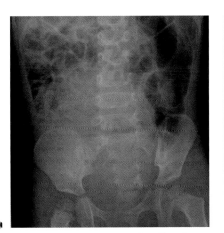 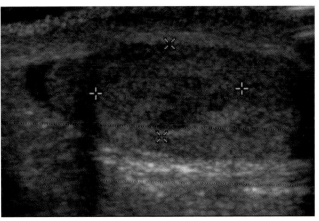

b

Fig. 3.84a, b   Teratoma. Plain film shows a soft-tissue mass arising from the pelvis with a calcific density inferiorly (**a**). This is confirmed on longitudinal US (**b**).

■ Further Reading

Avni FE, Hall M, Janssens F. Urinary tract infection. In R, ed. Pediatric uroradiology. New York: Springer, 2001

Baker LA, Sigman D, Mathews RI, Benson J, Docimo SG. An analysis of clinical outcomes using color Doppler testicular ultrasound for testicular torsion. Pediatrics 2000;105:604–607

Blask AR, Sanders RC, Rock JA. Obstructed uterovaginal anomalies: demonstration with sonography. Part I. Neonates and infants. Radiology 1991;179:79–83

Blask AR, Sanders RC, Rock JA. Obstructed uterovaginal anomalies: demonstration with sonography. Part II. Teenagers. Radiology 1991;179:84–88

Buckus ML, Mack LA, Middleton WD, et al. Testicular microlithiasis: imaging appearances and pathologic correlation. Radiology 1994;192:781–785

Blickman JG. Pediatric radiology, the requisites. 3rd ed. St. Louis: Mosby, 2009

Brodeur GM, Pritchard J, Berthold F, et al. Revisions of the international criteria for neuroblastoma diagnosis, staging, and response to treatment. J Clin Oncol 1993;11:1466–1477

Carty H, Brunelle F, Stringer DA, Kao SCS, eds. Imaging children, vol. I. London: Churchill Livingstone, 2005.

Cast JE, Nelson WM, Early AS, et al. Testicular microlithiasis: prevalence and tumor risk in a population referred for scrotal sonography. Am J Roentgenol 2000;175:1703–1706

Ciftci AO, Bingöl-Koloğlu M, Senocak ME, et al. Testicular tumors in children. J Ped Surg 2001;36:1796–1801

Cohen HL, Eisenberg P, Mandel F, Haller JO. Ovarian cysts are common in pre-menarchal girls: a sonographic study of 101 children 2–12 years old. Am J Roentgenol 1992;159:89–91

Darge K, Grattan-Smith JD, Riccabona M. Pediatric uroradiology: state of the art. Pediatr Radiol 2010 Apr 21 [Epub ahead of print]

Dubinsky TJ, Chen P, Maklad N. Color-flow and power Doppler imaging of the testes. World J Urol 2004;16(1):35–40

Garel L, Dubois J, Grignon A, et al. US of the pediatric female pelvis: a clinical perspective. Radiographics 2001;21:1393–1407

Gargollo P, Borer G. Contemporary outcomes in bladder exstrophy. Curr Opin Urol 2007;17(4):272–280

Graif M, Itzchak Y. Sonographic evaluation of ovarian torsion in childhood and adolescence. AJR 1988;150:647–649

Grattan-Smith D, Jones RA. MR urography in children. Ped Radiol 2006;36:1119–1132

Groff DB. Pelvic neoplasms in children. J Surg Oncol 2001;77:65–71

Hellerstein S, Linebarger JS. Voiding dysfunction in pediatric patients. Clin Pediatr (Phila) 2003;42:43–49

Howman-Giles R, Shaw PJ, Uren RF, Chung DK. Neuroblastoma and other neuroendocrine tumors. Semin Nucl Med 2007;37:286–302

Jaramillo D, Lebowitz RL, Hendron WH. The cloacal malformations: radiologic findings and imaging recommendations. Radiology 1990;177:441–448

Jung SE, Lee JM, Rhas SE, et al. CT and MR imaging of ovarian tumours with emphasis on differential diagnosis. Radiographics 2002; 22:1305–1325

Kuhn J, Slavis T, Haller J. Caffey's pediatric diagnostic imaging. 10th ed. St. Louis: Mosby, 2004

Lang IM, Babyn P, Oliver GD. MR imaging of paediatric uterovaginal anomalies. Pediatric Radiology 1999;29:163–170

Leenen AS, Riebel TW. Testicular microlithiasis in children: sonographic features and clinical implications. Pediatr Radiol 2002,32(8): 575–579

Lonergan GJ, Rice RR, Suarez ES. Autosomal recessive polycystic kidney disease: radiologic-pathologic correlation. Radiographics 2000; 20:837–855

Lowe LH, Isuani BH, Heller RM, et al. Pediatric renal masses: Wilms tumor and beyond. Radiographics 2000;20:1585–1603

Luker GD, Siegel MJ. Pediatric testicular tumors: evaluation with gray-scale and color Doppler US. Radiology 1994;191:561–564

Mäkelä E, Lahdes-Vasama T, Rajakorpi H, Wikström S. A 19-year review of paediatric patients with acute scrotum. Scand J Surg 2007;96(1):62–66

McAndrew HF, Pemberton R, Kikiros CS, Gollow I. The incidence and investigation of acute scrotal problems in children. Ped Surg Int 2002;18:435–437

McHugh K. Renal and adrenal tumours in children. A review. Cancer Imaging 2007;5(7):41–51.

McHugh K, Stringer D, Herbert D, Babiak CA. Simple renal cysts in children: diagnosis and follow-up with US. Radiology 1991; 178:383–385

Paltiel HJ, Rupich RC, Babcock DS. Maturational changes in arterial impedance of the normal testis in boys: Doppler sonographic study. AJR 1994;163:1189–1193

Parisi MT, Greene MK, Dykes TM, Moraldo TV, Sandler ED, Hattner RS. Efficacy of metaiodobenzylguanidine as a scintigraphic agent for the detection of neuroblastoma. Invest Radiology 1992;27:768–773

Reinhold C, Hricak H, Forstner R, et al. Primary amenorrhea: evaluation with MR imaging. Radiology 1997;203:383–390

Rescorla FJ. Malignant adrenal tumors. Semin Pediatr Surg 2006; 15(1):48–56

Riccabona M, Avni FE, Blickman JG, Dacher JN, Darge K, Lobo ML, et al. Imaging recommendations in paediatric uroradiology: minutes of the ESPR workgroup session on urinary tract infection, fetal hydronephrosis, urinary tract ultrasonography and voiding cystourethrography, Barcelona, Spain, June 2007. Pediatr Radiol 2008;38(2):138–145

Riccabona M, Avni FE, Blickman JG, Dacher JN, Darge K, Lobo ML, et al. Imaging recommendations in paediatric uroradiology. Minutes of the ESPR uroradiology task force session on childhood obstructive uropathy, high-grade fetal hydronephrosis, childhood haematuria, and urolithiasis in childhood. ESPR Annual Congress, Edinburgh, UK, June 2008. Pediatr Radiol 2009;39(8):891–898

Riccabona M, Avni FE, Dacher JN, Damasio MB, Darge K, Lobo ML, et al. ESPR uroradiology task force and ESUR paediatric working group: imaging and procedural recommendations in paediatric uroradiology, part III. Minutes of the ESPR uroradiology task

force minisymposium on intravenous urography, uro-CT and MR-urography in childhood. Pediatr Radiol 2010;40(7):1315–1320

Rorschneider WK, Wierich A, Rieden K, et al. US, CT and MR imaging characteristics of nephroblastomatosis. Pediatr Radiol 1998;28:435–443

Rufini V, Calcagni ML, Baum RP. Imaging of neuroendocrine tumors. Semin Nucl Med 2006;36(3):228–247

Stallion A. Vaginal obstruction. Semin Ped Surg 2000;9:128–134

Tannous WN, Azouz EM, Homsy YL, Kiruluta HG, Grattan-Smith D. CT and ultrasound imaging of pelvic rhabdomyosarcoma in children. A review of 56 patients. Pediatr Radiol 1989;19:530–534

Taylor GA, Guion CJ, Potter BM, Eichelberger MR. CT of blunt abdominal trauma in children. AJR 1989;153:555–559

Velchik MG, Alavi A, Kressel HY, Engelman K. Localization of pheochromocytoma: MIGB, CT and MRI correlation. J Nucl Med 1989;30: 328–336

Weber DM, Rösslein R, Fliegel C. Color Doppler sonography in the diagnosis of acute scrotum in boys. Eur J Ped Surg 2000;10:235–241

Wittenberg AF, Tobias T, Rzeszotarski M, Minotti AJ. Sonography of the acute scrotum: the four T's of testicular imaging. Curr Probl Diagn Radiol 2006;35(1):12–21

Woolf AS, Price KL, Scambler PJ, Winyard PJ. Evolving concepts in human renal dysplasia. J Am Soc Nephrol 2004:15:998–1007

Wright NB, Smith C, Rickwood AM, Carty HM. Imaging children with ambiguous genitalia and intersex states. Clin Radiol 1995;50:823–829

Yagan N. Testicular US findings after biopsy. Radiology 2000;215: 768–773

Yazbeck S, Patriquin HB. Accuracy of Doppler sonography in the evaluation of acute conditions of the scrotum in children. J Pediatr Surg 1994;29:1270–1272

4 Skull, Intracranial Space, and Vertebral Column

Intracranial Abnormalities

The Orbits

Orbital Calcification

Orbital Masses

Nasal Cavity

The Nares and Nasal Passages

Paranasal Sinuses

Oral Cavity

The Pharynx

→

The Jaw and Teeth

The Neck

The Salivary Glands

Thyroid Gland

The Temporal Bone

Normal Variants

Congenital Anomalies

Syndromes Associated With Ear Anomalies

→

The Pediatric Vertebral Column

Anomalies of Vertebral Body Shape and Size

Anomalies of the Spinal Canal and Neural Arches

Anomalies of the Intervertebral Foramina

Alterations in Bone Structure

→

The Spinal Canal and Its Contents

Sutures and Fontanelles

The width of the sutures is highly variable in neonates; therefore, measurements are not reliable. Plain film, ultrasound (US), and computed tomography (CT) can be used for assessment of sutural patency.

The coronal suture is the first to manifest widening in response to increased intracranial pressure (ICP; upper limit of normal above 2 years of age is 2 mm). With an expanding mass in the occipital region, the lambdoid suture is the predominant suture affected. The principal sutures remain visible in adulthood as fine, interdigitated, radiolucent lines. The mendosal suture closes during the first months of life. Metopic fusion (frontal suture) may normally occur as early as 3 months of age, and complete fusion occurs by 9 months of age. The suture remains open after the age of 2 years in approximately 5% of cases.

In the occipital bone at birth, three primary sutures can be identified. Occipital and innominate sutures start to fuse at the age of 0 to 3 years, and complete closure is at 4 years. The mendosal suture may be open until 6 years of age.

Craniosynostosis: The premature closure of sutures during the first 3 years of life can lead to cranial growth abnormalities (see "Craniosynostosis"). Sutural fusions occurring after 3 years of age are usually of no clinical importance. "Passive" premature synostosis results from the rapid shunting of hydrocephalus and is occasionally associated with microcephaly.

Accessory sutures: These may occur unilaterally or symmetrically in the posterior parietal bones and occipital squamae.

Wormian bones: These are most often idiopathic, occurring most commonly in the lambdoid and occipitomastoid sutures.

The author would like to thank R. Nijland and T. de Jong for their assistance in preparing this section.

The differential diagnosis includes cleidocranial dysostosis, osteogenesis imperfecta, and hypothyroidism. The following normal structures may be mistaken for fractures:

- Mendosal suture, metopic suture, synchondroses at the skull base (intersphenoidal, spheno-occipital, and posterior intraoccipital synchondroses), accessory sutures
- Fibrous strips in the parietal bones of young infants; these faint radiolucent lines (unilateral or symmetric) disappear within a few weeks.

The fontanelles and the timing of their bony fusion are as follows:
- Anterior fontanelle: 12–15 months
- Anterolateral fontanelle: by 3 months
- Posterior fontanelle: by 2 months
- Posterolateral fontanelle: by 2 years.

Accessory fontanelles (also called cranium bifidum) occur in the midline, as follows:
- Metopic fontanelle in the frontale suture
- An additional fontanelle below the metopic fontanelle at the level of the glabella
- Parietal fontanelle in the posterior sagittal suture
- Large, often symmetrical parietal "foramina" are considered a normal variant.

Premature closure of the anterior fontanelle:
- May be a normal harmless variant if the coronal and sagittal sutures are patent.
- Is pathologic if there is any premature sutural fusion; there is possible associated bulging of the fontanelle.
- May be mimicked by a fontanelle (inca) bone (harmless variant).

Delayed closure of the anterior fontanelle often implies defective ossification when associated with marked suture widening and wormian bones.

Table 4.1 Widening of the sutures	
Diagnosis	**Findings**
Physiologic	Wide sutures can occur in premature infants (especially during growth spurt), in neonates, and in young infants. The coronal suture is most commonly affected. Cranial size and growth are normal.
Pathologic	Accelerated growth of the sutural connective tissue without concurrent ossification; ICP rise causes suture diastasis without prominent sutural interdigitations; spread occurs within 24–48 h in young infants and within 2 wk in older children. Gradual pressure rise is marked by elongated, ill-defined, sutural interdigitations.
Leukemia	Increased ICP due to infiltration of meninges, often with concomitant calvarial and sellar destruction.
Metastatic neuroblastoma ▷ *Fig. 4.1*	Bone destruction at the sutural edges, often involving other areas of the calvaria as well.
Trauma	Cranial injury, rupture of sutural connective tissue, diastatic sutural fracture.

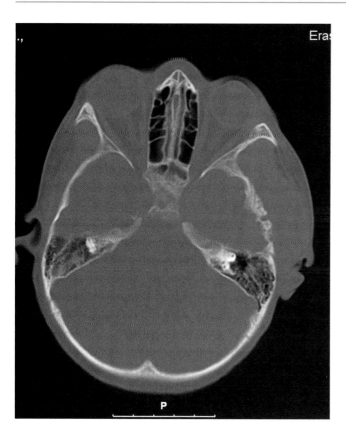

Fig. 4.1 Metastatic neuroblastoma with bone destruction involving the left coronal suture region.

Widened Sutures as a Symptom of Defective Ossification

In this instance, no signs of increased ICP are present. Usually, the suture has sharp edges without prominent interdigitations. Suture widening is often associated with numerous wormian bones and a persistent fontanelle.

Rare causes of widened sutures include the following:
- Pseudotumor cerebri, brain edema of unknown cause, post-traumatic with headache and papilledema: normal US, CT, and magnetic resonance imaging (MRI) findings

- Superior sagittal sinus (SSS) thrombosis: diagnosed by US (Doppler), CT, or MRI
- Vitamin A toxicity or deficiency
- Hyperparathyroidism
- Long-term use of steroid medication
- Long-term prostaglandin E_1 therapy
- Lead poisoning.

Table 4.2 Widening of the sutures as a symptom of defective ossification

Diagnosis	Findings
Florid rickets	Indistinct suture margins, generally obscured osseous structures.
Hypothyroidism, untreated	Delayed closure of fontanelles, often numerous wormian bones.
Osteogenesis imperfecta	Numerous wormian bones are generally present; thinned calvarial bones.
Cleidocranial dysostosis ▷ *Fig. 4.2, p. 294*	Persistent, large anterior fontanelle, numerous wormian bones.
Hypophosphatasia	Widely patent fontanelles, widened sutures.
Long-term prostaglandin E_1 therapy	Widely patent fontanelles.
Pycnodysostosis	Persistent anterior fontanelle, wormian bones, and osteosclerosis.
Menke syndrome (kinky hair syndrome)	Numerous wormian bones, microcephaly.
Progeria	Extremely rare condition of premature aging.
Zellweger syndrome ▷ *Fig. 4.3a, b, p. 294* ▷ *Fig. 4.4a, b, p. 295*	Facial manifestations, wide sutures, hypotonia, developmental delay, hepatomegaly, peripheral retinal pigmentation.
Hallermann-Streiff syndrome (oculomandibulo-dyscephaly)	Delayed closure of fontanelles. Syndrome is characterized by birdlike face, micropthalmia, cataracts, micrognathia, beaked nose, abnormal dentition, hypotrichosis, cutaneous atrophy, and proportional small stature.

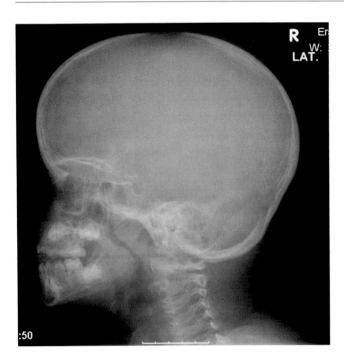

Fig. 4.2 Cleidocranial dysostosis in 4-year-old boy. Note the persistent open anterior fontanelle.

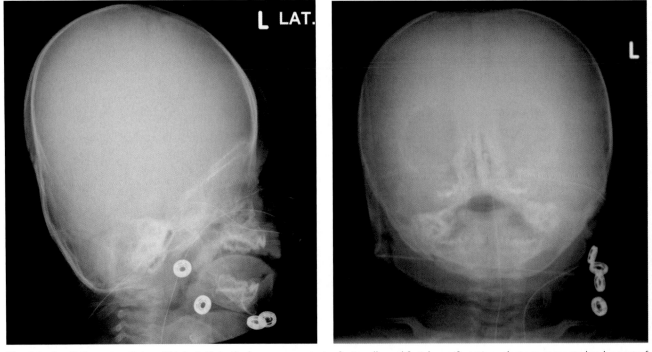

a

Fig. 4.3a, b Epilepsy in a 2-day-old infant. Note the large open anterior fontanelle and facial manifestations that are suspected to be part of Zellweger syndrome.

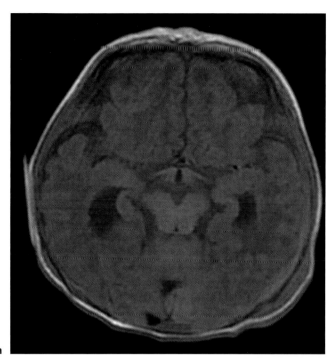
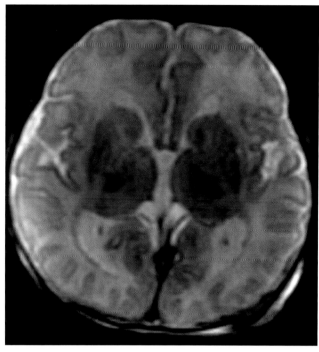

a   b

Fig. 4.4a, b   Subependymal heterotopia as part of Zellweger syndrome on T1- and T2-weighted brain images of the same patient as **Fig. 4.3**.

Linear Lucencies

Linear structural discontinuities may be observed at the level of the inner table, outer table, or diploë, or may entail the full thickness of the calvaria.

Table 4.3   Linear lucencies

Diagnosis	Findings
Normal vascular channels	Tortuous course, branching, with sclerotic and smooth borders and little radiographic contrast; different from the straight or zig-zag pattern of sharp fracture lines.
Arteries	Middle meningeal artery (inner table) located behind the coronal suture, often the superior and occipital branching is radiographically visible. The superficial and posterior temporal arteries run vertically in the temporal squama (outer table); they are rarely visible but can mimic a fracture. The supraorbital artery courses vertically in the outer table.
Veins	The broad sphenoparietal groove of the bregmatic vein (a meningeal vein) is clearly visible as it runs downward from the bregma in the inner table, taking a rather tortuous course behind and parallel to the coronal suture. The channels of the meningeal vessels become better visible at a later (school) age.
Venous sinuses	Inner table is traversed by broad, deep, nontortuous channels that appear by approximately 3 y of age. The sagittal sinus drains occipitally into the confluence sinus (torcula herophili) along with the transverse sinus and straight sinus (not visible). The right transverse sinus is often wider than the left.
Diploic veins	These vessels typically have a stellate configuration in the parietal bone and form "varix nodes" or "lakes" that appear as radiolucencies. Several fine diploic veins are sometimes visible in the frontal squama of infants.
Emissary veins	These connect the venous sinuses with the extracranial veins. They show a well-defined "vermiform" configuration in the calvaria and perforate it through smooth-edged foramina: the frontal (supraorbital) emissary vein; the mastoid emissary vein; the occipital emissary vein, which traverses one or more foramina in the midline at the internal occipital protuberance; and the parietal emissary vein, which traverses small, rarely visible, parietal foramina next to the sagittal suture in the posterior third. Emissary veins are uncommon in the area of the former metopic suture but may occur along its course to a point above the crista galli.
Abnormal vascular channels Diploic hyperplasia in hemolytic anemia and cyanotic heart disease ▷ Fig. 4.5a–c, p. 296	Vascular channels are widened and show increased tortuosity.
Craniostenosis	Markedly wide and deep vascular channels.

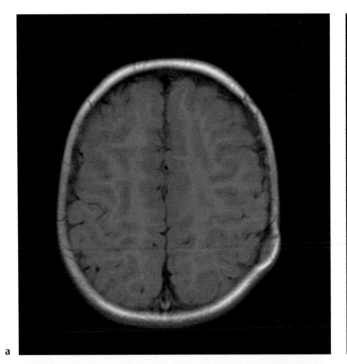

a

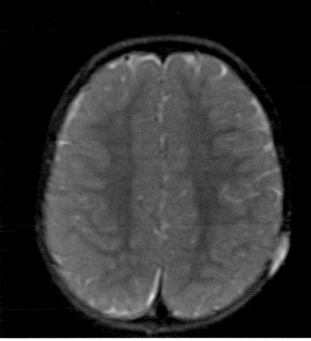

b

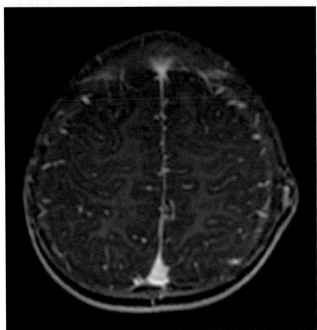

c

Fig. 4.5a–c   Sinus pericranii. (a) The lump in the left parieto-occipital region of 2-year-old boy is thought to be a dermoid. On T1-weighted image, it is isointense to gray matter. **(b)** On T2-weighted image, it is hyperintense. **(c)** There is little enhancement after gadolinium (Gd).

■ Fractures

In **normal fracture union**, the fracture line widens slightly and is thus more "visible" around 3 to 5 days after trauma, then its margins become indistinct. This is due to osteoclastic resorption of the debris, followed by osteoblastic repair.

Fracture malunion ("growing" fracture, see **Fig. 4.9a–c**) is marked by progressive widening of the fracture line (most common with burst fractures) and a protracted "hematoma" (cerebrospinal fluid [CSF] pulsations) with bridging of the fracture site by connective tissue, due to a dural tear.

Lines that mimic a fracture include the following:
- Metopic suture
- Posterior intraoccipital synchondrosis
- Mendosal suture
- Accessory suture in the parietal bone
- Wormian bones

Nonlinear Lucencies, Single or Multiple

Table 4.4   Nonlinear lucencies

Diagnosis	Findings	Comments
Emissary veins	Round smooth-bordered "holes" in the calvaria, marginal sclerosis, typical anatomic location.	An unusually large emissary vein at an atypical site is suspicious for an angioma or highly vascular intracranial tumor. Imaging best with CT or MRI.
Diploic venous lakes	Round, oval lucency in the diploë with corticated margins, occasional central phlebolith, single or multiple. Inner and outer tables are thinned but intact.	Frequently parietal or occipital adjacent to the transverse sinus. Lakes of unusual size or number may signify an angioma or meningioma. Imaging best with CT or MRI.
Pacchionian granulations	Resemble diploic venous lakes, often with a feeding vascular channel. Erosion of the inner table. Possible central phlebolith.	Occasional thinning and bulging of the outer table, typically in the parasagittal and frontal regions. Seldom noted before 9 y of age.
Large cisterna magna	Erosion of the inner table at the center of the inferior occipital squama, similar to a venous lake or larger.	Findings similar to arachnoid cysts and superficial gliomas.
Arachnoid cyst	Localized bulging and thinning of the calvaria.	Involvement of occipital squama closely resembles a large cisterna magna.
Enlarged parietal foramina ▷ *Fig. 4.6a, b*	Paramedian defects adjacent to the posterior third of the sagittal suture. Location matches that of the parietal fontanelle.	May communicate across the midline. Familial occurence, relatively common in patients with craniosynostoses. No correlation with brain malformations.
Encephaloceles; cranium bifidum (accessory fontanelle)	Round to oval defects with smooth margins, variable size, and no marginal sclerosis. Located in the midline, usually frontal or occipital, sometimes sphenoidal or frontoethmoidal, rarely in the area of the parietal fontanelle; temporal occurrence is very rare.	The soft-tissue mass over the defect is typical. Skull defect without herniation means cranium bifidum. May coexist with dysplastic corpus callosum and Chiari malformation.
Pneumatization of the crista galli	Aerated crista galli should not be mistaken for a frontal encephalocele.	

(continues on page 298)

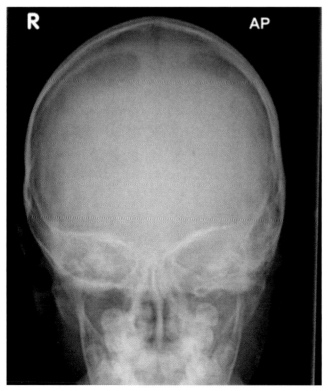
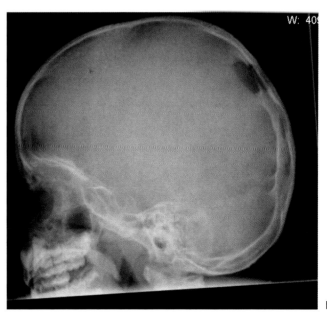

Fig. 4.6a, b   **Parietal foramina** in a healthy 5-year-old boy.

Table 4.4   (Cont.) Nonlinear lucencies

Diagnosis	Findings	Comments
Epidermoid and dermoid	Indistinguishable on skull films, US, CT, or MRI. Epidermoids are more common. Round or oval defect in the diploë with smooth, well-corticated margins, often located near the lateral canthus or suture. CT and MRI best techniques to rule out intracranial extension.	Spontaneous resolution is common, further growth rare. Together with Langerhans cell histiocytosis (LCH), the most commonly encountered skull lesions in the pediatric population.
Langerhans cell histiocytosis ▷ *Fig. 4.7a, b* ▷ *Fig. 4.8a–c*	Single or multiple defects, rounded or irregular, of highly variable size. "Geographic skull." No marginal sclerosis.	Bone scan shows a cold lesion with increased uptake at its edges. Other skeletal foci should be ruled out.
Fibrous dysplasia (FD), aneurysmal bone cyst	Cyst degeneration may occur within an existing FD lesion, manifesting as acute clinical deterioration. Cyst degeneration occurs most commonly in the sphenoid and frontal bones. Appearance ranges from a simple lesion to aneurysmal bone cyst. In aneurysmal bone cyst, CT shows the cystic lesion in the diploë, with predominantly inward expansion. Fluid-fluid levels may be seen on both CT and MRI; the latter can also show bleeding within the cyst.	Cyst degeneration may occur spontaneously within the FD lesion years after the initial diagnosis. Cavarial aneurysmal bone cyst is rare, with only 3% to 6% of cases occurring in this anatomic location.
Metastatic neuroblastoma or extension of leukemia in the diploë	Multiple small and irregular defects with ill-defined margins; may coalesce.	Neuroblastoma may produce isolated defects and suture widening.
Leptomeningeal cyst (growing fracture) ▷ *Fig. 4.9a–c*	Calvarial defect after traumatic dural laceration; irregular; sharp edges with marginal sclerosis.	Detection weeks to months after the fracture event, due to cerebrospinal fluid (CSF) pulsations.
Older cephalhematoma	Irregular osteolysis of the outer table.	Best depicted on CT.
Previous craniectomy	Initially smooth defect that acquires irregular borders with healing. Central sequestrum may be present.	
Neurofibromatosis (NF)	Extensive cranial defects associated with underlying dural ectasia. Best detected on CT.	Besides defects in the cranium, also at the level of the sphenoid wing.
Osteomyelitis	Moth-eaten defects in the cranium. Sequestrum formation rarely seen.	May be a complication of a craniectomy.
Hyperparathyroidism	Disseminated ill-defined lucencies mixed with faint calcifications. Generalized demineralization of the calvaria, sometimes with calcifications in the falx and tentorium.	Generally secondary (renal osteodystrophy) resorption of the dental laminae dura. Secondary hyperparathyroidism may cause or result in brown tumors, especially in the facial bones.

(continues on page 300)

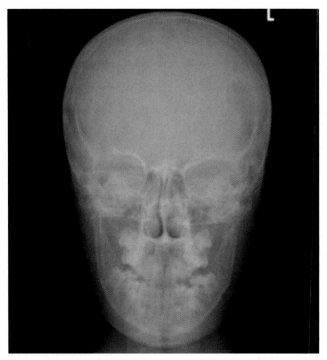
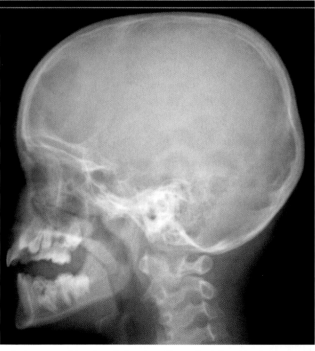

a

Fig. 4.7a, b   Langerhans cell histiocytosis. (a) A 10.5-year-old girl with a lytic mass with sclerotic borders above the left orbit characteristic for LCH. **(b)** Lateral view of same patient.

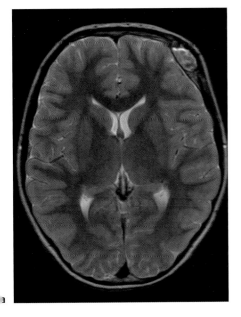
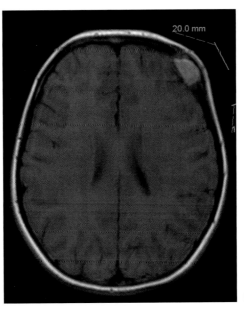

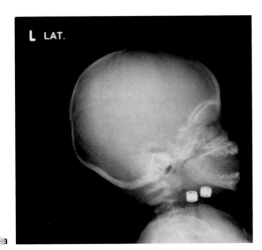

Fig. 4.8a–c   Langerhans cell histiocytosis (LCH). (**a**) T2-weighted image shows an inhomogeneous mass with hyperintense and hypointense signal intensity involving the diploë in the left os frontale. (**b**) T1-weighted image shows a homogeneous mass with hyperintense signal intensity. (**c**) This sagittal T1-weighted image after contrast shows extensive enhancement of the mass with meningeal enhancement.

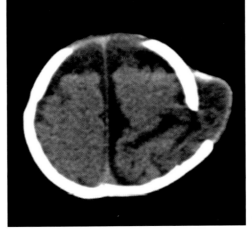

Fig. 4.9a–c   Leptomeningeal cyst. (**a**) A 3-month-old boy after a fall from stairs. His head hit the tile floor. A fracture is seen on the right parieto-occipital side. (**b**) CT several weeks later: the fracture is "growing." Note the herniation of brain tissue through the fracture site due to dura rupture. (**c**) CT bone setting: "growing" distance between the fracture parts.

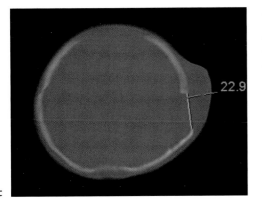

Table 4.4   (Cont.) Nonlinear lucencies

Diagnosis	Findings	Comments
Hemangioma ▷ *Fig. 4.10a–c*	May present as a progressive mass. A plain X-ray of the skull, cranial CT, or MRI may show an intraosseous, osteolytic lesion.	Intraosseous cavernous hemangiomas are a rare finding in the calvarium. These are benign tumors arising from the intrinsic vasculature of the bone.
Primary calvarial tumors	Plain films and CT demonstrate an osteolytic mass surrounded by the sclerotic rim within the diploic space. MRI can be used for the evaluation of the intracranial and intraosseous extensions of the tumor. It can be very difficult to differentiate it from other osteoblastic tumors or from osteoid osteoma. Malignant tumors, like sarcomas, may also occur in the calvaria.	Osteoblastoma is an uncommon primary bone tumor that usually involves the vertebrae and the long bones. This tumor rarely develops in the calvaria, showing a preference for the temporal and frontal bones.
Giant cell tumor	Can occur in the skull, principally in the sphenoid and temporal bones. Radiographically, the tumors appear osteolytic and radiolucent without a sclerotic border.	Rarely occurs in patients under 20 y of age.

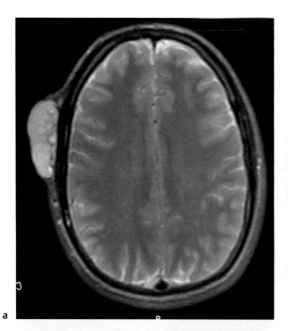

a

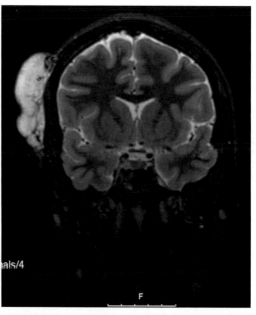

b

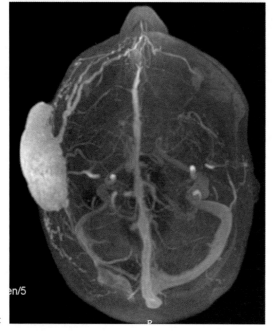

c

Fig. 4.10a–c   Hemangioma. (a, b) A 7-year-old boy with a vascular malformation involving skin and subcutical region. No intracranial component is noted. In the T2-weighted image with characteristics of a hemangioma, note the signal voids. **(c)** Arterial supply of hemangioma via the right external carotid artery.

Craniosynostosis

Craniosynostosis is a premature fusion of cranial sutures in infants that may lead to profound changes in craniofacial shape. These changes are a result of anatomic differences between the calvarial unit and skull base portion of the skull. Growth within the craniofacial skeleton is based on two key concepts: displacement and bone remodeling. Calvaria growth in the infant requires rapid and symmetrical displacement of each of the large bones (frontal, parietal, and occipital) of the skull along with osseous deposition along the sutures and within the bone matrix. Concomitant with these growth patterns is endocranial and ectocranial remodeling of the skull bones. Each of these patterns changes rapidly in infancy, continues into childhood, and in some cases continues even into adulthood. Following closely and symmetrically behind calvarial growth is skull base and facial growth. In the growth sequence, the anterior fossa completes its growth first, followed by the posterior and middle fossa. During this growth cycle, the skull base and face follow in form to the calvaria. When the three skull base fossae are examined individually, a unique growth pattern develops within each one. The anterior fossa relies on the growth at the sphenoid, ethmoid, and frontal bones primarily using the growth at the sphenofrontal and sphenoethmoidal sutures. Growth is rapid in this area up to about 7 years of age. The middle fossa continues its growth for an even longer period, into the teenage years, with the sphenopetrosal and petro-occipital synchondroses being most affected. The posterior fossa also continues an active growth pattern into childhood and the adolescent years. The intraoccipital synchondroses complete their growth in childhood, with the spheno-occipital synchondroses remaining active into adolescence. Concomitant to this skull base growth pattern is the growth rate of the facial skeleton. Growth within the face continues until well into the adolescent era, with a spurt that occurs during puberty. Critical angulation patterns of the maxilla are finalized in adolescence and closely follow the pattern of growth of the anterior fossa. As a result, if there is any form of premature fusion of any of the skull base sutures and synchondroses, these premature fusions can lead to significant alterations of the skull and facial alignment, resulting in a variety of different craniofacial anomalies. Head shape depends on which sutures are prematurely synostosed, the order in which they synostose, and the timing at which they synostose. Craniosynostosis may be of prenatal or perinatal onset or may occur later during infancy or childhood. The earlier synostosis occurs, the more dramatic the effect on subsequent cranial growth and development. The later synostosis occurs, the less the effect on cranial growth and development. Synostosed skulls with almost normal-shaped skulls have been observed. Therefore, skull and facial morphogenesis is a complex and multifactorial development, some of which we are only just beginning to understand.

The so-called single-suture synostoses (e.g., scaphocephaly) rarely involve the skull base and its concomitant sutures. There are two potential exceptions to this rule: plagiocephaly, which is due to premature closure of one of the coronal sutures, and trigonocephaly, where there is a premature closure of the metopic suture.

Most craniosynostoses are congenital and manifest themselves predominantly during the period of intense cranial growth (birth through 3 years of age). Along with a small posterior fossa, cerebellar crowding occurs; Chiari malformation is a not uncommon finding associated with all these factors. Measurements of the foramen magnum typically show small aperture openings and other asymmetries. Angiographic studies have also shown significant alterations in the venous outflow patterns at the skull base, which can lead to intracranial venous hypertension. Venous hypertension is thought to be secondary to narrowing of the skull base foramina, particularly in the area of the jugular bulb. These skull base abnormalities are felt to be an important cause of hydrocephalus seen especially in syndromal craniosynostosis. Today, concepts about the pathophysiology of complex syndromic craniosynostoses have shifted from mechanical models involving tension forces of the dural structures to a molecular signalling disorder model. Mutations of the fibroblast growth factor receptors 1, 2, and 3, as well as of the *TWIST* and *MSX2* genes, are commonly associated with the different phenotypes of this group of autosomal dominant (AD) malformations. Significant brain abnormalities have been reported in all syndromes. However, whether these abnormalities are secondary to the bone disease or primary (e.g., callosal agenesis) is still controversial. Recent evidence suggests that a white matter defect might be a primary disorder.

■ Radiographic Signs

Craniosynostosis is initially manifested on radiographs by straight, narrow, sharp-edged sutures with marginal sclerosis. Later, the sutures become partially or entirely bridged by bone. Cranial growth is deviated in the direction of the prematurely fused suture. On three-dimensional (3D) CT, better appreciation of the small posterior fossa, cerebellar crowding, and sometimes associated Chiari malformation is possible. Also, narrowing of the skull base foramina, particularly in the area of the jugular bulb, which may give rise to intracranial hypertension, is better evaluated on CT. Additional structural intracranial abnormalities are easily shown on CT. For the surgeon, 3D CT is an excellent tool for preoperative and postoperative assessment in patients with complex craniosynostosis.

Secondary synostoses result from decreased ICP after shunting of hydrocephalus and only rarely result in microcephaly. This type of fusion does not produce craniosynostosis.

Skull deformity may also be the result of various metabolic diseases and skeletal disorders, such as the following:
- Vitamin D deficiency rickets (healed)
- Vitamin D–resistant forms of rickets
- Hypophosphatasia
- Idiopathic hypercalcemia
- Mucopolysaccharidosis (MPS)
- Primary hyperthyroidism
- Hypothyroidism due to hormonal overdose

Table 4.5 Types of plagiocephaly

Types of Sutures	Synostosed	Relative Frequencies
Synostotic anterior plagiocephaly	Unilateral coronal	Less common than bilateral coronal synostosis
	Unilateral frontosphenoidal without coronal synostosis	Very rare
	Unilateral frontozygomatic without coronal synostosis	Very rare
Synostotic posterior plagiocephaly	Unilateral lambdoid	Rare
Deformational anterior plagiocephaly	No sutures synostosed	Formerly common; now uncommon
Deformational posterior plagiocephaly	No sutures synostosed	Common

Table 4.6 Craniosynostosis

Diagnosis	Findings	Comments
Premature fusion of one frontal-parietal (coronal) suture (plagiocephaly) ▷ *Fig. 4.11a–d*	Anteroposterior (AP) skull film: cranium smaller on the affected side, with a thinner calvaria, temporal bone prominence, and increased convolutional markings. Sagittal and lambdoid sutures deviate toward the affected side; crista galli and falx may also be deviated. The orbit is enlarged with an elevated superolateral rim. The lesser sphenoid wing and planum sphenoidale slope laterally upward. The petrous bone is more horizontal. Lateral view: fused suture limb is not visualized or appears as a thin, sharp-edged fissure; terminates inferiorly as a linear density in the elevated lesser sphenoid wing; middle fossa is expanded.	External appearance: Unilateral frontal flattening with apparent widening of the palpebral aperture. Even bilateral coronal synostosis can cause asymmetry if areas of the suture fuse at different times.
Premature fusion of one frontal-parietal suture and ipsilateral frontal-sphenoid suture ▷ *Fig. 4.12a–d, p. 304*	See above, with the exception of a smaller orbit and contralateral deviation of the skull base.	Best appreciated on 3D CT reconstructions.
Premature fusion of the lambdoid and/or mendosal suture ▷ *Fig. 4.13a, b, p. 305*	AP skull film: deep posterior fossa, asymmetric petrous pyramids. Lateral view; increased occipital convolutional markings, occipital flattening, anterior displacement of petrous pyramid.	Rare craniosynostosis coexists with premature fusion of other sutures.
Premature fusion of sagittal suture (dolichocephaly) ▷ *Fig. 4.14a–c, p. 305*	Frontal region narrow, calvaria small and elongated. Sagittal suture is narrow in young infants with sharp edges and partial ossification. Anterior fontanelle is very small. Other sutures are otherwise normal, with no signs of increased ICP. Head size is macrocephalic but sometimes normal.	Normal development. Optic nerve atrophy is very rare. No signs of increased ICP. The orbits appear quite large due to the projection effect (elongated skull); in some cases, the enlargement is real.

(continues on page 306)

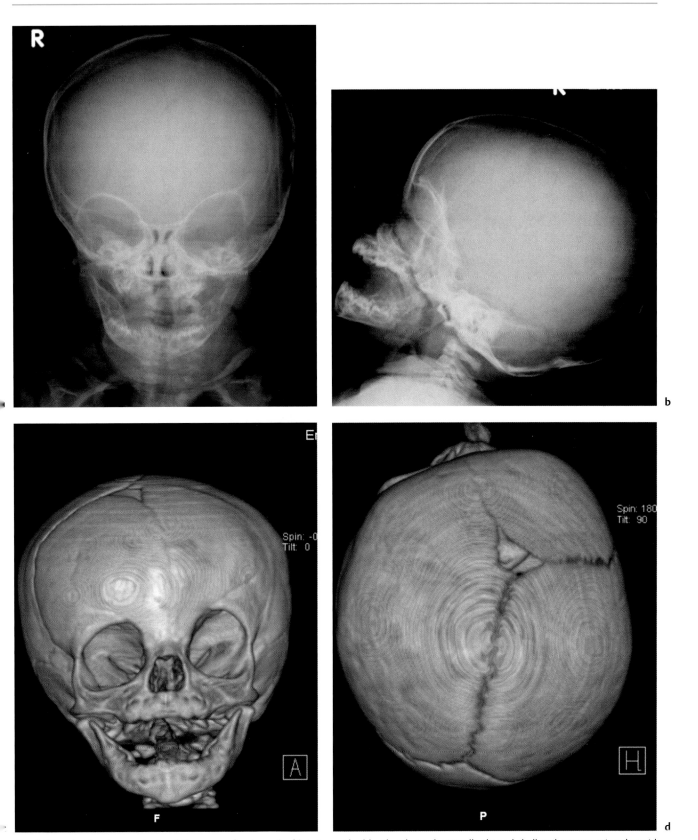

Fig. 4.11a–d   Craniosynostosis of the coronal suture. (a, b) A 6-month-old girl with an abnormally shaped skull and asymmetric sphenoid wing. **(c, d)** 3D rendering shows a craniosynostosis of the left coronal suture.

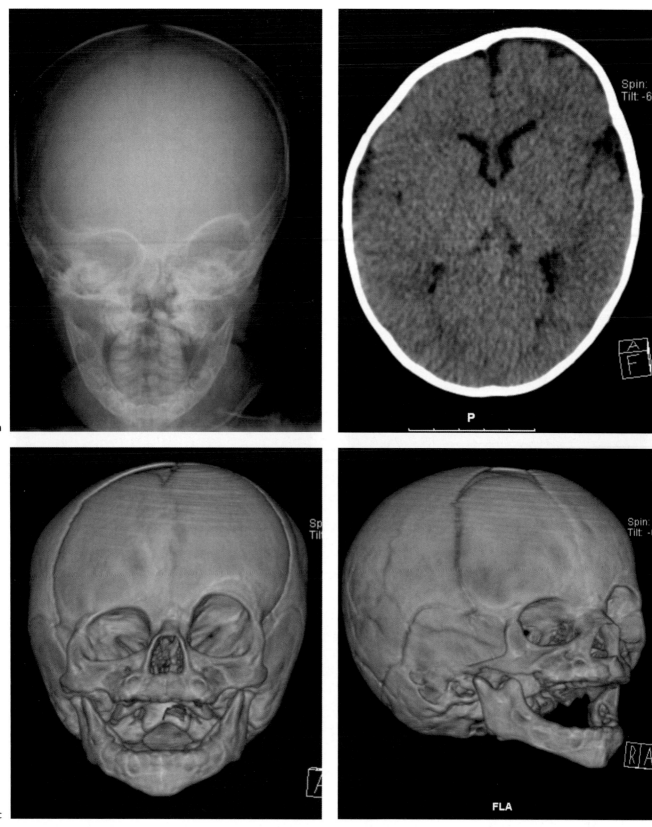

Fig. 4.12a–d Craniosynostosis. (a) A 5-month-old boy with an abnormally shaped skull. Closed right-sided coronal suture and synostosis of the right frontosphenoid suture result in a small right orbit. **(b)** On CT, note the flattening of the forehead on the right side. **(c, d)** 3D rendering shows the closed right-sided coronal suture and synostosis of the right frontosphenoid suture, resulting in a small right orbit.

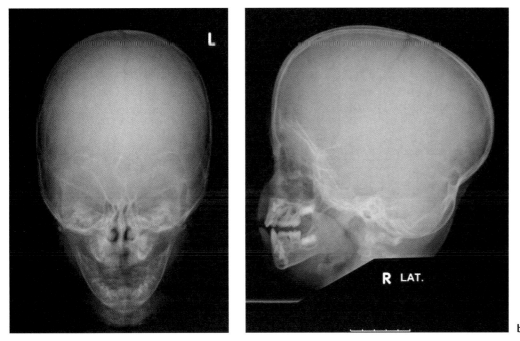

Fig. 4.13a, b Craniosynostosis of both lambdoid sutures. (**a**) Multiple dysmorphic characteristics in an 8-month-old boy with an abnormally shaped skull and scalloping of the calvaria. (**b**) Lateral view. Note underdevelopment of the occipital region and posterior fossa due to early closure of lambdoid sutures.

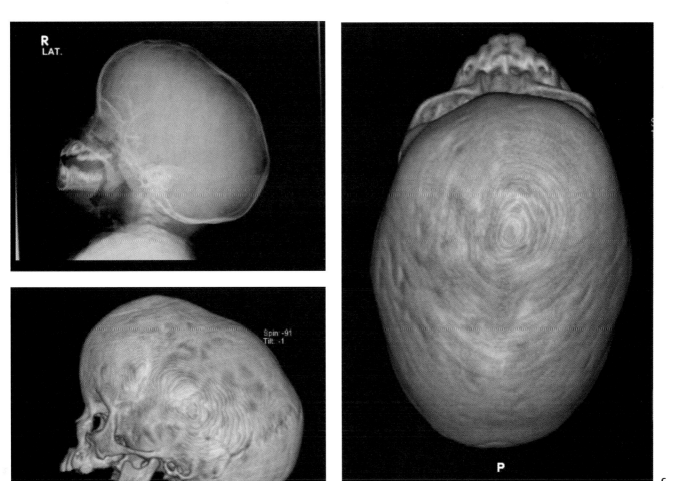

Fig. 4.14a–c Dolichocephaly. (**a**) An 18-month-old boy with an abnormally shaped skull and scaphocephaly with frontal impressions due to craniosynostosis of sagittal suture. (**b**) 3D rendering shows the impressions probably due to increased ICP. (**c**) 3D rendering shows the synostosis of the sagittal suture.

Table 4.6 (Cont.) Craniosynostosis

Diagnosis	Findings	Comments
Premature fusion of metopic suture (trigonocephaly) ▷ *Fig. 4.15a–c*	Small, keel-shaped frontal bone with hyperostosis. Metopic suture is fused. Elliptical orbits with decreased interorbital distance (hypotelorism). Coronal suture bows anteriorly toward the small anterior fontanelle. Head size normal; no signs of increased ICP.	Recent studies show cognitive impairment may be due to abnormal development of frontal lobe. Metopic suture is a normal finding in children up to 2 y of age (15% of cases); it is patent by the age of 20 y in 3% of cases (metopism).
Coronal and sagittal synostosis	Often, there is no pronounced calvarial deformity, though ICP symptoms can become very severe.	If the sutures ossify at different times, the first suture to fuse determines the calvarial configuration (see sagittal and cranial synostosis).

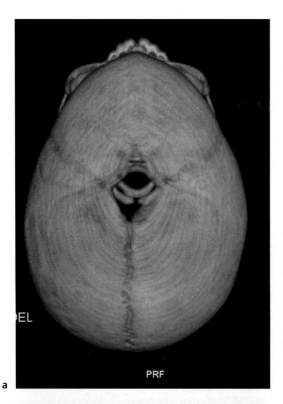

a

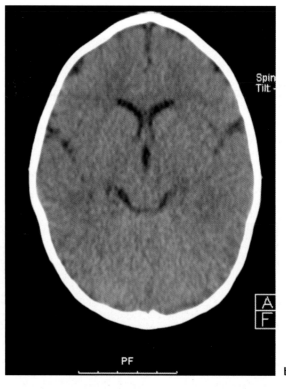

b

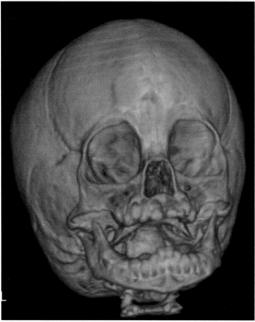

c

Fig. 4.15a–c Trigonocephaly. (**a**) A 10-month-old girl with trigonal shaped head because of an early closure of the metopic suture. (**b**) Note also the hypoplastic aspect of the frontal lobes. (**c**) Hypotelorism because of the early closure of the metopic suture.

Table 4.7 Syndromal craniosynostosis

Diagnosis	Findings	Comments
Acrocephalosyndactyly type I (Apert syndrome) ▷ *Fig. 4.16a–c*	Coronal synostosis, marked cranial deformity even in neonates. Accessory fontanelles in the frontal and parietal regions. Hypertelorism, maxillary hypoplasia; later, progressive signs of increased ICP are best visualized with CT or MRI. Absence of olfactory bulbs and tracts, midline fusion of olfactory tubercles, incomplete development of the olfactory tubercle and hippocampus and abnormal pyramidal tracts and decussation have been described. Also abnormal corpus callosum, septal defects, gyral abnormalities, seldom gray matter heterotopia, hypoplastic white matter, and megalencephaly.	Coronal synostosis is rarely unilateral. Marked bony and soft-tissue syndactyly of hands and feet. AD inheritance. Mental deficiency in Apert syndrome may be related to limbic structures' abnormality.
Acrocephalosyndactyly II (Carpenter syndrome)	Skull as in Apert syndrome, may include craniosynostosis due to fusion of all sutures.	Extremely rare. Postaxial polydactyly, variable syndactyly. Obesitas, male hypogonadism, and mental retardation have been reported. It is autosomal recessive.

(continues on page 308)

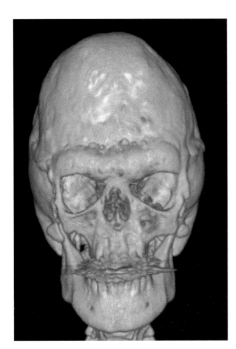

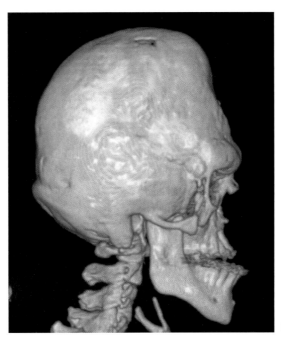

b

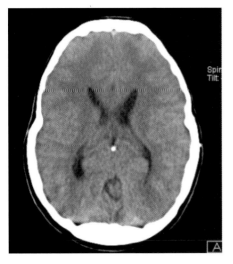

Fig. 4.16a–c Acrocephalosyndactyly type I. (a, b) CT rendering images show underdeveloped frontal calvarium and maxilla in an 18-year-old girl with Apert syndrome. **(c)** Note the thinning of the inner surface of the vault due to raised ICP.

Table 4.7 (Cont.) Syndromal craniosynostosis

Diagnosis	Findings	Comments
Acrocephalosyndactyly type III (Saethre-Chotzen syndrome)	Craniosynostosis may involve the coronal, lambdoid, or metopic sutures, with late closing of fontanelles and parietal foramina, thus associating hyperostosis with ossification defects. CT and/or MRI findings are described from normal to mega cisterna magna, abnormal gyral structures, and atrophy (enlarged subarachnoid spaces).	Characterized by brachycephaly with maxillary hypoplasia, prominent ear crus, and cutaneous syndactyly; shallow orbits with eyelid ptosis; other bony abnormalities are common. Children present with a flat forehead, low set hairline, and facial asymmetry with syndactyly involving the second and third fingers and the third and fourth toes, with small distal phalanges. Mental deficiency is classically uncommon. Hypotonia, seizures, and pyramidal signs have been described.
Acrocephalosyndactyly type V (Pfeiffer syndrome)	Very few imaging descriptions in the literature. In subtype I and III, ventriculomegaly and short concave clivus. Chiari type I may be present. In subtype II hydrocephalus and small posterior fossa may be seen. Subtype II is also characterized by the cloverleaf skull shape.	Subdivided into three subtypes. Subtype I is the classical, milder form with bicoronal synchondrosis, brachycephaly and flat face, hypertelorism, and mild syndactyly with broad thumbs and great toes; it is AD, with occasional mental deficiency. Subtypes II and III are sporadic and much more severe, with marked ocular proptosis and central nervous system (CNS) involvement, elbow ankylosis, and congenital heart disease. The survival rate is usually but not always poor.
Crouzon syndrome, craniofacial dysostosis ▷ *Fig. 4.17a, b*	All forms of craniosynostosis can occur, even fusion of all sutures with extreme signs of increased ICP. Hypoplasia or agenesis of the corpus callosum may be seen. Nonprogressive ventriculomegaly is common. In 70%, Chiari type I is present.	May occur without hydrocephalus. AD. Brachycephaly with underdevelopment of the midface, especially the maxilla. No deformities of the hands and feet. Mental deficiency is common.
Muenke craniosynostosis	Coronal synostosis, mild maxillary hypoplasia. Hypertelorism. CT and MRI findings in majority are unremarkable. Mild degree of chronic tonsillar herniation with normal looking posterior fossa has been reported.	Uncommon. AD. Mental deficiency common.
Cloverleaf skull or Kleeblattschädel	Trilobular skull with craniosynostosis. Coronal, lambdoid, and metopic sutures may be closed with bulging of the cerebrum through an open sagittal suture or through open squamosal sutures. Synostosis of sagittal and squamosal sutures with cerebral eventration through a widely patent anterior fontanelle may also be observed.	Severity varies and different sutures may be involved.

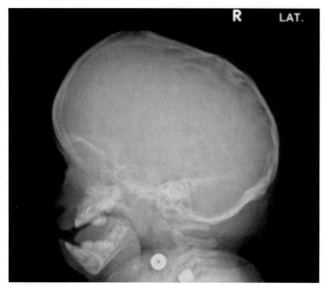
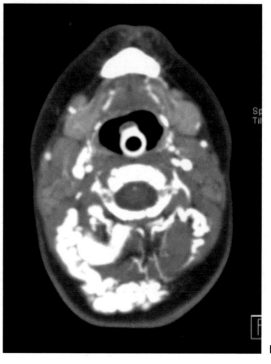

Fig. 4.17a, b Crouzon syndrome. (a) Crouzon syndrome in a 14-month-old boy; note the hypoplasia of the maxilla and the calvarial scalloping. **(b)** This intravenous contrast-enhanced CT (CECT) shows the venous collaterals because of intracranial venous obstruction.

The Skull Base

The skull base is one of the most complex regions of the human body because of its intricate network of neural, vascular, and lymphatic structures. An additional complexity exists in the pediatric population because of the postnatal maturation of the skull base. This may lead, among other things, to misinterpretations of sutures and synchondroses as fractures. This section will focus not on skull base maturation itself, but on the more important aspects of diagnosis, differential diagnosis, and diagnosis pitfalls in pediatric patients with lesions of the skull base using conventional X-ray, CT, or MRI of the skull and skull base.

Extensive involvement and guidance by the pediatric radiologist is important to both surgeon and oncologist because it provides an exact assessment of the topography, degree of vascularization, and extent of the lesion for the appropriate surgical or radio-oncologic planning.

CT can detect lesions and fractures, using ultrathin slices, 3D reconstructions, and contrast medium administration, even with a recently introduced CT-angiography (CTA) technique. Regarding tumorous lesions, MRI is superior to CT due to its better soft-tissue contrast and the possibility of choosing a variety of parameters emphasizing different types of tissues and substances. Another important advantage of MRI, especially in children, is its lack of radiation burden.

Table 4.8 Pathology at the skull base

Diagnosis	Findings
Nonneoplastic tumors	
Arachnoidal cyst	See arachnoid cysts, p. 344
Cephalocele ▷ *Fig. 4.18a–e, p. 310*	Occurs usually at the midline. The most common basal cephalocele is the sphenopharyngeal type. CT can show the bony defect. CTA can show the relation to vascular structures around the cephalocele. MR is better to depict the extent and content of the cephalocele and accompanying (midline) structure abnormalities.
Benign tumors	
Cholesterol granuloma	MRI is the imaging modality of choice. The tumor has increased signal intensity on T1 and T2 sequences with a hypointense rim that represents expanded cortical bone and hemosiderin peripheral deposits.
Epidermoid	Most common at the cerebellopontine angle cisterns and parasellar region. Epidermoids are typically extra-axial lesions, like arachnoid cysts. On CT, epidermoids appear hypoattenuating with possible marginal calcifications. On MRI, the tumor is hypointense on T1 and hyperintense on T2, with no significant contrast enhancement (CE). There is usually some internal heterogeneity, which is best seen in the proton-density and FLAIR images, and this could help distinguish these cysts from arachnoid cysts, which they closely mimic. DWI is the most helpful imaging sequence in diagnosing an epidermoid cyst. Epidermoid tumors demonstrate an ADC that is similar to that of gray matter and lower than that of CSF. In contrast, arachnoid cysts or other cystic intracranial lesions do not show restricted diffusion and follow the CSF signal on DWI and ADC maps. Epidermoids often show encasement of vessels without displacement.
Lipoma	A lipoma is thought to result from a maldifferentiation of the primitive meninx. The majority of lipomas are located around the corpus callosum. On CT, a lipoma appears exactly the same as subcuteous fat: homogeneous hypoattenuation. On MRI, a lipoma has a signal intensity compatible with subcutaneous fat on all sequences.
Schwannoma/neurofibroma	Schwannomas usually arise from the vestibular division of the eighth cranial nerve. Acoustic schwannoma may occur either sporadically or as part of a clinical complex in NF2. In the latter situation, patients usually present at an earlier age and sometimes with bilateral tumors. Sporadic or non-NF2 vestibular schwannomas are very rare in children. On CT, the lesion is hypodense and may show homogeneous enhancement. On MRI, the lesion is hypointense on T1 and hyperintense on T2 and show marked enhancement after Gd. Schwannoma and neurofibroma are indistinguishable by neuroimaging.

(continues on page 311)

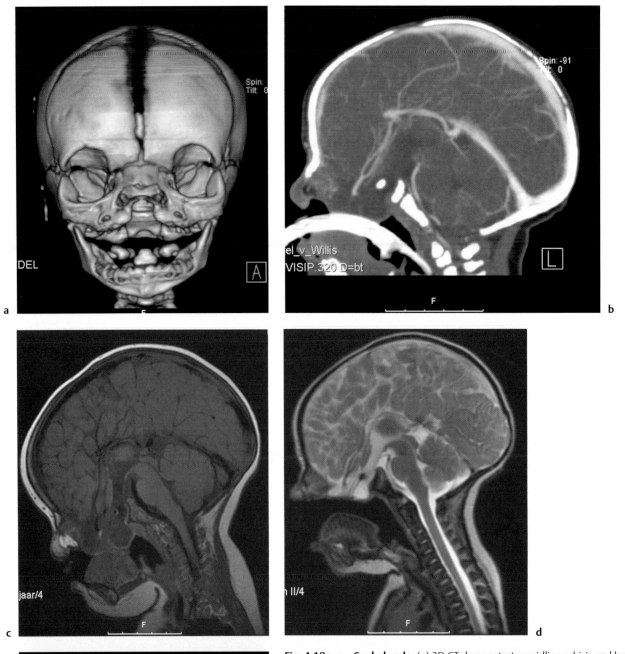

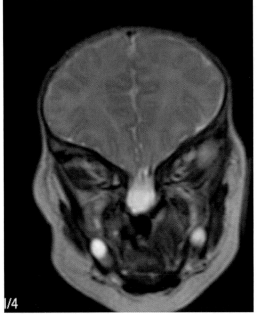

Fig. 4.18a–e   Cephalocele. (a) 3D CT demonstrates midline schisis and bulging of soft tissue in the oronasal pharynx in a 3-month-old boy. **(b)** Sagittal reconstruction of a CTA. The pericallosal arteries are herniating through the encephalocele. T1 **(c)** and T2 **(d, e)** MRI shows a frontal nasal encephalocele including herniation of the pituitary gland.

Table 4.8   (Cont.) Pathology at the skull base

Diagnosis	Findings
Benign tumors (cont.)	
Meningioma ▷ *Fig. 4.19a–c*	Pediatric meningiomas are rare, comprising less than 5% of all pediatric brain tumors and less than 2% of all meningiomas. Risk factors for the development of meningiomas include a history of radiation therapy or a diagnosis of NF2. MRI is the imaging modality. The lesion is iso-/hypointense on T1 and hyperintense on T2 with occasional cysts and calcifications. The lesion shows a marked homogeneous enhancement after Gd. On CT, the demarcated exostosis of bone in the area of the lesion is better seen than on MRI.
Glomus tumor	Benign but locally aggressive tumors, destroying the bones of the skull base with a moth-eaten appearance at CT. MRI shows signs of a vascular tumor and a mixture of multiple punctate and serpentine signal voids, due to high-flow intratumoral vessels and intratumoral hemorrhage, producing the characteristic salt-and-pepper appearance. It is a rare tumor in children.
Malignant tumors	
Rhabdomyosarcoma ▷ *Fig. 4.20a–c, p. 312*	Rhabdomyosarcomas at the skull base, by virtue of an often parameningeal location, show an invasive behavior. They can extend intracranially and produce neoplastic meningitis. The four anatomic sites showing this potential are the nasopharynx/nasal cavity, the middle ear, the paranasal sinuses, and the infratemporal fossa/pterygopalatine space. Most patients are under 10 y old at diagnosis (72%) and present with skull base erosion, cranial nerve palsy, and intracranial extension.
Chondrosarcoma	Usually more lateral in location than a chordoma. Otherwise, see chordoma, discussed subsequently.
Chordoma	Originate from embryonic remnants of the primitive notochord and are located in the midline, near the clivus. On CT, chordoma typically appears as a centrally located, well-circumscribed, expansile soft-tissue mass with extensive lytic destruction of the clivus. On MRI, the tumor is heterogeneous with an intermediate to low signal on T1 with foci of hyperintense signal due to ossified fragments of the skull base, tumor calcifications, collections of proteinaceous fluid, or hemorrhage. On T2, a chordoma has high signal intensity and septa of low signal intensity. Slight enhancement after Gd.
Metastatic disease	Rare in the pediatric population. May mimic a meningioma or schwannoma. Often surrounded by peritumoral edema.

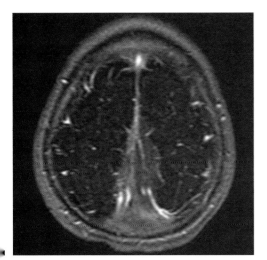
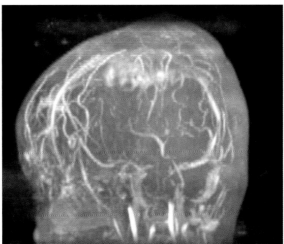

b

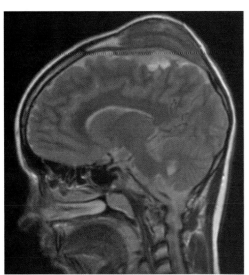

Fig. 4.19a–c   Meningioma. (a) A 9-year-old girl with a destructive lesion of the calvaria due to an intraosseous meningioma in the midline and paramedian left. Tumor shows invasion of the SSS. Note the swollen cortical veins due to impaired venous drainage of the sinus. **(b)** 3D map of contrast-enhanced MRA show the involvement of the SSS. **(c)** Sagittal T2 image shows the involvement of the diploic space. Note the relative low signal intensity of the tumor.

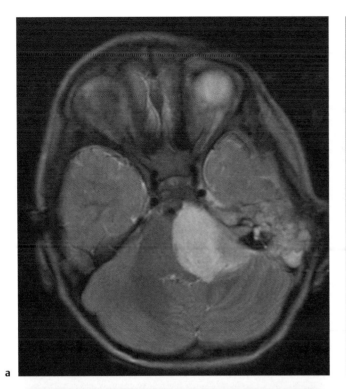

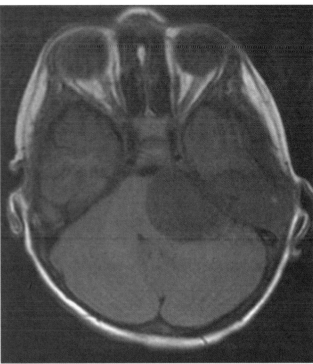

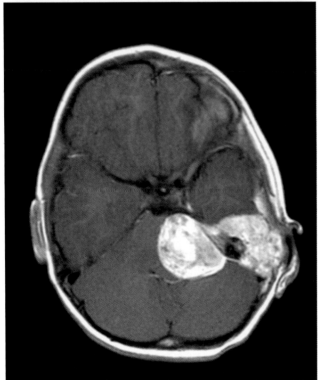

Fig. 4.20a–c Rhabdomyosarcoma. (a) A 4-year-old boy with progressive neurologic deterioration due to compression of the brainstem. The tumor is located in the left mastoid with cerebellopontine expansion, histologically an embryonal rhabdomyosarcoma. Note the high signal intensity on this T2-weighted image. **(b)** On this axial T1-weighted image, the tumor is hypointense. **(c)** Intense contrast enhancement (CE) on this Gd-enhanced T1 sequence is noted.

Table 4.9   Sclerosis and hyperostosis of the skull base

Diagnosis	Findings
Physiologic	In prematures and neonates.
Chronic infection	Mastoiditis, inflammation of the apex of the petrous bone. Mucocele. Sinusitis complicated with surrounding osteomyelitis, known as Pott puffy tumor at the level of the frontal sinus.
Fibrous dysplasia ▷ *Fig. 4.21a, b* ▷ *Fig. 4.22*	See **Table 4.4** and skeletal dysplasia in **Table 4.9**

(continues on page 314)

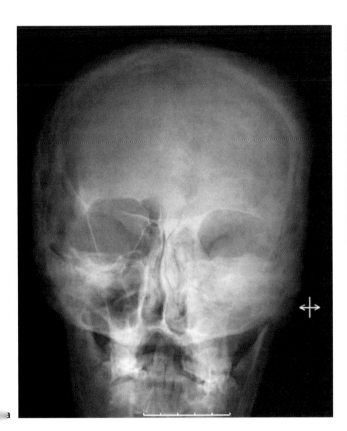

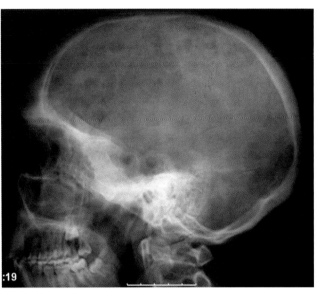

Fig. 4.21a, b   McCune-Albright syndrome in a 15-year-old girl involving the left side of the vault and skull base.

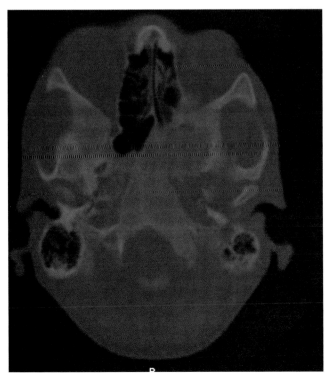

Fig. 4.22   McCune-Albright syndrome in a 16-year-old boy. CT shows a ground-glass aspect of the clivus and sphenoid region on the left. Foramina are smaller and there is aplasia of the left part of the sphenoid sinus.

Table 4.9   (Cont.) Sclerosis and hyperostosis of the skull base

Diagnosis	Findings
Hemolytic anemias	Hemolytic anemia may cause hyperplasia of the bone marrow as well as hyperostosis of the entire calvarial bone.
Hyperparathyroidism	Bone changes are primarily due to high bone turnover, often combined with a mineralization defect leading to increased bone fractures and bone deformities. Although rarely considered, the craniofacial skeleton represents one of the peculiar targets of this complex metabolic disease whose more dramatic pattern is a form of leontiasis ossea.
Mucopolysaccharidosis ▷ *Fig. 4.23a–d* ▷ *Fig. 4.24*	MPS may cause sclerosis and enlargement of the skull.

(continues on page 315)

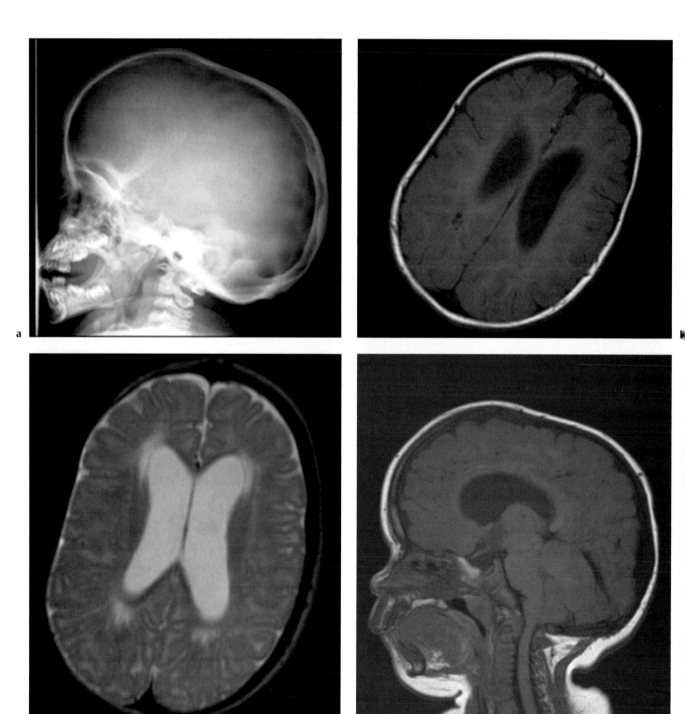

Fig. 4.23a–d   Mucopolysaccharidosis. (a) Macrocephaly of 2-year old girl with Hurler syndrome (MPS I). **(b)** Enlarged perivascular spaces are hypointense on T1 image in the same patient. **(c)** Enlarged perivascular spaces are hyperintense on T2 image; fluid contains mucopolysaccharides. Note the hydrocephalus. **(d)** Sagittal T1-weighted image of same patient shows a narrow foramen magnum.

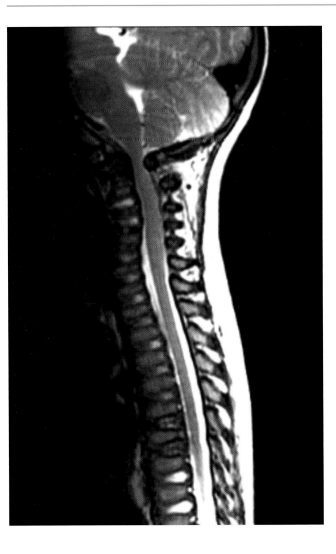

Fig. 4.24 Mucopolysaccharidosis type IV (Morquio syndrome) in 2-year-old boy with compression on the myelum at the cranio-cervical junction.

Table 4.9 (Cont.) Sclerosis and hyperostosis of the skull base

Diagnosis	Findings
Vitamin D toxicity Fluorosis Idiopathic hypercalcemia Hyperphosphatasia	
Tumors	
Skeletal dysplasias	These include osteopetrosis, pycnodysostosis, sclerosteosis, craniometaphyseal dysplasia (Pyle disease), FD, hyperostosis corticalis generalisata/endosteal hyperostosis (van Buchem disease), Camurati-Engelmann disease, frontometaphyseal dysplasia, dysosteosclerosis, and hyperostosis cranialis interna. Only FD has a pagetoid pattern with ground-glass appearance on CT. On MRI, the affected bone areas show low to intermediate signal on T1, heterogeneous signal on T2, and heterogeneous enhancement. In all other diseases, the affected bone sites show low signal intensity on T1 and T2 and no enhancement.
Osteopathia striata ▷ *Fig. 4.25a–d, p. 316*	Rare skeletal dysplasia characterized by longitudinal striations of the long bone dia- and metaphyses and sclerosis of the cranial vault and base. Typical physical presentations of this disorder are a squarelike skull, frontal bossing, flat nasal bridge, palate abnormalities, and hearing loss. Mental retardation is present in many patients with osteopathia striata with cranial stenosis.

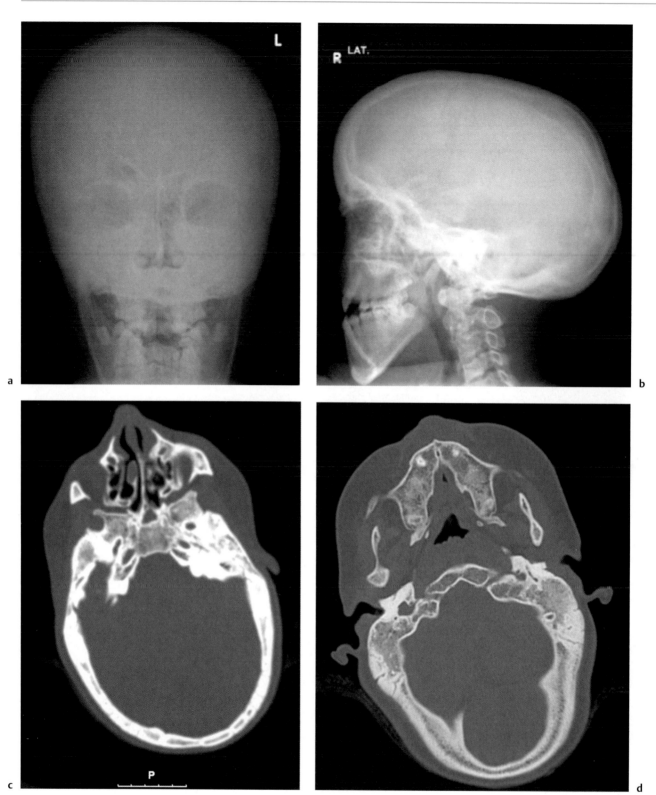

Fig. 4.25a–d   Osteopathia striata. (a) A 16-year-old girl showing macrocephaly and a dense vault and skull base. **(b)** Lateral view. **(c, d)** CT showing the dense skull base and vault.

Table 4.10 The enlarged sella

Diagnosis	Findings	Comments
Chronically elevated ICP ▷ *Fig. 4.26*	Enlarged sella without changes in contour and structure. Sometimes with an empty sella appearance.	Triventricular hydrocephalus due to obstruction at the aquaduct as a result of tumor compression, postinfection, or posthemorrhage. May also occur in (non)syndromal craniosynostosis.
Parasellar mass effect		
Glioma of the optic nerve and hypothalamus	Enlarged sella with changes in contour and structure. Hypothalamic and optic chiasm glioma are sometimes indistinguishable.	MRI is the imaging modality of choice.
Suprasellar cysts	Part of a cystic form of a craniopharyngioma or glioma, or arachnoid cyst.	MRI is the imaging modality of choice.
NF/neuroma/schwannoma	Enlargement is rare. The most frequent schwannoma is of the trigeminal nerve.	
Chordoma	May extend into the sellar region, destructing the floor and dorsum sellae.	

(continues on page 318)

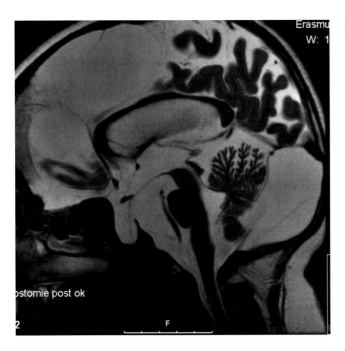

Fig. 4.26 Empty sella on a sagittal T2-weighted image. Note also the retrocerebellar arachnoid cyst.

Table 4.10   (Cont.) The enlarged sella

Diagnosis	Findings	Comments
Intrasellar mass effect		
Rathke cleft cyst ▷ *Fig. 4.27a–c*	Located between the anterior and intermediate lobes of the pituitary gland. Almost always intrasellar in location. On MRI, the signal intensity depends on its content. If the protein content is less than 15%, the cyst is hypointense on T1 and hyperintense on T2. Between 15%–25%, the cyst may be hyperintense on T1 and T2. In more than 25%, it may be hyperintense on T1 and hypointense on T2. Rim enhancement may be seen.	Rarely symptomatic, unless larger than 1 cm. MRI is the imaging modality of choice.
Craniopharyngioma	Look for density (CT) or signal intensity (MRI) differences in the cystic parts of the mass, due to special "motor oil" content.	Most common intrasellar tumor. CT may be helpful for identifying calcifications.
Hypophyseal tumors ▷ *Fig. 4.28a–d*	Adenoma is most common sellar/parasellar mass. Macroadenoma (> 1 cm) causes visual disturbance or hypopituitarism. Usually erosion of the bottom of the sella. Rarely invasive with extension into the sphenoid sinus. Macroadenoma may also give parasellar extension into the cavernous sinus.	Presentation near puberty. MRI is the imaging modality of choice.

(continues on page 320)

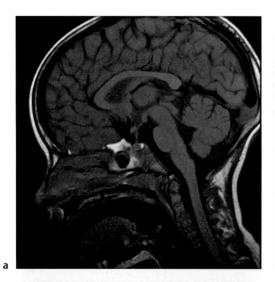

a

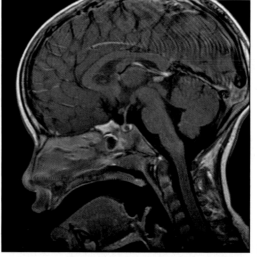

b

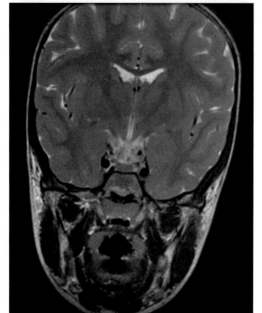

c

Fig. 4.27a–c   Rathke's cleft cyst. (a) A 4-year-old girl with familial growth hormone deficiency. MRI shows a Rathke cleft cyst. **(b)** Sagittal T1-weighted image after contrast shows no enhancement consistent with a Rathke cleft cyst. **(c)** Coronal T2-weighted image of same patient.

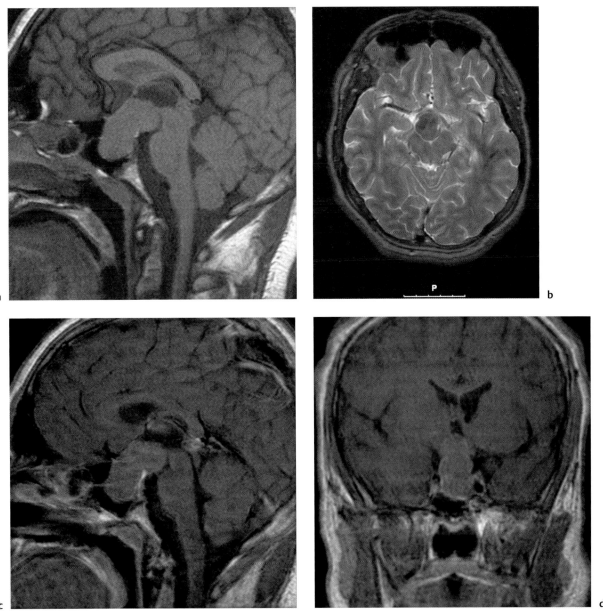

Fig. 4.28a–d   Hypophyseal tumors. (a) A 16-year-old boy with visual impairment due to a prolactin-producing macroadenoma with suprasellar extension. Note the enlargement of the sella and disruption of the sellar diaphragm. (**b**) Note the compression on the optic chiasm on this T2 image. (**c**) Note the lack of enhancement of the macroadenoma on this T1 image. (**d**) Note the thin wall enhancement of the macroadenoma and the compression on the optic chiasm.

Table 4.10   (Cont.) The enlarged sella

Diagnosis	Findings	Comments
Intrasellar mass effect (cont.)		
Germinoma ▷ *Fig. 4.29a–c*	Thirty-five percent are intra-/suprasellar. Usually large at presentation. On CT, the mass is well-marginated and isodense to hyperdense to brain parenchyma with homogeneous enhancement. On MRI, the mass is hypointense to isointense to gray matter on T1 and hyperintense on T2 and shows intense enhancement after Gd. CSF spread and systemic metastasis is possible.	Clinical presentation includes diabetes insipidus, visual disturbances, and panhypopituitarism.
Meningioma	Rare in children.	
Metastasis	Leukemia and lymphoma do occur.	Most patients die before becoming symptomatic, but diabetes insipidus may occur.
Untreated hypothyroidism	Massive enlargement without destruction.	Enlargement due to reactive response of hypophysis.
Empty sella syndrome (ESS) ▷ *Fig. 4.26, p. 317*	MRI shows a flattened gland with increased CSF within the sella turcica. Enlargement and erosion of the sella may be seen. Normal position differentiates ESS from arachnoid cyst.	The causes of ESS may be high ICP, neglected or improperly treated hydrocephalus, and suprasellar arachnoid cyst. Primary ESS has also been described.

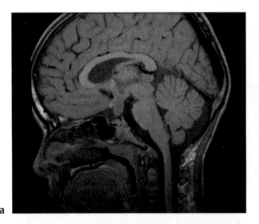
a

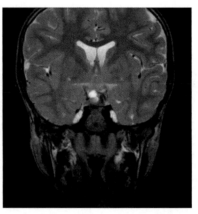
b

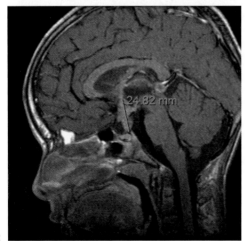
c

Fig. 4.29a–c   Germinoma. (**a**) A 9-year-old boy with diabetes insipidus and thyroid-stimulating hormone and growth hormone deficiency. The space occupying the process in the suprasellar region is most consistent with a germ cell tumor on this T1-weighted image. (**b**) T2-weighted image shows a solid and cystic component. (**c**) Sagittal T1 image shows minimal CE.

Table 4.11   The small sella

Diagnosis	Findings	Comments
Normal variant, decreased hypophyseal function	There are several syndromes with genetic mutations involving the development of the pituitary gland that may give a hypoplastic sella. There are, for example, bone morphogenetic proteins like fibroblastic growth factor that influence the sella development, but also transcription factors, and signaling proteins like sonic hedgehog are important for the development of the pituitary gland.	
After relief of elevated ICP, growth hormone deficiency, Prader–Willi syndrome		
Chiari malformation		
Fibrous dysplasia ▷ *Fig. 4.30*		
Myotonic dystrophy		
Primary dysplasia		

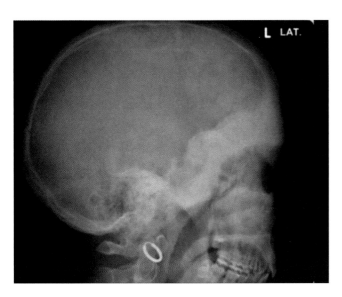

Fig. 4.30   Camurati-Engelmann disease in a 15-year-old boy with polyostotic FD; note the small sella.

Table 4.12   Changes in contour and shape of the sella

Diagnosis	Findings	Comments
Rickets	Size of sella is normal. Sella less dense on X-ray and CT as a result of demineralization.	Density returns to normal after treatment.
Chronically elevated ICP	Sella enlarges, and dorsum sellae becomes shorter and angulated.	
Leukemia	Demineralization detectable on X-ray and CT.	
Nasopharyngeal tumors	Rarely seen, but tumor may cause destruction of the sella.	
LCH	Demineralization, may progress to destruction.	
Transsphenoidal encephalocele	Defect in the sellar floor as a result of persistence of the craniopharyngeal canal or developmental failure of multiple ossification centers. MRI is necessary to show the extension and herniation of the encephalocele. Bony defect best shown on CT.	Associated anomalies are midline defects like agenesis of the corpus callosum, cleft palate, and hypertelorism. Nasal obstruction.
Chordoma	See **Table 4.8,** Pathology of the skull base.	

Intracranial Abnormalities

■ Imaging Methods

Ultrasonography

Brain US plays a central role in the detection and management of neonatal disease in the preterm and term infant. Although a morphological study, by using high-frequency transducers it remains the cornerstone of neonatal intracranial imaging. Pulsed and color Doppler scans provide additional information and improve the diagnostic and prognostic accuracy of US. The value of Doppler techniques may be found in, for example, the demonstration of flow within the aqueduct of Sylvius, visualization of patency of the terminal veins and venous sinus, demonstration of Doppler spectrum fluctuations, and recognition of low or abnormally high blood flow.

Particular features of normal brain US in the neonate should be recognized and reported using a systematic approach, as outlined here

Starting with a coronal approach, it is easy to pick up asymmetric abnormalities through the anterior fontanelle and, if patent, the posterior fontanelle. Subsequent parasagittal images should incorporate the midline to the outer border of the cortex. Additionally, one can look at the asterion for interpreting abnormalities at the brainstem and cerebellum. With this total imaging approach, one can rule out abnormalities at the midline and can assess if the abnormality is infra- or supratentorial in location. Is it bi- or unilateral? Are the central and peripheral CSF spaces normal? Are there abnormalities of the gyri and sulci? If there is a focal lesion, is it hemorrhagic? Also, repeating the US examinations can help to focus the differential diagnosis or give a better insight into the neurologic outcome.

In extreme prematurity, one may see some specific abnormalities that occur with a higher incidence, like cerebral hemorrhage and its different patterns (intraventricular hemorrhage and periventricular hemorrhagic infarction) and periventricular leukomalacia (PVL). Especially in these infants, repeated US examinations (until near term) are important to rule out the development of cystic PVL.

Computed Tomography Scan

CT has no prominent place in imaging of preterm and term infants, except for ruling out intracranial calcifications or (sub)acute bleeding due to (birth) trauma.

Magnetic Resonance Imaging

MRI improves the radiologist's ability to assess brain development and to detect anomalies of brain formation. In contrast to US and CT, MRI allows the assessment of brain development by analysis of the effects of myelination of the pediatric brain in both T1 and T2 modes. A continuously evolving pattern will normally be seen up to the age of 2 years. During prematurity, MRI provides excellent detail of the immature brain with good delineation of the cortex, white matter, and central gray matter structures. The cortex is seen as high signal intensity on T1-weighted imaging and low signal on T2-weighted imaging, reflecting its high cellular density. At 24 weeks gestational age, the surface of the brain appears smooth apart from the parieto-occipital fissure, central sulci, cingulate sulci, calcarine sulci, and very wide sylvian fissures. Sulcation and gyration develop at different rates in different regions of the brain. At any given age prior to term, the folding of the central sulcus is the most advanced, followed by the medial occipital lobe. The parietal lobe is the next most advanced, followed by the frontal and posterior temporal lobes. The anterior temporal region is the least well developed structure. At term, the cortex has extensive folding with the formation of tertiary sulci. Familiarity with this evolution of signal changes allows an estimation of the approximate stage of brain development. Although high-resolution multiplanar MRI is not better than those images acquired with US, using high-frequency transducers, MRI provides good anatomic detail, with excellent distinction between gray and white matter. This technique allows improved detection of many abnormalities of brain formation, some of which were previously detectable only at autopsy. These malformations and their imaging characteristics are discussed subsequently.

Table 4.13 Abnormalities in preterm infants

Diagnosis	Findings
Intraventricular–periventricular hemorrhagic disease ▷ *Fig. 4.31*	Classification in four grades: Grade I: hemorrhage in subependymal space Grade II: subependymal hemorrhage with bleeding into normal or minimally dilated ventricles Grade III: subependymal hemorrhage with blood in dilated ventricles Grade IV: similar to grade III hemorrhage, with hemorrhage in the adjacent brain parenchyma. The hemorrhage may be entirely intraparenchymal without ventricular involvement. Extremely rare.
Periventricular hemorrhagic infarction ▷ *Fig. 4.31*	This entity used to be considered a sequela of Grade III. The subependymal hemorrhage at the caudal-thalamic groove blocks the terminal vein and its drainage area, resulting in a venous infarction. It is much more frequent than a Grade IV hemorrhage. Even a Grade I hemorrhage can cause a venous infarction. On MRI, the periventricular hemorrhage is shown as a fan-shaped structure due to obstructed medullary veins; it is of low signal intensity on T2-weighted imaging.
Posthemorrhagic ventricular dilatation ▷ *Fig. 4.32a, b*	This affects approximately 36% of preterm infants with intraventricular hemorrhage, but resolves in 65% of affected infants. US can demonstrate the onset of ventricular dilatation and determines its progression or resolution. The pulsed Doppler scan may give additional information by demonstrating an increased resistance index in the presence of increased ICP.

(continues on page 324)

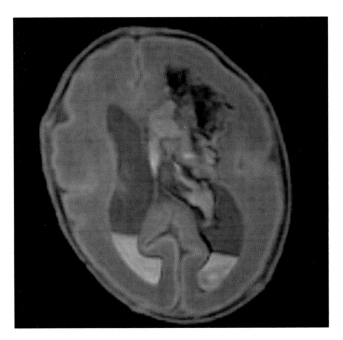

Fig. 4.31   Obstructive hydrocephalus in an 8-day-old boy, born at 32 weeks, due to germinal matrix bleeding Grade II on the right side and Grade III on the left side. Note also the hemorrhagic venous infarct in the left frontal lobe that is hypointense on the T1-weighted image due to hemosiderin.

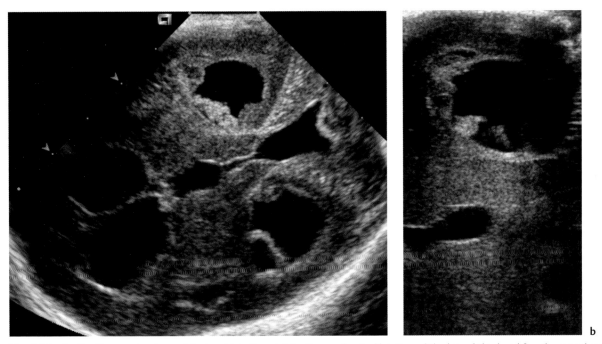

b

Fig. 4.32a, b   Posthemorrhagic ventricular dilatation. (a) Posthemorrhagic dilatation of the lateral third and fourth ventricle in a preterm infant demonstrated on US. Note thickening of the ependyma. **(b)** Note the hemorrhagic clots in the occipital horn.

Table 4.13   (Cont.) Abnormalities in preterm infants

Diagnosis	Findings
PVL ▷ *Fig. 4.33a–d*	The sonographic diagnosis of PVL depends on the detection of abnormal periventricular parenchyma and diagnosis is difficult. Equal or higher echogenecity than the choroid plexus is abnormal. In equivocal cases, recognition of the optic radiation may be helpful. If the optic radiation is not visible (due to surrounding hyperechogenicity), there is another indication of PVL. MRI may be helpful, especially if there is a hemorrhagic component. As a special MRI sequence, DWI will link PVL to areas of high signal intensity, representing restricted diffusion, before cysts are shown on US. On US, the pattern may show a lateral extension with spiculated margins, high hyperechogenicity with sharp margins, organization in clusters, butterfly appearance on coronal images, and extensive density with scattered punctate regions. Repeat the US examination to rule out development of cysts. When macrocysts appear, with their progressive confluent extension, the diagnosis is easy, but this is rare. Most often, there are microcysts, which are more difficult to detect even if surrounded by hyperechoic white matter. They appear between day 8 and day 25 after any type of echodensity. Their recognition is important because they are correlated with a suboptimal clinical outcome.

(continues on page 325)

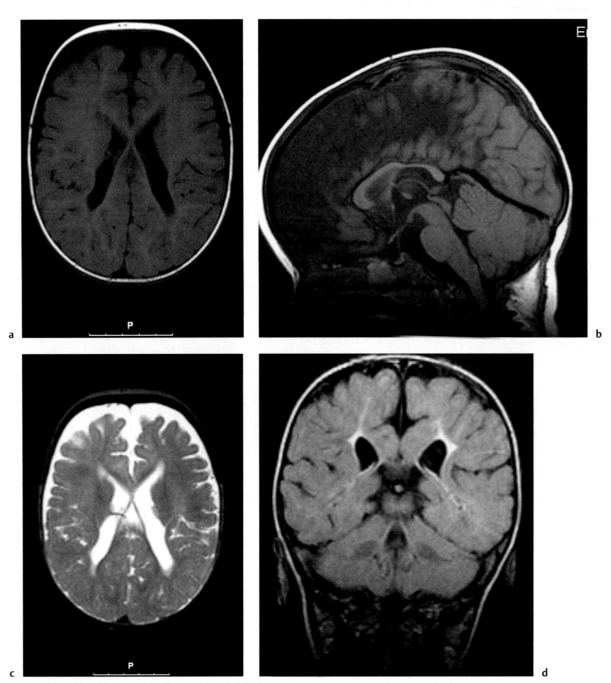

Fig. 4.33a–d   Periventricular leukomalacia. (a) Classic PVL in a premature 14-month-old infant with spastic tetraplegia. Note the irregular wall of the ventricles and the periventricular white matter loss visible on this T1-weighted image. **(b)** Thin corpus callosum is due to white matter loss. **(c)** Axial T2-weighted image: note again the irregular wall of the ventricles, periventricular white matter loss, and prominent CSF spaces. **(d)** Coronal fluid-attenuated inversion recovery (FLAIR) image shows periventricular gliosis.

Table 4.13   (Cont.) Abnormalities in preterm infants

Diagnosis	Findings
Brain infarction ▷ *Fig. 4.34a–d* ▷ *Fig. 4.35a, b, p. 326*	Unilateral infarction is more common on the left side (61%) than on the right (32%), whereas in 7% bilateral arterial distribution infarcts can occur. The majority of strokes involve the middle cerebral artery. Brain infarction is not uncommon in preterm infants with a gestational age of 34 wk, with an incidence of 7/1000, compared to an incidence of 1/4000 in full-term infants. Lenticulostriate infarcts appear to be especially common in the preterm population and can be well visualized by US and MRI.
Cerebellar hemorrhage	Observed in 10%–25% of very-low-birth-weight preterm infants at postmortem examination and is associated with traumatic birth, injury from overly tightly applied ventilator masks, and supratentorial hemorrhage. On MRI cerebellar hemorrhage is more frequently seen than with US. Morbidity is high for infants with large supratentorial and cerebellar hemorrhages.
Hypoxic/anoxic insult ▷ *Fig. 4.36a, b, p. 326*	In the premature infant, the white matter is damaged and this encephalopathy is often accompanied by peri-intraventricular hemorrhage. Gray matter is predominantly involved in the term baby.
Porencephalic cyst ▷ *Fig. 4.37a, b, p. 327*	Hypoechoic area on US as a result of hypoxic, ischemic insult or bleeding. On MRI the area has, on all sequences, the signal intensity of CSF. A true porencephalic cyst has to communicate with the ventricle.
Meningitis/encephalitis ▷ *Fig. 4.38a, b, p. 327* ▷ *Fig. 4.39, p. 328* ▷ *Fig. 4.40a–c, p. 328*	On US, hyperechoic areas near the brain surface; the arachnoid may be thickened with increased echogenicity due to increased cell count and/or proteins. In encephalitis, the subcortical white matter is also involved. Cystic degeneration or destruction of the affected white matter may occur, even quite rapidly (within a couple of days). MRI is the best technique to show the extent of brain damage.
Abscess/ventriculitis ▷ *Fig. 4.41a–c, p. 329*	Ventriculitis is easily detected by US, especially if intraventricular septa are present. In most of the cases, the ependyma is thickened. Abscess formation may be a complication of meningitis. MRI may be helpful in differentiating between bleedings, infarction, or tumors. A dark rim on T2-weighted images is characteristic for abscess formation.

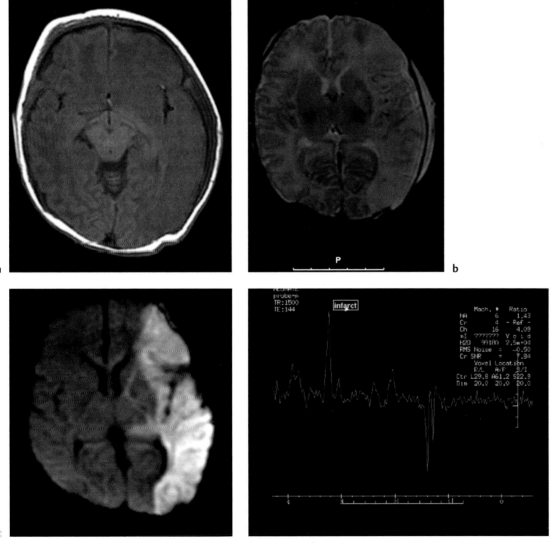

Fig. 4.34a–d   Brain infarction. A 5-day-old boy with seizures due to a parietal and frontal infarct in the left medial cerebral artery distribution. Note the loss of gray and white matter differentiation and swelling of the left temporal lobe on the T1-weighted image (**a**) and (**b**) the T2-weighted image. (**c**) The infarct in the left medial cerebral artery distribution area presents as a hypersignal intensity on this DWI. (**d**) Note the deep, double peak at 1.33 ppm, presenting lactate due to severe ischemia in this area.

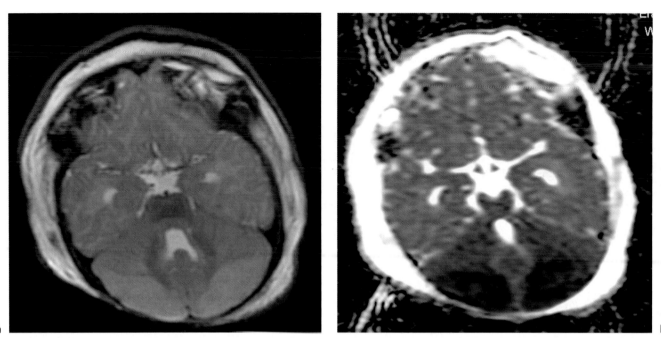

a   b

Fig. 4.35a, b Brain infarction. (**a**) A 10-month-old boy with hypotensive period during craniotomy resulting in cerebellar infarcts on both sides, presenting as hyperintense zones on T2-weighted images. (**b**) Apparent diffusion coefficient (ADC) map shows the infarcted areas as hypointense.

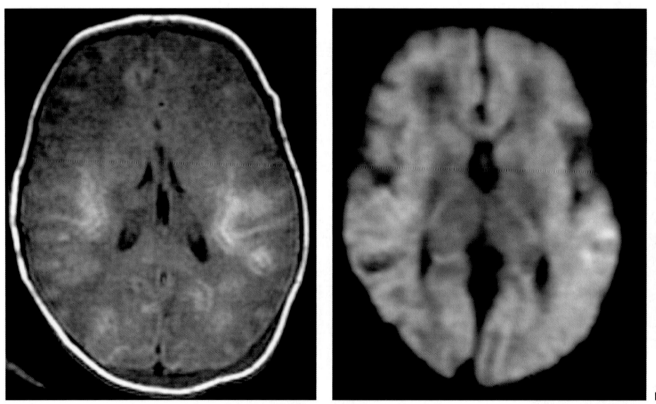

a

Fig. 4.36a, b Hypoxic/anoxic insult. (**a**) T1-weighted image shows cortical involvement with a hemorrhagic component in a term infant with a history of severe asphyxia. (**b**) DWI shows destruction of the whole cortex.

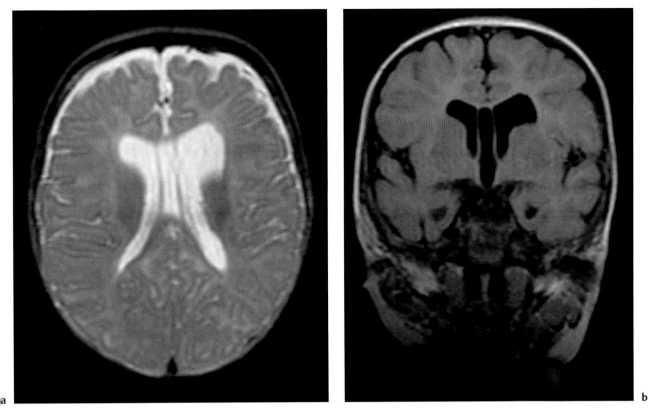

Fig. 4.37a, b   Porencephalic cyst. (a) A 9-month-old boy with an old infarction of the head of the left caudate nucleus. **(b)** Coronal FLAIR image shows that the old infarction of the head of the left caudate nucleus has the signal intensity of CSF.

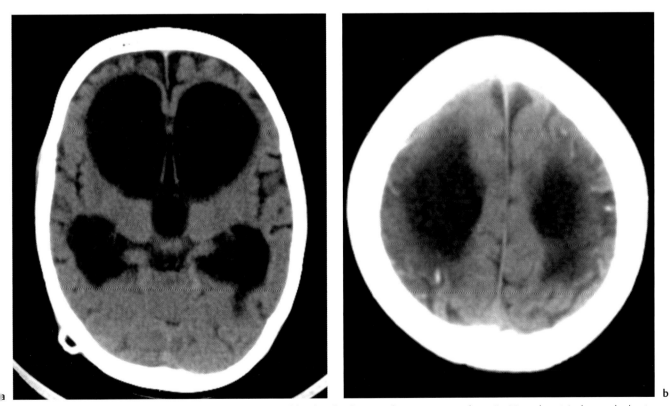

Fig. 4.38a, b   Meningitis/encephalitis. (a) CT of a 7-year old girl with a history of a pneumococcal meningitis and ventriculomegaly due to parenchymal loss and calcification frontoparietal. **(b)** Note the calcifications.

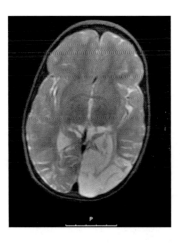

Fig. 4.39   Occipital encephalitis/infarction (on the left side) due to herpes simplex CNS infection in 3-year-old girl.

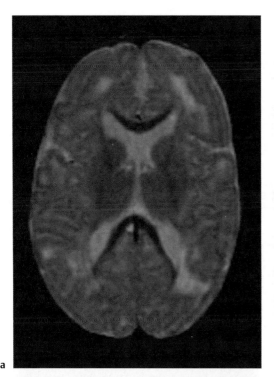

a

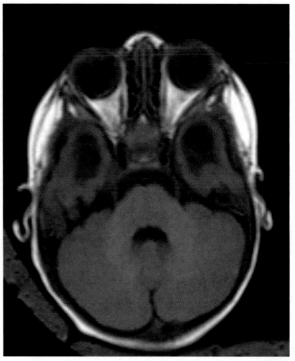

b

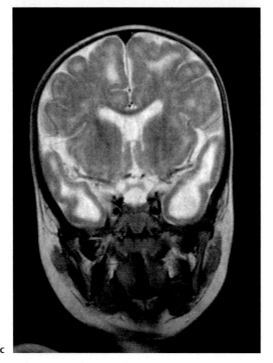

c

Fig. 4.40a–c   Meningitis/encephalitis. (a) A 14-month-old girl with failure to thrive and proven cytomegalovirus (CMV) infection resulting in periventricular leukodystrophy. **(b)** CMV infection resulting in periventricular cysts in the temporal lobes that are hypointense on this T1-weighted image. **(c)** CMV infection resulting in subcortical leukomalacia in the frontal and temporal lobes.

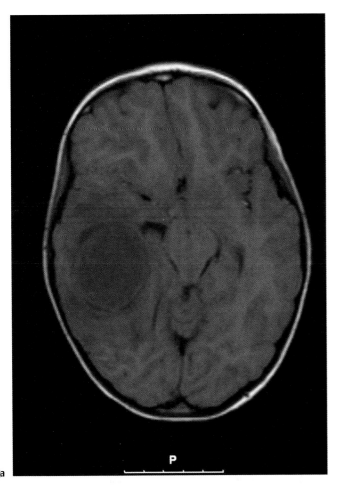

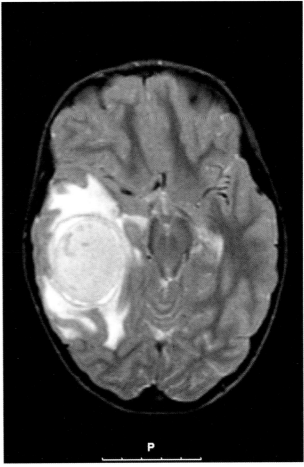

a

b

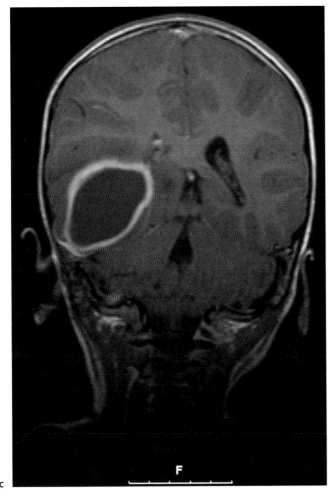

Fig. 4.41a–c   Abscess/ventriculitis. (a) A 6-year-old girl diagnosed with a temporoparietal abscess on the right side, visible on this T1 image as an inhomogeneous, hypointense, well-circumscribed lesion with a thick wall. **(b)** The abscess wall has a low signal intensity on this T2-weighted image. Extensive peripheral edema is noted. **(c)** Coronal T1-weighted image after Gd shows a ring-enhanced lesion, diagnosed as a right temporoparietal abscess.

c

Table 4.14 Abnormalities of brain formation

Diagnosis	Findings	Comments
Callosal agenesis ▷ *Fig. 4.42a–c* ▷ *Fig. 4.43a–c*	On US, abnormalities of the corpus callosum can be difficult to identify. Indirect signs of callosal anomalies on US include lack of visualization of the cavum septi pellucidi, enlarged atria and occipital horns resulting in a teardrop configuration of the lateral ventricles, a high-riding third ventricle, and radiating medial hemispheric sulci. On MRI, abnormalities of the corpus callosum are more easily detected.	More than three-quarters of patients with callosal agenesis have additional CNS anomalies, and two-thirds have additional extra-CNS anomalies. Associations with callosal agenesis include Chiari type II malformation, Dandy-Walker malformation, gray matter heterotopia, holoprosencephaly, schizencephaly, and encephaloceles.
Holoprosencephaly ▷ *Fig. 4.44a, b, p. 332*	MRI is the imaging modality of choice. *Alobar:* Absence of falx, interhemispheric fissure, septum pellucidum, and superior sagittal sinus. Thalami are fused. Single monoventricle. Approximately 90% have severe facial abnormalities, the most severe is cyclopia. *Semilobar:* Partial development of falx, interhemispheric fissure, and superior sagittal sinus. Septum pellucidum is absent. Thalami may be fused. Thirty percent have facial abnormalities. *Lobar:* Midline structures almost normal. Septum pellucidum is absent. Rostral brain may show some midline deficiencies; posterior aspect of the brain is normal. May have severe facial abnormalities.	Different types of holoprosencephaly exist, representing a continuous spectrum. The most severe type is alobar, followed (in decreasing severity) by semilobar, and the lobar type. Semilobar most common type. Alobar usually lethal.

(continues on page 332)

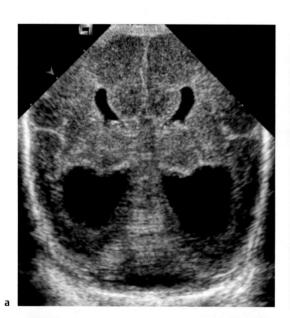

a

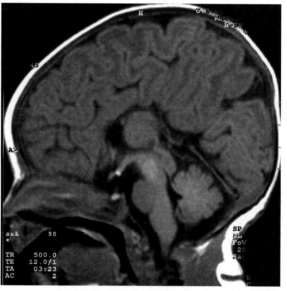

b

Fig. 4.42a–c Callosal agenesis. (a) Coronal US shows callosal agenesis on the medial side of the frontal horns (the Probst bundles). **(b)** Sagittal T1-weighted image shows that the sulci are reaching the roof of the third ventricle wall due to absence of the corpus callosum. **(c)** Note the colpocephaly due to the absence of the corpus callosum on the CT.

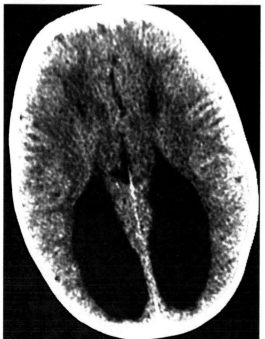

c

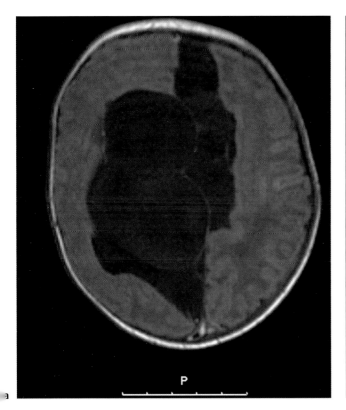

a

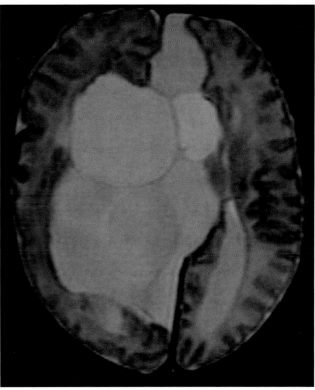

b

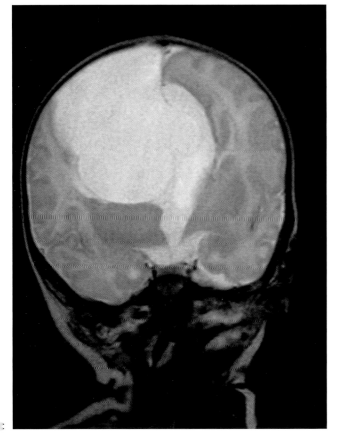

Fig. 4.43a–c **Macrocephaly** in a 7-day-old boy. T1 (**a**) and T2 images (**b, c**) show callosal agenesis and noncommunicating interhemispheric cysts.

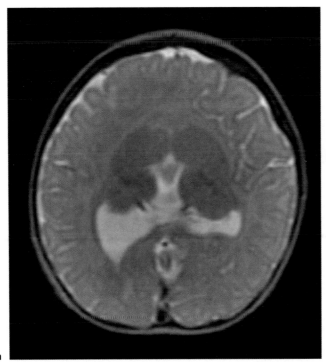
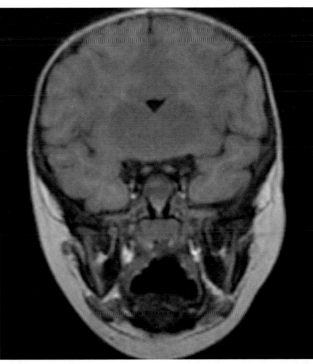

Fig. 4.44a, b Holoprosencephaly. (a) An 18-month-old boy with semilobar holoprosencephaly. Axial T2-weighted image shows fusion of the frontal lobes. (b) Coronal FLAIR image shows fusion of the frontal lobes and partial fusion of thalami.

Table 4.14 (Cont.) Abnormalities of brain formation

Diagnosis	Findings	Comments
Septo-optic dysplasia	Third ventricle and thalami are normal. Also corpus callosum is present. Thin optic chiasm.	Some consider septo-optic dysplasia as a variant of lobar holoprosencephaly.
Cephaloceles	CT is the modality to show the bone defect; MRI is the best technique to confirm presence of brain tissue in a cephalocele.	Can occur anywhere in the cranial vault, but most commonly in the midline at the occiput, skull base, or vertex. The most common basal cephalocele is the sphenopharyngeal type.
Chiari malformations ▷ *Fig. 4.45*	Chiari malformation is more a MRI diagnosis than a US one. *Chiari type I:* cerebellar tonsils below foramen magnum > 5 mm, small posterior fossa, 50% asymptomatic, 50% hydromyelia, no myelomeningocele (MMC). *Chiari type II:* Cerebellar tonsils and part of vermis below foramen magnum. Dorsal medulla descends behind cervical spinal cord, kinking medullocervical junction. Beaking of tectum, hydrocephalus, small posterior fossa, strawlike fourth ventricle, and 100% associated with MMC. *Chiari type III:* occipital cephalocoele involving cerebellar tissue with traction on brainstem. *Chiari type IV:* Chiari type II with vanishing cerebellum.	All Chiari types are the result of lack of expansion of fourth ventricle with consequent hypoplasia of the posterior fossa.
Dandy-Walker complex	Hypoplasia of the vermis, a pseudocystic fourth ventricle, upward displacement of the tentorium, and torcular and AP enlargement of the posterior fossa. A Blake pouch cyst has also been referred to as Dandy-Walker variant. Although US can easily identify severe Dandy-Walker malformations, it is generally more limited in distinguishing mild forms of vermian hypoplasia from a mega cisterna magna or an arachnoid cyst than MRI.	A cerebellar vermis with three groups of lobes and two main fissures, identified on sagittal MRI T2 images, not only has the greatest chance not to be associated with other malformations but also to have a favorable neurocognitive outcome. On the contrary, a deeply dysgenetic vermis with only two or one recognizable lobes is not only constantly associated with other brain malformation but also with poor prognosis.

(continues on page 333)

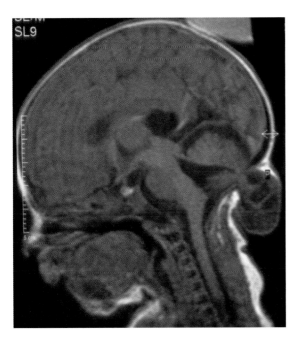

Fig. 4.45   Chiari malformation. Sagittal T1-weighted image shows an occipital cephalocele involving cerebellar tissue with traction on the brainstem consistent with a Chiari type III malformation.

Table 4.14   (Cont.) Abnormalities of brain formation

Diagnosis	Findings	Comments
Cerebellar anomalies ▷ *Fig. 4.46* ▷ *Fig. 4.47a–c, p. 334*	Cerebellar, vermian hypoplasia: focal and generalized hypoplasia (Dandy-Walker continuum with enlarged fourth ventricle, pontocerebellar hypoplasia with normal fourth ventricle). *Cerebellar dysplasia:* • Focal vermian dysplasia with molar tooth sign (Joubert and Joubert-like syndromes) • Rhombencephalosynapsis • Generalized dysplasia: (congenital muscular dystrophies, CMV, lissencephaly with reelin [RELN] gene mutation, lissencephaly with agenesis of corpus callosum and cerebellar dysplasia, associated with diffuse cerebral polymicrogyria and diffusely abnormal foliation).	
Spectrum of neuronal migration anomalies	MRI is superior to US in identifying schizencephaly, lissencephaly, polymicrogyria, and gray matter heterotopia.	Epilepsy is often present in patients with cortical malformations and tends to be severe, although its incidence and type vary in different malformations.

(continues on page 335)

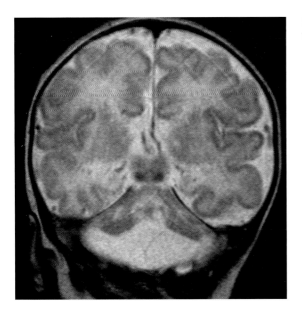

Fig. 4.46   Cerebellar anomaly. A term infant with clonic seizures. Coronal T2-weighted image shows cerebellar hypoplasia.

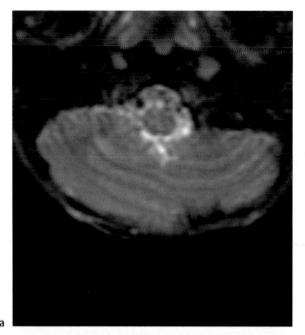

a

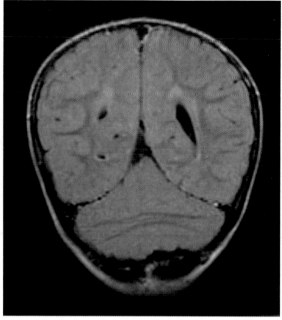

b

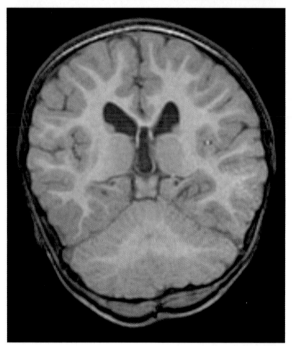

c

Fig. 4.47a–c   Cerebellar anomaly. (a) A 2.5-year-old boy with difficulty maintaining his balance as well as impaired motor function and a hypotonic neck. Note the fusion of both cerebellar hemispheres on this axial T2-weighted image, compatible with the diagnosis of rhombencephalosynapsis. **(b)** Coronal FLAIR image. **(c)** Coronal T1 gradient echo sequence.

Table 4.14   (Cont.) Abnormalities of brain formation

Diagnosis	Findings	Comments
Periventricular nodular heterotopia (PNH) ▷ *Fig. 4.48*	Appears as nodules that are isointense to the gray matter and are located along the ventricular walls.	PNH is a malformation of neuronal migration in which a subset of neurons fails to migrate into the developing cerebral cortex. X-linked PNH is mainly seen in females and is often associated with focal epilepsy. Filamin A mutations have been reported in all familial cases and in about 25% of sporadic patients. A rare recessive form of PNH due to ARGEF2 gene mutations has also been reported in children with microcephaly, severe delay, and early seizures.
Lissencephaly (also known as agyria, smooth brain) and subcortical band heterotopia ▷ *Fig. 4.49, p. 336* ▷ *Fig. 4.50, p. 336*	Classic lissencephaly is associated with the shallow appearance of the sylvian fissures, reduced number or complete absence of additional sulci for the expected gestational age of the fetus, absence of normal multilayered appearance of the brain, and a large thick band of arrested neurons within the developing white matter. Autosomal recessive lissencephaly with cerebellar hypoplasia, accompanied by severe delay, hypotonia, and seizures, has been associated with mutations of the *RELN* gene. X-linked lissencephaly with corpus callosum agenesis and ambiguous genitalia.	Disorders of neuronal migration represent a malformative spectrum resulting from mutations of either *LIS1* or *DCX* genes. *LIS1* mutations cause a more severe malformation in the posterior brain regions. Most children have severe developmental delay and infantile spasms, but milder phenotypes are on record, including posterior SBH owing to mosaic mutations of *LIS1*. *DCX* mutations usually cause anteriorly predominant lissencephaly in males and SBH in female patients. Mutations of *DCX* found in male patients with anterior subcortical band heterotopia (SBH) and in female relatives with normal brain MRI in genotypic males are associated with mutations of the *ARX* gene. Affected boys are severely delayed and show seizures with suppression-burst electroencephalogram. Early death is frequent. Carrier female patients can have isolated corpus callosum agenesis.
Schizencephaly ▷ *Fig. 4.51, p. 336*	Schizencephaly appears as a gray matter–lined cleft extending from the ventricle to the subarachnoid space. Closed-lip schizencephaly is characterized by gray matter–lined lips that are in contact with each other (type I). Open-lip schizencephaly has separated lips and a cleft of CSF, extending to the underlying ventricle (type II).	The etiology is unclear, although a primary malformation secondary to a neuronal migrational anomaly is considered most likely. Familial cases of schizencephaly have been reported, suggesting a possible genetic origin within a group of neuronal migration disorders. Heterozygous mutations of the *EMX2* have been reported in cases with schizencephaly. However, early prenatal injury, such as that associated with drug abuse or abdominal trauma, has also been reported to be associated with schizencephaly, possibly from a vascular insult or resulting from CMV infection. Therefore, the appearance of schizencephaly is likely to be secondary to multiple factors, leading to a final common manifestation of abnormal neuronal migration.
Polymicrogyria ▷ *Fig. 4.52, p. 336* ▷ *Fig. 4.53, p. 337*	Polymicrogyria appears as localized and/or generalized absence of normal sulcation with multiple abnormal infoldings of the affected cortex.	Among several syndromes featuring polymicrogyria, bilateral perisylvian polymicrogyria shows genetic heterogeneity, including linkage to chromosome Xq28 in some pedigrees, AD or recessive inheritance in others, and an association with chromosome 22q11.2 deletion in some patients. About 65% of patients have a severe form of epilepsy. Recessive bilateral frontoparietal polymicrogyria has been associated with mutations of the *GPR56* gene.

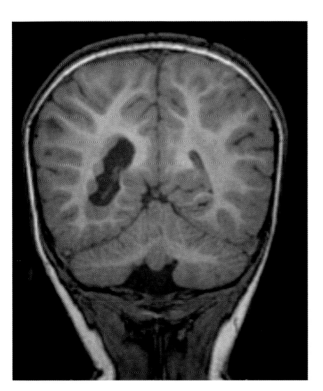

Fig. 4.48   Periventricular nodular heterotopia. Coronal T1-weighted image shows periventricular noduli in a 2-year-old girl.

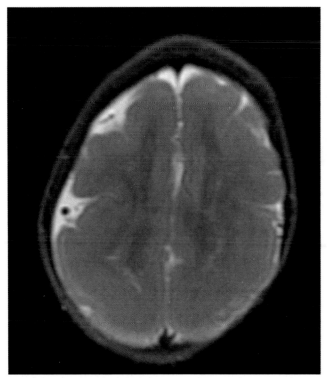

Fig. 4.49 Miller-Dieker lissencephaly syndrome. A 3-year-old boy with mental retardation. This axial T2-weighted image shows few sulci, a cell-sparse zone, and that the parietal-occipital is more affected than frontal, which is compatible with Miller-Dieker syndrome.

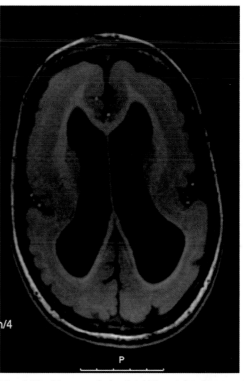

Fig. 4.50 Lissencephaly. Axial T1-weighted image shows a band of heterotopia in a 9-year-old girl.

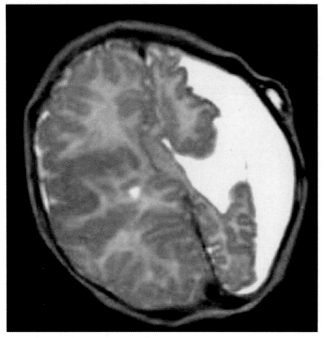

Fig. 4.51 Schizencephaly. Axial T2-weighted image shows an open lip schizencephaly in an 8-month-old boy with motor delay and early hand preference.

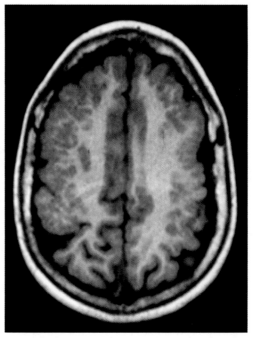

Fig. 4.52 Bilateral polymicrogyria is visible on this axial T1-weighted image.

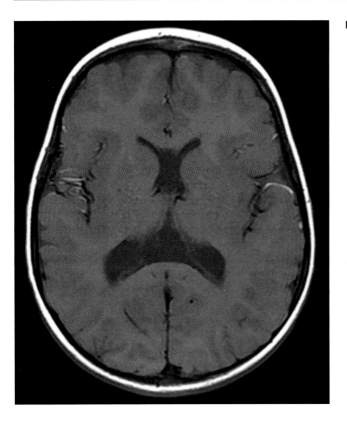

Fig. 4.53   Bilateral perisylvian polymicrogyria.

Table 4.15   Intracranial hemorrhage

Diagnosis	Findings	Comments
Grade I–IV intracranial hemorrhage	See **Table 4.13** abnormalities in premature infants	
Venous infarction	See **Table 4.13** abnormalities in premature infants	
Intraparenchymal hemorrhage, acute ▷ *Fig. 4.54a–c, p. 338*	Logistic CT is the best imaging method. In infants with patent fontanelle, US may also be used. MRI can be used, especially as the FLAIR sequence can pick up acute hemorrhages.	
Intraparenchymal hemorrhage, subacute ▷ *Fig. 4.55a–c, p. 339*	MRI is the modality of choice because it will best show the time at which different bleedings occurred. May be of significance in child abuse and shaken baby syndrome.	

(continues on page 340)

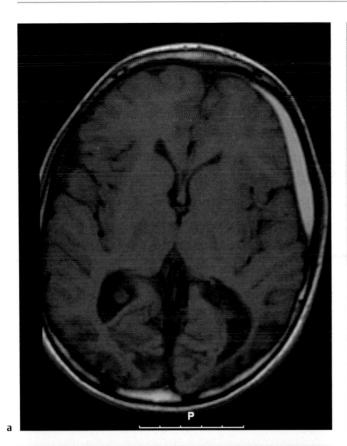

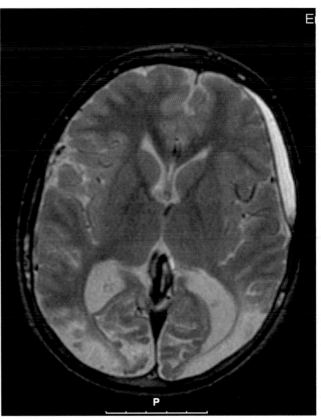

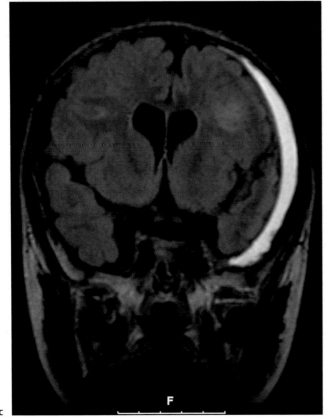

Fig. 4.54a–c Intraparenchymal hemorrhage, acute. A 9-year-old boy with an epidural hematoma (EDH) at the left frontal side and infarcts in the occipital lobes based on child battering. It shows high signal intensity on T1- (**a**) and T2-weighted (**b**) image due to extracellular methemoglobin. (**c**) EDH with high signal intensity on a FLAIR image in the same patient.

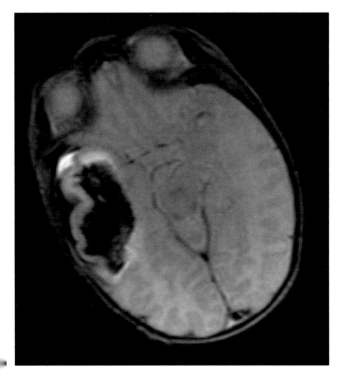

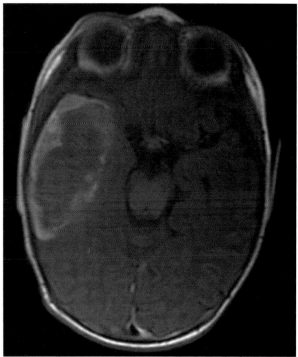

b

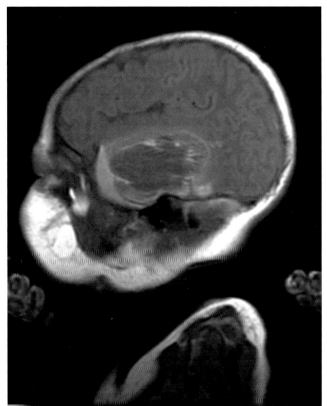

Fig. 4.55a–c Intraparenchymal hemorrhage, subacute. (a) A 4-day-old girl term neonate with postpartum bleeding from umbilical cord and pulmonary arrest/irregular breathing. This T2-weighted image shows parenchymal bleeding involving almost the entire right temporal lobe. **(b)** On the T1-weighted image, the bleeding is hyperintense at the periphery and isointense centrally, compatible with intra- and extracellular methemoglobin. **(c)** Sagittal T1-weighted image shows the extent of the bleeding in the right temporal lobe.

Table 4.15 (Cont.) Intracranial hemorrhage

Diagnosis	Findings	Comments
EDH ▷ *Fig. 4.56*	EDHs are hemorrhagic collections located between the inner table of the skull and the dura. Because the dura is tightly adherent to the inner table at cranial suture sites, EDHs do not typically cross cranial suture lines (unlike subdural hematomas [SDHs], which can freely cross these sites) unless the dura is lacerated. Whereas the extension of SDHs is restricted by the falx cerebri and tentorium cerebelli, EDHs can freely extend across these sites.	On occasion, EDH cannot be detected on CT because of its small size and may be first seen on MRI. The changes in density on CT and of signal intensity of EDH on MRI follow the same temporal progression as that of SDH.
SDH ▷ *Fig. 4.57a–c* ▷ *Fig. 4.54a–c, p. 338*	Acute SDHs located over the cerebral convexity appear as a hyperintense crescent-shaped collection with a sharp margin between the collection and adjacent brain. Alternatively, SDHs can have a biconvex (lentiform) shape like that of a typical EDH. SDHs undergo a typical temporal evolution on both CT and MRI. On CT, acute SDHs are characteristically hyperdense, with a few exceptions. At first, in the setting of severe anemia, acute SDHs can be isodense with gray matter. SDHs that are only a few hours old can have a mixed appearance of both hyperdense and hypodense regions because of the presence of uncoagulated blood before clot formation. Also, in neonates it can be difficult to differentiate SDH from the more dense aspect of fetal hemoglobin especially at the transverse sinus level. On MRI in the first few days, while blood is in the stage of intracellular deoxyhemoglobin, the SDH is isointense to gray matter on T1-weighted images and hypointense on T2-weighted images. SDHs become hyperintense on T1-weighted images after a few days because of blood in the stage of intracellular methemoglobin. After approximately the first week, with lysis of red blood cells and production of extracellular methemoglobin, SDHs become hyperintense on both T1- and T2-weighted images, a finding that may persist for many months. Thereafter, the pattern will be iso- or hypointense on T1 and hypointense on T2 due to hemosiderin, especially on T2* sequence.	SDHs most commonly occur at one of three locations: along the cerebral convexities, the falx cerebri, and the tentorium cerebelli. Child abuse should be ruled out, especially in cases of SDH with different densities, due to different timing of SDH. There is an important differential diagnosis, especially metabolic disease like Menkes disease and Glutaric aciduria type I and D-2-hydroxyglutaric aciduria.
Acute SDH		Acute SDHs are often seen after trauma and are frequently associated with a skull fracture. The term *acute subdural hematoma* is generally meant to refer to an SDH that is a few days old, whereas subacute is generally meant to refer to SDHs that are more than a few days but less than a few weeks old.
Chronic SDH ▷ *Fig. 4.57a–c*	Chronic SDH typically appears homogeneously hypodense relative to gray matter as red blood cells lyse and a proteinaceous fluid remains. When fresh hemorrhage occurs into a chronic SDH, a bilayered appearance typically results, with a hypodense layer (because of chronic hemorrhage) in the less dependent position and a hyperdense component (because of acute hemorrhage) in the dependent position.	The term *chronic subdural hematoma* generally refers to an SDH that is more than a few weeks old.
Subarachnoid hemorrhage (SAH) ▷ *Fig. 4.58a–c, p. 342*	CT is generally considered more sensitive than MRI in the detection of SAH. However, a number of recent articles have suggested that SAH is also readily detected on proton-density, T2-weighted MRI, but is best seen on FLAIR images.	A small amount of SAH is often seen after head trauma. Common sites of SAH include basilar cisterns such as the prepontine, ambient, interpeduncular, and perimesencephalic cisterns. It is rare in the pediatric population, but SAHs do occur due to rupture of aneurysms.

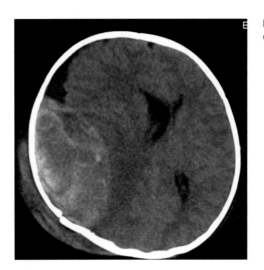

Fig. 4.56 Epidural hemorrhage. A 4-month-old boy who has fallen down the stairs. CT shows a right EDH with midline shift and fracture.

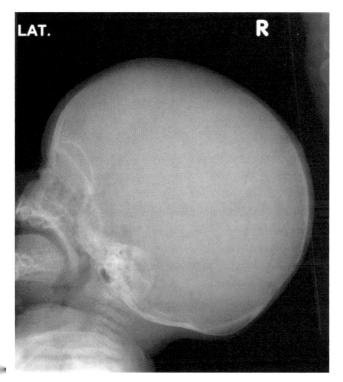

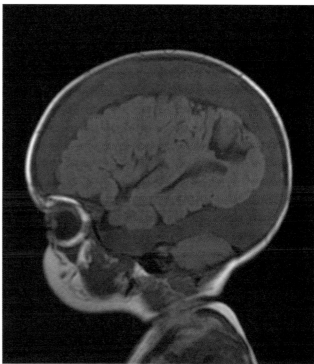

b

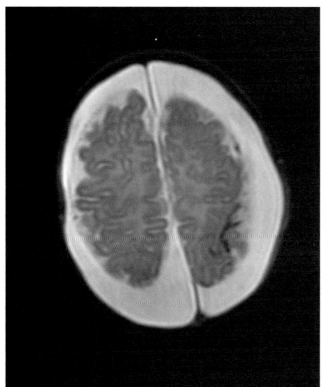

Fig. 4.57a–c   Subdural hematoma. (a) Multiple sharply demarcated lines are suspicious for fractures in child abuse. **(b)** Sagittal T1-weighted image showing subdural effusion with higher signal than CSF due to old bleeding and occipital parenchymal loss due to old bleeding or infarct. **(c)** T2-weighted image shows subdural effusion and old bleeding in the left hemisphere.

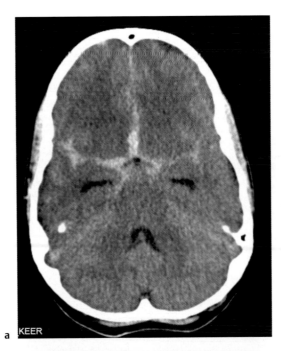

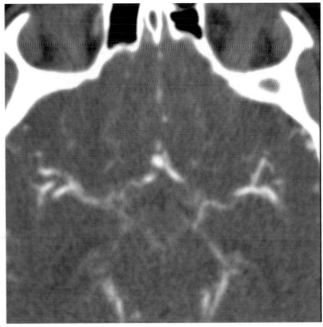

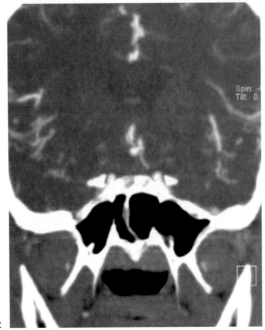

Fig. 4.58a–c   Subarachnoid hemorrhage. (**a**) A 12-year-old girl with an acute on-set of headache. CT shows subarachnoid blood at the basal cisterns, with the maximum of blood at the the A1 and M1 level on the right. (**b**) CTA shows an aneurysm at the A1/A2 level on the left. (**c**) Coronal reconstruction of the CTA confirms an aneurysm at the A1/A2 level on the left.

Table 4.16   Cystic structures

Diagnosis	Findings	Comments
Choroid plexus cyst (CPC) ▷ *Fig. 4.59a–c*	Best seen on US as a rounded hypoechoic mass of varying size. On MRI, hypointense on T1- and hyperintense on T2-weighted images.	CPCs are more common in fetuses with chromosomal aneuploidies, particularly trisomy 18.
Subependymal pseudocyst (germinal matrix cyst)		Subependymal pseudocysts are found in 5% of all neonates. When isolated, they have a good prognosis and regress spontaneously within a few months. However, associated anomalies are frequent and in such cases the prognosis is poor. They can be of infectious, vascular, metabolic, or chromosomal origin.
Dilatation of the cavum septum pellucidum	Expanded cystlike cavum septum pellucidum, may extend dorsally, called "et vergae."	Cavum septi pellucidi may serve as a significant marker of cerebral dysfunction manifested by neurodevelopmental abnormalities while the cavum et vergae alone does not identify individuals at risk for cognitive delays.

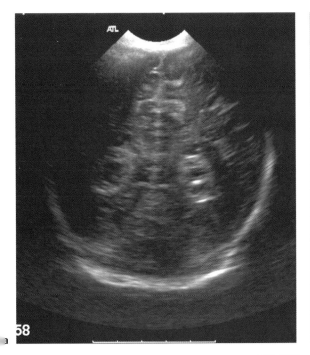

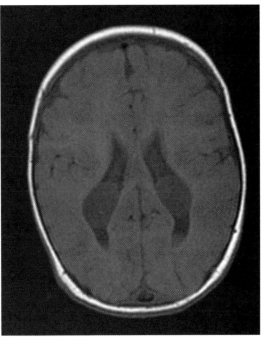

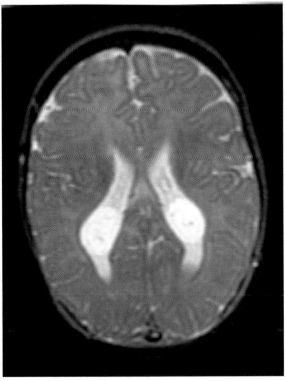

Fig. 4.59a–c **Choroid plexus cyst.** (a) A 7-month-old girl diagnosed with bilateral CPC. (b) The bilateral CPC is hypointense on T1-weighted image. (c) The lesions are hyperintense on T2-weighted image.

■ Arachnoid Cysts

Arachnoid cysts are nontumorous intra-arachnoid fluid collections that account for approximately 1% of all intracranial space-occupying lesions. Arachnoid cysts can be congenital cysts (also called "true" arachnoid cysts, which occur most commonly) or secondary arachnoid cysts. Congenital cysts should be differentiated from other types of cysts that result from CSF sequestration due to inflammatory or following traumatic processes, hemorrhage, chemical irritation, and tumors; these are called secondary arachnoid cysts. In congenital arachnoid cysts, the wall contains arachnoid cells connected with unchanged arachnoid matter; in secondary cysts, the loculations of CSF are surrounded by arachnoid scarring. Congenital arachnoid cysts are developmental anomalies in which splitting or duplication of the primitive arachnoid membrane in the early embryonal life leads to collection of clear CSF-like fluid. The majority of arachnoid cysts (90%) are found in supratentorial locations, while 10% are located in the posterior fossa. The most common supratentorial site is the middle cranial fossa (60%; **Fig. 4.60**). Other sites include the quadrigeminal plate, sellar region, and convexity.

Diagnostic evaluation should include not only the initial identification of intracranial arachnoid cysts but also the detection of mass effect, determination of the type of communication between cyst and subarachnoid space, and recognition of the presence, location, and severity of obstructive hydrocephalus and cisternal block. During patency of the sutures and fontanelles, US is the imaging modality. MRI is best suited to rule out other brain abnormalities and can be used to identify a possible communication with the central ventricles or subdural space using cine phase-contrast MRI.

Differential diagnosis includes the following:
- Intraventricular cysts (e.g., colloid cysts)
- Intraparenchymal cystic structure (e.g., parasitic infections, cystic metastases)
- Porencephalic cysts
- Craniopharyngioma
- Holoprosencephaly
- Agenesis of corpus callosum with interhemispheric cysts
- Dandy-Walker complex (posterior fossa cysts).

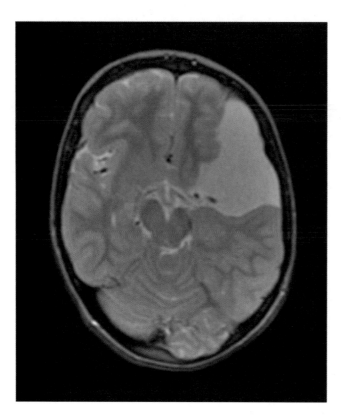

Fig. 4.60 **Arachnoid cyst** in the left perisylvian region in a 7-year-old boy.

■ Hydrocephalus

Hydrocephalus is a disturbance of formation, flow, or absorption of CSF that leads to increased intracranial CSF volume. Acute hydrocephalus occurs over days, subacute hydrocephalus develops over weeks, and the chronic form over months or years. Conditions such as cerebral atrophy and focal destructive lesions also lead to an abnormal increase of CSF in the brain, but in these cases this is due to loss of cerebral tissue and passive filling of the resulting space(s) with CSF. If a communication exists with the ventricular system, such as a lesion, it is defined as porencephaly. If only the ventricles are prominent due to surrounding loss of brain tissue, it is named ventriculomegaly.

There are two different types of hydrocephalus:
1. Communicating hydrocephalus occurs when full communication exists between ventricles and subarachnoid space. It is caused by overproduction of CSF (rarely), defective absorption of CSF (most often), or venous drainage insufficiency (occasionally). Defective absorption of CSF is the most common presentation in infancy and early childhood and is also known as benign external hydrocephalus. It is a self-limiting absorption deficiency with raised ICP and enlarged subarachnoid spaces. The infants often present with macrocephaly. The ventricles usually are not enlarged significantly, and equilibrium or resolution within 1 year is the rule. The communicating type is more common and usually occurs in adults, owing to interference with absorption of CSF at the level of the arachnoid villi. This is often a result of an adhesive process at this level, whether caused by prior infection, hemorrhage, or neoplastic involvement.
2. Noncommunicating hydrocephalus occurs when CSF flow is obstructed within the ventricular system or in its outlets to the arachnoid space, resulting in ventricular/subarachnoid space dilatation. The noncommunicating or obstructive type is far more prevalent in children, with obstruction to CSF flow occurring at any point within the ventricular system. The most common causes of hydrocephalus in children include neonatal hemorrhage, Chiari malformations, and aqueductal stenosis.

Hydrocephalus can be progressive or stable. Stable hydrocephalus is defined as stabilization of known ventricular enlargement, probably secondary to compensatory mechanisms. These patients may decompensate, especially following minor head injuries. It is important to distinguish progressive from stable hydrocephalus because of therapeutic implications.

Normal CSF production is 0.20 to 0.35 mL/min; a majority is produced by the choroid plexus, which is located within the ventricular system, mainly the lateral and fourth ventricles. Normal route of CSF from production to clearance is the following: from the choroid plexus, the CSF flows to the lateral ventricle, then through the foramen of Monro to the third ventricle, the aqueduct of Sylvius, the fourth ventricle, the two lateral foramina of Luschka and the medial located foramen of Magendie, the subarachnoid space, the arachnoid granulations, the dural sinus, and finally into the venous drainage system.

ICP rises if production of CSF exceeds absorption. This occurs if CSF is overproduced, resistance to CSF flow is increased, or venous sinus pressure is increased, or a combination of all three. CSF production falls as ICP rises. Compensation may occur through transventricular absorption of CSF and also by absorption along nerve root sleeves. Temporal and frontal horns dilate first, often asymmetrically. This may result in elevation of the corpus callosum, stretching or perforation of the septum pellucidum, thinning of the cerebral mantle, or enlargement of the third ventricle downward into the pituitary fossa (which may cause pituitary dysfunction).

Hydrocephalus may have major implications in the daily life of a child because it may impair development of cognitive function. This can be the result of untreated hydrocephalus and it may persist after treatment. Untreated hydrocephalus can also cause visual loss and may persist after treatment. Shunt dependence occurs in 75% of all cases of treated hydrocephalus and in 50% of children with communicating hydrocephalus, all with a risk of shunt complications and repeated hospitalizations for scheduled shunt revisions or for treatment of shunt dysfunction.

Imaging modalities to assess increased ICP in children are radiography, US with or without Doppler, CT, and/or MRI (**Table 4.17**).

If a child has an enlarged head circumference and other signs of increased ICP, one has to rule out hydrocephalus and its causes.

If the fontanelle is still open, US is the imaging modality of choice. One can measure the ventricular size, ventricular ratios, or ventricular volume. Hemorrhages and hematoma can be picked up easily. Detection of malformations and tumors may be hampered due to their location, especially in the posterior fossa.

CT can also assess the size of ventricles and other structures. Especially in follow-up cases for drain dysfunction. Low-dose CT is a good imaging option as it is easily available and quick because of its near ubiquitous presence and scan speed. With the use of multidetector CT imaging, it is now also possible to make reconstructions in multiple planes. Less differentiation between gray and white matter and its radiation burden means that many institutions favor MRI above CT. Another advantage of MRI over CT is the possibility to check for flow voids in the ventricle and aqueduct and see if a therapeutic intervention, like third ventriculostomy, is still functioning adequately.

CT and MRI criteria for acute hydrocephalus include the following:
- Size of both temporal horns is greater than 2 mm, and the sylvian and interhemispheric fissures are not visible. In the absence of hydrocephalus, the temporal horns should be barely visible.
- The ratio between the maximum width of the frontal horns and the internal diameter from inner-table to inner-table at this level should be greater than 0.5 in the presence of hydrocephalus.
- The ratio of the largest width of the frontal horns to maximal biparietal diameter (i.e., Evans ratio) is more than 30% in acute hydrocephalus.
- Transependymal absorption is translated on images as periventricular low density on CT and as hypointense on T1 and hyperintense on T2 in MRI.
- Ballooning of frontal horns of lateral ventricles and third ventricle (i.e., "Mickey Mouse" ventricles) indicates aquaductal obstruction.
- Upward bowing of the corpus callosum on sagittal MRI indicates acute hydrocephalus.

CT and MRI criteria for chronic hydrocephalus include the following:
- The temporal horns may be less prominent than in acute hydrocephalus.
- The third ventricle may herniate into the sella turcica.
- The sella turcica may be eroded.
- Macrocrania (i.e., occipitofrontal circumference > 98th percentile) may be present.
- Corpus callosum may be atrophied (best appreciated on sagittal MRI).

Table 4.17   Imaging findings of increased ICP in children

Radiography

Generalized findings:
- Abnormal calvarial enlargement.
- Sutural changes may appear within 24–48 h after an abrupt ICP rise in infants or within 1–2 wk in older children: ill-defined margins, elongated sutural interdigitations, suture widening.
- Increased inner-table convolutional markings in the frontal and parietal regions; a useful marker in craniosynostosis.
- Secondary sellar abnormalities; enlarged, deformed, demineralized dorsum sellae, from approximately 5 y of age.

Individual signs:
- Calvarial "bulging," generalized or unilateral.
- Shallow orbits due to anterior displacement of greater sphenoid wings; orbital roofs short and steep; steep lateral slope of lesser sphenoid wings.
- Downward convexity of the cribriform plate; scalloping of the clivus; widening of vascular grooves (sinuses, emissary veins); increased basal angle; calcifications due to infection or tumor.

US

Acute ICP increase:
- Ill-defined cerebral surface features, increased parenchymal echogenicity, reduced or absent vascular pulsations.

Chronic ICP increase:
- Lateral ventricular margins are round and smooth with loss of normal contour; ventricular enlargement usually starts in the occipital horn region; effacement of cerebral gyri
- Extra-axial CSF spaces and cisterns diminished in size.

Doppler US

- Negative diastolic peak in the sampled artery
- Normal flow restored after decompression.

Table 4.18   Congenital causes of hydrocephalus

Diagnosis	Findings	Comments
Aqueductal stenosis ▷ *Fig. 4.61*	Progressive dilatation of the lateral ventricles and third ventricle. MRI preferable to CT.	Responsible for 10% of all cases of hydrocephalus in newborns.
Dandy-Walker malformation ▷ *Fig. 4.62a–c* ▷ *Fig. 4.63, p. 348* ▷ *Fig. 4.64, p. 348*	Hypoplasia of the vermis, cystic dilated fourth ventricle communicating with a retrocerebellar cyst and upward displacement of the tentorium, torcular and lateral sinuses, and AP enlargement of the posterior fossa.	Hydrocephalus in 80% of cases. Affects 2%–4% of newborns with hydrocephalus. It is frequently associated with genetic anomalies, brain malformations (anomalies of gyration, gray matter heterotopias, meningoceles, corpus callosum agenesis), or systemic malformations (heart, orthopedic, intestinal, urogenital and facial anomalies).
Chiari malformation ▷ *Fig. 4.65, p. 348* ▷ *Fig. 4.66, p. 348*	Herniation of cerebellar tonsils below the level of foramen of magnum in Chiari type I. Usually progressive hydrocephalus, mainly involving the occipital horns in Chiari type II. Large massa intermedia. Cerebellar vermis is displaced downward through the enlarged foramen magnum. Enlarged third ventricle, relative aqueduct stenosis with dorsal beaking of mesencephalon.	Chiari type I shows hydrocephalus in 7% of cases. Commonly associated with syringomyelia as a result of deranged CSF dynamics at craniovertebral junction and upper cervical canal. Chiari type II is associated in 97% of cases with MMC.
Agenesis of the foramen of Monro or atresia of the lateral ventricle	Progressive dilatation of the lateral ventricle.	Extremely rare.
Congenital toxoplasmosis	Hydrocephalus often results from the granulomatous meningeal or ependymal reaction that can cause aquaductal stenosis and communicating hydrocephalus. Intracranial calcifications can be seen.	Chorioretinitis and convulsions are the typical presentation of classic congenital toxoplasmosis.
Syndromes with hydrocephalus	Dilatation of third and lateral ventricles due to aqueduct stenosis. MRI preferable to CT to pick up the additional brain abnormalities.	This is an X-linked hydrocephalus accounting for 7% of cases in males. It is characterized by stenosis of the aqueduct of Sylvius, severe mental retardation, and in 50% by an adduction-flexion deformity of the thumb. Another AD periventricular heterotopy gene exists, distinct from the previously described X-linked and autosomal recessive forms. Affected individuals have severe developmental delay and may have radiographic findings of hydrocephalus.

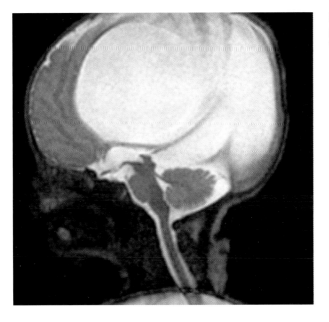

Fig. 4.61   Aqueductal stenosis. Sagittal T2-weighted image of a 3-day-old girl with macrocephaly due to hydrocephalus. Note the open beak aspect of the anterior part of the aquaduct due to aqueductal stenosis.

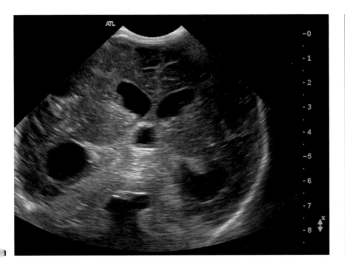

a

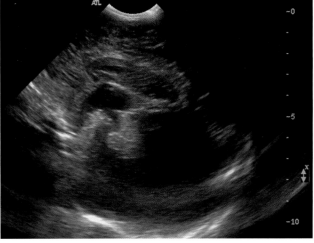

b

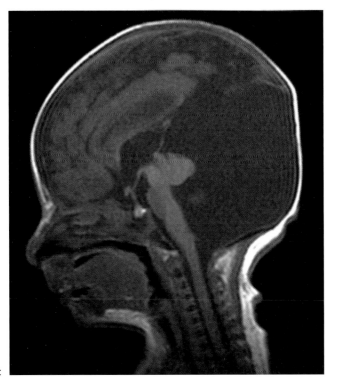

c

Fig. 4.62a‒c   Dandy-Walker malformation. (a, b) Coronal and sagittal cranial US scans show Dandy-Walker malformation with hydrocephalus. **(c)** Sagittal T1 image of the same patient. Note enlarged posterior fossa.

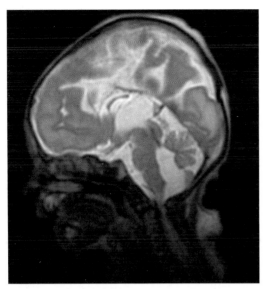

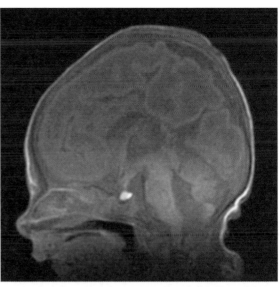

Fig. 4.63   Dandy-Walker variant. A premature girl, born at 33 weeks, who is a monochorionic twin with an enlarged fourth ventricle. MRI on day of birth shows callosal agenesis and a Dandy-Walker variant.

Fig. 4.64   Dandy-Walker variant shown on a sagittal T1-weighted image of the same patient as in **Fig. 4.63**.

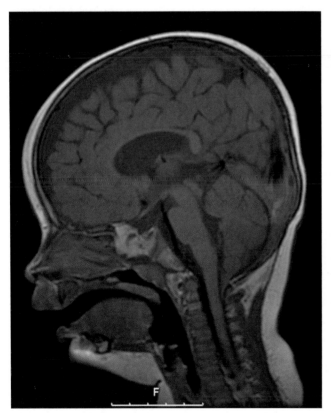

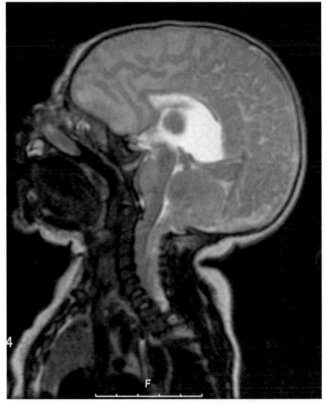

Fig. 4.65   Chiari type I malformation. Sagittal T1-weighted image shows a tonsillar herniation of the cerebellum with normal position of the fourth ventricle compatible with the diagnosis of Chiari type I malformation.

Fig. 4.66   Chiari type II malformation shown on sagittal T2-weighted image. Note the abnormal lower position of the cerebellar tonsils (midcervical level).

Table 4.19   Acquired causes of hydrocephaly

Diagnosis	Findings	Comments
Mass lesions ▷ *Fig. 4.67* ▷ *Fig. 4.68a, b* ▷ *Fig. 4.69a, b, p. 350* ▷ *Fig. 4.70, p. 350* ▷ *Fig. 4.71a, b, p. 351* ▷ *Fig. 4.72a–d, p. 351*	May be tumors, cysts, abscesses, hematomas, or vascular malformations.	Account for 20% of all cases of hydrocephalus in children. Tumors can cause blockage anywhere along the CSF pathways. The most frequent tumors associated with hydrocephalus are ependymoma, subependymal giant cell astrocytoma, choroid plexus papilloma (CPP), craniopharyngioma, pituitary adenoma, hypothalamic or optic nerve glioma, hamartoma, and leptomeningeal tumor spread.

(continues on page 352)

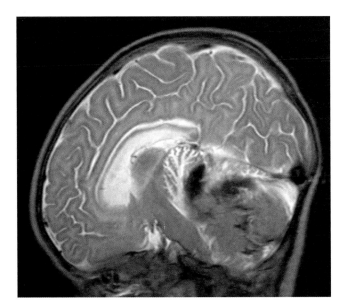

Fig. 4.67   Obstructive hydrocephalus due to a cerebellar tumor shown on sagittal T2-weighted image of an infant.

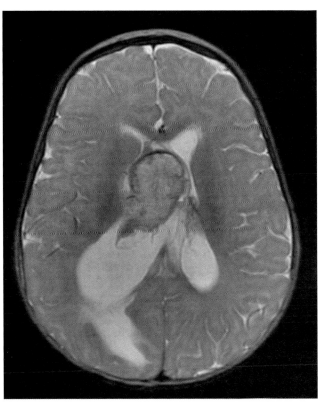

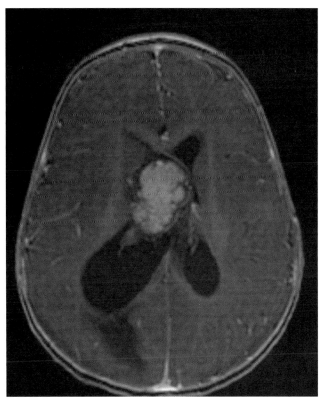

b

Fig. 4.68a, b   Choroid plexus papilloma. (a) Axial T2-weighted image of a 7-month-old boy shows obstruction of the lateral ventricles. Dilatation could also be due to increased CSF production, caused by a CPP. **(b)** Axial T1-weighted Gd-enhanced image in the same patient.

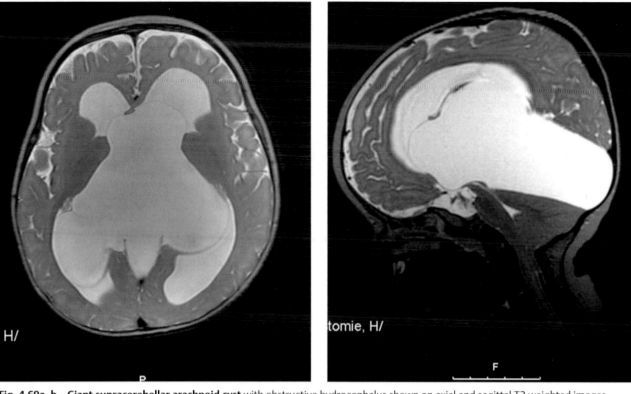

a

b

Fig. 4.69a, b   Giant supracerebellar arachnoid cyst with obstructive hydrocephalus shown on axial and sagittal T2-weighted images.

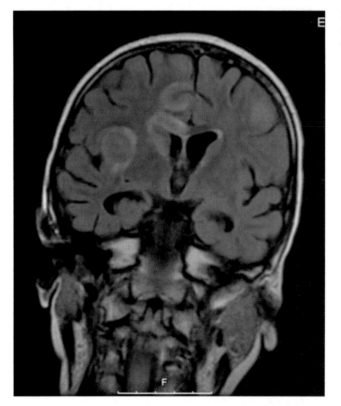

Fig. 4.70   *Aspergillus* abscesses and ventriculitis, as shown on coronal FLAIR images, causing hydrocephalus in this immunocompromised 4-year-old boy.

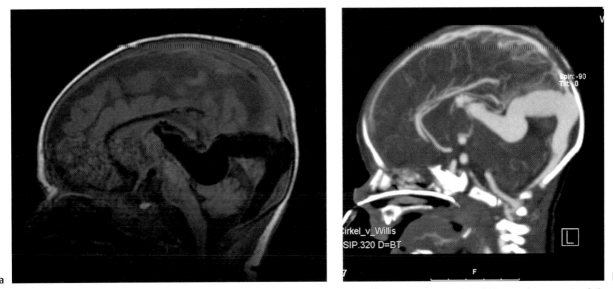

Fig. 4.71a, b   Compression on aqueductal region due to vein of Galen malformation in an 8-day-old boy with congestive failure, demonstrated on a sagittal T1 MRI (**a**) and CTA (**b**).

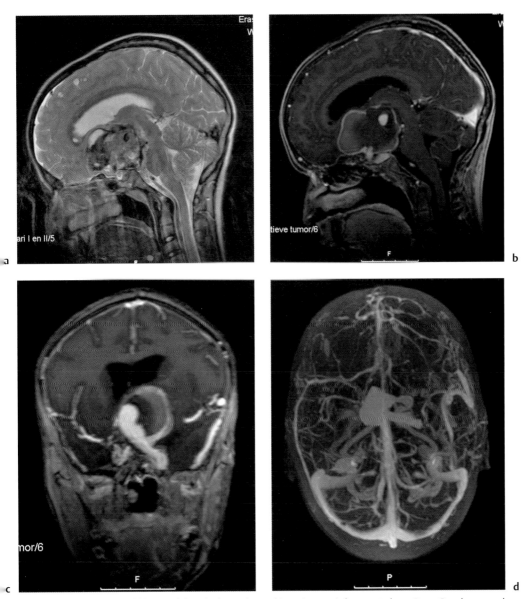

Fig. 4.72a–d   A 9-year-old boy with headache and visual impairment is known to have Parre-Romberg syndrome. T2 and T1 after contrast and MRA demonstrate **hydrocephalus due to obstruction, caused by a giant aneurysm** of the left internal carotid artery (ICA)—not to be confused with a suprasellar tumor mass such as a craniopharyngioma.

Table 4.19   (Cont.) Acquired causes of hydrocephaly

Diagnosis	Findings	Comments
Intraventricular hemorrhage ▷ *Fig. 4.73a, b*	Progressive dilatation of ventricles filled with blood. Not always symmetrical.	May be due to rupture of fragile vessels of the choroid plexus or breakthrough of intraventricular germinal matrix bleeding (Grade 3) predominantly in prematurity. In older children, head injury or rupture of a vascular malformation may be the cause.
Infections	Outlet obstruction of the fourth ventricle, the cisterna magna, the tentorial notch, or subtentorial CSF pathways. Progressive dilatation of all ventricles. MRI preferable to CT.	Meningitis (especially bacterial) and, in some geographic areas, cysticercosis can cause hydrocephalus.
Increased venous sinus pressure ▷ *Fig. 4.74* ▷ *Fig. 4.75*	Dilatation of the ventricles and subarachnoid space. Obstruction at the convexity. Impaired reabsorption of CSF.	Venous thrombosis. It may also be the mechanism in some cases of craniostenosis or achondroplasia.
Iatrogenic	Dilatation of the ventricles and subarachnoid space.	Hypervitaminosis A, by increasing secretion of CSF or by increasing permeability of the blood–brain barrier, can lead to hydrocephalus. Postoperative complication.

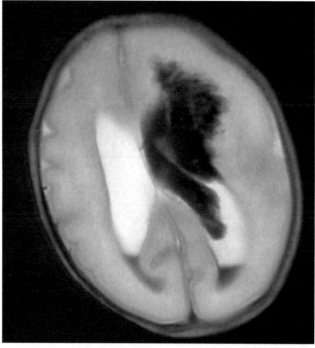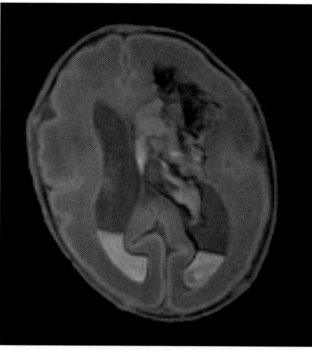

Fig. 4.73a, b An 8-day-old boy, born at 32 weeks, with **obstructive hydrocephalus due to germinal matrix bleeding** grade II on the right side and grade III on the left. Additionally, in the left frontal lobe, a venous infarction is seen; it is hypointense on T2 and hyperintense on T1 due to hemorrhage.

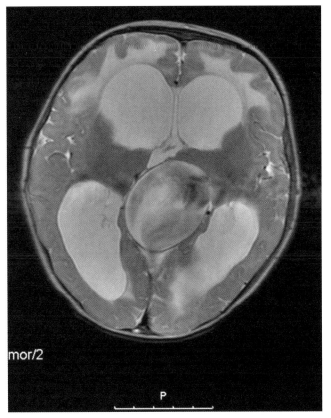

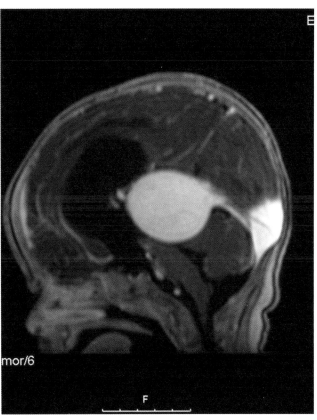

Fig. 4.74 Axial T2-weighted image of a 6-month-old boy with macrocephaly. Hydrocephalus is caused by compression on the aqueduct and **increased venous sinus pressure** due to a vein of Galen malformation.

Fig. 4.75 Sagittal Gd-enhanced T1-weighted image of the same patient as **Fig. 4.74** shows the venous malformation. Note the enlarged confluens due to **increased venous sinus pressure**.

Shunt Complications

The main therapy for hydrocephalus is diversion of CSF via a ventricular shunt to decompress the ventricles. These shunts are meant to prevent or reverse brain damage that may occur secondary to increased ICP. Placement of the proximal end of the drain is with its proximal tip within the cerebral ventricular system, usually within the bodies of the lateral ventricles or at the foramen of Monro. The location of the distal end of the catheter is more variable, terminating usually within the peritoneal cavity, as its lining is a highly efficient site of absorption. Other distal sites for catheter tip placement include the superior vena cava, the right atrium of the heart, and within the pleural space. Lumbar–peritoneal shunts are also being used. Ventriculoperitoneal (VP) shunts are, however, prone to complications, with failure rates as high as 40% within the first year after placement and 50% within 2 years. Shunt failure may be the result of infection, which is thought to occur in 8.1% of patients. Noninfectious causes of shunt failure include shunt obstruction and mechanical failure due to disconnection or fracture. In addition,

specific intra-abdominal causes of mechanical failure have been reported, including the development of a pseudocyst, which is a loculated CSF collection causing obstruction at the distal end of the catheter.

Imaging is essential, and this includes low-dose CT scan or MRI of the brain if US is not possible and an additional so-called shunt series in patients with rapid onset of signs of increased ICP. In other cases, a shunt series alone is sufficient and if this is normal, an additional US of the abdomen may be indicated. Radionuclide CSF clearance study is only indicated in special cases. Imaging evaluation includes an assessment of catheter position, ventricular size and configuration, and any change thereof. Findings may include an obvious increase in ventricular size; a more subtle increase in dilatation with rounding of the temporal horns, frontal horns, or third ventricle; asymmetric or disproportionate ventricular dilatation; edema or cysts about the ventricles or along the catheter; a decrease or loss of the sulci, fissures, or cisterns; reduced gray-white matter differentiation; a shift of the midline markers; or other signs of impending or frank herniation.

Table 4.20 Signs of shunt complications

Diagnosis	Findings	Comments
Increased ICP	Skull film: suture widening. US or CT/MRI: progressive increase in ventricular size.	Clinical signs of increased ICP, increasing head circumference in neonates and infants. Suture widening.
Obstructed ventricular catheter	US: location of tip of drain intracranially and in abdomen in case of a VP drain. Shunt series: disconnection or kinking. CT/MRI: Location of tip of drain, severity of distension of ventricles. Need for baseline scan, MRI or low-dose CT scan after ventricular catheter placement.	Plugging of the drain by choroid plexus, brain tissue, or clotted blood. Catheter may be malpositioned in brain parenchyma.
Disconnection of ventricular catheter or Rickham reservoir at the valve ▷ *Fig. 4.76* ▷ *Fig. 4.77*	Visible on plain films as part of the shunt series.	Be aware of radiolucent connection parts. Inadequate length for the growing child is a common reason for shunt dysfunction.
Obstructed peritoneal catheter	Abdominal radiograph: kinking, malposition in the abdominal wall, mass around tip. US: CSF pseudocyst at the catheter tip.	Other distal shunt complications are hernia, hydrocele, ascites, intestinal volvulus and obstruction, viscus or peritoneal perforation, and neoplastic or infectious seeding.

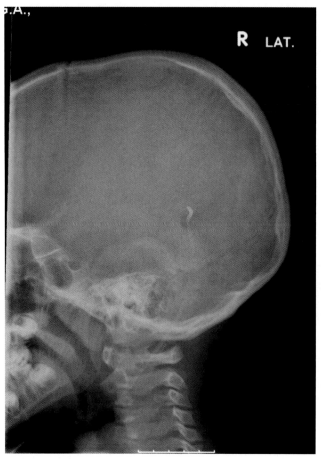

Fig. 4.76 Ventriculoperitoneal drain. Progressive hydrocephalus and stenosis of the aqueduct in an 8-year-old boy with headache and vomiting. No drain disconnection is noted at this level.

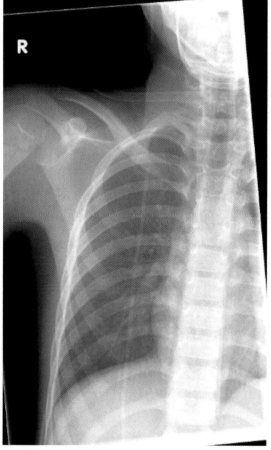

Fig. 4.77 Ventriculoperitoneal drain. Drain disconnection is shown at the neck/thorax level.

Table 4.21   Intracranial complications of ventricular drainage

Diagnosis	Findings	Comments
Slitlike ventricle ▷ *Fig. 4.78*	US or CT/MRI: ventricular collapse due to overshunting.	Recurrent headaches. In majority clinically asymptomatic.
Subdural effusion ▷ *Fig. 4.79*	Parenchymal shrinkage. May result in SDH due to rupture of subdural veins. On MRI, a subdural fluid collection may be seen with different signal intensity due to blood products in different stages of breakdown (see subsequent discussion).	
SDH, intraventricular hemorrhage; transtentorial herniation of brain tissue	US or CT. MRI is better for timing the hemorrhage.	
Isolated dilatation of the fourth ventricle	US or CT. MRI is better for imaging posterior fossa and herniation of cerebellum or brainstem through foramen magnum.	After shunting, due to obstruction of fibrous tissue or postinfectious tissue.
CSF leakage	US, CT, or MRI. Leakage through the drain trajectory especially after a third ventriculostomy procedure, or subcuteous in case of disconnection at the valve of the Rickham reservoir.	
Craniosynostosis and seizures	Craniosynostosis best seen on 3D CT.	

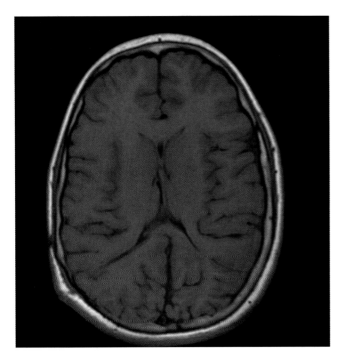

Fig. 4.78 Axial T1-weighted image shows **slitlike ventricles** due to overdrainage. Note the VP shunt had its tip at the level of the atrium of the right lateral ventricle.

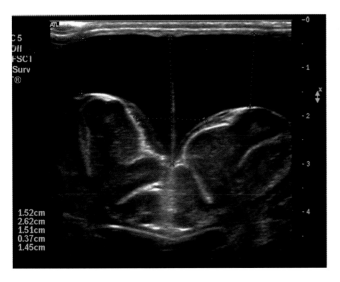

Fig. 4.79 **Subdural effusion** and small subarachnoid spaces shown on coronal US image.

■ Brain Tumors and Their Differential Diagnosis

Brain tumors are the second most common neoplasm after leukemia. Infra- and supratentorial tumors occur in equal numbers, however, there are age related differences: supratentorial tumors occur more often within the first 2 to 3 years of life, whereas infratentorial tumors reach their peak between 4 and 10 years. After the tenth year, infra- and supratentorial tumors occur with equal frequency.

For neuroimaging, one can use US (during the neonatal period), CT, or MRI. CT may have a role in screening and can diagnose hydrocephalus as well as most supratentorial and even posterior fossa tumors, but a major drawback is the radiation dose. MRI is far superior to CT once a tumor is identified and is the method of choice for follow-up. Certain tumors that generally seed to the CSF axis require baseline and sequential assessments of the neuraxis with gadolinium-enhanced MRI of the brain. This approach allows identification of relapse in the absence of clinical signs and symptoms and is recommended for children with medulloblastomas, primitive neuroectodermal tumors, ependymomas, malignant gliomas, pilocytic astrocytomas, and germinomas. While there is still controversy as to whether surveillance spinal MRI is necessary, there are studies that have demonstrated that surveillance imaging is associated with improved survival.

In addition to conventional MRI sequences, newer techniques are available, like diffusion-weighted imaging (DWI) and magnetic resonance spectroscopy (MRS). These may improve the accuracy of the differential diagnosis of the brain tumor, but up until now have not replaced histology.

Studies show that signal characteristics on DWI and ADC maps correlate well with tumor grade. High-grade lesions were shown as hyperintense on DWI and as hypointense on ADC maps. The routine use of DWI in all newly diagnosed pediatric brain tumors could give insight into the aggressiveness of the lesion and may be helpful to the pediatric neurosurgeon preoperatively in the differentiation of brain tumors and in predicting prognosis.

MRS has been used to identify tumors, distinguish tumors from radiation necrosis, determine the degree of malignancy, and identify the tumor extension beyond that seen on traditional enhanced MRI. Solid brain tumors typically have a decreased or absent N-acetylasparate (NAA), elevated choline and, at times, elevated lactate and lipid peaks. The choline/NAA ratio is usually increased in pediatric brain tumors, while NAA/choline and NAA/creatinine ratios are decreased. MRS has also been used to study response to radiation in children with pontine gliomas.

Today, neuroimaging, with its new and rapidly evolving techniques, permits the neuroradiologist and neuro-oncologist to monitor initial response to therapy, duration of response, and site of failure. In addition to diagnosing primary brain tumors and leptomeningeal dissemination, neuroimaging helps to identify and quantify the long-term consequences of radiation and chemotherapy. With the advent of magnetic resonance angiography (MRA), children irradiated for midline tumors can be monitored for the development of radiation vasculopathy (moyamoya disease) without having to undergo invasive angiography. As neuroimaging techniques improve, quantification of normal white matter volumes will allow investigators to better understand long-term declining neurologic status, which is sometimes seen after cranial irradiation and chemotherapy.

A special group of brain tumors is seen during the first year of life. The presentation is an increased head circumference due to hydrocephalus and/or rapid tumor growth.

These tumors can be easily imaged with US, but for a better delineation (if clinically relevant) MRI should be used. This brain tumor group includes:

- Superficial cerebral astrocytoma (usually frontal and with dural enhancement)
- PNET
- Teratoma
- CPP/carcinoma
- Ependymoma
- Medulloblastoma
- Desmoplastic infantile ganglioglioma (usually frontal or parietal)

Table 4.22 Brain tumors

Diagnosis	Findings	Comments
Astrocytic tumors ▷ *Fig. 4.80* ▷ *Fig. 4.81* ▷ *Fig. 4.82* ▷ *Fig. 4.83* ▷ *Fig. 4.84, p. 358*	Depends on location, grade, and composition of the tumor. Most tumors have a solid component with peripheral cystic changes. The solid part enhances and the cystic part consists of nonenhancing, nonneoplastic glial tissue.	Most common primary brain tumor in children. Two groups: the diffuse astrocytomas with higher grades are more common in adults and the second more heterogeneous group more frequent in children, including pilocytic astrocytoma, pleomorphic xanthoastrocytoma, and subependymal giant cell astrocytoma.
Brainstem gliomas ▷ *Fig. 4.85, p. 358* ▷ *Fig. 4.86, p. 358*	On CT, a hypodense, partially enhancing mass. Calcifications and hemorrhage are uncommon. On MRI, hypointense on T1 and hyperintense on T2, with variable and often minimal or absent enhancement.	Ten to twenty percent of all pediatric brain tumors. Short clinical history (< 6 mo), cranial nerve deficits at diagnosis, pontine location, greater tumor volume, ill-defined margins, peritumoral edema, and ring enhancement correlate with poor outcome. Most important factor for prognosis is whether or not the tumor is focal or diffuse.
Glioblastoma multiforme ▷ *Fig. 4.87, p. 358* ▷ *Fig. 4.88, p. 359* ▷ *Fig. 4.89, p. 359*	Ill-defined and heterogeneous tumor with surrounding edema and mass effect. Hemorrhage is common. Enhancement is heterogeneous with thick rim and central necrosis. Often involves corpus callosum. CSF spread in 20%.	Seven percent of all childhood brain tumors. Biphasic, peaks around 4–5 y and 11–12 y. Ninety percent are supratentorial. Frontal most common location.

(continues on page 359)

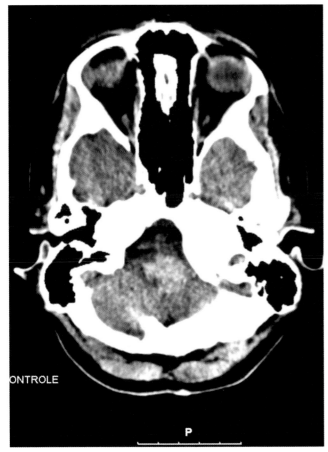

Fig. 4.80   CT of a 12.5-year-old girl with a low-grade **astrocytoma in the brainstem** at the medulla-oblongata level.

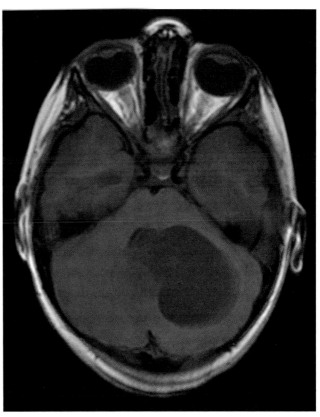

Fig. 4.81   **Astrocytoma** in a 4-year-old girl with an abducens paresis due to a solid tumor with cystic component in the posterior fossa. On T1-weighed image the solid and cystic part of the tumor is hypointense.

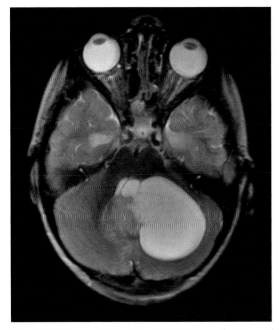

Fig. 4.82   Same patient as **Fig. 4.81**. Note, on the T2-weighted image, the different signal intensities of the cystic components and the lack of perifocal edema.

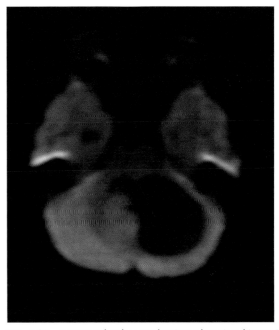

Fig. 4.83   A tumor that has predominant low signal intensity on the trace map of this DWI suggests that it is a low-grade tumor, such as a **pilocytic astrocytoma**.

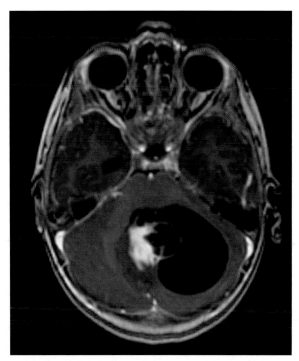

Fig. 4.84 Pilocytic astrocytoma shows strong enhancement of the solid part of the tumor and of the cystic tumoral wall. The cystic component in the left cerebellar hemisphere does not enhance and may not be a tumoral cyst.

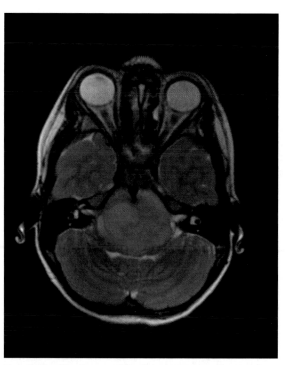

Fig. 4.85 Classic pontine glioma suspected in a 6.5-year-old girl with headache for 1 week and bilateral papilledema and left-sided abducens nerve paresis. It is slightly hyperintense to gray matter on the T2-weighted image; note the basilar encasement.

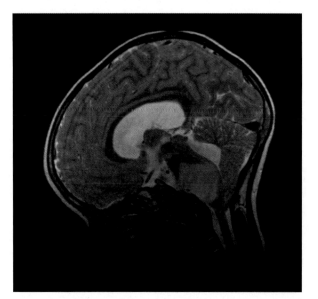

Fig. 4.86 Brainstem glioma. Note enlargement of brainstem due to diffuse infiltration on the T2-weighted image.

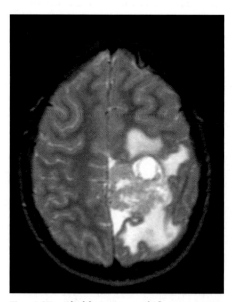

Fig. 4.87 Glioblastoma multiforme. An 11-year-old boy with abducens (VI) paresis, hydrocephalus, and peripheral edema. Tumor with cystic and solid components is in the left hemisphere.

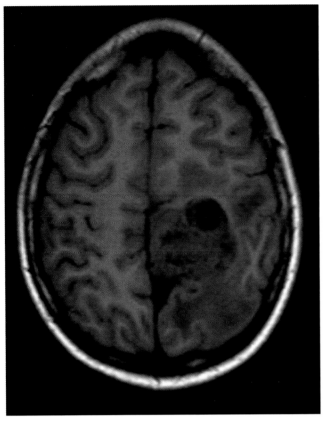

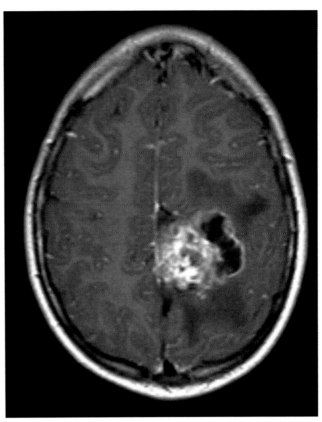

Fig. 4.88   Glioblastoma multiforme. T1-weighted image shows an inhomogeneous tumor with isointense solid parts and hypointense cystic parts.

Fig. 4.89   Glioblastoma multiforme. T1-weighted image after Gd shows inhomogeneous enhancement.

Table 4.22   (Cont.) Brain tumors

Diagnosis	Findings	Comments
Primitive neuroectodermal tumor (PNET) ▷ *Fig. 4.90, p. 360* ▷ *Fig. 4.91, p. 360*	On CT, the tumor is heterogeneous and well-circumscribed. Solid component hyperdense due to high cellularity and high cellular nucleus-to-cytoplasm ratio. On MRI, signal intensity on T1 and T2 is heterogeneous due to hemorrhage, calcifications, and cystic changes. Relatively little peritumoral edema. Solid component enhances homogeneously, heterogeneously, or not at all.	Second most frequent pediatric tumor (20%). The classic PNET is a medulloblastoma (see subsequent discussion), making up 85% of this group of tumors. The rest (15%) is supratentorial.
Medulloblastoma ▷ *Fig. 4.92, p. 360* ▷ *Fig. 4.93, p. 360*	Hyperdense mass with sharp margins on CT; on MRI iso- to hyperintense on T2-weighted images. Signal on T2-weighted images may be heterogeneous due to calcification, cyst, necrosis, hemorrhage, and vascular voids. In approximately 80%, the tumor is in the midline	Cerebellar PNET, most commonly arising at the middle and inferior portions of the anterior vermis. Most common posterior fossa tumor in children. At initial diagnosis, approximately 40% have leptomeningeal metastases. In adolescents and young adults, the tumor is usually located in the cerebellar hemispheres.

(continues on page 361)

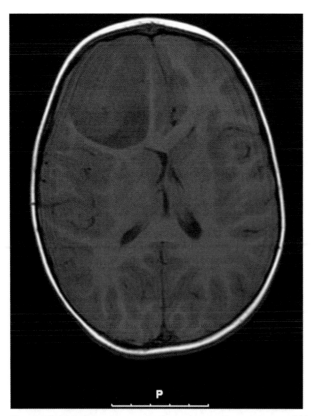

Fig. 4.90 Primitive neuroectodermal tumor in a 2.5-year-old boy with a space-occupying process right frontal lobe. He has nausea, vomiting, and confusion and an intra-axially located tumor involving the cortex with solid and cystic components.

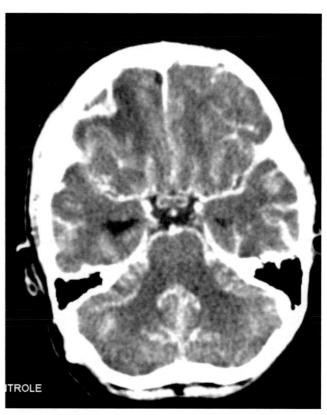

Fig. 4.91 Primitive neuroectodermal tumor. Note, on this CECT, the pathological enhancement of the meninges infra- and supratentorially.

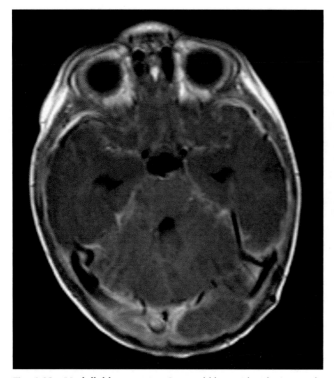

Fig. 4.92 Medulloblastoma in a 2-year-old boy with enhancing subarachnoid spaces due to leptomeningeal metastases.

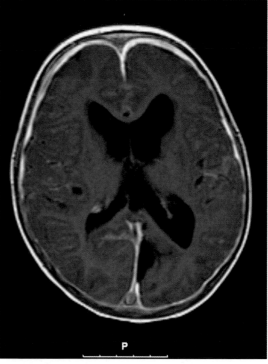

Fig. 4.93 Medulloblastoma. Note the pathological enhancement of the dura.

Table 4.22   (Cont.) Brain tumors

Diagnosis	Findings	Comments
Ependymoma ▷ *Fig. 4.94* ▷ *Fig. 4.95* ▷ *Fig. 4.96, p. 362* ▷ *Fig. 4.97, p. 362* ▷ *Fig. 4.98, p. 362*	On CT, the tumor is isodense and, in 50%, partially calcified and has a variable enhancement. Tumor margins often irregular and ill-defined due to infiltration of surrounding tissues. On MRI, signal intensity often variable due to calcifications, cysts, and hemorrhage.	Arising from ependymal cells lining the ventricles and central canal of spinal cord. Approximately 70% are infratentorial. Tumor tends to invade the cerebellopontine angle through the foramen of Luschka and the cisterna magna through the foramen of Magendie, often causing hydrocephalus.
Ganglion cell tumors ▷ *Fig. 4.99, p. 362*	On CT usually hypodense, well circumscribed with little or no mass effect, and peripheral in location. On MRI, the imaging findings are nonspecific.	Most tumors are composed of a mixture of ganglion cells and glial elements. May occur anywhere in the neural axis, commonly in the temporal lobe. Seizures are the most common presentation. Within the cerebellum, dysplastic gangliocytoma may occur, known as Lhermitte-Duclos disease. One tumor type usually presents in the first year of life: desmoplastic infantile ganglioglioma. Seizures and macrocephaly are the most common presentations.
Dysembryoplastic neuroepithelial tumor	On CT, the tumor is usually well circumscribed and hypodense with a cystic appearance. On MRI, the lesion is hypointense on T1 and hyperintense on T2. No peritumoral edema. Thinning of the inner table may be seen.	Locations: intracortical, multinodular, and supratentorial. The most frequent location is the temporal lobe. Present as partial complex seizures.
Oligodendrogliomas	On CT, usually well circumscribed, hypodense, partially calcified in a cortical or subcortical location. On MRI, the tumor is hypointense on T1-weighted images and hyperintense on T2-weighted images.	Approximately 95% occur in the cerebral hemispheres, favoring the frontal lobes. In the pediatric population, tumor calcification, enhancement, and peritumoral edema occur less frequently.

(continues on page 363)

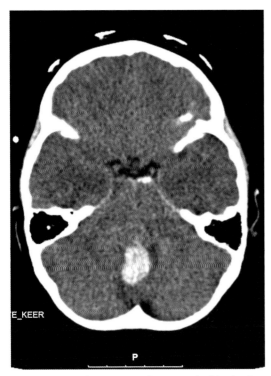

Fig. 4.94   Ependymoma. CT of a 20-month-old girl with an infratentorial hyperdense mass in the midline due to bleeding in an ependymoma.

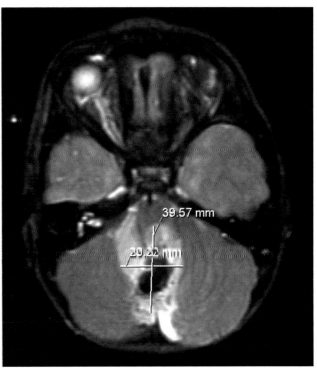

Fig. 4.95   Ependymoma. MRI of the same patient as **Fig. 4.94** shows an infratentorial mass in the midline, centrally hypointense on this T2-weighted image due to bleeding in the ependymoma. A more hyperintense extension of the tumor at the dorsal part of the brainstem and in the foramen of Luska on the right is noted.

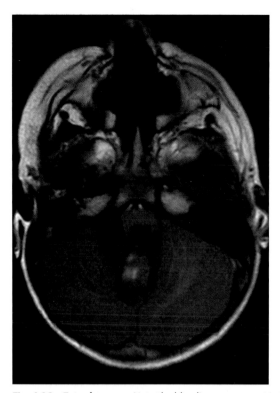

Fig. 4.96 Ependymoma. Note the bleeding component in the tumor on this T1-weighted image.

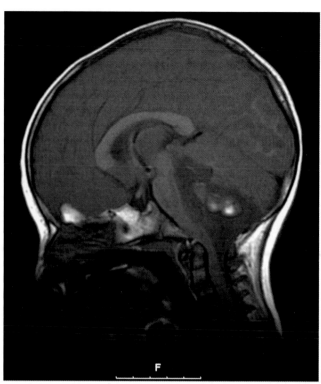

Fig. 4.97 Ependymoma. Sagittal image confirms the infratentorial mass in the midline that is centrally inhomogeneous iso-/hyperintense on this T1-weighted image because of bleeding in an ependymoma. A more hypointense extension of the tumor at the dorsal part of the brainstem results in compression of the brainstem against the clivus. Note the extension of the tumor through the foramen of Magendie.

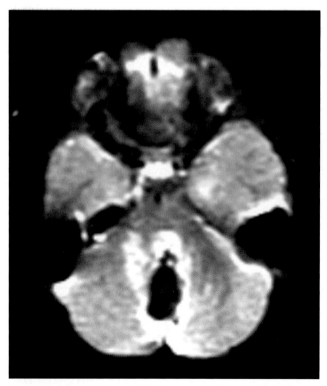

Fig. 4.98 Ependymoma. DWI shows central hypointensity due to bleeding; the more hyperintense extension of the tumor of the dorsal part of the brainstem and in the foramen of Luska on the right favors the ependymoma diagnosis.

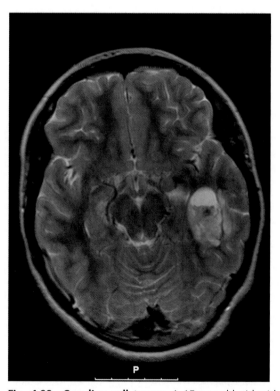

Fig. 4.99 Ganglion cell tumor. A 15-year-old girl with a space-occupying process in the left temporal lobe with daily headaches, occasionally with dizziness, and problems finding the right words, but no nausea or visual impairment. On this T2-weighted image, the lesion is suspected to be a ganglioglioma.

Table 4.22   (Cont.) Brain tumors

Diagnosis	Findings	Comments
Choroid plexus tumors	On CT, isodense to hyperdense intraventricular tumor with punctate calcifications and marked homogeneous enhancement. Most common at the trigone region. On MRI, hypo- to isointense on T1 and heterogeneous on T2, with areas of signal loss due to calcifications and vascular flow voids. Bifocal lesions occur in 14% of cases. No distinction between CPP and CPC. Parenchymal invasion and metastatic nodules in the ventricles are suggestive for CPC.	Seventy percent consist of CPP; the rest are CPCs. CPP commonly presents within the first year of life. In children, usually in the lateral ventricle; in adults, more in fourth ventricle. Principal symptom is increased ICP secondary to hydrocephalus.
Atypical teratoid/rhabdoid tumors (ATRT)	Radiologic presentation includes multiple prominent cystic and necrotic areas associated with an inhomogeneous contrast-enhancing solid component.	ATRT is most common in the pediatric age group, 94% of whom are 5 y of age or less at diagnosis. They may arise anywhere in the CNS. The distribution is as follows: 52% in the posterior fossa (the cerebellum being the predominant site); 39% supratentorial; 5% in the pineal region; 2% in the spine; and 2% are multifocal.
Craniopharyngiomas ▷ *Fig. 4.100a–c*	The rule of 90s: 90% cystic, 90% calcify, 90% enhance. Calcifications are curvilinear and along the periphery of the tumor. Enhancement of solid component and cyst wall distinguish it from epidermoids (no enhancement). On CT, heterogeneous enhancement, with solid and cystic parts and calcifications. On MRI, cysts are often hyperintense on T1 and hypo- or hyperintense on T2, depending on protein concentration and the presence of free methemoglobin.	Most common nonneuroepithelial tumor in children. Ninety-four percent are suprasellar, but they can be entirely intrasellar or intraventricular within the third ventricle. Often involve adjacent structures causing impairment of vision, disturbance of endocrine control, and sometimes involvement of memory and cranial nerves. Peak age is between 10 and 20 y.

(continues on page 364)

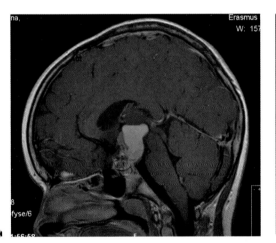
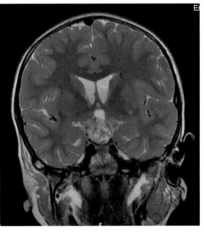
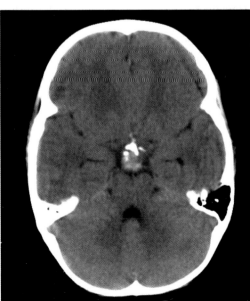

Fig. 4.100a–c   Craniopharyngioma in a 7-year-old girl with visual impairment. (**a**) On CT, chunks of calcification are visible. (**b**) On T1-weighted image, the tumor has high signal intensity because of "motor oil" content. (**c**) T2-weighted image shows small cysts, all of which are compatible with the diagnosis of craniopharyngioma.

Table 4.22 (Cont.) Brain tumors

Diagnosis	Findings	Comments
Pineal region tumors ▷ *Fig. 4.101* ▷ *Fig. 4.102* ▷ *Fig. 4.103* ▷ *Fig. 4.104* ▷ *Fig. 4.105*	On CT, germ cell tumors (GCTs) and pineal cell tumors (PCTs) are hyperdense, often well-circumscribed. On MR, GCTs are slightly hypo- to isointense on T1 and iso- to hyperintense on T2. Hemorrhage and cysts may be seen. In tumors with a teratoma component, the imaging characteristics on CT and MRI are those of fat. Calcifications do occur. Factors pointing to a high degree of malignancy are necrosis, hemorrhage, local invasion, and CSF spread.	Ten percent of all pediatric brain tumors. Most tumors are GCTs (50%–70%). The rest are PCTs (15%–30%). Nonneoplastic lesions do occur, like PCTs, arachnoid cysts, lipoma, and (epi-) dermoid. Of GCTs, the majority (65%) are germinoma. CSF spread is seen in 8%–18% of cases. Parinaud syndrome (paralysis of upward gaze) in 50%–75% of cases. Peak age for germinoma 10–15 y.
Hypothalamic hamartoma	CT is not a good imaging modality, because the lesion is isodense to brain and does not enhance. On MRI, the mass is well circumscribed, nonenhancing, and has a signal intensity on T1 and T2 comparable to gray matter. Uncommonly, the mass may have large cystic components. No calcifications.	Congenital nonneoplastic heterotopias containing ectopic rests of gray and white matter. Located at the tuber cinereum or mamillary bodies. Clinical presentation consists of precocious puberty and less commonly seizures, especially gelastic type. Often associated abnormalities include polymicrogyria, heterotopia, callosal agenesis, and facial and heart anomalies. Association with extracranial anamolies is known as Pallister-Hall syndrome.

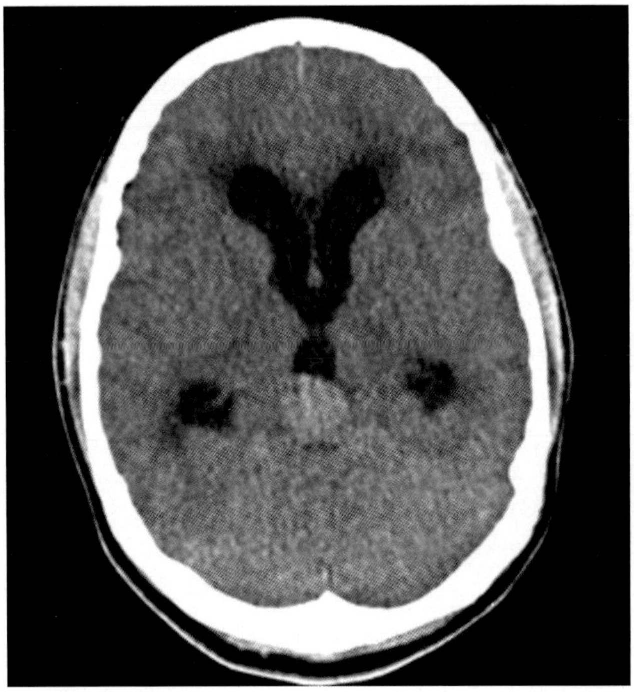

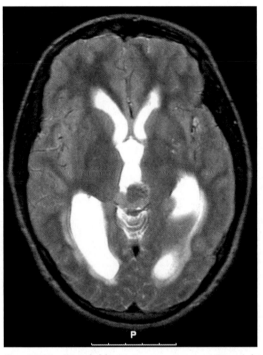

Fig. 4.101 Pinealoblastoma in a 13-year-old girl presenting with a headache. CT shows a dense midline tumor at the pineal gland region. Also note the triventricular ventricular dilatation.

Fig. 4.102 Pinealoblastoma, as seen on a T2-weighted image of the midline tumor in the pineal gland region, shows a relative high signal intensity, suggesting a highly cellular tumor with triventricular hydrocephalus with transependymal leakage. The hypointense areas suggest calcification or hemorrhage.

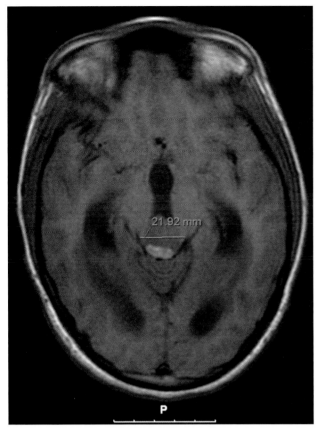

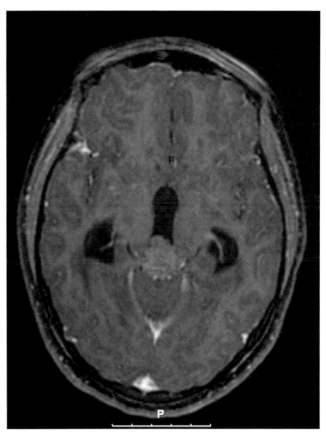

Fig. 4.103 Pinealoblastoma. As seen on T1-weighted image, the midline tumor in the pineal gland region shows a relatively high signal intensity, suggesting calcification or hemorrhage.

Fig. 4.104 On Gd-enhanced T1-weighted image, the midline **pineal region lesion** enhances homogeneously.

Fig. 4.105 This sagittal Gd-enhanced T1-weighted image shows a **pineal region lesion**. Note the increased pressure on the posterior fossa and the tonsils herniating through foramen magnum.

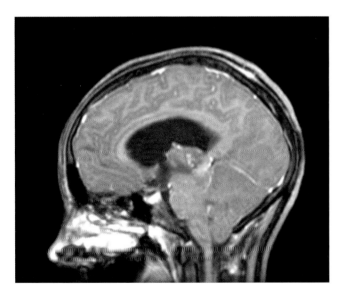

Table 4.23 "Secondary" intracranial tumors

Diagnosis	Findings	Comments
Neuroblastoma ▷ *Fig. 4.106* ▷ *Fig. 4.107* ▷ *Fig. 4.108* ▷ *Fig. 4.109* ▷ *Fig. 4.110* ▷ *Fig. 4.111*	On plain CT, there is bony destruction with soft-tissue mass. On bone window, there is a sunburst appearance. After contrast, there is patchy enhancement. On MRI, isointense on T1-weighted and hyperintense on T2-weighted images. Bony part is hypointense on T2. Postcontrast marked enhancement, and better delineation of meningeal involvement.	Classical areas are lateral orbital ridge with exophtalmos.
Metastases ▷ *Fig. 4.112, p. 368* ▷ *Fig. 4.113, p. 368*	Nonspecific mass lesion. If hemorrhagic, think of metastasis of neuroblastoma and melanoma.	Rare. Seen in association with Wilms tumor, clear cell sarcoma, Ewing sarcoma, osteosarcoma, and rhabdomyosarcoma.
Leukemia	Leukemic infiltrates often hemorrhagic, with surrounding edema. Postcontrast moderate to marked enhancement on CT and MRI.	

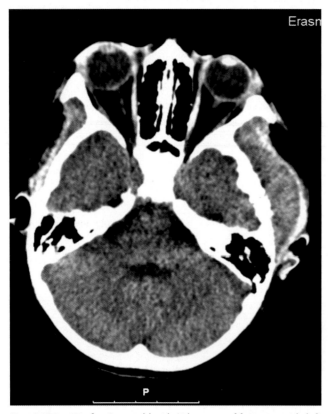

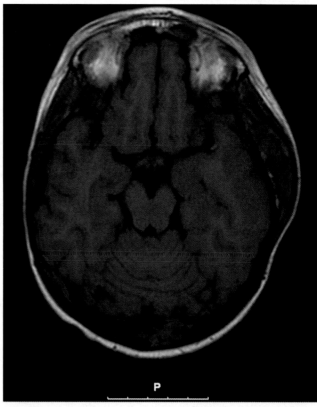

Fig. 4.106 CT of a 5-year-old girl with a **neuroblastoma** with left temporal with bone involvement.

Fig. 4.107 MRI of the same patient in **Fig. 4.106** with a **neuroblastoma**: a left temporal soft-tissue mass that is isointense on this T1-weighted image.

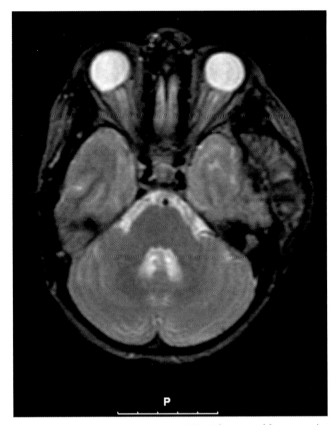

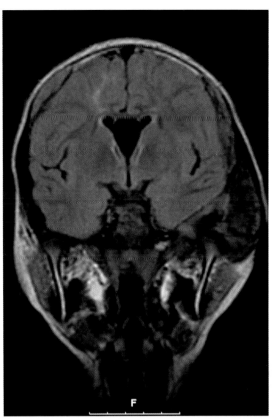

Fig. 4.108 Same patient as in **Fig. 4.106** with a **neuroblastoma**: the left temporal mass is inhomogeneous and iso-/hypointense on this T2-weighted image.

Fig. 4.109 Same patient as in **Fig. 4.106** with a **neuroblastoma**: on this coronal FLAIR image, the left temporal soft-tissue metastasis is inhomogeneous and iso-/hypointense. Note also the bone metastases in the right and left frontal bone.

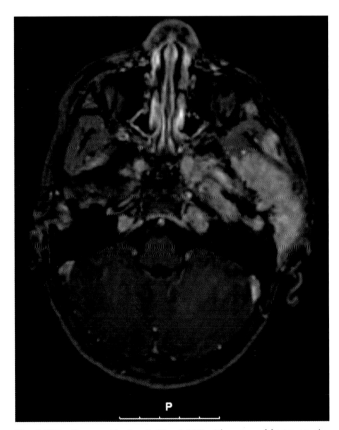

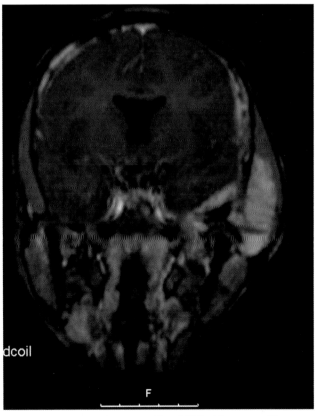

Fig. 4.110 Same patient as in **Fig. 4.106** with a **neuroblastoma**: the neuroblastoma metastasis at the left temporal site shows diffuse enhancement. Note also the pathological enhancement of the left part of the skull base.

Fig. 4.111 Same patient as in **Fig. 4.106** with a **neuroblastoma**: note also the pathological enhancement of the skull base and leptomeninges (coronal image).

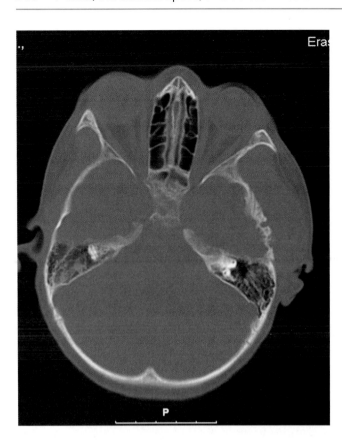

Fig. 4.112 CT of a 5-year-old girl with a **neuroblastoma and bone metastases**, presenting as abnormal, hyperostoic temporal bone with lytic lesions on the left. Note also the accompanying soft-tissue component.

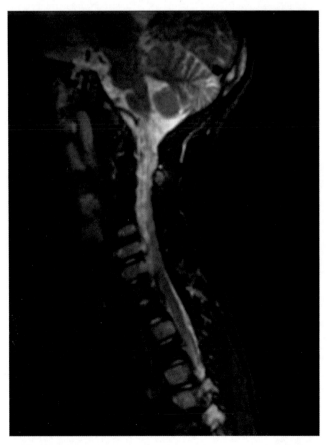

Fig. 4.113 A 5-year-old girl with a **neuroblastoma and bone metastases**, presenting as abnormal, hyperintense cervical and thoracic vertebrae on this short inversion-time inversion-recovery image.

The Orbits

Table 4.24 Small orbit

Diagnosis	Findings	Comments
Anophthalmia/microphthalmia	CT/MRI: proportionate decrease in size of orbit on all imaging modalities. Absent ocular tissue in anophthalmia. Small complete globe in simple microphthalmia; small abnormal globe with coloboma in complex micropthalmia. Globe size abnormalities may be associated with intracranial abnormalities.	Micropthalmia may be associated with coloboma, congenital infections, retinopathy of prematurity, or persistent hyperplastic primary vitreous (PHPV). May see hypertelorism or hyperplastic ethmoid air cells.
Postenucleation/radiotherapy	CT: orbital growth ceases. May get thickening of the orbital walls with time.	Get a greater degree of deformity in younger children.
Fibrous dysplasia	Radiograph/CT: sclerotic ground-glass appearance with thickening and resultant decreased orbital size.	When also involving adjacent facial bones, there is leonine appearance (leontiasis ossea).
Osteopetrosis/thalassemia/ severe anaemia	Radiograph/CT: due to hyperostosis.	
Mass effect from expansile process in adjacent sinus ▷ Fig. 4.114	CT/MRI: orbital walls are displaced causing deformity and decreased size.	Usually mucocoele or tumor.

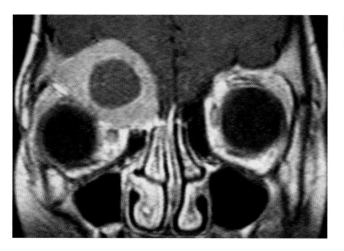

Fig. 4.114 Mass effect from expansile process in adjacent sinus. T1-weighted postcontrast coronal MRI shows right frontal ossifying fibroma displacing orbital roof.

Table 4.25 Enlarged orbit

Diagnosis	Findings	Comments
Macrocephaly/hydrocephalus	All imaging modalities: spurious enlargement due to large skull.	Bilateral and symmetric.
Buphthalmos ▷ Fig. 4.115, p. 370	Radiograph/CT: asymmetrical enlargement with characteristic globe appearance. Need to exclude tumor.	(see **Table 4.29**)
Orbital space-occupying lesion	All imaging modalities: degree of enlargement related to rate of growth of lesion.	Orbital enlargement not uncommon.
NF ▷ Fig. 4.116, p. 370	Radiograph/CT: elevation of lesser wing of sphenoid and associated dysplasia giving "bare orbit" appearance. Also, see widening of the optic canal.	Usually unilateral. Need MRI to assess for associated optic glioma.

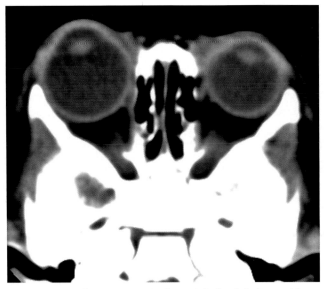

Fig. 4.115   Axial noncontrast CT shows right **buphthalmos** with en-larged, elongated right globe.

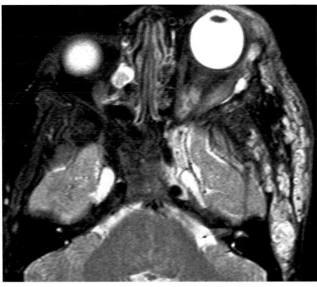

Fig. 4.116   T2 axial MRI shows left **buphthalmos, sphenoid wing dysplasia, and frontotemporal plexiform neurofibroma** showing the characteristic "target" sign appearance (hyperintense periphery/ hypointense center) in NF1.

Table 4.26   Hypertelorism

Diagnosis	Findings	Comments
Micro-/anophthalmia	Due to compensatory enlargement of ethmoid air cells.	(see **Table 4.24**)
Craniosynostosis ▷ **Fig. 4.117**	In bicoronal synostosis and related syndromes (Apert, Crouzon, and Pfeiffer syndromes).	
Greig syndrome	Dolichocephaly, anomalies of facial bones and extremeties.	Mental retardation.
Fibrous dysplasia	Involving ethmoid air cells with characteristic findings.	(see **Table 4.31**)
Midline facial defects/ cephalocoeles ▷ **Fig. 4.118** ▷ **Fig. 4.119**	CT: thin-slice axial and coronal shows defect in frontal bone. MRI: assessment of cranial contents and associated brain abnormalities.	

- Interorbital distance is greater than normal.
- Mild hypertelorism occurs in multiple syndromes (cleidocra-nial dysostosis/trisomy 13/Hurler syndrome/thalassemia).
- It may be isolated, familial, and of no clinical significance.

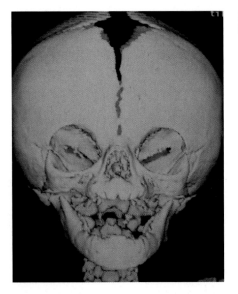

Fig. 4.117   Coronal 3D CT shows **bicoronal synostosis** with harlequin eye appearance and hypertelorism.

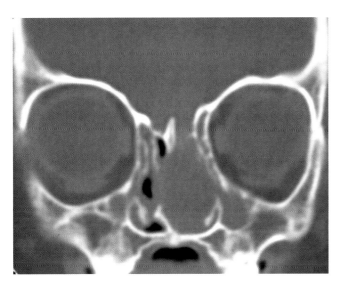

Fig. 4.118 Coronal CT (bone window) shows **nasoethmoidal cephalocele**, a defect in the left frontal bone with herniation of intracranial contents into left ethmoid air cells and resultant hypertelorism.

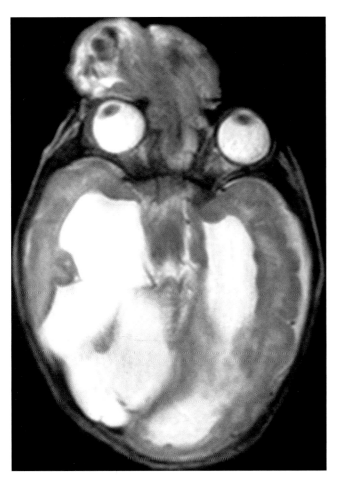

Fig. 4.119 T2 axial MRI shows hypertelorism due to **nasofrontal cephalocele**.

Table 4.27   Hypotelorism

Diagnosis	Findings	Comments
Down syndrome	Small calvarium and hypoplastic maxillae.	
Metopic and sagittal synostosis ▷ **Fig. 4.120**	Radiographs/CT: characteristic skull shape with premature fusion of metopic and sagittal sutures.	May see hypoplastic ethmoid sinuses.
Holoprosencephaly	CT/MRI: Midline malformation. Alobar is most severe.	Associated with midface hypoplasia.

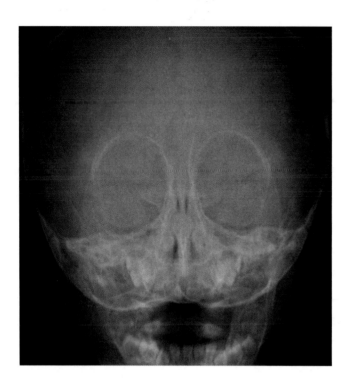

Fig. 4.120 AP skull radiograph shows **metopic synostosis** with medial and upward angulation of the orbits and hypotelorism.

Table 4.28   Microphthalmia

Diagnosis	Findings	Comments
Congenital	CT/MRI: Small globe (see **Table 4.24**). MRI is best imaging modality to assess internal structure of globe, ocular contents, and brain.	Many chromosomal abnormalities: sporadic, AD, recessive, and X-linked forms. One-third of cases have associated cranial malformations. Consider genetic counseling.
Congenital infections (rubella, CMV, syphilis)	CT: Small globe that may contain calcification. Usually have other manifestations of disease; therefore, CT brain indicated to assess for calcification.	Uni- or bilateral.
Persistent hyperplastic primary vitreous	CT: High-density vitreous. No calcification.	Leukocoria at birth (see **Table 4.30**).
Retinopathy of prematurity	Leukocoria.	Appropriate clinical history (see **Table 4.30**).
Trauma ▷ **Fig. 4.121**	All imaging modalities: small, shrunken, distorted globe.	Appropriate history.
Phthisis bulbi	CT: small calcified globe.	End result of destructive process.
Maternal exposure (alcohol, benomyl, thalidomide, retinoic acid, lysergic acid diethylamide [also known as LSD], hydantoin)	Small globe that may contain normal anatomic structures or be malformed.	Correlate with clinical history.
Surgery	Imaging findings depend on cause of surgery.	Appropriate history.

- Globe with total axial length < 2 standard deviations below mean for age
- Less than 19 mm in 1 year old and < 21 mm in adult

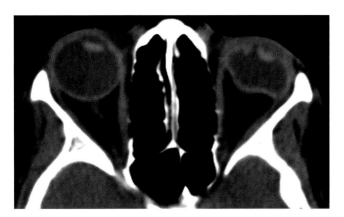

Fig. 4.121 Posttrauma axial noncontrast CT shows distorted small left globe due to rupture.

Table 4.29 Macrophthalmia/buphthalmos

Diagnosis	Findings	Comments
Isolated buphthalmos ▷ *Fig. 4.115, p. 370*	Enlarged globe, proptosis, and eyelid swelling without raised pressure.	
Congenital glaucoma	CT/MRI: enlarged, elongated globe with clinical finding of increased pressure—primary and bilateral in 80%.	Child < 3 y. Medical or surgical treatment indicated. If not treated, follow-up imaging will show progressive decrease in size of globe.
Axial myopia	Enlargement of AP diameter of the globe.	Present with visual impairment. Older children.
Colobomatous macrophthalmia	Syndrome of macrophthalmia, coloboma, and microcornea.	AD.
Phakomatoses (NF1 and Sturge-Weber syndrome) ▷ *Fig. 4.116, p. 370*	CT: Enlarged, elongated globe. Look for sphenoid wing dysplasia and plexiform neurofibroma in NF and characteristic intracranial appearances in Sturge-Weber syndrome.	NF: it was thought that plexiform neurofibroma infiltrates angle of ciliary body. Occurs in 50%. Sturge-Weber syndrome: angiomatous change in ciliary body or angle of anterior chamber.
Intraocular mass	Enlarged globe with intraocular mass.	(see **Table 4.33**)
Staphyloma	CT: focal bulge posteriorly with thinning of the sclera.	Infections, scleritis, trauma, and glaucoma predispose to development of focal bupthalmos.

- Globe is larger than normal for age.
- Greater than 12 mm in infants.
- Greater than 23.5 mm in the mature globe.

Table 4.30   Leukokoria

Diagnosis	Findings	Comments
Retinoblastoma ▷ *Fig. 4.122* ▷ *Fig. 4.123*	CT: Non-contrast–enhanced CT (NECT) best for identifying calcification. CECT sees variable enhancement of noncalcified portion of mass and normal sized/enlarged globe. MRI: Best for extraocular and intracranial disease. Mass hyperintense on T1 and hypointense on T2 relative to vitreous. Postcontrast heterogeneous enhancement. Image whole brain to assess for pineal (trilateral) and suprasellar (quadrilateral) disease.	Calcification rarely seen in other lesions in children < 3 y. Unilateral in 75%. Bilateral and multifocal in 25% is more often familial and must be screened for pineal and suprasellar involvement.
PHPV ▷ *Fig. 4.124*	NECT: Microphthalmia, small irregular lens, no calcification, and hyperdense vitreous chamber. Abnormal vitreal tissue may enhance. Linear hyperdensity extending from retina to lens represents Cloquet canal and persistent hyaloid artery. MRI: High-signal vitreous on T1 and T2, fluid levels as a result of hemorrhage. Also demonstrates canal as previously.	Presents in infancy with leukocoria, microphthalmia, and cataract. Sporadic disease unilateral; bilateral usually part of multisystem syndrome.
Coats disease ▷ *Fig. 4.125*	CT: High-density vitreous, no calcification, and is indistinguishable from noncalcified retinoblastoma. Vitreous contains wing-shaped retinal detachment. MRI: superior for subretinal effusion—high signal on T1 and T2.	Usually boys, unilateral. Present from birth but present near end of first decade when retina detaches and vision deteriorates.
Retinopathy of prematurity	CT: Noncalcified, retrolental, hyperdense mass that may be associated with retinal detachment. May be calcified and microphthalmic if chronic. MRI: findings nonspecific.	Uni- or bilateral in setting of appropriate medical history.
Toxocara canis infection	CT: opaque vitreous or a localized irregular, nonenhancing retinal mass. No calcification.	Present at approximate 6 y. History of close contact with dogs and positive serology are suggestive.
Retinal astrocytoma	CT/MRI: intraocular mass(es) with or without exudative retinal detachment, hemorrhage, and calcification.	Rare; isolated or in association with tuberous sclerosis or less commonly NF or retinitis pigmentosa. May be bilateral.
Retinal hemangioma	CT/MRI: Hemorrhage and often retinal detachment. Post-CE of retina.	Rare.
Medulloepithelioma	CT/MRI: markedly enhancing tumor that may erode the orbital wall or induce hyperostosis.	Rare tumor located anterior to the iris. Occasionally may arise next to the optic nerve. Lack of calcification helps differentiate it from retinoblastoma.
Retinal dysplasia/Norrie disease	CT: microphthalmia and dense vitreous with blood-fluid level. Often also have calcification and retinal detachment.	X-linked recessive, have seizures, mental deficiency and deafness by age 4 y.

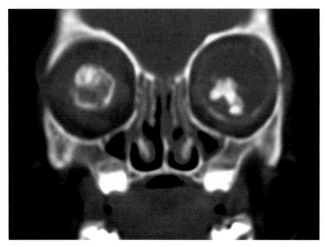

Fig. 4.122   Coronal CT (bone window) shows bilateral calcified intraocular masses consistent with **retinoblastomas**.

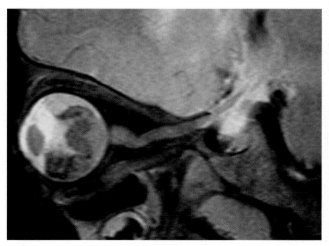

Fig. 4.123   T2-weighted fat-saturated sagittal oblique MRI shows intraocular mass with extension into proximal optic nerve and showing T2-weighted hypointensity in keeping with calcification—traits that are characteristic of a **retinoblastoma**.

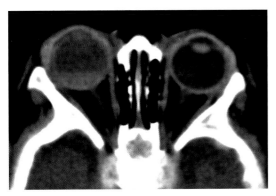

Fig. 4.124 Persistent hyperplastic primary vitreous. Axial noncontrasted CT shows high-density fluid level in PHPV due to hemorrhage within the right eye.

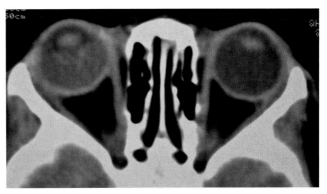

Fig. 4.125   Axial noncontrast CT shows high-density vitreous without focal mass or calcification in **Coats disease** of the right eye.

Table 4.31   Orbital sclerosis

Diagnosis	Findings	Comments
Fibrous dysplasia	Radiograph/CT: sclerosis, hyperostosis, and bone expansion of one or both orbits. Characteristic ground-glass appearance.	May also have exophthalmos.
LCH	Radiograph/CT: in the healing phase previously lucent lesion will show sclerosis.	Skeletal survey may show other characteristic bone lesions.
Chronic osteomyelitis	Radiograph/CT: sclerosis adjacent to chronically infected frontal sinus.	
Osteoma	Radiograph/CT: Well circumscribed sclerotic lesion in frontal sinus. Orbital roof can be displaced and sclerotic.	
Osteopetrosis	Radiograph/CT: sclerosing dysplasia with widespread bone involvement.	Skeletal survey will show characteristic appearance of long bones and spine.
Infantile cortical hyperostosis (Caffey disease)	Radiograph/CT: thickening and sclerosis of predominantly upper and lateral orbital walls.	Skeletal survey will show other areas of involvement especially mandible (see **Table 4.45**).
Radiotherapy	Radiograph/CT: sclerosis posttargeted radiotherapy.	Correlate with history.

Orbital Calcification

Table 4.32   Pitfalls: lens density, foreign bodies, and projection of intracranial calcification

Diagnosis	Findings	Comments
Retinoblastoma ▷ **Fig. 4.122**	Radiograph/CT: Uni- or bilateral. Greater than 95% calcifcation. Globe normal size or enlarged.	(see **Table 4.30**)
Cataract	CT: calcification in lens and limbus.	
Retinopathy of prematurity	CT: calcification of vitreous body if chronic.	Uni- or bilateral (see **Table 4.30**).
Phthisis bulbi	Radiograph/CT: small shrunken calcified globe.	
Vascular malformation	Radiograph/CT: ateriovascular malformation or hemangioma with calcified phleboliths.	Calcify rarely (see **Table 4.30**).
Optic nerve head drusen	CT: dystrophic calcification related to optic nerve heads.	Idiopathic and asymptomatic.

Orbital Masses

Table 4.33   Globe

Diagnosis	Findings	Comments
Retinoblastoma ▷ *Fig. 4.122, p. 374* ▷ *Fig. 4.123, p. 374*	Radiograph/CT: usually calcified mass in child < 3 y.	(see **Table 4.30**)
Hemangioma	CT/MRI: usually intra-/extraconal but may spread to involve globe. Best imaged with MRI to assess extent.	(see **Table 4.35**)
Melanoma	MRI: T1 hypointense mass related to choroids, which enhances with contrast. CT: enhancing mass.	Older children/teenagers. Best imaged with MRI.

Table 4.34   Intraconal/involving muscle cone

Diagnosis	Findings	Comments
Optic nerve glioma ▷ *Fig. 4.126a, b*	MRI: Best to evaluate extent. Mass isointense/slightly hyperintense to normal white matter on T1 and T2 and shows prominent CE. Causes fusiform enlargement of nerve, which is buckled and kinked.	One-third in the setting of NF1 and characteristically bilateral.
Hemangioma	CT/MRI: usually extraconal but some lesions intraconal.	(see **Table 4.35**)
Inflammatory pseudotumor	CT/MRI: unilateral or bilateral uveoscleral thickening with enhancement, an enhancing retro-ocular mass, or enlargement of extraocular muscles, tendons, and lacrimal gland.	Idiopathic disorder with inflammatory, lymphoid infiltration of intraorbital tissues.
Lymphoma and metastases	CT/MRI: Lymphoma: diffuse infiltration of entire intraconal region. Shows slight to moderate enhancement. Metastases: neuroblastoma/rhabdomyosarcoma, usually also with extraconal and orbital wall involvement.	Lymphoma best imaged with MRI.
Hematoma	CT: Hyperdense if acute. CT best for evaluating fractures.	If traumatic, assess for foreign body.
Rhabdomyosarcoma ▷ *Fig. 4.127* ▷ *Fig. 4.128*	CT/MRI: May be primary or secondary. Usually intraconal or involving muscle but may extend extraconal and intracranial. MRI best for extent: T1 iso-/hypointense relative to muscle and T2 hyperintense. Degree of enhancement varies. Enhanced scans in coronal plane best for evaluating intracranial extension.	Usually embryonal subtype.

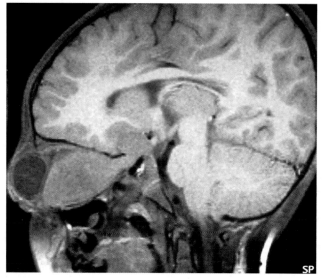
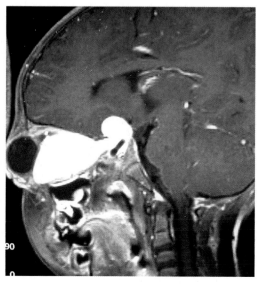

Fig. 4.126a, b   T1-weighted sagittal oblique pre- (**a**) and postcontrast (**b**) MRI: a right **optic nerve glioma** with fusiform enlargement of the nerve, which shows marked enhancement postcontrast.

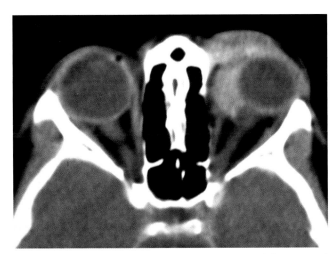

Fig. 4.127 Axial postcontrast CT shows enhancing left intraconal mass with anteromedial, extraconal extension. The biopsy proved **rhabdomyosarcoma**.

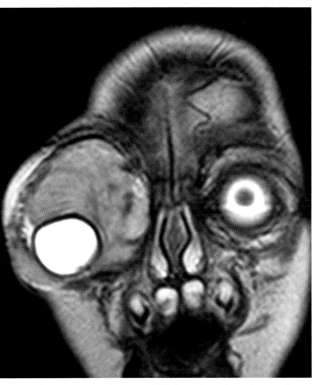

Fig. 4.128 T2-weighted coronal MRI shows large hyperintense **intraconal rhabdomyosarcoma** causing marked proptosis.

Table 4.35 Extraconal

Diagnosis	Findings	Comments
Dermoid/epidermoid ▷ *Fig. 4.129, p. 378*	CT/MRI: well-demarcated, anterior extraconal mass with fatty, fluid, or mixed contents. Majority superolateral related to frontozygomatic suture. CT shows osseous remodelling ± fine calcification in cyst wall.	MRI if features are not diagnostic or suspect deep extension into sinuses, masticator space, or intracranially.
Teratoma ▷ *Fig. 4.130, p. 378*	MRI: best for assessing extent. CT: best for showing calcification. Usually complex with cystic and solid elements, composed fat/fluid/calcium and soft tissue. Often marked expansion of the orbit and displacement of the globe.	Benign but cause severe progressive proptosis in infancy. Transspatial.
Capillary hemangioma	MRI is imaging modality of choice to show extent especially if suspected intracranial extension. Use enhanced T1 and T2, axial, and coronal planes. T1 iso- or hypointense, showing diffuse intense enhancement postcontrast. T2 heterogeneous/hyperintense with frequent flow voids. MRA unhelpful as vascular component is at capillary level. CT: slightly hyperdense homogeneous mass with intense enhancement.	Usually present before 6 mo. Only imaged if symptomatic or fail to involute.
Lymphatic, venous, and venolymphatic malformations	MRI best to show extent; use fat-saturated axial and coronal sequences. See multilocular, transspatial, variably enhancing mass. Fluid-fluid levels with signal corresponding to age of blood products. Pure lymphatic malformation is nonenhancing. Venolymphatic variable.	Present in childhood with progressive, slow-growing mass. Usually extraconal but often transspatial. Include brain imaging for associated intracranial abnormalities especially in venolymphatic malformations.
Malignancy (lacrimal gland/lymphoma/leukemia) ▷ *Fig. 4.131, p. 378*	Primary lacrimal gland malignancy rare and associated with bony destruction. Lymphoma/leukemia: well-defined high-density mass involving lacrimal gland or isolated soft-tissue mass.	May present with exophthalmos (see **Table 4.36**).
Orbital cellulitis/subperiosteal abscess ▷ *Fig. 4.132, p. 378*	CECT: thickening and edema of orbital soft tissues representing cellulitis and/or phlegmon. Low-density, rim-enhancing area represents subperiosteal abscess. Usually extraconal but can extend intraconally. Procure axial and coronal images.	Need brain imaging (CT or MRI) to evaluate intracranial complications of sinusitis. MRI more sensitive.

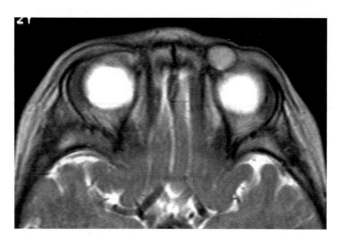

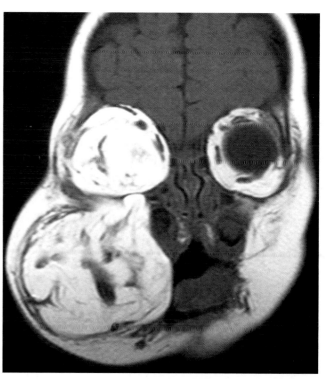

Fig. 4.129 T2-weighted axial MRI shows hyperintense medial extraconal mass related to frontoethmoidal suture, which is characteristic of a **dermoid cyst**.

Fig. 4.130 T1-weighted coronal MRI shows a large right extraconal mass with extension into right maxillary sinus and face. It is hyperintense on T1 with focal hypointensity in keeping with fat and calcification, which is characteristic of a **teratoma**.

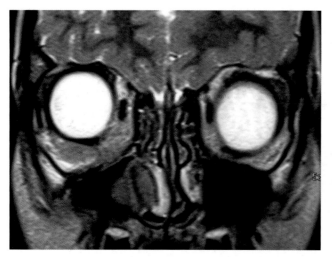

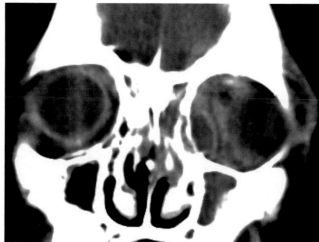

Fig. 4.131 T2 coronal MRI shows an intermediate signal intensity, inferior, extraconal mass, with a second mass seen centered on right maxillary sinus; biopsy proved it to be **lymphoma**.

Fig. 4.132 Orbital cellulitis/subperiosteal abscess. Peripheral rim-enhancing medial subperiosteal collection displacing the left globe laterally on coronal postcontrast CT. Note also the opacification of the left ethmoid and maxillary sinuses.

Table 4.36 Orbital wall

Diagnosis	Findings	Comments
Metastases/lymphoma/ leukemia ▷ *Fig. 4.133*	Radiograph/CT: show defect or destruction often not confined to orbits. CT/MRI shows adjacent soft-tissue mass and exophthalmos.	Most common causes are neuroblastoma, hematological malignancy, rhabdomyosarcoma, and Ewing sarcoma.
Extension from lacrimal gland/tumor	Radiograph/CT/MRI: Localized wall expansion adjacent to tumor. Lesions have a sclerotic rim.	
Spread of adjacent infection	CT: usually subperiosteal abscess but if longstanding may cause destruction of orbital wall.	Wall involvement usually due to aggressive pathogen particularly aggressive fungal sinus infections such as mucormycosis and aspergillosis (see **Table 4.35**).
Adjacent tumor	CT: ethmoid or maxillary antral tumors invade by direct extension.	
Mucocoele	Radiograph/CT: Bony expansion of adjacent sinus, which protrudes into orbit. Sinus may be sclerotic if chronically infected. Contains nonenhancing soft tissue.	Present with unilateral proptosis. Most common is frontal sinus with palpable mass in superomedial orbit.
LCH	Radiograph/CT: Single or multiple lytic lesions with beveled edges and adjacent soft-tissue mass. Often have exophthalmos. MRI needed if sphenoid bone involved and present with diabetes insipidus.	Need skeletal survey to look for other bone lesions.

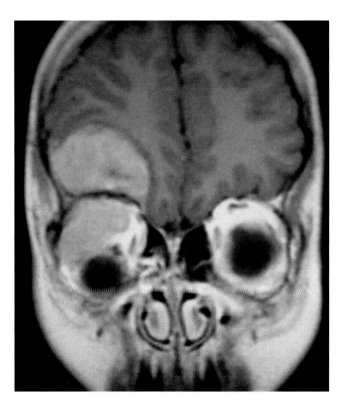

Fig. 4.133 T1-weighted coronal postcontrast MRI shows enhancing right extraconal mass with intracranial extension characteristic of **neuroblastoma metastases**.

Nasal Cavity

The Nares and Nasal Passages

Table 4.37   Opacification

Diagnosis	Findings	Comments
Choanal atresia/stenosis ▷ *Fig. 4.134*	CT: measure width of both posterior choanae at maximum stenosis and width of the inferoposterior vomer, which is abnormally widened.	Most common congenital abnormality of nasal cavity. Bony/membranous/mixed. Severe respiratory compromise if bilateral. Choanal airspace < 0.34 cm. Inability to pass nasogastric tube 3–4 cm into nose.
Foreign body ▷ *Fig. 4.135*	Lateral/AP radiograph: visible it radiopaque + soft-tissue swelling.	
Hypertrophied nasal turbinate ▷ *Fig. 4.136*	Lateral radiograph: soft-tissue mass encroaching on nasopharynx. Coronal CT/MRI: Asymmetry of turbinates is well demonstrated. No demonstrable air between wall and turbinate.	Can cause nasal airway obstruction. May be physiological nasal cycle.
Polyp ▷ *Fig. 4.137*	Radiograph: vague soft-tissue density in nasal fossa. CT/MRI: discrete single or multiple broad-based masses.	Uncommon in children. Associated with cystic fibrosis. If multiple, does not destroy septa.
Ossifying fibroma ▷ *Fig. 4.138*	CT: expansile, well-circumscribed lesion that ossifies starting around the periphery with central nonossified fibrous tissue.	Grows aggressively and may recur postsurgery.
Neoplasm (malignancy)	Extension into nasal cavity from sinus/pharyngeal/orbital tumor.	(see **Table 4.39**)

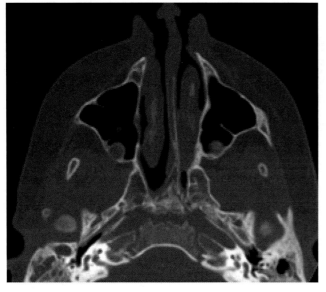

Fig. 4.134 Axial CT (bone window) shows left posterior **choanal atresia**.

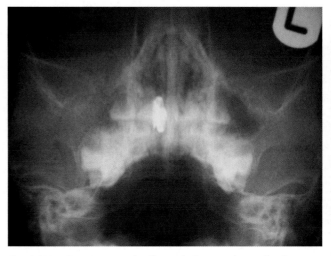

Fig. 4.135 Occipitomental radiograph shows right nasal radiopaque **foreign body**.

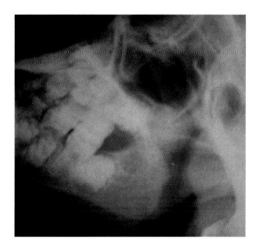

Fig. 4.136 Lateral radiograph of the nasopharynx shows a soft-tissue mass projected over the nasopharynx representing **hypertrophy of nasal turbinate**.

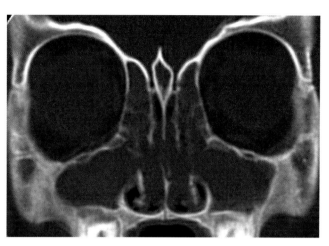

Fig. 4.137 Coronal CT (bone window) shows bilateral nasal, maxillary, and ethmoid sinus opacification in **polyposis**.

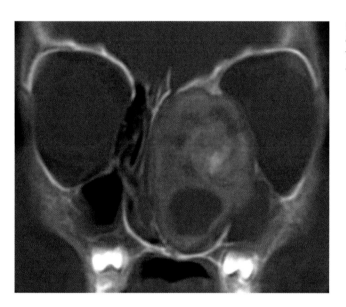

Fig. 4.138 Coronal CT (bone window) shows a well-circumscribed, expansile osseous lesion with a central nonossified portion centered in the left ethmoid sinus and nasal passage, which has the characteristic appearance of an **ossifying fibroma**.

Paranasal Sinuses

Table 4.38   Small/absent sinuses

Diagnosis	Findings	Comments
Congenital absence	Absence of frontal sinuses in 5% of population.	
Cretinism	Delayed/decreased pneumatisation of sinuses.	
Down syndrome	Absent frontal sinuses in 90%.	
Kartegener syndrome	Absent frontal sinuses.	
Fibrous dysplasia	Due to overgrowth of bony wall.	
Hemolytic anemia ▷ *Fig. 4.139, p. 382*	Overgrowth of bony wall.	
Postsurgery	Post Caldwell Luc operation.	

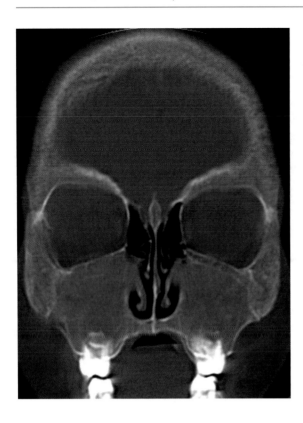

Fig. 4.139 Hemolytic anemia. Coronal CT (bone window) shows expanded marrow cavities and diploic space causing a "hair-on-end" appearance and obliteration of sinuses in thalassemia.

Table 4.39 Opacification of paranasal sinuses

Diagnosis	Findings	Comments
Sinusitis—acute and chronic	Radiograph/CT/MRI: homogeneous opacification, mucosal swelling or air-fluid levels. May see bony sclerosis or destruction if chronic.	CT important to assess for anatomic variations prior to functional endoscopic sinus surgery. Use low-dose coronal scans. Also useful to look for complications.
Trauma ▷ Fig. 4.140	Radiograph: soft-tissue swelling, maxillary sinus opacification, ± air-fluid level. CT: axial and coronal planes to visualize fracture.	
Polyp/retention cyst	Radiograph: Opacification of single maxillary antrum. Soft-tissue mass in anterior nasopharynx on lateral view. CT: homogeneous soft-tissue masses with smooth margins, outlined by air (e.g., mucocoele).	Sequelae of sinonasal inflammation.
Tooth bud	Radiograph: usually caused by projection and overlap. CT: shows true ectopic tooth bud within maxillary sinus.	
Osteoma	Radiograph/CT: well-defined bony density. Mainly in frontal sinuses; rarely ethmoid and maxillary.	Assess for Gardner syndrome.
Mucocoele ▷ Fig. 4.141	CT/MRI: appearance varies with water and mucoid content. Shows peripheral enhancement, distinguishing it from neoplasm. Exhibits mass effect on adjacent structures and often expands into orbit.	Due to obstruction of sinus ostium. Most commonly frontal and ethmoid sinuses.
Primary malignancy ▷ Fig. 4.142a, b	CT/MRI: MRI preferred due to superior soft-tissue contrast and to show intracranial extension. Need pre- and postcontrast studies.	Lymphoma, rhabdomyosarcoma, nasopharyngeal carcinoma, malignant histiocytoma.
Metastases	CT: usually neuroblastoma and is associated with soft-tissue mass.	
Juvenile angiofibroma	CT: isointense or low-density mass with widening of pterygopalatine fossa and bowing of posterolateral maxillary sinus. Marked CE. MRI: T1 hypointense, T2 hyperintense with flow voids and avid enhancement. Can show cysts, cavitation, and hemorrhage.	Benign, most common in adolescent boys.
Osteomyelitis	Radiograph/CT: sclerosis and destruction of sinus wall in setting of infection.	Usually frontal sinus.
Fibrous dysplasia ▷ Fig. 4.143	CT: depends on fibrous vs. osseous component. Varies from radiolucent to ground-glass. Unilocular/multilocular lesion, well-defined margin. MRI: sharply demarcated mass, variable signal intensity, diffuse CE.	
Ossifying fibroma ▷ Fig. 4.114, p. 369 ▷ Fig. 4.138, p. 381	CT/MRI: expansile lesion with prominent areas of nonossified fibrous tissue. Can be lytic, expansile containing calcification, and show cortical erosion.	

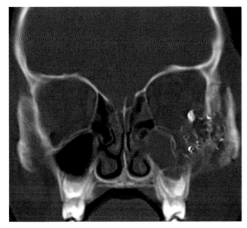

Fig. 4.140 Coronal CT (bone window) shows comminuted fractures involving the lateral orbital wall and floor due to a **gunshot wound** (note bullet fragments) with opacification of the left maxillary sinus.

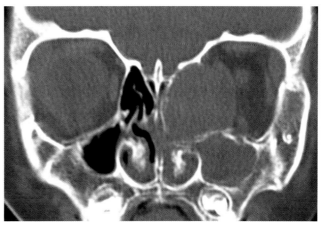

Fig. 4.141 A left **ethmoid mucocele** obstructing the ostiomeatal complex with resultant opacification of the left maxillary sinus on a coronal CT (bone window).

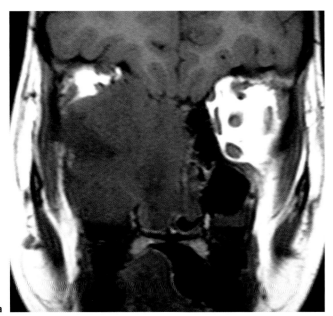

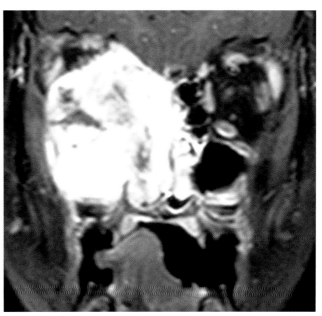

Fig. 4.142a, b T1-weighted coronal pre- (**a**) and postcontrast (**b**) MRI shows a T1-hypointense mass arising in the right maxillary sinus with extension into nose, orbit, and intracranially. The mass shows marked CE and is characteristic of a **rhabdomyosarcoma**.

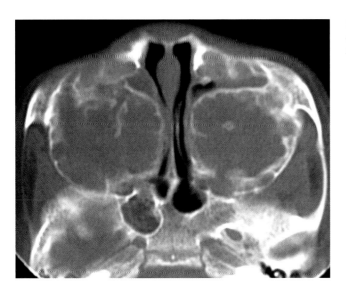

Fig. 4.143 Bilateral symmetrically expanded maxillary sinuses with central fibrous component in keeping with **fibrous dysplasia** on an axial CT (bone window).

Oral Cavity

The Pharynx

Table 4.40   Pharyngeal/prevertebral soft-tissue swelling

Diagnosis	Findings	Comments
Normal: anterior buckling (expiration ± flexion) in the ear lobe	Lateral radiograph: "pseudothickening"—if neck not adequately extended or flexed may get artificially thickened soft tissue in younger children.	
Adenoid tonsil ▷ *Fig. 4.144*	Lateral radiograph: soft-tissue pad in posterior nasopharynx causing narrowing of airway. Sagittal MRI: Soft-tissue mass in nasopharynx. High signal on T2.	If enlarged, causes obstructive sleep apnea. If > 12 mm, it is abnormal.
Palatine tonsil ▷ *Fig. 4.145*	Lateral radiograph: prominent soft-tissue mass overlying posterior inferior aspect of soft palate. MRI: bilateral enlarged high signal masses on T2.	If enlarged, causes obstructive sleep apnea.
Trauma/hematoma ± fracture ▷ *Fig. 4.146*	Lateral radiograph: prevertebral soft-tissue swelling is greater than the width of vertebral body ± fracture, ± spondylolothesis. Atlas dens interval (ADI) may be > 5 mm. Basion-dens interval may be > 12 mm. Power ratio > 1 in atlantoccipital dissociation. Sagittal MRI: prevertebral soft-tissue swelling/hematoma. Retroclival hematoma and blood between basion and dens implies apical/alar ligament disruption. Check tectorial ligament and posterior ligaments. May have associated cord edema.	Prepontine blood seen on NECT should alert to possible cervical spine injury with retroclival hematoma; urgent MRI is indicated even in face of normal lateral cervical spine radiograph.
Epiglottitis	Lateral radiograph: (patient upright) enlargement of epiglottis and thickening of aryepiglottic folds. CT (rarely indicated): enlarged, edematous epiglottis and aryepiglottic folds.	Medical emergency—complete airway obstruction may occur at any time. "Thumb" sign.
Retropharyngeal abscess ▷ *Fig. 4.147* ▷ *Fig. 4.148*	Lateral radiograph: widening of retropharyngeal soft tissue, ± gas, or air-fluid level. Loss of normal cervical lordosis. CECT: identifies extent of disease and drainable collections, which are hypodense with rim enhancement.	Cellulitis more common than abscess. Mass effect on the airways may cause respiratory compromise.
Foreign body	Lateral radiograph: only if radiopaque.	May require contrast swallow postremoval to check for leak.
Lingual thyroid	CT: hyperdense, well-circumscribed mass at base of tongue that enhances strongly with contrast. MRI: T1—increased signal compared to tongue. T2—increased signal. Enhances with contrast. Nuclear medicine (NM): positive technetium-99m pertechnetate uptake confirms ectopic thyroid.	A 1–3 cm well-circumscribed, round/ovoid, midline/paramedian tongue base mass. Important to look for normal cervical thyroid tissue, which may be absent.
Lymphadenopathy	US: oval homogenous nodes of varying sizes, ± central hypoechogenicity if forming abscess CECT: well-defined homogenous masses with variable enhancement; ± linear enhancement of hilum of node; ± ring enhancement with hypodense center representing phlegmon or early abscess; ± perinodal fat stranding. MRI: homogenous signal intensity unless suppurative.	Nonneoplastic enlargement of nodes may be reactive or associated with infection. Waldeyer ring may be enlarged. Important to assess adjacent jugular vein for thrombosis.

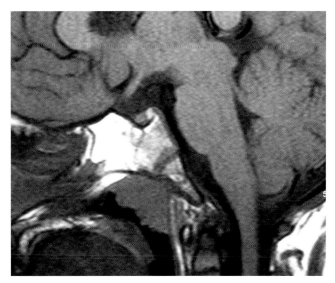

Fig. 4.144 T1 midline sagittal MRI of nasopharynx shows posterior nasopharyngeal soft-tissue isointense mass consistent with an **adenoid tonsil**.

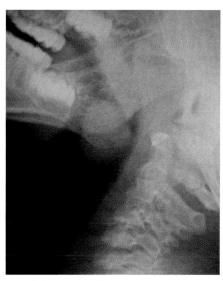

Fig. 4.145 Nasopharyngeal soft-tissue mass consistent with **a palatine tonsil** on lateral radiograph of neck.

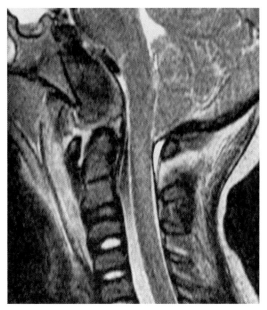

Fig. 4.146 T2 midline sagittal MRI neck shows a large hypointense retroclival **hematoma displacing an intact tectorial ligament posttrauma**. Note increased basion-dens interval and prevertebral soft-tissue edema.

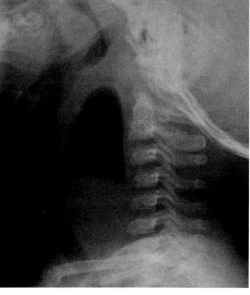

Fig. 4.147 Lateral radiograph of the neck shows massive prevertebral soft-tissue swelling with prominent air-fluid level consistent with a **retropharyngeal abscess**.

Fig. 4.148 Retropharyngeal abscess. Axial postcontrast CT of suprahyoid neck shows left ring-enhancing abscess with hypodense center in prevertebral space displacing the carotid sheath laterally and causing mild airway compression.

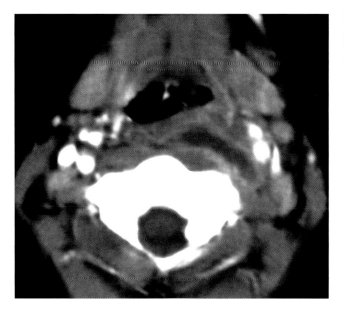

The Jaw and Teeth

Table 4.41 Cystic lesions: dental

Diagnosis	Findings	Comments
Periodontal/radicular cyst/ periapical cyst	Radiograph (panorex): well-circumscribed radiolucency around apex of tooth surrounded by thin rim of cortical bone.	Most common cyst. Associated with carious teeth. If large may displace teeth.
Dentigerous/follicular cyst ▷ *Fig. 4.149*	Plain radiograph/panorex/CT: well-defined unilocular cyst, which incorporates the crown of the unerrupted tooth.	Vary in size. More common in mandible. If maxillary, may project into antrum.
Odontogenic keratocyst/ primordial cyst **Multiple indicates Gorlin syndrome**	Radiograph/CT: expansile cystic lesion, uni-multiloculated, smooth/scalloped border, ± impacted tooth.	Characteristically in body/ramus of mandible. Often recurs. Aggressive.
Residual cyst		A cyst that remains or develops after surgical removal of a tooth.

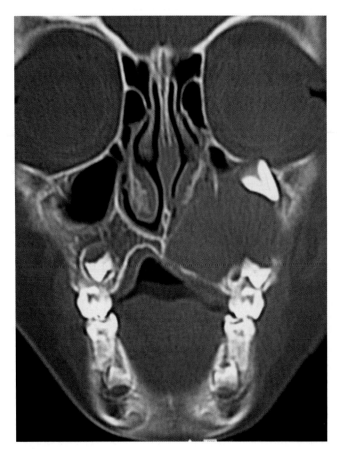

Fig. 4.149 Left dentigerous cyst with opacification of adjacent maxillary sinus on coronal CT of face (bone window).

Table 4.42   Cystic lesions: nondental

Diagnosis	Findings	Comments
Fissural cyst	Radiograph/panorex: round or ovoid midline cyst near anterior palatine papilla.	Unusual in children. Developmental cyst in incisive canal. Often incidental.
Aneurysmal bone cyst	Radiograph/panorex: large, multiloculated. CT: cystic, expansile, multiple fluid-fluid levels.	More common in females. Rapidly growing, painless.
Giant cell granuloma	Plain radiograph/CT: Expansile, multilocular radiolucent lytic lesion with tiny bone septa traversing lesion. Contains intralesional mineralization. Enhances postcontrast. MRI: T1 and T2 hypointense, enhances postcontrast.	Rare, benign, slow-growing lesion in mandible/maxilla. Present with swelling and pain. Teeth and root displacement occurs.
LCH ▷ Fig. 4.150	Radiograph/CT: Lytic destructive bone lesion with resorption of lamina dura resulting in floating teeth appearance. Associated heterogeneously enhancing soft-tissue mass. MRI: T1 iso-/hypointense mass, T2 hyperintense, variable CE.	
Hemangioma	Radiograph/CT: Radiolucent area traversed by trabeculae forming various sized cavities. If trabeculae arranged in radiating pattern, then sunburst appearance.	Rare. Rapid proliferation phase followed by slower involution phase.
Metastasis	Radiograph/CT: fairly well-defined, lytic mass with soft-tissue component.	
Bone cyst due to trauma/injury	Radiograph/panorex: slightly irregular cyst with poorly defined borders and scalloped margins between the roots.	Often incidental. May regress spontaneously.
Fibrous dysplasia ▷ Fig. 4.151	CT: Depends on fibrous vs osseous component. Varies from radiolucent to ground-glass. Uni-/multilocular lesion, well-defined margin. MRI: sharply demarcated mass, variable signal intensity, diffuse CE.	Pain, swelling, and displacement of teeth. Active growth in childhood. Malignant transformation in polyostotic variant described.

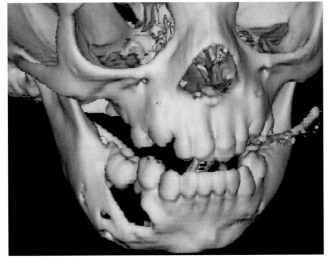

Fig. 4.150   Right mandibular bone destruction with floating tooth characteristic of **Langerhans cell histiocytosis** on 3D CT reconstruction of face.

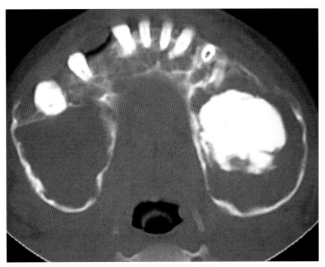

Fig. 4.151   Axial CT of mandible (bone window) showing a diffuse, expansile, ground-glass bone lesion with large osseous component on left, which is characteristic of **fibrous dysplasia**.

Table 4.43   Tumor/tumorlike lesions

Diagnosis	Findings	Comments
Burkitt lymphoma ▷ *Fig. 4.152*	Radiograph: Poorly-defined destructive, mottled bone lesion with root resorption and loss of lamina dura of developing teeth. Associated cortical loss. CT: destructive soft-tissue mass with extension into surrounding soft tissue. MRI: diffuse infiltration, heterogenous mass with CE.	African variant most common childhood malignancy in Africa. African Burkitt strongly associated with Epstein-Barr virus (EBV).
LCH ▷ *Fig. 4.150, p. 387*	Radiograph/CT: Lytic destructive bone lesion with resorption of lamina dura resulting in floating tooth appearance. Associated heterogeneously enhancing soft-tissue mass. MRI: T1 iso-/hypointense mass, T2 hyperintense, variable CE.	
Osteosarcoma	Radiograph/CT: lytic bone destruction with ill-defined margins (osteolytic type) or areas of sclerosis (osteoblastic type) with aggressive periosteal reaction, ± sunburst effect, ± cortical breakthrough, and ± calcification/osteoid formation. MRI: heterogeneous mass. NM: increased uptake, identifies other bone lesions.	Prone to recurrence and metastases.
Rhabdomyosarcoma	CT: Soft-tissue mass with variable but diffuse CE, + bone erosion. May extend to involve mandible depending on site. MRI: T1 isointense, T2 hyperintense, variable but diffuse CE.	Forty percent occur in head and neck May extend intracranially.
Leukemia	Radiograph/CT: loss of lamina dura, varying degree of lytic bone destruction.	
Odontoma ▷ *Fig. 4.153*	Radiograph/panorex: initially radiolucent then calcified, with the calcified portion separated from expanded cortex by a radiolucent zone ± impacted, unerupted tooth.	Benign tumor made up of various components of teeth (enamel, dentin, cementum, pulp). Located between roots of teeth. May be associated with unerupted tooth.
Metastasis	Radiograph/CT: fairly well-defined, lytic mass with soft-tissue component.	
Cementoma: **cementifying fibroma**	Radiograph/panorex: Early—well-circumscribed, well-demarcated radiolucent lesion with no internal radiopacities. Late—contains internal radiopacities.	Slow growing: 1–2 cm.
Benign cementoblastoma **(true cementoma)** ▷ *Fig. 4.154*	Well-defined, dense radiopaque material attached to tooth root with surrounding radiolucent zone.	Rare. Mandibular first molar most frequently involved.

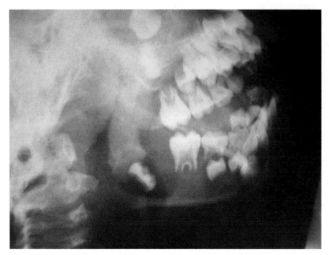

Fig. 4.152   Burkitt lymphoma with floating tooth and loss of lamina dura and cortical resorption on oblique radiograph of mandible.

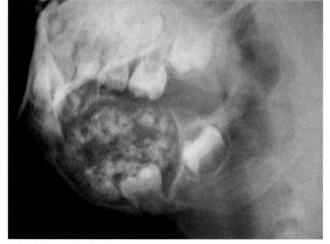

Fig. 4.153   Oblique radiograph of mandible showing expanded radiolucent lesion with calcification and unerupted tooth consistent with an **odontoma**. Note how the calcified portion is separated from the cortex by a radiolucent zone.

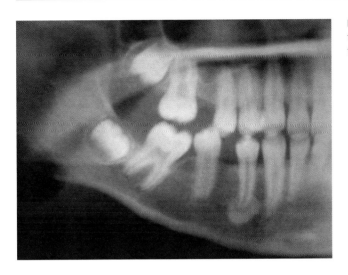

Fig. 4.154 Well-defined dense radiopaque material attached to tooth root is characteristic of a **true cementoma** on panorex view of the right mandible.

Table 4.44 Floating teeth

Diagnosis	Findings	Comments
LCH ▷ *Fig. 4.150, p. 387*	Radiograph/CT: Lytic destructive bone lesion with resorption of lamina dura resulting in floating tooth appearance. Associated heterogeneously enhancing soft-tissue mass. MRI: T1 iso-/hypointense mass, T2 hyperintense, variable CE.	
Metastasis	Radiograph/CT: aggressive bone destruction, no periosteal reaction/calcification.	
Leukemia	Radiograph/CT: loss of lamina dura, varying degree lytic bone destruction. CT: permeative bone destruction. MR: T1—leukemic infiltrate of low signal replacing normal fatty marrow. T2—increased signal.	
Burkitt lymphoma ▷ *Fig. 4.152*	Radiograph: Poorly defined destructive, mottled bone lesion with root resorption and loss of lamina dura of developing teeth. Associated cortical loss. CT: destructive soft-tissue mass with extension into surrounding soft tissue. MRI: diffuse infiltration, heterogenous mass with CE.	African variant most common childhood malignancy in Africa. African Burkitt strongly associated with EBV.
Desmoplastic fibroma	Radiograph/CT: destructive, expansile mass, contains lacelike calcification.	Aggressive, high recurrence rate.

Table 4.45 Hyperostosis/sclerosis/destruction

Diagnosis	Findings	Comments
Osteomyelitis	Radiograph: sclerosis or mixed sclerotic/lucent.	Primary chronic osteomyelitis: nonsuppurative, noninfectious. Actinimycosis occurs in mandible.
Infantile cortical hyperostosis (Caffey disease) ▷ *Fig. 4.155, p. 390*	Radiograph: periosteal thickening, dense laminated subperiosteal new bone formation of mandible, may cause mandibular asymmetry.	
Fibrous dysplasia ▷ *Fig. 4.151, p. 387*	CT: Depends on fibrous vs. osseous component. Varies from radiolucent to ground-glass. Uni-/multilocular lesion, well-defined margin. MRI: sharply demarcated mass, variable signal intensity, diffuse CE.	
Camurati-Engelmann disease	Radiograph: sclerosis of base of the skull (BOS) ± cranial vault and facial bones.	
Van Buchem disease	Radiograph: osteosclerosis and hyperostosis of mandible, endosteal sclerosis of cranium.	

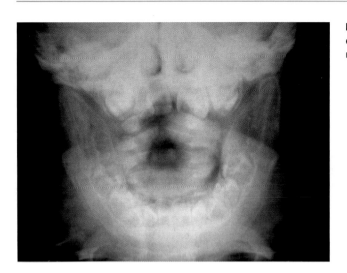

Fig. 4.155 AP radiograph of mandible shows diffuse periosteal thickening of mandible with dense laminated subperiosteal new bone formation, which is characteristic of **Caffey disease**.

Table 4.46 Congenital abnormalities: affecting size and symmetry

Diagnosis	Findings	Comments
Down syndrome	Radiograph: hypoplasia of the facial bones and sinuses, short hard palate, hypotelorism, dental abnormalities (delayed tooth eruption, anodontia).	
Pierre Robin syndrome ▷ *Fig. 4.156*	Radiograph: mandible hypoplasia, obtuse mandibular angle, cleft palate.	
Alcohol embryopathy	Radiograph: mandible hypoplasia, microcephaly.	Growth retardation.
DiGeorge syndrome	Radiograph: mandible hypoplasia, hypertelorism.	Thymic aplasia.
Crouzon syndrome	Radiograph: premature closure any/all sutures, hypoplasia of the maxillomalar facial mass, recession malar bone, short and distorted zygomatic arches.	
MPS (Hurler syndrome)	Radiograph: short wide mandible with obtuse angle, short rami, and flat/concave condyles. Premature closure of sutures, thickened calvarium at base, J-shaped sella.	
Mandibulofacial dysostosis	Radiograph: hypoplasia/agenesis of malar bones, cleft palate.	Abnormality of first and second pharyngeal pouch, groove and arch structures.
Seckel syndrome	Radiograph: hypoplasia maxilla and mandible, microcrania, hypertelorism.	"Bird-headed appearance."
Acrofacial dysostosis	Radiograph: mandible hypoplasia, craniosynostosis.	
Melnick-Needles syndrome	Radiograph: mandible hypoplasia, BOS sclerosis.	
Goldenhar syndrome	Radiograph: hypoplasia maxilla ± mandible and temporal bones.	Usually unilateral.
Caffey disease ▷ *Fig. 4.155*	Radiograph: periosteal thickening and dense, laminated, subperiosteal new bone formation of mandible causing mandibular asymmetry.	Mandible, clavicles, and ribs most commonly involved.
Trisomy 13/15	Radiograph: mandible hypoplasia.	
Trisomy 17/18	Radiograph: mandible and maxilla hypoplasia, J-shaped sella, thin calvaria.	
Pyknodysostosis ▷ *Fig. 4.157*	Radiograph: mandible hypoplasia, obtuse or absent angle of mandible, wormian bones, dental abnormalities.	Generalized osteosclerosis.
Hallermann-Streiff syndrome	Radiograph: mandible hypoplasia, anterior displacement of temporomandibular joint, brachycephaly.	
Campomelic dysplasia	Radiograph: mandible hypoplasia, antegonal notching of mandible, macrocephaly.	
Metaphyseal chondrodysplasia (Jansen type)	Radiograph: mandible hypoplasia with irregular mineralization, brachycephaly, platybasia.	
Russell-Silver syndrome	Radiograph: mandible hypoplasia.	Two-thirds have partial or total asymmetry of face, small triangular face.
Rubenstein-Taybi syndrome	Radiograph: mild retrognathia, mandible hypoplasia, cleft palate.	

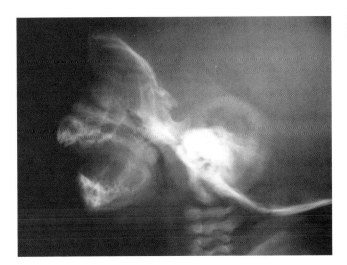

Fig. 4.156 Lateral radiograph of face shows mandibular hypoplasia in a patient with **Pierre Robin syndrome**.

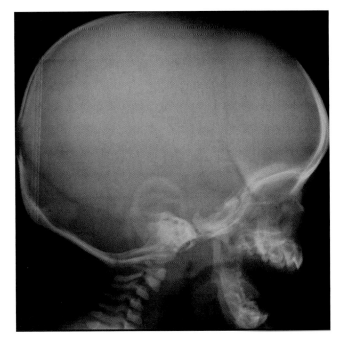

Fig. 4.157 Mandibular hypoplasia with absent angle of mandible in a patient with **pyknodysostosis**. Note the osteosclerotic bones on lateral radiograph of skull and face.

The Neck

Table 4.47   Midline masses

Diagnosis	Findings	Comments
Thyroglossal duct syst ▷ *Fig. 4.158*	US/CT/MRI: midline cystic mass embedded in infrahyoid strap muscles. Hypodense/intense and anechoic unless infected. If calcified or has solid elements, needs work-up for malignancy.	Most present < 10 y. US confirms normal thyroid gland. CT/MRI if cyst suprahyoid or infected.
Ectopic thyroid	CT/MRI: Well-circumscribed midline or paramedian tongue mass with density/intensity similar to normal thyroid tissue. Can be multifocal.	May expand rapidly during puberty. Assess normal thyroid tissue as lingual thyroid is only functioning tissue in 75% of cases.
Dermoid/epidermoid	CECT: cystic, well-demarcated mass containing fluid (epidermoid) or fat/fluid (dermoid). MRI: Use fat-saturated techniques to diagnose dermoid.	Unusual before 5 y of age. Usually involve floor of mouth but if large, can protrude inferiorly.
Lymph node	US: typical node appearances.	(see **Table 4.49**)
Cervical thymus	US/MRI: midline or on the left.	(see **Table 4.49**)
Extension of plunging ranula ▷ *Fig. 4.159*	US/CT: cystic. MRI: Thin-walled cyst with intermediate signal on T1 and high signal on T2. Bulk of the lesion is in submandibular space with characteristic connection to the floor of the mouth.	

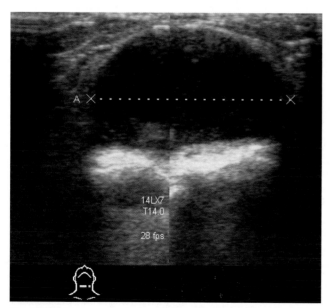

Fig. 4.158 Transverse US of neck shows a hypoechoic midline cystic lesion consistent with a **thyroglossal duct cyst**.

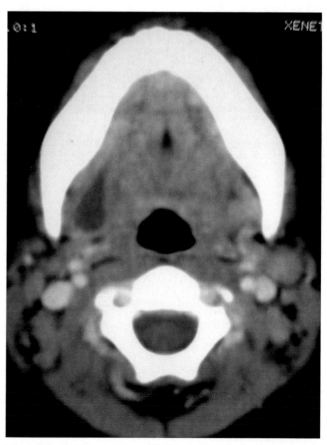

Fig. 4.159 Axial postcontrast CT of the neck at the level of the angle of the mandible shows a right nonenhancing hypodense cystic lesion in the submandibular space consistent with a **plunging ranula**.

Table 4.48   Lateral cystic masses

Venolymphatic malformations ▷ *Fig. 4.160* ▷ *Fig. 4.161*	MRI: T2 for extent and fluid levels, postcontrast T1 with fat saturation for enhancing septations and venous elements. CT: shows phleboliths.	Usually identified at or soon after birth. US helpful initially to direct further imaging. 1. Lymphatic malformation—transspatial cystic mass uni- or multilocular. 2. Venous malformation—enhancing mass with calcifications. 3. Lymphaticovenous—cystic and enhancing transspatial lesion.
Branchial cleft cyst	US: demonstrates location, usually hypoechoic. CT/MRI: demonstrate infection with enhancing wall/increased attenuation and signal.	Cystic mass posterolateral to submandibular gland, lateral to carotid space, anterior or anteromedial to SCM muscle.
Abscess ▷ *Fig. 4.162, p. 394*	US/CT/MRI: fluid-filled mass with irregular, thick enhancing wall and low-density/-intensity center. If involving thyroid, think of fourth branchial pouch anomaly.	Present with symptoms and signs of infection.
Thymic cyst	US/CT/MRI: Nonenhancing, low attenuation, hypo-/anechoic left lateral neck cyst closely associated with carotid sheath. Solid components rare, represent aberrant thymic/parathyroid tissue.	Can occur anywhere along thymopharyngeal duct but left lateral infrahyoid neck at level of thyroid gland is most common.
Laryngocoele	Radiograph: shows air-filled lateral structure. Best imaged with CT or MRI, which show unilocular air or fluid-filled cyst. Lies within the submandibular space.	Occur as a result of increased intraglottic pressure. Increase in size with Valsalva.
(Para)Thyroid cyst	Usually colloid cyst.	(see **Table 4.53**)
Varix of jugular vein	US: expanded jugular vein with Doppler flow.	Best seen during straining, coughing, or crying.

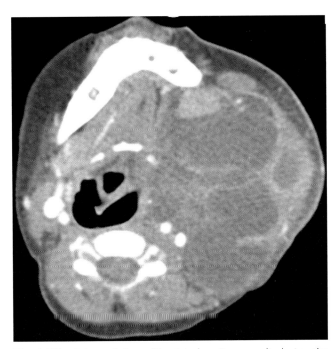

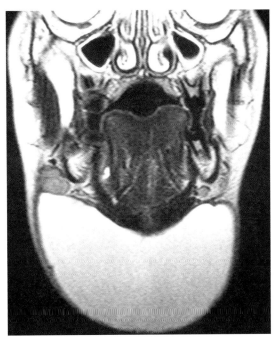

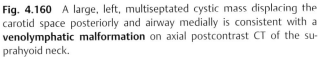

Fig. 4.160 A large, left, multiseptated cystic mass displacing the carotid space posteriorly and airway medially is consistent with a **venolymphatic malformation** on axial postcontrast CT of the suprahyoid neck.

Fig. 4.161 A large hyperintense cystic mass without septations is consistent with a **venolymphatic malformation** on T2 coronal MRI of the face and neck.

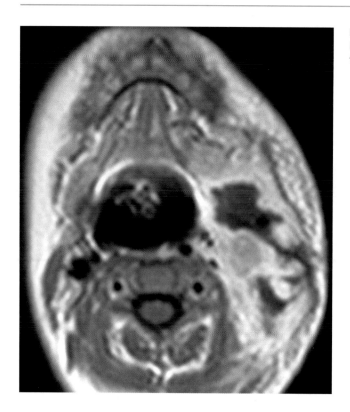

Fig. 4.162   T1 axial postcontrast MRI of the suprahyoid neck shows left neck swelling with marked enhancement of soft tissues and a central rim-enhancing hypointense area consistent with an **abscess**.

Table 4.49   Lateral solid masses

Diagnosis	Findings	Comments
Fibromatosis colli ▷ *Fig. 4.163a, b*	US: Focal mass in or diffuse enlargement of the middle/lower third of affected SCM muscle. Variable echogenicity. CT: enlarged muscle without discrete mass. MRI: Usually iso-/hypointense to normal muscle on T1. T2 variable but usually hypointense at area of maximal enlargement probably due to fibrosis.	Infant with torticollis tilting head to same side and rotating head toward opposite side.
Lymph nodes/lymphoma ▷ *Fig. 4.164*	US: Oval nodes increased in size and number. Central hypoechogenicity in suppuration. CECT: best to differentiate cellulitis/phlegmon/abscess and assess extent of disease in suspected malignancy. MRI: T1 low/intermediate signal; T2 high signal.	Findings nonspecific and depend on clinical scenario; often rely on tissue diagnosis.
Teratoma ▷ *Fig. 4.130, p. 378*	CT/MRI: Large and infiltrative with multiple cystic and solid elements. Contain fat and calcification. Both modalities show extent and components.	Usually < 1 y; may cause significant airway and feeding compromise.
Neuroblastoma	CT/MRI: Well-defined mass lying posterior to the vascular sheath and occasionally extending into the cervical spinal canal. MRI is best for delineating extent of tumor and spinal and intracranial extent.	Less than 5% occur in the neck. Need chest and abdomen CT as part of initial work-up to rule out abdominal primary.
Hemangioma	US: well-defined mass with prominent vessels. MRI: Best for extent. T1 isointense to muscle with intense enhancement postcontrast; T2 hyperintense with multiple flow voids.	Characteristic presentation; therefore, imaging indicated if suspect deep extension, pretreatment, or to assess treatment response.
Rhabdomyosarcoma	CT: heterogeneous lesion with or without osseous destruction. MRI: isointense to muscle on T1, hyperintense on T2 and show enhancement postcontrast.	May be a primary lesion or related to metastatic adenopathy that is present in 50% of patients. Forty percent occur in head and neck.
Fibrosarcoma/sarcoma	CT/MRI: Heterogeneously enhancing soft-tissue mass. Usually less intense and homogeneous enhancement than hemangioma. May show osseous destruction.	Often with regional lymph node involvement. Need chest CT for metastatic surveillance.

(continues on page 396)

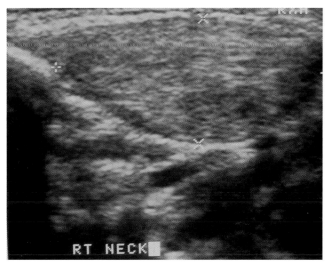
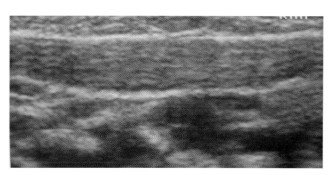

Fig. 4.163a, b   Longitudinal US of SCM muscle shows diffuse enlargement of muscle characteristic of **fibromatosis colli** (**a**) and normal side for comparison (**b**).

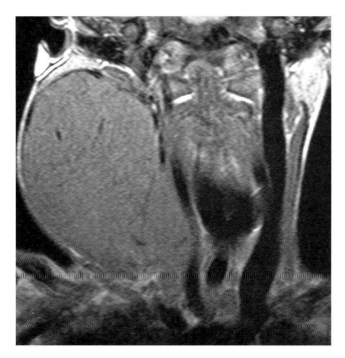

Fig. 4.164   T2 coronal MRI of the neck shows a large right isointense mass displacing the jugular vein and airway to the left; it was proven by histology to be **lymphoma**.

Table 4.49 (Cont.) Lateral solid masses

Diagnosis	Findings	Comments
Hematoma	US: Imaging findings depend on age of bleed. Acute bleed hyperechoic, less echogenic in 96 h, and eventually anechoic. Usually well defined but may become irregular if blood escapes into adjacent structures. Differentiate from tumor by absence of flow.	Usually due to trauma, anticoagulation, or coagulopathy.
Neurofibroma/plexiform neurofibroma ▷ *Fig. 4.165*	MRI: T2 hyperintense with hypointense center (target sign). Heterogeneous CE.	MRI best for tumor extent, especially when close to spine. Assess for other manifestations of NF.
Brachial plexus schwannoma	MRI: Well-circumscribed, fusiform, T2 hyperintense enhancing mass between anterior and middle scalene muscles. T1 isointense. CT: Isodense to muscle, calcification uncommon, moderate enhancement. Smooth, corticated widening of bony neural foramen.	Painless, slow-growing mass in neck. May be indistinguishable from neurofibroma.
Cervical thymus	CT/MRI: At cervicothoracic junction, midline or to the left. Mimics appearance of normal thymus on all imaging modalities, and MRI may show connection with the mediastinal thymus.	Incomplete thymic descent, usually asymptomatic but may cause dysphagia.

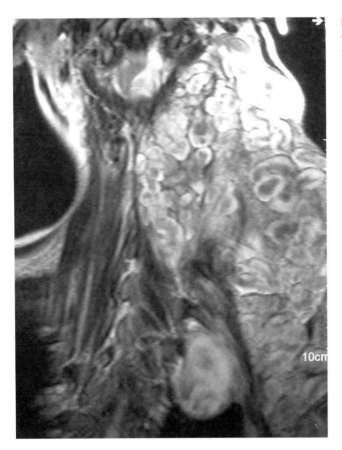

Fig. 4.165 Massive left **plexiform neurofibroma** on T2 coronal MRI of the neck. Note multiple target lesions with hyperintense periphery and hypointense center.

The Salivary Glands

Table 4.50   Unilateral masses

Diagnosis	Findings	Comments
Pleiomorphic adenoma	US: solid, well-defined, homogeneous, hypoechoic mass ± echogenic foci, with calcification. CT: If small, well-marginated homogeneously enhancing ovoid mass. If large, enhances inhomogeneously with foci necrosis/hemorrhage ± calcification. MRI: depending on size, homogeneous or heterogenous low signal on T1 and high signal on T2 with mild to moderate enhancement. NM: cold lesion.	Third most common benign salivary gland tumor in children. Sixty to ninety percent occur in parotid gland. Hard painless mass.
Hemangioma ▷ *Fig. 4.166*	US: focal/diffuse, heterogenous, hypoechoic soft-tissue mass with prominent vascular flow. CT/MRI with contrast: diffuse CE of well-defined mass.	Most common benign tumor of salivary gland in children. Capillary/cavernous/hemangioendothelioma. Identify shortly after birth with rapid growth then slow spontaneous involution.
Lymphangioma	US: cystic mass with thin septa ± solid elements; ± fluid-fluid levels; ± vascularization in septa or solid portions. CT: Low-density, poorly circumscribed cystic mass that may be uni- or multilocular, ± fluid-fluid levels. No enhancement. MRI: T1 hypoisointense, T2 hyperintense, no CE (unless mixed vascular component).	Second most common salivary gland tumor in children. Involve adjacent structures commonly (i.e., trans-spatial). Sixty-five percent present at birth.
Warthin tumor (papillary cystadenoma lymphomatosum)	US: well-defined, hypoechoic, cystic mass or masses. CT: Solitary well-circumscribed ovoid mass with poor enhancement. Thirty percent have cystic component. No calcification. MRI: solid/cystic lesions with minimal enhancement. NM: hot lesion.	Occurs only in parotid gland: superficial lobe. Twenty percent are multiple lesions. Ten percent are bilateral. Most common multifocal salivary tumor.

(continues on page 398)

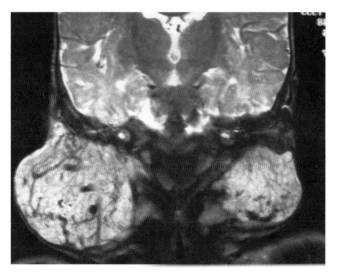

Fig. 4.166 Bilateral large hyperintense parotid masses with flow voids are consistent with bilateral **parotid hemangiomas** on this T2 coronal fat-saturated MRI of the face and neck.

Table 4.50   (Cont.) Unilateral masses

Diagnosis	Findings	Comments
Mucoepidermoid carcinoma ▷ *Fig. 4.167*	US: unifocal, heterogenous, ill-defined margins. CT: enhancing inhomogenous mass. MRI: heterogenous signal and heterogenous enhancement.	Sixty percent of malignant salivary tumors are mucoepidermoid or acinic cell carcinoma. Majority arise in parotids. Associated with rapid growth, facial nerve paralysis, and lymphadenopathy Low-grade: well-defined. High-grade: ill-defined shaggy margins, invasive.
Rhabdomyosarcoma	Extension into glands from other sites.	(see **Tables 4.39** and **4.49**)
Sialectasis ▷ *Fig. 4.168* ▷ *Fig. 4.169*	US: calculi are echogenic foci with posterior shadowing. ± ductal dilatation, ± inflammation. Sialogram: punctuate dilatation of the salivary ducts. T2 MRI: foci of high signal intensity throughout the gland.	Ninety percent involve submandibular gland. Majority of calculi are radiopaque and may be ductal/intraglandular.
Abscess (*Staphylococcus aureus*) ▷ *Fig. 4.170*	US: well-defined hypoechoic mass with surrounding edema/induration. CECT: rim-enhancing, thick-walled cystic mass. MRI: rim enhancement of abscess, high signal on T2.	Local tenderness and fever.
Ranula ▷ *Fig. 4.159, p. 392*	US: cystic mass in floor or mouth, ± echoes and septa. CT: thin-walled unilocular hypodense lesion with thin enhancing wall. MRI: low signal on T1 and high signal on T2 with wall enhancement.	Specific type of mucocele that originates in the sublingual gland—may be simple (i.e., within gland and lined by epithelium or diving ranula when simple cyst becomes large and ruptures into submandibular space creating a pseudocyst).

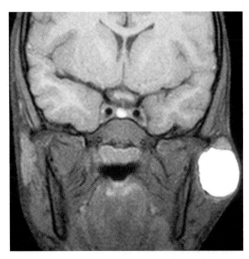

Fig. 4.167   T1 coronal fat-saturated MRI of the parotid glands shows a well-defined, hyperintense left parotid mass; it was proven by histology to be **mucoepidermoid carcinoma**.

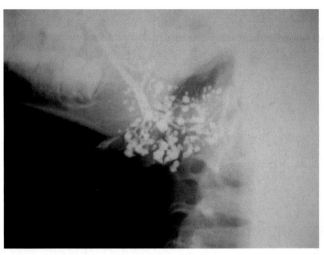

Fig. 4.168   Sialogram of submandibular gland shows multiple dilated salivary ducts, which is consistent with **sialectasis**.

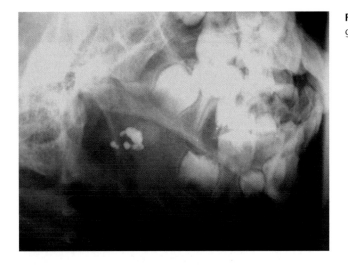

Fig. 4.169   **Sialectasis** with radiopaque calculi in submandibular gland on an oblique radiograph of the mandible.

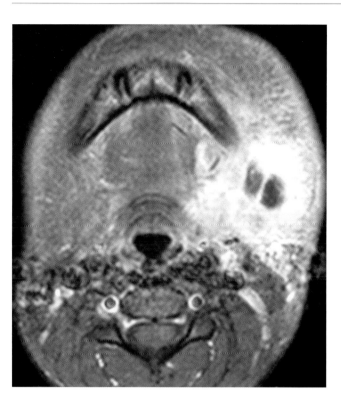

Fig. 4.170 Submandibular abscess with left hypointense rim enhancing on T1 axial fat-saturated postcontrast MRI. Note the surrounding soft-tissue swelling and enhancement.

Table 4.51 Bilateral masses

Diagnosis	Findings	Comments
Infection: mumps, parotitis, MOTTS, tuberculosis, cat scratch (*Bartonella*)	US: enlarged, hypoechoic, heterogenous glands, ± hypoechoic collections, indicating abscess formation. CT: hyperdense glands with mild enhancement MRI: T2—diffuse high signal ± areas focal high signal. T1 with contrast—moderate enhancement, enlarged gland.	Viral parotitis is a clinical diagnosis. Suppurative parotitis often bilateral in neonates.
Human immunodeficiency virus lymphoproliferative disorder ▷ *Fig. 4.171*	US: multiple hypo-/anechoic cysts with thin septa in gland. CT: Thin rim-enhancement of cystic lesions; heterogenous enhancement of solid lesions. MRI: T1—low signal intensity cysts with thin rim enhancement. T2—multiple high signal intensity round lesions.	Multiple solid and cystic lesions within enlarged glands. Often associated cervical adenopathy and tonsillar hyperplasia.
Sjögren's disease	US: enlarged heterogenous glands with multiple hypoechoic areas, ± small echogenic foci that represent mucous plugs in dilated ducts/walls of ducts. CT: enlarged hyperdense and heterogenous glands, ± calcification with heterogenous enhancement, solid and mixed solid-cystic components. T2 MRI: High signal intensity cystic foci. Size depends on stage. Heterogenous CE.	Chronic inflammation and destruction of gland. Increased risk of developing lymphoma in gland. Juvenile type < 20-y-old men, may resolve spontaneously at puberty.

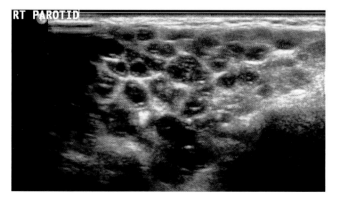

Fig. 4.171 Human immunodeficiency virus lymphoproliferative disorder with multiple hypoechoic/anechoic cysts of varying sizes on longitudinal US of right parotid gland.

Thyroid Gland

Table 4.52   Enlarged thyroid

Diagnosis	Findings	Comments
Goiter	US: Diffusely enlarged hypoechoic gland with increased vascularity. If multinodular, goiter is enlarged and asymmetrical with several focal nodules of mixed echogenicity.	Correlate with antibody results and NM.
Hemiagenesis	US: unilateral, more common on left.	Due to hypertrophy of single lobe or dysfunction.
Thyroiditis	US: Findings depend on stage, usually diffuse or focal hypoechogenicity and enlargement of both lobes. Doppler shows no increased vascularity.	Clinical signs of thyrotoxicosis in 50%.

Table 4.53   Thyroid mass

Diagnosis	Findings	Comments
Cyst (usually colloid)	US: hypo-/anechoic mass. If any solid component, requires work-up for thyroid malignancy. MRI: may appear bright on T1 due to hemorrhage, colloid, or high protein.	Uncommon in young children. True thyroid cysts are rare.
Abscess ▷ *Fig. 4.172*	US: hypoechoic or anechoic mass, ± internal echoes if infected. CT: rim-enhancing mass with central low density.	Rare. Suggests congenital pyriform sinus fistula—correlate with barium swallow or fistulogram.
Adenoma	US: Either increased or decreased echogenicity. Classically have hypoechoic halo around isoechoic mass.	Uncommon. May be single or multiple. May be hyper- or nonfunctioning.
Carcinoma ▷ *Fig. 4.173*	US: Primary imaging modality showing either solid or cystic mass usually hypoechoic but may have hyperechoic calcification. Cervical lymphadenopathy seen in 90%.	Rare. Ninety percent are papillary; three-quarters of cases occur in females. Neck and chest CECT and bone scan are required for staging.

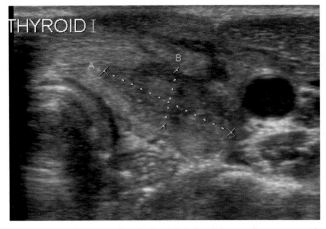

Fig. 4.172   Abscess with a fairly well-defined, hypoechoic mass with internal echoes on transverse US of left thyroid.

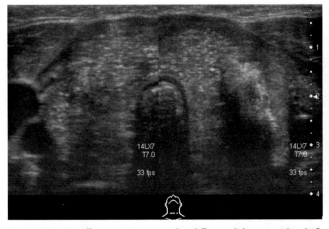

Fig. 4.173   Papillary carcinoma with a diffuse solid mass with calcification involving both lobes on transverse US of the thyroid gland.

The Temporal Bone

Technical Factors

Plain films are almost obsolete in imaging of the ear. Sometimes, a Stenvers view is requested to verify the course of electrodes of an electronic inner ear implant. In all other cases, CT is the preferred imaging modality to depict the petrous bone. Due to the large density differences between air, soft tissue, and bone, thin slices can be acquired for an isotropic data set with great anatomic detail from which multiplanar re-formations can be constructed in any desired plane, obviating a data acquisition in a second plane.

MRI is used to evaluate the inner ear and the retrocochlear auditory pathway in sensorineural hearing loss. It is also valuable for the imaging of tumors in and around the petrosal bone. DWI can be of value to diagnose cholesteatoma.

Normal Variants

Knowledge of normal variants prevents confusion and a possible incorrect diagnosis. Normal variants are also important to report if they can cause a risk during operative procedures.

Table 4.54   Normal variants

Diagnosis	Findings	Comments
Cochlear cleft ▷ Fig. 4.174	Especially in children. Lucency lateral to apical turn.	
Lucent periotic zone in infants		No retrofenestral otosclerosis.
Incudal "hole" ▷ Fig. 4.175, p. 402	Lucency in incus body.	Partial volume effect.
High jugular bulb	Jugular bulb above the caudal level of the posterior semicircular canal.	Frequently a diverticulum of the jugular bulb.
Fatty marrow in petrous apex ▷ Fig. 4.176, p. 402	High signal intensity on T1 and T2 turbo spin echo.	Can be misinterpreted as a lesion, especially when unilateral. Compare signal intensity with subcutaneous fat.
Bulging sigmoid sinus ▷ Fig. 4.177, p. 402	Anterior impression in posterior surface of mastoid.	To be avoided during mastoidectomy.
Pseudofractures	Cochlear aqueduct, petromastoid canal.	Be aware of sutures.

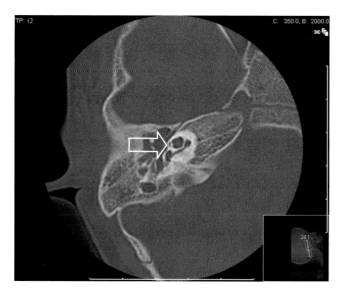

Fig. 4.174 Lucent line at the cochlear apex, a so-called **cochlear cleft** (arrow). This is seen in the majority of young children, and its incidence decreases with advancing age.

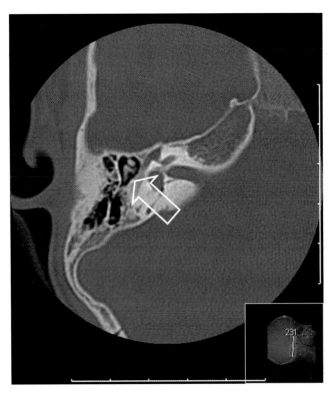

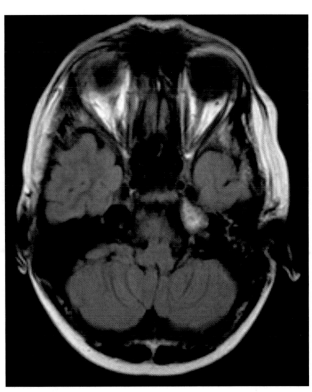

Fig. 4.175   CT examination for suspected cholesteatoma in an 8-year-old boy. The lucency in the body of the incus (arrow) is a **partial volume effect of the space between the short and long process of the incus** and not a focal erosion.

Fig. 4.176   High signal intensity in the left **petrous apex is consistent with fatty bone marrow** on a T2 FLAIR sequence in a 13-year-old boy. This could be mistaken for a petrous apex lesion.

Fig. 4.177   **Bulging sigmoid sinus** (arrow); knowledge of this normal variant can prevent accidental laceration at operation.

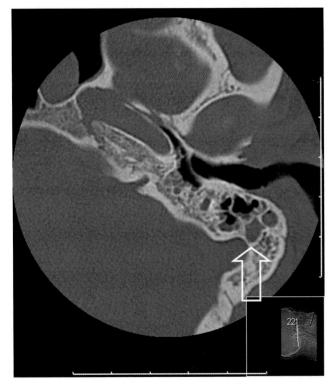

Congenital Anomalies

During embryonic development, the external and middle ear are derived from the first and second branchial groove and pouch. The inner ear is derived from surface ectoderm. Its development starts in the third week and is completed around the twelfth week. In the majority of children with congenital sensorineural hearing loss, no anatomic anomaly is demonstrated. Combined anomalies of external, middle, and inner ear occur in approximately 10% of patients.

In external ear atresia, it is important to note whether the atretic plate is composed of soft tissue or bone. The extent of ossicular chain malformation can differ from a fusion of the mallear head and the incudal body to a small clump of malformed chain. Bilateral external ear canal atresia is often associated with a syndrome, while unilateral atresia is usually nonsyndromal.

The lateral semicircular canal develops last. In malformations of the semicircular canals, the lateral canal is most commonly affected.

The vestibular aqueduct is widened when its diameter is larger than the diameter of the posterior semicircular canal, which corresponds with a diameter at its midpoint of 1.5 mm. It is almost always associated with cochlear modiolar deficiencies.

Absence of the cochlear nerve is rare. The internal auditory canal can be narrowed, but it can also occur with an internal auditory canal of normal diameter. On heavily T2-weighted images perpendicular to the internal auditory canal, the anteroinferiorly located cochlear nerve is absent.

Table 4.55   Congenital anomalies of the external and middle ear

Diagnosis	Findings	Comments
External ear atresia	Membranous atresia.	Often with external auditory canal stenosis.
	Bony atresia.	Usually also middle ear anomalies.
	Ossicular chain anomalies, contracted middle ear.	Spectrum from isolated mallear fusion to lateral wall to absence of chain.
	Anterior position of mastoidal part of facial nerve canal.	Important if surgery is contemplated.

Table 4.56   Congenital inner ear anomalies

Diagnosis	Findings	Comments
Large vestibular aqueduct ▷ Fig. 4.178a, b	Diameter is larger than diameter of the posterior semicircular canal.	Search for cochlear malformation, especially absence of bony modiolus.
Mondini malformation	Incomplete partition of cochlea.	
Michel malformation	No cochlea/single cavity.	Rare.
Deformed lateral semicircular canal	Can be fused with vestibule.	Common among inner ear anomalies.
Absence of cochlear nerve ▷ Fig. 4.179, p. 404	No nerve seen on MRI.	Inferior and superior vestibular nerve split at the fundus.

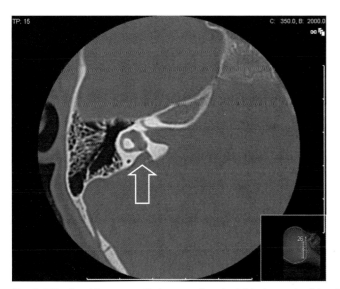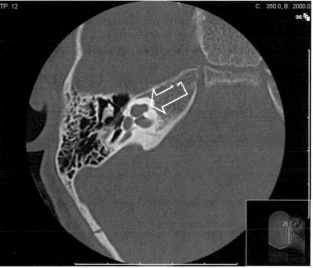

b

Fig. 4.178a, b   A **large vestibular aqueduct** is visible (arrow in **a**) in a 5-year-old boy with a perceptive (sensorineural) hearing deficit. A large vestibular aqueduct is visible (arrow in **a**). The cochlea is malformed with an absent cochlear modioli (arrow in **b**).

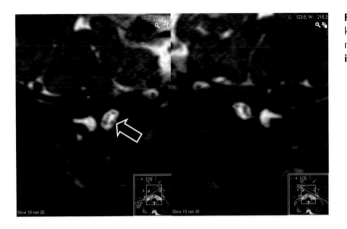

Fig. 4.179   A 16-month-old boy with a left-sided deafness of unknown cause. On the right side, a normal cochlear nerve is visible (arrow) on the T2-weighted image. On the left side, the **cochlear nerve is absent**. The facial nerve and vestibular nerves are present.

Syndromes Associated With Ear Anomalies

A large number of syndromes are associated with ear anomalies, with different importance. The list is too long to repeat here. An overview is provided by Lachman and Taybi. The most important syndromes are listed in **Table 4.57**.

Table 4.57   Syndromes with ear anomalies

Diagnosis	Findings	Comments
Charge syndrome ▷ *Fig. 4.180a, b*	Fused semicircular canals and vestibule.	
Apert syndrome	Large vestibule, short and deformed lateral semicircular canal (SCC).	Upward angulation of petrous apex with eustachian tube dysfunction.
Crouzon syndrome	Large vestibule; short and deformed lateral SCC; dehiscent jugular bulb.	Upward angulation of petrous apex with eustachian tube dysfunction.
Treacher Collins syndrome ▷ *Fig. 4.181a, b*	Hypoplastic/aplastic external ear canal and tympanic cavity.	Hypoplasia of mandibular neck, concave horizontal.
Hemifacial microsomia		
Goldenhar syndrome (oculoauriculovertebral dysplasia)	External auditory canal atresia/dysplasia.	Deformed auricle.
Branchiootorenal syndrome	Hypoplastic apical cochlear turn, large vestibular aqueduct, deformed SCCs.	
Osteopetrosis	Narrow internal auditory canal, narrow facial nerve canal.	Sclerotic skull base.
Osteogenesis imperfecta	Lucencies around inner ear.	Resembles severe otospongiosis.
Achondroplasia ▷ *Fig. 4.182*	Dehiscent jugular bulb.	

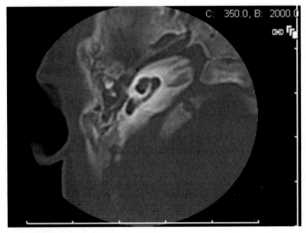
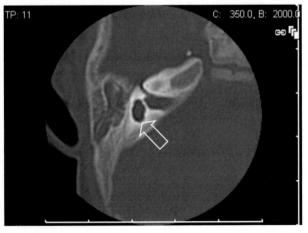

a   b

Fig. 4.180a, b   **Charge syndrome** is a fusion of the vestibule and the semicircular canals (arrow).

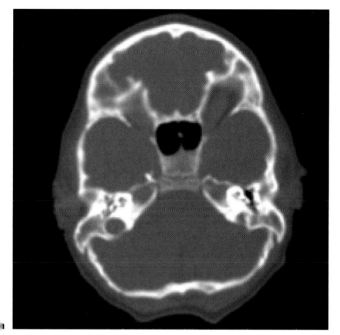

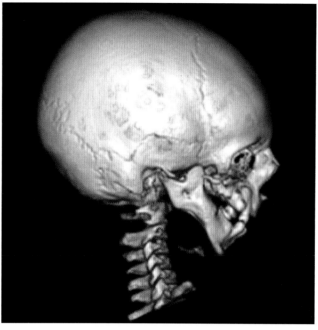

b

Fig. 4.181a, b   Treacher Collins syndrome. (a) A 5-year-old boy with bilateral atresia of the external ear canal. **(b)** 3D reconstruction shows an interrupted zygomatic arch, a hypoplastic mandible, and absence of the orifice of the external ear canal.

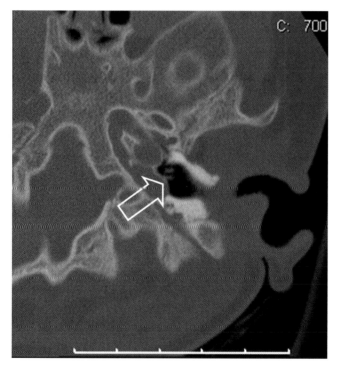

Fig. 4.182   Achondroplasia in a 1-year-old girl. Severe venous bleeding occurred during placement of a tympanostomy tube. CT demonstrates absence of the bony septum between jugular bulb and middle ear cavity (arrow). The tympanostomy tube, which is not visible on this image, was placed at a later point in time.

■ Conductive Hearing Loss

Conductive hearing loss can have a multitude of causes. Blockage of the external ear canal is visible for the otolanryngologist, although the medial extension of lesions can be obscured. Exostoses are often multiple, and osteomas are often single.

Many middle ear anomalies cause conductive hearing loss. Fluid in the middle ear can be serous, glue, pus, or blood. Ossicular chain disruption can be traumatic or iatrogenic. Erosion of the ossicles can be caused by cholesteatoma but also by chronic otitis media. Otosclerosis can lead to fixation of the foot plate of the stapes or impingement of a bony spur of the fissula ante fenestram on the ossicular chain. Middle ear masses can cause immobilization of the ossicles.

Table 4.58 Conductive hearing loss

Diagnosis	Findings	Comments
External ear canal		
External ear canal obstruction	Cerumen, foreign body, exostose, osteoma.	Exostoses often in swimmers/surfers. Exostoses multiple, osteoma isolated.
Middle ear		
Acute otitis media	Opacified middle ear.	Imaging rarely performed.
Glue ear	Opacified middle ear; few air bubbles.	Imaging rarely performed, retracted eardrum, tympanostomy tubes.
Hematotympanum	Opacified middle ear	Posttraumatic, resolves after several weeks. History.
Ossicular disruption	(see **Table 4.63**, trauma)	
Tympanosclerosis ▷ *Fig. 4.183a, b*	Calcified foci in tympanic cavity/tympanic membrane.	In chronic otitis media, sclerotic mastoid.
Chronic otitis media	Sclerotic mastoid, (partly) opacified mastoid cells/tympanic cavity.	Ossicular chain erosion may be present.
Cholesteatoma ▷ *Fig. 4.184*	Ossicular chain disruption, especially lenticular process and stapedial superstructure. Mass may be evident but can be obscured by surrounding fluid/granulomatous tissue.	Note labyrinth fistula, erosion of tegmen. Diffusion-weighted MRI can be helpful.
Cholesterol granuloma		(see **Table 4.61**, blue eardrum)
Otosclerosis ▷ *Fig. 4.185*	Thickened stapedial foot plate; lytic lesion in front of oval window (fissula ante fenestram; lucencies around inner ear.	Productive bony spurs can encroach on ossicles.
Paraganglioma		(see **Table 4.61**, blue eardrum)
Tumors	Middle ear mass.	Rare.

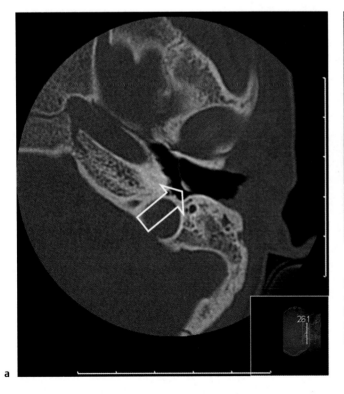

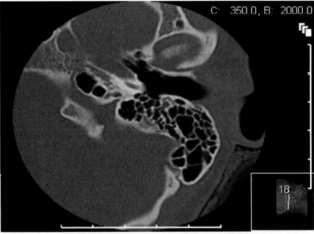

Fig. 4.183a, b Tympanosclerosis. (**a**) An 11-year-old girl with conductive hearing loss. The thickened and calcified focus (arrow) in the tympanic membrane is a sign of tympanosclerosis (also named myringosclerosis). (**b**) Normal ear for comparison. The eardrum is hardly visible.

a

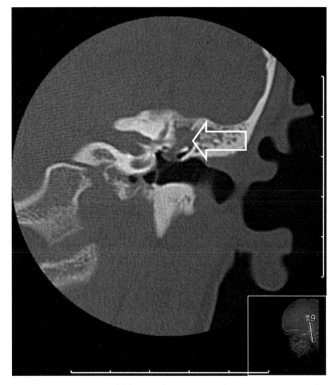

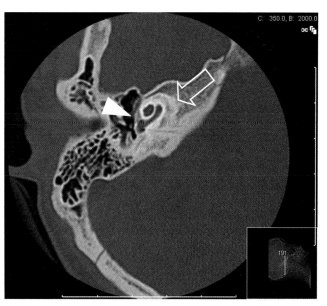

Fig. 4.184   A 9-year-old boy with a mass in the epitympanum. The distal long process of the incus is eroded (arrow). A **cholesteatoma** was operatively removed.

Fig. 4.185   A 14-year-old girl with conductive hearing loss. There is a large focus of **otosclerosis** in front of the oval window at the fissula ante fenestram (arrowhead) and a lucent ring around the cochlea (arrow).

■ Sensorineural Hearing Loss

Sensorineural hearing loss can be caused by cochlear or retrocochlear anomalies. Retrocochlear anomalies are imaged with MRI.

Table 4.59   Sensorineural hearing loss

Diagnosis	Findings	Comments
Cochlear anomalies		
Congenital anomalies (see Table 4.3)	Cochlear/vestibular malformation.	Often no abnormalities detected.
Otosclerosis ▷ *Fig. 4.185*	Thickened stapedial foot plate; lytic lesion in front of oval window (fissula ante fenestram; lucencies around inner ear).	Often symmetric and easily overlooked. Lytic zone around cochlea, so-called fourth ring of Valvassori.
Posttraumatic ▷ *Fig. 4.190, p. 411*	Fracture line through inner ear.	Obvious from history.
Retrocochlear anomalies		
Schwannoma ▷ *Fig. 4.186a, b, p. 408*	Intermediate on T1, hyperintense on T2. Strong enhancement after Gd. Centered over internal auditory canal.	Rare in children, NF2.
Meningioma	Intermediate on T1, hypo- to hyperintense on T2, strong enhancement after Gd.	Rare in children, NF2.
	Obtuse angles.	
Brain lesions	Brainstem glioma, hemangioblastoma, multiple sclerosis.	
Absence of cochlear nerve	See previous discussion of congenital anomalies, this table.	

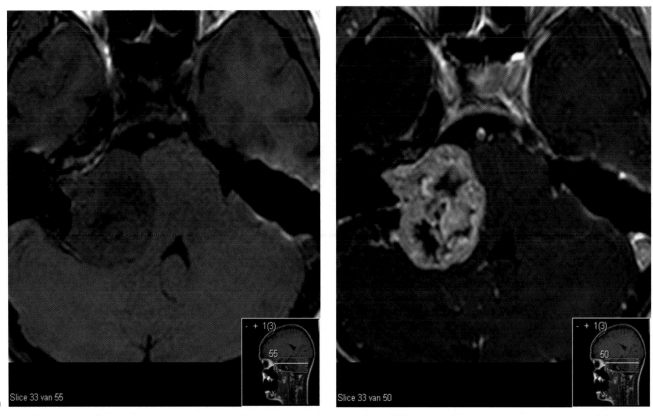

a

Fig. 4.186a, b   Schwannoma. (a) An 18-year-old girl with minor hearing loss on the right side. On MRI, a large schwannoma is found. **(b)** Strong enhancement after intravenous contrast with some cystic parts. The patient has no other diseases.

■ The Opacified Middle Ear

The middle ear can be opacified by a multitude of disease states. CT is nonspecific. Serous fluid, pus, blood, and cholesteatoma have the same attenuation on thin-slice CT. The presence of bony erosion favors cholesteatoma, but erosion can be seen in chronic inflammation.

Table 4.60   The opacified middle ear

Diagnosis	Findings	Comments
Serous otitis media	Opacified middle ear. Retracted eardrum.	
Acute otitis media	Opacified middle ear. Intracranial abscess, empyema. Sinus thrombosis.	Coalescence of air cells in advanced stage.
Chronic otitis media	Sclerotic mastoid. Partly or completely opacified middle ear. Ossicular chain erosion possible.	MRI: low T1, high T2, Gd enhancement, low DWI.
Posttraumatic		(see **Table 4.62**)
Cholesteatoma ▷ *Fig. 4.187*	Displacement and/or erosion of ossicular chain, especially in long process of incus/scutum. Erosion of lateral semicircular canal, tegmen tympani.	MRI: low T1, high SI T2, Gd rim enhancement, high DWI, low ADC.
Postoperative state	Inflammation; recurrent cholesteaoma; fat obliteration of cavity; meningocele into operative cavity.	MRI helpful.

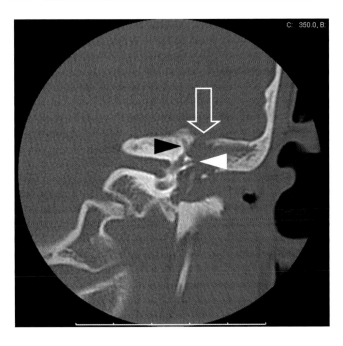

Fig. 4.187   Large cholesteatoma in an 11-year-old boy with erosion of the ossicular chain, lateral wall of the tympanic cavity, the tegmen tympani (arrow), the lateral semicircular canal (white arrowhead), and the superior semicircular canal (black arrowhead).

■ The Blue Eardrum

A blue eardrum can be caused by vascular structures like an aberrant ICA or dehiscent jugular bulb. Analysis of axial slices will show the vascular nature of the mass. A glomus jugulotympanicum is rare in the pediatric age group. A cholesterol granuloma leads to a complete opacification of the middle ear.

Table 4.61   The blue eardrum

Diagnosis	Findings	Comments
Cholesterol granuloma	CT: opacified middle ear, mass effect with erosion of tympanic cavity walls and ossicles. MRI: high signal intensity on T1 and T2, rim enhancement, low on DWI.	
Aberrant ICA	Soft-tissue mass in middle ear. On consecutive slices, follow to horizontal carotid canal.	Courses on promontory, do not confuse with glomus tympanicum.
Dehiscent jugular bulb ▷ Fig. 4.188	Mass in posterior middle ear; on consecutive slices follow to jugular bulb.	Root of jugular bulb partially absent.
Paraganglioma	Mass on promontory.	Rare in children.
Posttraumatic hematotympanum	Opacified middle ear.	History will tell.

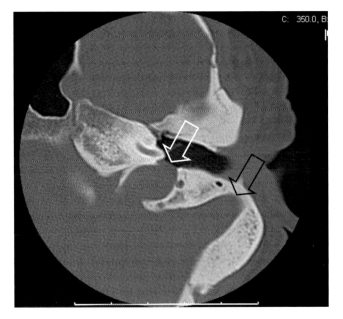

Fig. 4.188   Dehiscent jugular bulb (white arrow). Also, note the bulging sigmoid sinus (black arrow).

■ Trauma

Fractures of the temporal bone are classically divided into longitudinal and transverse fractures. Longitudinal fractures follow the long axis of the temporal bone, are the most common, and can cause ossicular chain disruption with conductive hearing loss and facial nerve paralysis. Sensorineural hearing loss is not common in longitudinal fractures. Transverse fractures run perpendicular to the long axis of the temporal bone and are less common, but often cause sensorineural hearing loss due to damage to the inner ear.

Fractures are frequently of a mixed type and a careful description of the course of the fracture(s) is required.

Table 4.62 lists the findings in conductive and sensorineural hearing loss but is to some extent artificial, as fractures are often of a mixed type.

Table 4.62 Posttraumatic findings

Diagnosis	Findings	Comments
Conductive hearing loss		
Ruptured tympanic membrane		Imaging mostly unnecessary, can show fracture of external auditory canal.
Hematotympanum	Opacified middle ear.	Posttraumatic, resolves after several weeks.
Ossicular disruption ▷ *Fig. 4.189a, b*	Incus luxation; isolated incudostapedial luxation; isolated incudomallear luxation; fracture of incus, fracture of stapedial crura.	Compare with contralateral side for subtle changes. Crural fractures difficult to demonstrate.
Sensorineural hearing loss		
Inner ear fracture ▷ *Fig. 4.190*	Fracture line crossing labyrinth or internal auditory meatus.	Often wide fracture line but can also be very subtle.
Labyrinth concussion	No fractures visible.	MRI can demonstrate blood in inner ear.
Facial nerve palsy	Fracture line crossing facial nerve canal; bony fragments impinge on facial nerve canal.	Palsy can be present without visible fracture.
CSF leakage	Fracture through tegmen tympani; through inner ear; herniation of cranial contents in middle ear.	Difficult diagnosis. MRI can be helpful; scintigraphy. Nasal liquorrhea via eustachian tube if tympanic membrane intact.

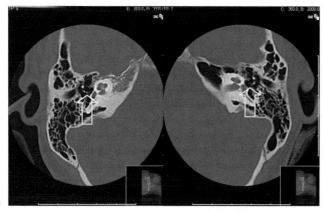
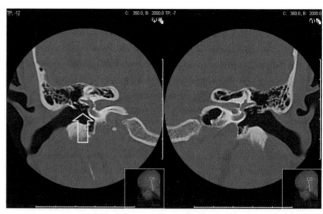

Fig. 4.189a, b Ossicular disruption in a 17-year-old girl with conductive hearing loss after a bicycle accident. On the axial images (**a**), the incudostapedial joint looks intact (arrow). On the coronal images (**b**), the lentiform process of the incus on the left projects beneath the stapedial head (arrow). Incudostapedial luxation was confirmed at operation. Also, a stapedial crural fracture was found.

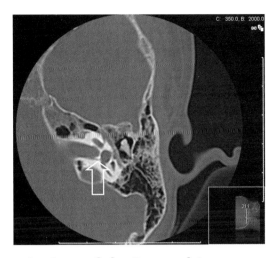

Fig. 4.190 A 7-year-old boy with left-sided deafness after skull base fracture. A **transverse fracture runs from the internal auditory canal to the vestibule** (arrow) and continues through the facial nerve canal.

■ Lesions of the Petrosal Apex

Lesions of the petrous apex are rare in children but cause great unrest. The petrous apex is pneumatized in one-third of adults. In children, the percentage increases with age. Asymmetric pneumatization is present in approximately 5%. Especially on MRI, the nonpneumatized petrous apex, containing fatty marrow, can simulate a mass.

Table 4.63 Lesions of the petrosal apex

Diagnosis	Findings	Comments
Fatty marrow in petrous apex ▷ *Fig. 4.176, p. 402*	High signal intensity on T1 and T2 turbo spin echo	Can be misinterpreted as a lesion, especially when unilateral. Compare signal intensity with subcutaneous fat.
Trapped fluid in petrous air cells	CT: opacified air cells. MRI: low on T1, high on T2.	
Cholesterol granuloma	Smooth expansive lesion. Often high intensity on both T1 and T2.	Can present with cranial nerve paralysis. Young to middle-aged adults.
Mucocele	CT: smooth expansive lesion. MRI: variable signal intensity on T1, bright on T2.	
Congenital cholesteatoma (epidermoid)	CT: smooth expansive lesion. Intermediate T1, high T2. Restricted DWI.	Rare, especially in childhood.
LCH	Lytic temporal bone lesion, mostly squama.	Affects mastoid process, temporal squama, middle ear. Less common in petrous apex. Bilateral involvement common.
Other tumors		Rhabdomyosarcoma most common (middle ear). Metastasis, lymphoma, lymphangioma.
Infection: apicitis ▷ *Fig. 4.191*	Destructive lesion apex; middle ear and mastoid opacified; enhancing walls, abscess can be present.	Gradenigo's triad: mastoiditis, sixth nerve palsy, deep facial pain (first branch fifth nerve).

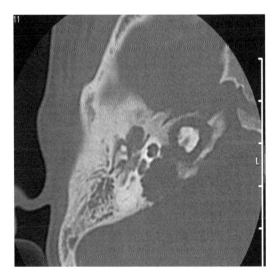

Fig. 4.191 Infection in a 6-year-old boy with a deaf right ear and chronic otitis media. CT shows a large destructive process of the petrous apex and labyrinth. Pathologic examination showed granulation tissue, but no organism was cultivated.

Vertebral Column Imaging Procedures

Standard radiographs in two projections are adequate in many situations. Additional obliques are often helpful in the cervical and lumbar regions (especially after neck trauma in adolescents and in low back pain if spondylolisthesis is found on the lateral image). In scoliosis, a frontal upright view, standing or seated, should be obtained if at all possible, plus a lateral image. Recumbent lateral bending films and perhaps recumbent traction (from above and below) belong to a more complete scoliosis evaluation to check flexibility of curves. Localized findings on conventional spine radiographs are confirmed with coned views or CT and MRI, as indicated.

US is suitable for examination of the lower spinal canal and motion of the spinal cord in infants, generally though 3 months of age. MRI images the marrow spaces and delineates the bones and soft tissues, including fatty tissue; this is the best method to examine the spinal cord and contents over 3 months of age. It can also be the best method in younger patients in certain situations.

CT shows structure of vertebral bone and allows effective 3D reconstruction.

Bone scanning is a sensitive indicator of altered metabolic activity of bone (infection, fracture, and tumor), as is positron emission tomography (PET) scanning.

The Pediatric Vertebral Column

The vertebral column consists of 7 cervical, 12 thoracic, and 5 lumbar levels, as well as 5 sacral segments and a few coccygeal levels. The dens, eventually attaching to the body of C2, replaces what would have been the body of C1.

Variants. In a series of 100 radiographs of patients aged between 4 months and 19 years, five complete lumbar vertebrae (without ribs) were present in 84% of cases, four in 5%, and six in 6%. A transitional vertebra with one side sacral and one side lumbar, or else a rib on what would be one side of L1, made up the remaining 5%. These variations are effects of hox genes and may also be seen in the VATER (vertebral, anal, cardiac, tracheo-esophageal, radial or renal) association.

Normal findings. A vertical midline cleft is normal in infants; the narrow interface lucency projects over the center of the vertebral body on frontal projections. The cleft progressively ossifies (fuses) caudocranially in thoracic levels in the first year of life. This line can persist as a laminar cleft at C1 and C7, and at the lower thoracic column; it then may serve as a marker to identify individuals. At L5, the cleft often does not fuse until age 10; thereafter, it is known as spina bifida occulta.

In neonates (**Fig. 4.192**) on the lateral image, the prenatal bone is relatively dense compared to the bone laid down in the first weeks of life, just adjacent to the denser end plates, which are cartilaginous zones of provisional calcification. The anterior arch of C1 may not ossify during the first year of life, but may be present at birth. The horizontal Hahn fissure, or vascular canal, causes the anterior midbody notch of the biconvex vertebral body, and gradually fades after the neonatal period. Similarly, the neurocentral synchondrosis (see **Figs. 4.192** and **Fig. 4.268**) may normally be unossified in early infancy. Anterior steplike projections extend out from the vertebral bodies of school-aged children. Ring apophyses appear in the unossified corner areas at approximately 10 years of age. Thoracic vertebral bodies may have mildly decreased height anteriorly and appear wedged. In the first year of life, the dens is connected to C2 body by a nonossified synchondrosis.

On frontal views of the chest, the cervical spine area often seems quite abnormal in infants, merely due to projection.

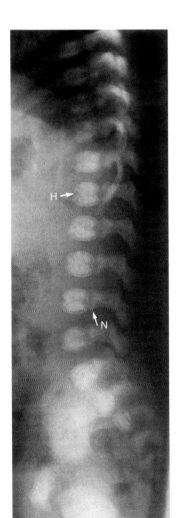

Fig. 4.192 Normal vertebral column of a neonate. Biconvex vertebral bodies, denser midbody structure with less dense newest bone adjacent to the endplates, and minimal lumbar lordosis are noted.
H Vascular fissure (Hahn)
N Neurocentral synchondrosis

Anomalies of Vertebral Body Shape and Size

■ Decreased Height

Generalized of Multiple Flattened Vertebrae (Platyspondyly)

In all cases of platyspondyly, it should be ascertained whether the dens is hypoplastic. A short dens predisposes to the dangerous atlantoaxial subluxation, particularly during sudden flexion or extension of the cervical spine (see, for example, **Fig. 4.200**).

Table 4.64 Neonatal platyspondyly

Diagnosis	Findings	Comments
Achondroplasia ▷ *Fig. 4.193*	Short rectangular vertebral bodies with vertically widened disk spaces, lumbar lordosis, and acute lumbar sacral angle anteroinferiorly. Narrowing of the distal lumbar spinal canal on the AP projection.	Short stature with short extremities and typical changes of the bony pelvis. Ice cream scoop en face proximal femurs in infancy. Occasional symptoms from narrow cervical spinal canal.
Thanatophoric dysplasia ▷ *Fig. 4.194*	Universal striking platyspondyly, much more severe than achondroplasia. Vertebrae appear like an "H" or a "U" on the frontal projection. European landline telephone receiver–shaped femora.	A member of the achondroplasia family, with much more severe enchondral slowing. This dysplasia, as implied by its name, is lethal. Survival can occur in the Torrance variant of thanatophoric dysplasia (straight femora).
Hypothyroidism ▷ *Fig. 4.195*	Vertebral body flattening, beaklike projection from the anteroinferior proximal lumbar bodies in infancy. Relatively dense bone normal in neonates.	Delayed skeletal age. Neonatal screening via thyroid stimulating hormone levels now detects early.
Osteogenesis imperfecta	One neonatal presentation as a result of intrauterine osteoporosis is collapse of many vertebral bodies.	Osteoporosis. Multiple fractures and healing or healed fractures elsewhere in the skeleton.
Spondyloepiphyseal dysplasia congenita	Pear shaped vertebral bodies with significant decrease in height, kyphoscoliosis, and irregular epiphyses.	Short trunk. Delayed ossification of pubic bones. A lethal form exists with thoracic dysplasia and pulmonary hypoplasia.
Hypophosphatasia	A neonatal lethal form has severe zones of rachitic-like changes and platyspondyly.	Phosphoethanolamine is excreted in the urine.
Congenital Cushing disease	Marked osteoporosis, fractures frequent.	Excessive steroids.
Achondrogenesis and homozygous achondroplasia	Variably deficient ossification of the axial skeleton.	Both are lethal dysplasias. Relatively large head.
Metatropic dysplasia	Universal platyspondyly. Wide clefts between the vertebral body and neural arches; older: kyphoscoliosis.	Rhizomelic shortening. Markedly widened metaphyses. Tubular bones have a dumbbell or diabolo shape.
Kyphomelic dysplasia	Relatively mild platyspondyly. Short long bones, some bowed, and ribs (often only 11 pairs).	Severe rhizomelic shortening, may have camptodactyly.
Hallermann-Streiff syndrome	Narrow long bones and thin calvarium; multiple wormian bones.	Oculomandibulofacial syndrome.
Osteoglophonic dysplasia	Multiple fibrous metaphyseal defects; platyspondyly with anterior projection; acromelic shortening.	Craniofacial dysostosis with fibrous metaphyseal defects.

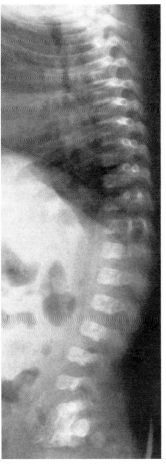

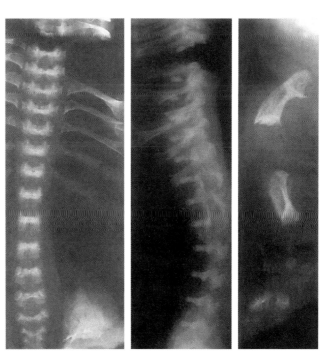

Fig. 4.193 Achondroplasia in a neonate. Lateral vertebral column: small vertebral bodies, widened intervertebral soft-tissue density spaces, thoracolumbar kyphosis, and sharply angled lumbosacral lordosis.

Fig. 4.194 Thanatophoric dysplasia in a neonate with marked short stature on postmortem radiographs: striking platyspondyly, short ribs, European telephone receiver–shape of the femur, and rhizomelia.

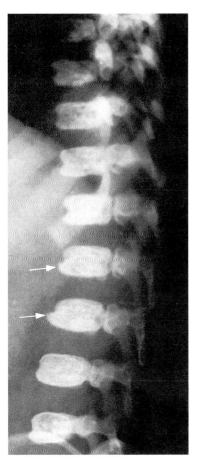

Fig. 4.195 Hypothyroidism in a neonate with rectangular small vertebral bodies and widened intervertebral soft-tissue density spaces. Hooklike anterior projection from the lower surface of L2 and L3 (arrows). Prominent soft-tissue density synchondrosis cleft between neural arches and the bodies. Striking Hahn vascular notches on midanterior bodies (courtesy of K. Koslowski, Sydney, Australia).

Table 4.65   Platyspondyly in older children

Diagnosis	Findings	Comments
Osteoporosis ▷ *Fig. 4.196* ▷ *Fig. 4.197a, b*	Generalized demineralization of bone with preservation of the cartilaginous zones of provisional calcification, including vertebral end plates (so that they are more conspicuous than normal). Multiple pathologic compression fractures. Thoracic vertebrae become flattened or anteriorly wedged; codfish (biconcave) vertebral deformity predominantly in the lumber region.	Many causes including steroid or heparin therapy, Cushing syndrome, idiopathic, sickle cell and other chronic anemias, leukemia, neuromuscular disease such as Duchenne muscular dystrophy, and homocystinuria.
Secondary (or primary) hyperparathyroidism ▷ *Fig. 4.198a, b*	If rickets is also present, the vertebral end plates (zones of provisional calcification) become difficult to see, which is the opposite of the situation in osteoporosis.	May also be a manifestation of renal osteodystrophy.
Osteogenesis imperfecta	Multiple (sometimes universal), flat, or biconcave (codfish) vertebrae. Demineralization (osteoporosis), compression fractures. Multiple wormian bones.	Blue sclerae. Clinical course quite variable depending on severity. Sometimes mistaken for child abuse.
Hypothyroidism ▷ *Fig. 4.195, p. 415*	Vertebral body flattening, beaklike projection from anterior inferior proximal lumbar vertebral bodies.	Delayed skeletal age. Multiple wormian bones in congenital hypothyroidism. Neonatal screening usually identifies congenital involvement.
NF1	May have platyspondyly, idiopathic or localized acute scoliosis, plexiform neuromas, and other spinal area tumors.	Café au lait spots.
Morquio syndrome ▷ *Fig. 4.199, p. 418* ▷ *Fig. 4.200a, b, p. 418*	Anterior midbody tonguelike projections off the lumbar vertebrae, hypoplastic dens.	MPS IV. Pectus carinatum. Increased urinary keratan sulfate. Spinal cord may become severely damaged from atlantoaxial subluxation related to the short dens. Normal or high intelligence.

(continues on page 419)

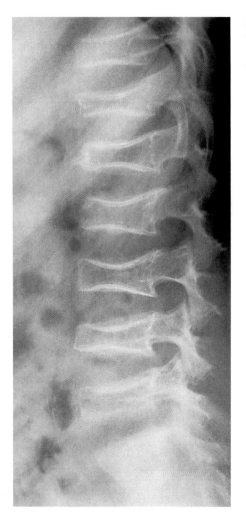

Fig. 4.196 Osteoporosis in a 13-year-old girl due to long-term steroid therapy for renal disease with simultaneously decreased body height and codfish vertebral shape. The end plates (zones of provisional calcification) maintain normal mineralization, and so appear strikingly dense compared to adjacent osteoporotic bone.

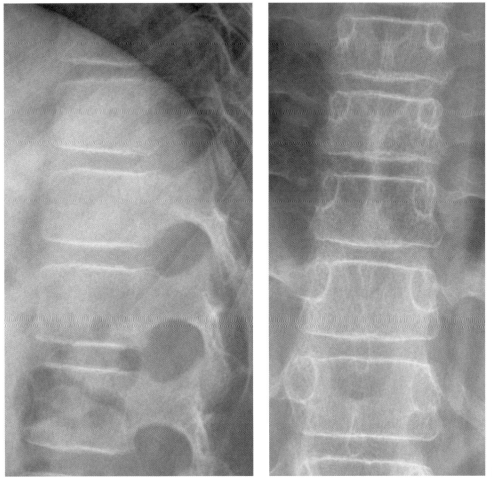

Fig. 4.197a, b **Osteoporosis** in 10-year-old boy with Duchenne muscular dystrophy. Lateral (**a**) and frontal (**b**) images show the osteoporosis pattern of demineralized bone leaving the normal density zones of provisional calcification (end plates) highly conspicuous. Pedicle cortices en face (**b**) are thin.

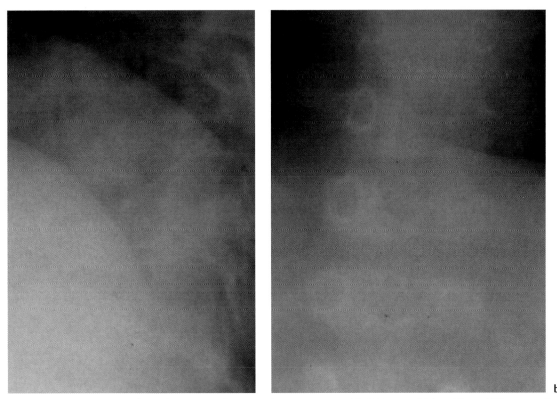

Fig. 4.198a, b **Hyperparathyroidism, secondary to rickets** in a 1-year-old child. Lateral (**a**) and frontal (**b**) images show the hyperparathyroidism and rickets pattern in contrast to **Fig. 4.197**. Because of the rickets, the end plates are quite inconspicuous as they are uncalcified. The pedicle cortices en face (**b**) are not thinned, but are somewhat washed-out, which is characteristic of hyperparathyroidism.

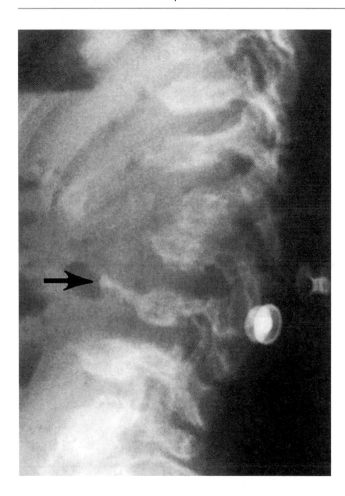

Fig. 4.199   Morquio syndrome. Irregular loss of height of vertebral body with tonguelike center anterior projection (arrow) in a 2.5-year-old girl.

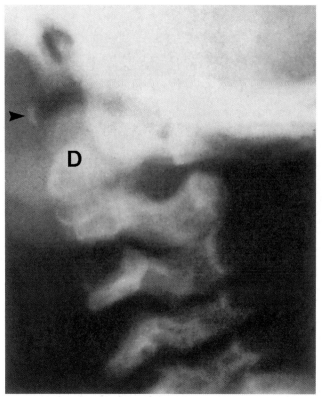

a

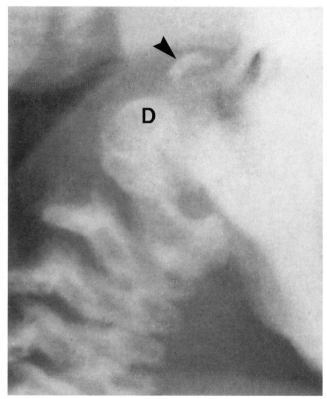

Fig. 4.200a, b   Atlantoaxial subluxation in Morquio syndrome in same patient as in **Fig. 4.198**. Cervical vertebral platyspondyly with short dens (D). The tip of the dens lies far below the anterior arch of C1 (arrowheads). (**a**) High position of the anterior arch of C1, in flexion. (**b**) Considerable atlantoaxial subluxation with (gentle) neck extension.

Table 4.65   (Cont.) Platyspondyly in older children

Diagnosis	Findings	Comments
Other MPS and heteroglycanoses	In most types, such as Hurler and Hunter syndromes, there is an anteroinferior beaklike projection from lower thoracic or upper lumber vertebrae.	The vertebral change resembles hypothyroidism. Skeletal changes are more pronounced in MPS I–H, i.e., Hurler syndrome. Diagnostic findings in urine help separate the types. Also includes most mucolipidoses.
Spondyloepiphyseal dysplasia tarda ▷ *Fig. 4.201*	Diminished height of the anterior portion of vertebral bodies. Bodies are middle and posteriorly biconvex. Occasional disk calcification.	Dysplastic femoral epiphyses, bilaterally symmetric, and also other epiphyses. Early onset of arthritis.
Progressive pseudorheumatoid dysplasia ▷ *Fig. 4.202*	Large limb joints look like JIA; vertebral bodies more like pseudoachondroplastic dysplasia.	A dysplasia and not an inflammatory condition. Rheumatoid factor normal, for example.
Treated (by transfusions) thalassemia major	May even be changes of scurvy; coarse trabeculae and wide diploic space of thalassemia may remain.	Anemia often quite pronounced.
Pyle disease	Biconcave platyspondyly. Abnormally wide diametaphyseal regions of long bones that lack normal concavity.	Familial metaphyseal dysplasia.
Spondylometaphyseal dysplasia, Kozlowski type ▷ *Fig. 4.203, p. 420*	Marked platyspondyly.	AD. Limitation of joint motion.
Kniest disease ▷ *Fig. 4.204, p. 420*	Multiple flattened vertebral bodies with irregular end plates. Coronal clefts in the midposterior vertebral bodies (common), spinal stenosis, kyphoscoliosis.	Spondyloepimetaphyseal dysplasia with widened metaphyses. Stiff, thickened joints. Myopia, deafness.
Dyggve-Melchior-Clausen dysplasia ▷ *Fig. 4.205, p. 420*	Vertebral bodies with anterior and posterior humps above and below ("Bactrian camel back"). Lacy iliac crests.	Short extremities, mental retardation. Similar changes with normal mental development indicates Smith-McCort syndrome.
Pseudoachondroplasia ▷ *Fig. 4.206, p. 420*	Vertebrae are biconvex in neonates; later diminished height with anterior wedging. End plates are irregular, as are epiphyses. Kyphoscoliosis.	A spondyloepiphyseal dysplasia. Short extremities, including hands and feet.
Stickler syndrome (arthro-ophthalmopathy)	Significantly low vertebral body height.	Marfan-like body habitus, progressive myopia, and retinal detachment. Epiphyseal dysplasia. Early onset of arthritis.
Dysosteosclerosis	Platyspondyly and osteosclerosis (punctate margins of vertebral bodies). Resorption of phalangeal tufts.	Multiple fractures.

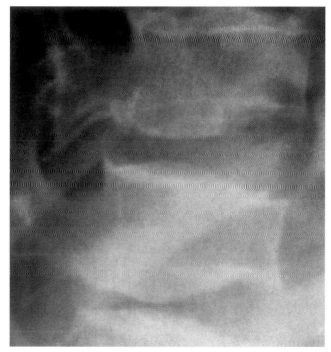
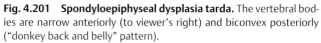
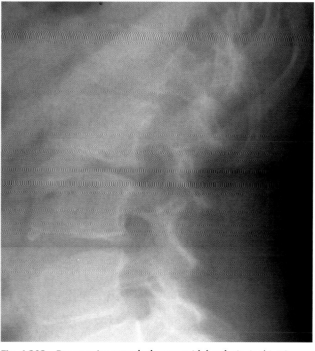

Fig. 4.201   Spondyloepiphyseal dysplasia tarda. The vertebral bodies are narrow anteriorly (to viewer's right) and biconvex posteriorly ("donkey back and belly" pattern).

Fig. 4.202   Progressive pseudorheumatoid dysplasia. In this 13-year-old girl, some of the typical deformed lower thoracic and upper lumbar vertebral bodies are noted (here, there is excessive convexity of the upper and lower posterior body with tapered anterior portions).

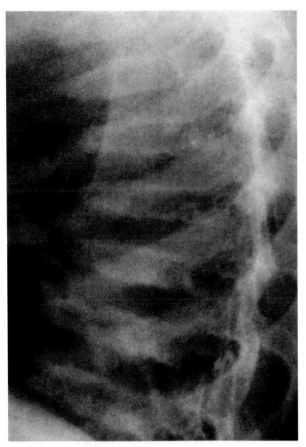

Fig. 4.203 Spondylometaphyseal dysplasia, Kozlowski type, showing short and sagittally elongated vertebral bodies.

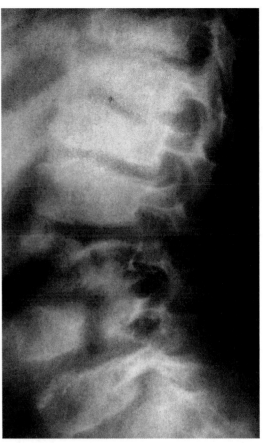

Fig. 4.204 Kniest disease. Short, sagittally long lumbar vertebral bodies with wavy upper and lower end plates and coronal cleft in L4 and forme fruste cleft in L3.

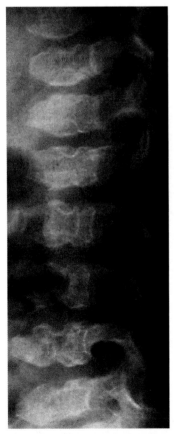

Fig. 4.205 Dyggve-Melchior-Clausen dysplasia. Vertebral bodies with anterior and posterior humps ("Bactrian camel back") of upper and lower margins; notches between the humps are concave toward the disks.

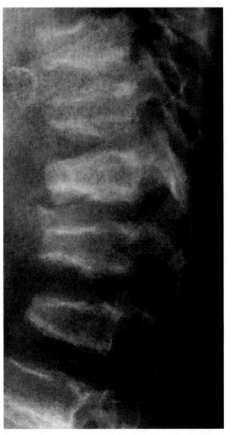

Fig. 4.206 Pseudoachondroplasia. The bodies have diminished height, and the end plates are irregular. Diminished height is most pronounced anteriorly.

Loss of Height in Single or Multiple Vertebral Bodies

Table 4.66   Loss of height in single or multiple vertebral bodies

Diagnosis	Findings	Comments
Spondylitis-diskitis (osteomyelitis) ▷ *Fig. 4.207a–d* ▷ *Fig. 4.278, p. 477*	The most common cause of decreased vertebral height with destruction in childhood. Early radiographic changes: decreased disk space and destruction of the adjacent end plate, with possible posterior displacement of vertebral body. Earlier positive findings on MRI or NM. Later, occasionally wedging or fusion in the healing phase. Rarely, central osteomyelitis in the vertebral body without disk space involvement.	Pyogenic bacteria, tuberculosis (starts anteriorly), brucellosis (also starts anteriorly). Also often no organism found. Differentiation from tuberculosis in early phase may be difficult: there is later calcification and gibbus formation in tuberculosis.
Fracture ▷ *Fig. 4.208, p. 422*	Many involve more than one vertebral body. Anterior wedging with decreased height (exception: a Chance fracture is transverse through body and arch, which may lead to "taller" vertebra). May be a nose-shaped projection from an anterior corner. Dense callus seen within the bone after 10 d. Disk spaces are maintained.	Caution: Lateral compression on frontal projection may be subtle. CT and MRI are indicated in comminuted fractures for position of fragments and spinal cord involvement, respectively.
Child abuse	Often fractures are multiple; spinous processes alone may be fractured. Many other typical fractures elsewhere in skeleton.	On chest images, look for paraspinal hematoma or rib fractures.
LCH (eosinophilic granuloma) ▷ *Fig. 4.209, p. 422*	Initial slight flattening, finally becoming vertebra plana. May affect single or multiple vertebral bodies. Arch elements less often affected; disk spaces intact. Regains height after the process is no longer active (the end plate zone of provisional calcification continues its enchondral bone growth).	Additional foci may be sought by bone scintigraphy, or, indeed, by PET scan. Typically painless in early stage.

(continues on page 423)

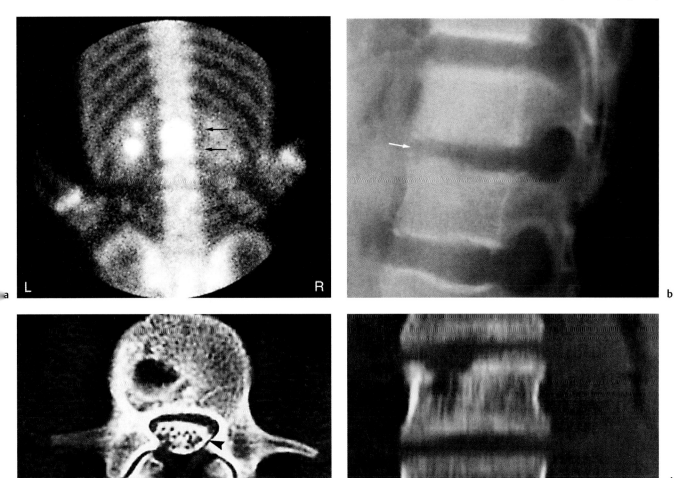

Fig. 4.207a–d   Osteomyelitis. (a) "Pioneer" bone scintigraphy shows increased activity at L2 and L3 (arrows). Radiograph at that time was normal. **(b)** Three weeks later, there is loss of height of the L2-L3 disk space (arrow). The adjacent end plates no longer show normal calcifi-cation. **(c)** A different patient with more advanced disease. CT shows destruction in the L3 body with no involvement of spinal canal (arrowhead). **(d)** Coronal reconstruction of **(c)** showing downward extension of the defect into the body and narrowing of the disk space.

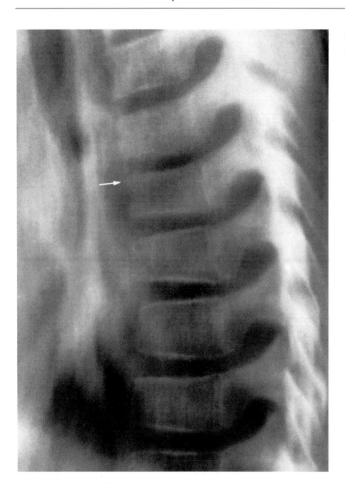

Fig. 4.208 Wedge-shaped **compression fractures** of the thoracic spine (tomogram). Arrow points out the beaklike projection.

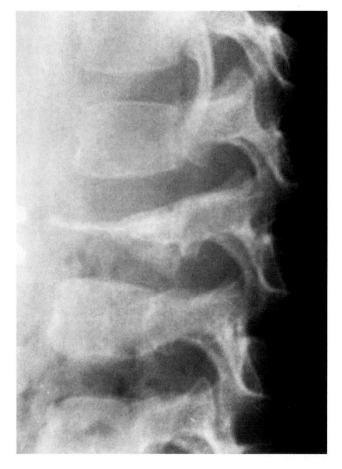

Fig. 4.209 Langerhans cell histiocytosis. Flattened vertebral body L2 with maintained disk spaces. One cervical body was also affected in this nearly 1-year-old boy.

Table 4.66   (Cont.) Loss of height in single or multiple vertebral bodies

Diagnosis	Findings	Comments
Leukemia	Osteoporosis, pathologic compression fractures. Disk spaces maintained.	Osteoporosis and vertebral compression can be the presenting findings of leukemia (may even simulate child abuse).
Sickle cell anemia ▷ *Fig. 4.228, p. 434*	Associated with the "Lincoln Log" notched indentation of middle, upper, and lower vertebral body margins.	Anemia. Look also for calcified gallstones.
Fibrous dysplasia ▷ *Fig. 4.210*	Flattening of a single vertebra can occur; may show scoliosis.	Café au lait spots, advanced bone age.
Following irradiation	Irregular growth disturbance.	Especially after radiation for renal or adrenal tumors. Dose-dependent (possible after 30 Gy; usual after 40 Gy).
Tumors, metastases ▷ *Fig. 4.211, p. 424*	Destruction and loss of height of one or more vertebral bodies. Disk spaces preserved. Pedicle destruction may occur.	Metastases: especially neuroblastoma (may be painless at first), rarely rhabdomyosarcoma, Wilms tumor, or Ewing sarcoma. Primary: Ewing sarcoma, may be sclerotic; vertebral body aneurysmal bone cyst, lucent and may collapse.
Chronic recurrent multifocal osteomyelitis	Associated sternal, clavicle, or long bone lesions.	May have acne or plantopalmar pustulosis (SAPHO [synovitis, *a*cne, *p*almoplantar pustulosis, *h*yperostosis, and *o*steitis] association). Many plasma cells but no organism on biopsy.
Fungal infection	Vertebral body destruction without disk space decrease.	One cause is disseminated coccidioidomycosis.
Tuberculosis and brucellosis ▷ *Fig. 4.212a, b, p. 424*	When vertebral body is affected, the anterior body typically loses height sooner than the posterior.	Tubercuosis: skin testing; brucellosis: contact with affected livestock.
Thalassemia major; Gaucher disease	Single vertebra can be affected.	

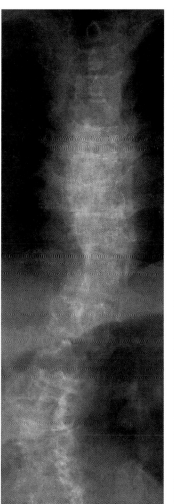 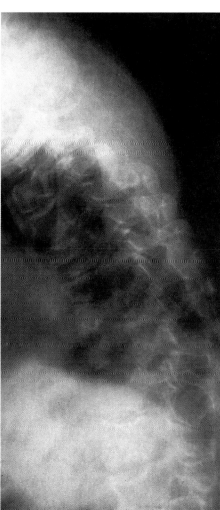

Fig. 4.210   Fibrous dysplasia. Severe disturbance of vertebral column with S-shaped scoliosis and the deformed bodies have some loss of height.

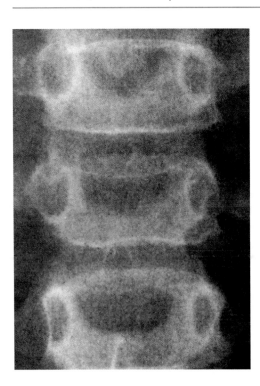

Fig. 4.211   Metastasis from Wilms tumor. Bowed downward depression of the upper end plate of a single vertebral body (initially unrecognized).

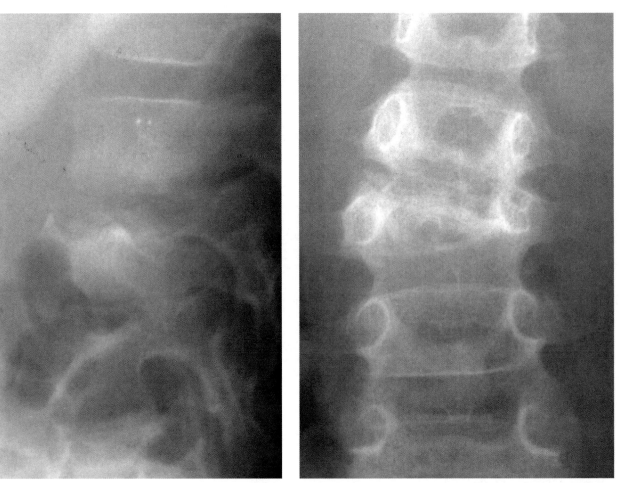

a

b

Fig. 4.212a, b   Tuberculosis. (a) Considerable loss of height of L3 body, with characteristic greater severity anteriorly. Loss of definition of upper end plate of L3 and part of lower end plate of L2. **(b)** Overall, the loss of height is greater on the left in this case.

True or Apparent Enlargement of the Vertebral Bodies

A compensatory increase in height occurs in vertebrae adjacent to a hemivertebra, acquired fused vertebrae after spondylitis, and in surgical posterior fusion in several types of scoliosis.

Table 4.67   Enlargement of the vertebral bodies

Diagnosis	Findings	Comments
Nonambulatory in early childhood: CNS impairment and neuromuscular disease ▷ Fig. 4.213	Tall or barrel-shaped vertebrae on the lateral image, predominantly in lower thoracic and the lumbar vertebrae.	May be already evident in neonates; changes increase with age and indicate that a child is not walking.
Polyostotic FD, Albright syndrome ▷ Fig. 4.214	Barrel-shaped vertebrae. Advanced bone age.	Café-au-lait spots.
Hox gene dependent increased height adjacent to hemivertebra	Although tilted, the disk height tends to be normal. Bodies adjacent to butterfly vertebrae similar have medial lengthening in compensation.	May be a part of VATER association.
Caudal regression syndrome	Sacral aplasia; may have vertical overgrowth of remaining lumber bodies.	May be associated with maternal diabetes.
Rachischisis	Vertebral bodies may be enlarged on frontal view; disk spaces decreased.	Spina bifida aperta, perhaps with associated Chiari type II malformation.
Scheuermann disease	At the kyphosis, bodies may have increased sagittal and coronal width, along with reduced height especially anteriorly.	Often familial.
Compression fracture	Enlargement can occur in width sagittally or coronally; callus after 10 d.	MRI for associated cord damage.
Mass in the spinal canal	Apparent increase in height on lateral image is caused by narrowing in the sagittal dimension.	MRI to show the mass.
Tumors and metastases; aneurysmal bone cyst	Vertebral elements may be expanded by tumor growth or else diminished by pathologic fracture or collapse.	Hemangioma, lymphangioma, giant cell tumor, osteoblastoma, and renal cell carcinoma are possibilities.

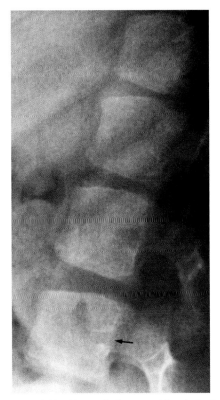

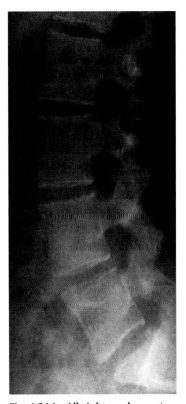

Fig. 4.213   Nonambulatory, with relatively tall lumbar vertebrae. A severely brain damaged 8-year-old child with motor delay. There is no vertical stress on the spine. There is an incidental striking posterior vascular fissure in L3 (arrow).

Fig. 4.214   Albright syndrome. In contrast to **Fig. 4.209**, the lumbar bodies may be relatively tall.

Table 4.68   Rarer syndromes with tall appearing vertebral bodies

Diagnosis	Findings	Comments
Pycnodysostosis	Relatively tall vertebral bodies. Bones abnormally dense and somewhat fragile.	Multiple wormian bones; obtuse angle of the mandible.
Kenny-Caffey syndrome ▷ *Fig. 4.215*	Tall vertebrae with hourglass shape. Gracile long bones.	Also known as tubular stenosis dysplasia.
Melnick-Needles syndrome	Relatively tall vertebral bodies with small lumbar disk spaces. "Twisted" ribs and long bones.	Also known as osteodysplasty.
Cartilage hair hypoplasia	Vertebral bodies look tall because of decreased transverse dimensions.	Also known as metaphyseal chondrodysplasia, McKusick type. Sparse, thin, light-colored hair.
Fuhrmann syndrome	Narrow tall vertebral bodies.	Bowed femurs; absent fibulas.
Freeman-Sheldon syndrome	Narrow tall vertebral bodies, including cervical. Some bodies may be flattened instead.	"Whistling face." Ulnar deviation of hands.
Hajdu-Cheney syndrome	Tall lumbar vertebral bodies with narrow disk spaces. Collapse may also occur. Bones dense. Osteolysis of terminal phalanges.	Also known as arthrodentosteodysplasia. Short stature. Multiple wormian bones.
Dolichospondylic dysplasia	High vertebral body dwarfism.	Gracile long bones, short stature.
3-M syndrome	Sagittally shorter lumbar vertebral bodies look tall. Slender ribs and tubular bones.	May be allelic with dolichospondylic dysplasia, which it resembles. The three "M"s represent the lead authors of the original description.

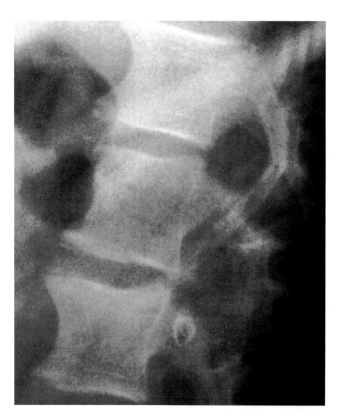

Fig. 4.215   Kenny-Caffey syndrome. Relatively tall vertebral bodies with an hourglass shape in a 16-year-old boy (courtesy of J. Dorst, Baltimore, MD).

■ Changes in the Shape of Single or Multiple Vertebral Bodies

Normal Shapes and Variants

Vertebral bodies appear relatively rectangular on the lateral radiograph. In school-aged children, smaller, rectangular, soft-tissue density (cartilage) gaps are present at the upper and lower corners of the anterior vertebral bodies; ossification of the ring apophyses within these gaps becomes evident at approximately 10 years of age. When ossification is significantly delayed, as may occur in multiple epiphyseal dysplasia (**Fig. 4.216**), the ossification of these ring apophyses is accordingly markedly delayed.

Single or multiple midthoracic or lower thoracic vertebral bodies may normally have mildly decreased height anteriorly (wedging). The angle between the upper and lower end plates (**Fig. 4.217**) can be up to 10°. **Table 4.69** shows the age distribution and frequency of this thoracic wedge shape in 100 healthy children. The angle was > 5° in 75 of the children. The midthoracic vertebrae are predominantly affected up to 13 years of age. In adolescents, wedging typically occurs in the lowest segments.

Anterior wedging and simultaneous vertebral flattening occurs in some of the rare dysplasias, including:
- Pseudoachondroplasia
- Spondylometaphyseal dysplasia, type Kozlowski
- Metatropic dysplasia

The anterior height also appears decreased with tall or barrel-shaped vertebral bodies associated with hypotonia. Among the unusual shapes are codfish vertebrae, butterfly vertebrae, anterior projections, and hourglass or spindle-shaped vertebrae.

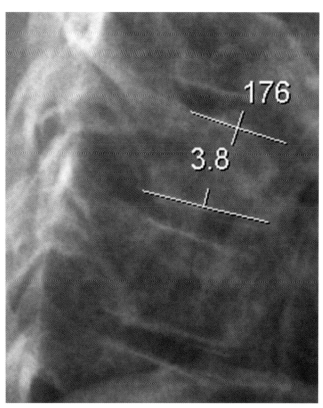

Fig. 4.217 Measurement of the angle of a physiologic wedged vertebra. The angle is 4° in this example and not pathologic.

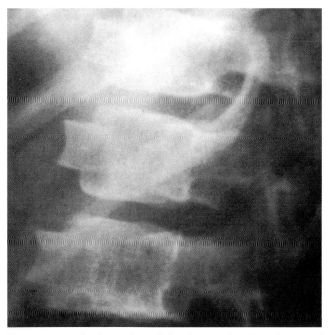

Fig. 4.216 Multiple epiphyseal dysplasia. Delayed ossification of the anterior ring apophyses yields "empty" anterior corners.

Table 4.69 Normal anterior wedging up to 10° in a thoracic vertebral body

Age	Frequency	Number of Patients
2 mo–2 y	15%	20
3–6 y	51%	21
7–10 y	67%	24
11–12 y	65%	17
13–17 y	53%	15

Table 4.70 Pathologic wedging of vertebral bodies

Diagnosis	Findings	Comments
Compression fractures	Single or multiple. Normal bone structure (except for callus after 10 d) and normal disk spaces.	Differentiation from pathologic wedging may be difficult, which is more of a problem in adults, where MRI may help by demonstrating normal or abnormal marrow cavity.
Spondylitis-discitis	Wedge deformity a possibility.	Positive bone scan.
Adolescent kyphosis (Scheuermann "disease") ▷ Fig. 4.218	Classically, at least three adjacent vertebral bodies are wedged. End plates are typically irregular with Schmorl nodes frequent. Schmorl herniation into bone has a sclerotic edge. In anterior Schmorl node, the herniation occurs between vertebral and ring apophysis (called a limbus vertebra).	Dramatic increase in kyphosis in puberty if not treated. Familial association is common. Thoracolumbar condition shows a straightening or reversal of the normal upper lumbar lordosis.
Congenital hemivertebrae and other segmentation anomalies	Posterior hemivertebra: triangular on the lateral view with apex anterior. Lateral hemivertebra: triangular of the frontal view with apex directed contralaterally.	Hox gene effects; may be part of syndromes. May be part of VATER association. Kyphosis or scoliosis results depending on orientation of the anomaly.
Vertebral body deformity in scoliosis	On frontal radiograph, relative narrowing of the vertebral bodies on the concave side of the scoliosis at and near the apex of the curve.	A consequence even of moderate idiopathic scoliosis. Rapid progression of scoliosis expected with unilateral vertical fusion of pedicles.
Asymmetric vertebral body loss of height in trauma, infection, leukemia, or localized tumor	Anterior or lateral wedging. The presence of destruction depends on the primary disease. MRI reveals the state of the marrow spaces.	One example is LCH at onset, with later flattening of the body into vertebra plana.
Wedged fusion of multiple vertebral bodies	Fusion after fractures, osteomyelitis, and tuberculosis, and possibly in severe Scheuermann "disease."	If posterior, tends to a gibbus configuration. Fusion in a solitary block vertebra suggests a congenital anomaly.
Achondroplasia	Anterior wedging at thoracolumbar region is frequent after infancy. Disk spaces maintained.	Associated mild scoliosis is less common.
NF1	Wedge deformity with kyphosis at one or more levels.	Multiple other bony abnormalities.
Growth disturbance postirradiation	Decreased vertebral body height on the side of the radiation.	Muscle hypoplasia may play a role in the development of scoliosis.
Melnick-Needles syndrome ▷ Fig. 4.219	Anterior wedging is one of many bony abnormalities.	Also known as osteodysplasty.

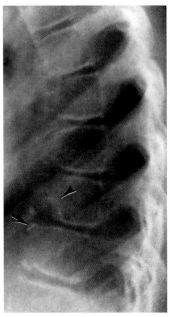

Fig. 4.218 Scheuermann "disease." Thoracic kyphosis, wedge-shaped vertebral bodies, large anterior Schmorl nodes (arrowhead) with sclerotic borders, and intact ring apophysis (arrow) in an 11-year-old-girl.

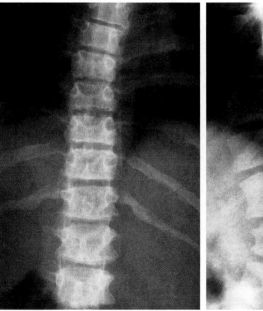
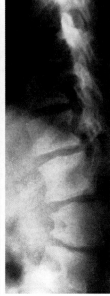

Fig. 4.219 Melnick-Needles syndrome. Irregularly tall vertebral bodies that are wedge-shaped at L2 level with classic rib changes.

Table 4.71   Deformity of vertebral body with anterior projection

Diagnosis	Findings	Comments
Normal variant in infants	Anteroinferior beaking at thoracolumbar junction is a frequent finding in normal infants.	Resolves as child gets older.
Muscular hypotonia	Anteroinferior beaking at thoracolumbar junction may be related to hyperflexion.	May also be seen in trisomy 21.
Congenital hypothyroidism ▷*Fig. 4.195, p. 415*	Anterior noselike projection along the inferior surface.	Delayed skeletal maturation.
MPS (dysostosis multiplex) excluding type IV ▷*Fig. 4.220* ▷*Fig. 4.221a, b, p. 430* ▷*Fig. 4.222, p. 430*	Oval vertebral bodies. Beaklike anteroinferior projection from the vertebral body, most common in lowest thoracic and upper lumbar regions. Posterior scalloping of the body may occur in lumbar region.	Most marked changes in type I-H (Hurler syndrom) and type VI (Maroteaux-Lamy syndrome). Milder changes in type II (Hunter syndrome). Only oval vertebral bodies in type III (Sanfilippo syndrome). Similar changes in many mucolipidoses.
Morquio disease ▷*Fig. 4.199, p. 418*	Platyspondyly with hypoplastic thoracolumbar vertebral bodies. Anterior tonguelike projection from midvertebral body in upper lumbar region or lower thoracic. Short dens.	MPS IV. Danger: the short dens predisposes to atlantoaxial dislocation and subsequent cord damage.

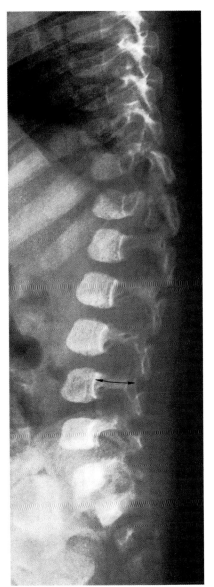

Fig. 4.220   Dysostosis multiplex (Hurler syndrome). Suggestive inferior anterior protrusion of bodies T11–L2. Widened lumbar spinal canal and posterior body concavity scalloping (arrow) in a 3-year-old boy.

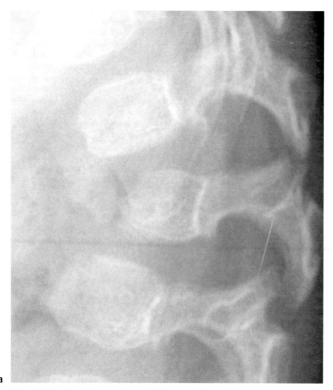

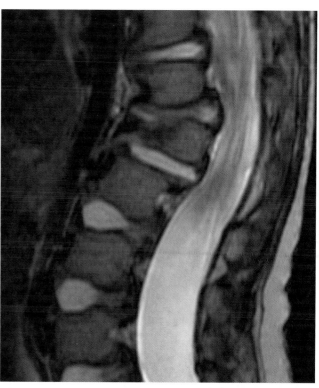

a

b

Fig. 4.221a, b Dysostosis multiplex. Hurler syndrome in a 1-year-old. (a) Upper lumbar (37°) kyphosis at a short body with anterior-inferior beaking, which is in retrolisthesis compared to the suprajacent and subjacent body. (b) T2 MRI shows associated posteriorly bulging disk and narrowed thecal sac

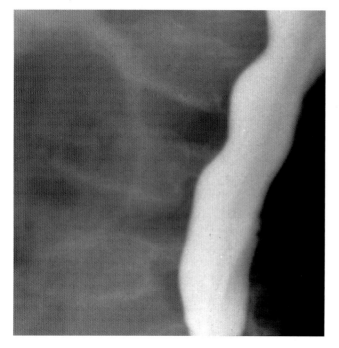

Fig. 4.222 Dysostosis multiplex. Anterior beaking of lumbar body in a 9-year-old child. Myelogram: lumbar spinal canal is widened beyond the contrast-filled thecal sac, perhaps by thickened meninges, with associated posterior body scalloping.

Vertebral Body Clefts

Table 4.72   Horizontal clefts

Diagnosis	Findings	Comments
Synchondrosis between the dens and the body of C2	Normal horizontal developmental cleft; can persist until the age of 7 y.	Examination of the dens on open mouth view as well as lateral.
Dens fracture	Up to the age of 7 y, the dens growth center is not fused and can be displaced traumatically at the synchondrosis.	Diagnosis is difficult without displacement. Look for soft tissue swelling anteriorly on lateral view.
Os odontoideum ▷ Fig. 4.223a, b	Isolated ossicle above a hypoplastic dens with a wide synchondrosis to it.	A traumatic cause is proposed by some experts (especially Fielding). Predisposes to atlantoaxial subluxation. Occasionally in Down syndrome.
Ossiculum terminale	Small ossicle above the tip of a nearly normal-sized dens.	No clinical significance. A normal variant ossification center.
Nutrient canal of bodies	Horizontal lucent zone or line in the center of the vertebral body associated with anterior or posterior notching of the contour. Most are incomplete fissures.	Normal, visible in infancy. They are longer and more obvious in hypothyroidism, osteoporosis, and diseases involving the bone marrow, such as anemia or leukemia.
Dens pseudarthrosis	Normal ossification early in childhood; ossification variant later in childhood.	Simulates fracture.
Chance (seatbelt) fracture	Transverse fracture of L1 or a neighboring level. Fracture passes through the body as well as the posterior arch. May see transverse split in pedicles en face on frontal image.	From impact in automobile collision while wearing lap belt.

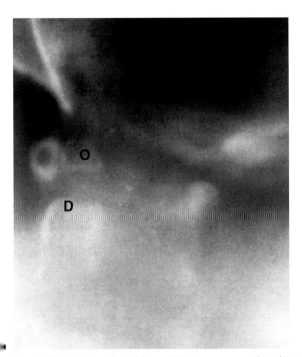 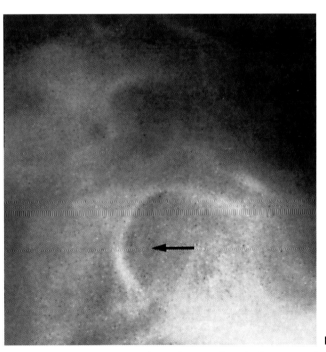

b

Fig. 4.223a, b   Os odontoideum (O). Accessory ossicle is directly posterior to the anterior arch of C1 and remote from the hypoplastic dens (D).

Vertical Clefts in the Vertebral Bodies (Midline)

Pitfalls

Midline vertical clefts in the posterior neural arch can mimic clefts in the vertebral bodies on frontal radiographs. Midline clefts in the anterior mandible, spaces between the first two incisors, and nonfusion of bilateral growth centers of the dens are other mimics (see **Table 4.73**).

Vertical Clefts in the Vertebral Bodies (Lateral Images)

Normal. A linear prenatal fissure (cleft) in the vertebral body can occasionally persist, more commonly in boys, into the first weeks of postnatal life. This may be caused by remains of notochord or be due to anterior and posterior growth centers that have not yet fused. This phenomenon is most often seen in the lower thoracic and upper lumbar bodies. Vertical vertebral clefts occur in some syndromes—their presence is of no structural importance (**Table 4.74**).

Table 4.73 Midline vertical clefts in vertebral bodies (frontal images)

Diagnosis	Findings	Comments
Butterfly vertebra ▷ *Fig. 4.224*	Complete or incomplete cleft in the center of the vertebral body—the body narrows as it approaches midline, like a bowtie or a butterfly.	May be isolated anomaly (perhaps hox gene effect) or part of a syndrome such as Alagille syndrome. Also seen in association with MMC, diastomatomyelia, neurenteric cyst, and anomalies of the lungs, gastrointestinal, or genitourinary tract.
Alagille syndrome	Butterfly and other vertebral anomalies, such as a more minor midline indentation than complete butterfly.	Paucity of the intrahepatic bile ducts. Jaundice; may show rickets as well. Medullary cystic kidney pattern.
Vertical vertebral body fracture	The body (or dens) then is coronally wider than normal.	May be caused by axial loading injury.
Spondylothoracic dysplasia; Jarcho-Levin syndrome	Complex vertebral anomalies with hemivertebrae, rib anomalies, and sometimes absent vertebral bodies.	Also known as spondylocostal dysostosis. Short neck. May benefit from vertical expandable prosthetic titanium rib surgery.
Aicardi syndrome	Butterfly and other vertebral anomalies.	Only in females. Failure to thrive, "salaam" spasms, hemihypertrophy.

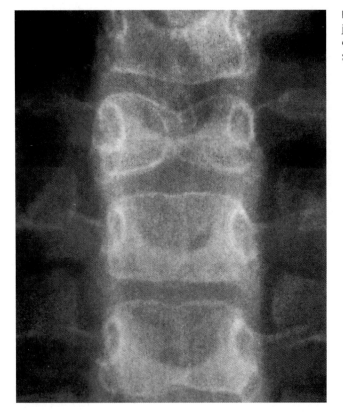

Fig. 4.224 Butterfly vertebra. Nonsyndromic anomaly in this subject; note the body above "protrudes" downward into the deformed disk space. The body two levels below shows a minimal butterfly shape.

Table 4.74 Vertical clefts in the vertebral bodies on lateral images

Diagnosis	Findings	Comments
Vertical vertebral body fracture	Also associated with compression fractures.	Usually due to hyperflexion during injury.
Multiple stippled epiphyses ▷ Fig. 4.225	Spinous process tips may be stippled. Several varieties of genetic abnormalities, as well as maternal warfarin exposure.	Also known as chondrodysplasia punctata. Becomes multiple epiphyseal dysplasia on follow-up.
Kniest disease	Associated platyspondyly and kyphoscoliosis. Coronal clefts early in childhood.	Megaepiphyses (the hip center ossifies late, however).
Larsen syndrome ▷ Fig. 4.226	Incompletely fused vertical clefts appearing as lateral butterfly vertebrae.	Many segmentation and alignment abnormalities of the cervical spine, including sometimes kyphosis.
Mucolipidosis II (I-cell disease)	Occasional vertebral body clefts. Dysostosis multiplex pattern in skeleton. Hyperparathyroidism at birth.	Hyperparathyroid bony change without rickets at birth, plus dysostosis multiplex, should be diagnostic.
Trisomy 13	Occasional coronal clefts.	Microcephaly, holoprosencephaly, and other anomalies.
Diastrophic dysplasia	Vertebral cleft with other vertebral anomalies, including severe cervical kyphosis. This kyphosis will be missed on frontal images alone.	Hitchhiker thumb is a characteristic limb finding.
Humerospinal dysostosis	Coronal clefts and rhizomelic shortening of the extremities, especially the humerus. Exaggerated lumbar lordosis.	Distal bifurcation of the humerus.
Weissenbacher-Zweymüller syndrome	Coronal clefts with platyspondyly.	Micrognathia, hearing loss.
Otospondylomegaepiphyseal dysplasia (OSMED)	Coronal clefts in infancy. May include relative platyspondyly and enlarged dens.	Often cleft palate.
Taybi-Lindner syndrome	Coronal clefts and severe microcephaly.	Cephaloskeletal dysplasia. (microcephalic osteodysplastic primordial dwarfism type I). Lethal in first year.
Dyssegmental dysplasia	Coronal clefts may be dramatic; oversized vertebral bodies; may have sagittal body clefts as well.	Rolland-Desbuquois syndrome.

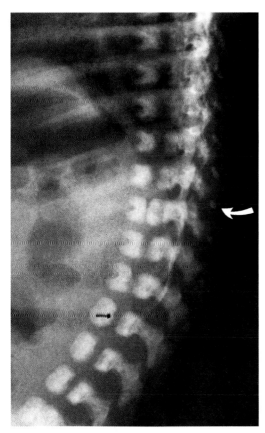

Fig. 4.225 Coronal (vertical) clefts (black arrow) in chondrodysplasia punctata. Multiple stippled epiphyses pattern in the posterior spinous processes (white arrow).

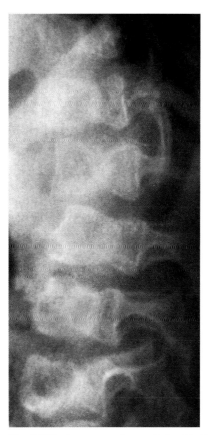

Fig. 4.226 Larsen syndrome. Lateral butterfly configuration vertebrae is residual from prior coronal clefts, which had been seen earlier in childhood.

Concave Deformities

Table 4.75 Concavity of the end plates

Diagnosis	Findings	Comments
Normal variant ▷ *Fig. 4.227*	Mild concavity of the end plates centered in the region of the nucleus pulposus of the intervertebral disk.	A faint manifestation of persistent notochord.
Osteoporosis ▷ *Fig. 4.196, p. 416*	Codfish vertebral deformity with or without overall loss of vertebral body height. Multiple vertebrae, especially lumbar.	Disks "want" to become spherical like a beach ball; vertebral bodies "want" disks to be flat like a pancake. In osteoporosis, end plates are less supported by bone than normal, so that the disks "win the battle of shape."
Sickle cell anemia ▷ *Fig. 4.228*	Presumably caused by infarction or vascular compromise in the end plate region. A definitely different pattern than that of osteoporosis. The peripheral portions of the end plates remain intact, leaving a "Lincoln Log" configuration.	Presumably, the vessels supplying the central end plate regions are smaller in diameter than peripheral, making them more susceptible to sickled red cells.
Metastatic disease	The concavity of one or both end plates can be the first sign of metastatic disease. Generally limited to one or a few vertebral bodies.	Neuroblastoma most common. Tumor-infiltrated bone decreases support for the end plate.
Gaucher disease	Changes can resemble those of sickle cell disease.	More severe vertebral collapse may cause compression of spinal cord (MRI).
Dyggve-Melchior-Clausen syndrome	The end plates are concave between the two "camel humps." Platyspondyly with relatively wide disk spaces.	Dens may be short, predisposing to atlantoaxial subluxation.

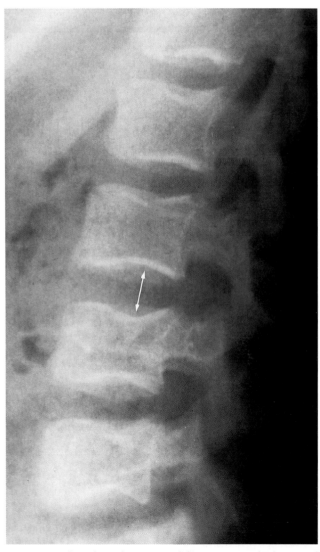

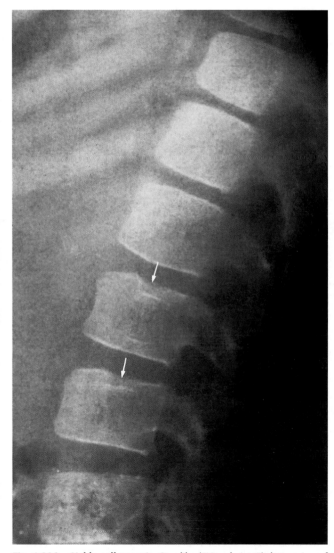

Fig. 4.227 Physiologic depression of the superior and inferior end plates that are associated with widened disk nucleus pulposi (arrow).

Fig. 4.228 Sickle cell anemia. Steplike ("Lincoln Log") depression of the end plates in the center of some vertebral bodies (arrows).

Table 4.76   Concavity that does not affect the entire end plate (superior or inferior)

Diagnosis	Findings	Comments
Schmorl nodes	Sclerotic borders except at the time of acute herniation of disk through weak area of end plate. Less commonly anterior, where it may form a limbus vertebra configuration.	An almost ubiquitous finding at least at one vertebral body in adolescence. Many Schmorl nodes are often a part of Scheuermann "disease."
Diskitis and osteomyelitis	The end plate indentation is initially unsharp and without sclerosis. Loss of height of the disk.	The defect enlarges over time; borders become sclerotic in the healing phase.
Brucellosis	Bony erosions at diskovertebral junction. May show vacuum phenomenon between disk and end plate.	Especially lower lumbar spine. Contact with infected animals.
Actinomycosis	Lytic defects, usually sparing disks.	Actinomycosis does not respect tissue planes and extends easily into neighboring tissues.

Triangular concavity of the end plates is a part of butterfly vertebrae, some vertebral clefts, and in burst fractures of vertebral bodies.
Irregular borders of the end plates are seen in many dysplasias and dysostosis with platyspondyly, in FD, and rarely in cartilage-hair hypoplasia and Stickler syndrome (arthro-ophthalmopathy).

Table 4.77   Anterior vertebral concavity

Diagnosis	Findings	Comments
Normal finding	Mild concavity with normal bone structure and borders, predominantly in the lower thoracic and upper lumbar vertebrae.	After infancy.
Vascular channel (Hahn) ▷ *Fig. 4.229*	Horizontal vascular channel in the anterior center of the vertebral body, causing a local depression in the contour. Especially seen in infants.	Can persist longer in hypothyroidism and sickle cell anemia; quite conspicuous in osteopetrosis and other dense vertebral conditions. If necessary, could confirm the vascular nature with MRA.
NF1	Anterior concavity of multiple vertebral bodies.	Associated idiopathic or acute, sharp scoliosis.
Trisomy 21	Anterior concavity occurs in young children. Spinal canal may be narrow behind the dens.	Down syndrome.
Tuberculosis	Excavation of the anterior body cortex from abscess below the anterior longitudinal ligament.	Can be initial location of vertebral tuberculosis.
Melnick-Needles syndrome ▷ *Fig. 4.219, p. 428*	Anterior concavity one of many misshapes of vertebral bodies possible.	Osteodysplasty.

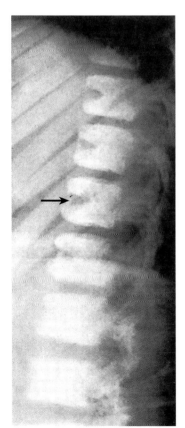

Fig. 4.229   Pyknodysostosis. Prominent anterior Hahn fissures (arrow) and poor definition of the posterior body margins in abnormally dense vertebrae; also, note the broad, dense ribs.

Table 4.78   Posterior vertebral concavity

Diagnosis	Findings	Comments
Normal finding	Mild posterior concavity in the lumbar vertebrae often seen.	
NF1 ▷ *Fig. 4.230* ▷ *Fig. 4.231a, b*	Posterior concavity of multiple vertebral bodies, associated with dural ectasia.	Associated idiopathic or acute, sharp scoliosis. Deformities associated with plexiform neurofibromas as well.
MPS	Concavity may be associated with meningeal (dural) thickening.	May be pronounced in Hurler syndrome. Can be seen in other mucopolysaccharidoses and heteroglycanoses.

(continues on page 437)

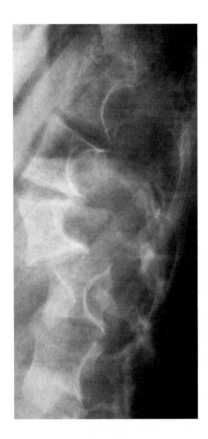

Fig. 4.230   Neurofibromatosis type 1. Marked widening of the spinal canal with posteriorly concave vertebral bodies, some of which are anteriorly displaced.

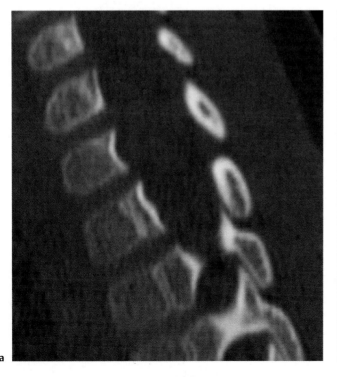

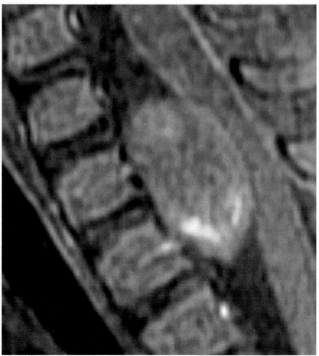

Fiq. 4.231a, b   Neurofibromatosis type 1. (**a**) Coronal reconstruction from CT shows widened spinal canal and concave posterior bodies. (**b**) T1 MRI image shows the ovoid neurofibroma that causes/explains the deformity seen on (**a**).

a

Table 4.78   (Cont.) Posterior vertebral concavity

Diagnosis	Findings	Comments
Achondroplasia and related dysplasias ▷ *Fig. 4.232a, b*	Associated with the narrow lumbar vertebral canal.	MRI useful to show effects on spinal cord and nerve roots. In hypochondroplasia, may be much milder concavity.
Lumbar spinal stenosis	Narrow canal sagittally and usually coronally as well.	May be seen without generally dysplasia or dysostosis. Will exaggerate the symptoms from minor disk protrusion.
Nonneoplastic expansile process in the spinal canal ▷ *Fig. 4.233a, b, p. 438* ▷ *Fig. 4.234, p. 438* ▷ *Fig. 4.280, p. 478*	Confirm and evaluate with MRI.	Syringomyelia, venous malformation (formerly hemangioma), and lipomatous masses, for example.
Spinal canal tumors	Slow-growing masses including cysts and intraspinal vascular malformations or hemangiomas.	Masses can be intramedullary, intradural, or extradural.
Cockayne syndrome	Ovoid vertebral bodies, may be posterior concave. May have intervertebral calcifications.	Exaggerated thoracic kyphosis. Microcephaly. Osteoporosis.

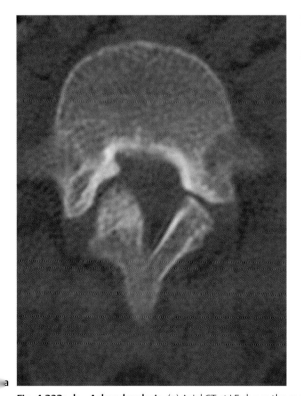
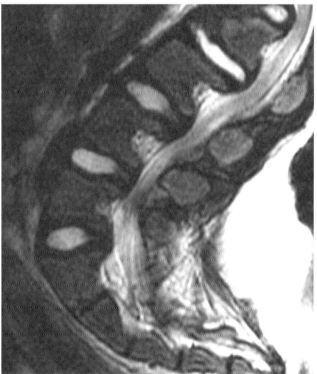

Fig. 4.232a, b   Achondroplasia. (a) Axial CT at L5 shows the markedly narrow spinal canal with short pedicles and somewhat short laminae. **(b)** T2 sagittal MRI shows the narrowing of spinal canal and cauda equina. Disks already bulge posteriorly somewhat in this 10-year-old boy.

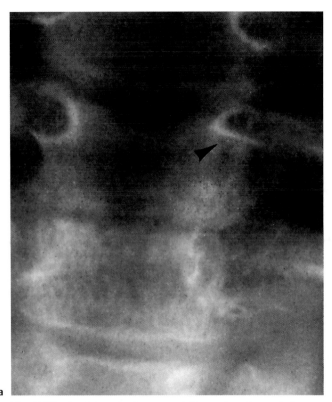

a

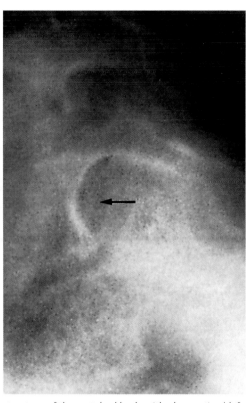

b

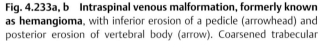

Fig. 4.233a, b   Intraspinal venous malformation, formerly known as hemangioma, with inferior erosion of a pedicle (arrowhead) and posterior erosion of vertebral body (arrow). Coarsened trabecular structure of the vertebral body with obscuration/deformation of pedicle and transverse process.

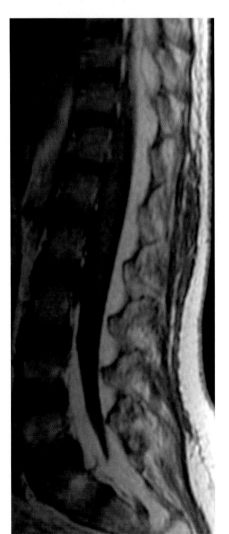

Fig. 4.234   Considerable fat in the spinal canal demonstrated in this 8-year-old child with urinary retention on T1-weighted MRI. The fat is bright signal as is subcutaneous fat and is in contrast to the somewhat narrowed thecal sac.

Concavities Anteriorly and Posteriorly (Spindle or Hourglass Shape)

The following concavities occur in neonates:
- Pyknodysostosis
- Melnick Needles syndrome
- Kenny-Caffey syndrome

Biconvex Vertebral Bodies

Biconvex vertebral bodies refer to convexity upward of upper body margin and downward of lower body margin.

Normal. In neonates and young infants, the vertebral bodies are conspicuously biconvex. If prominent, they may be associated with delay of ring apophysis ossification.

Meningomyelocele. Biconvex vertebral bodies associated with rachischisis.

Hypothyroidism. Vertebral bodies are biconvex associated with delayed bone development.

Cleidocranial dysplasia/dysostosis. Biconvex vertebral bodies, patent neurocentral synchondroses, and multiple clefts in the neural arches indicate cleidocranial dysplasia/dysostosis.

Spondyloepiphyseal dysplasia, tarda form. Biconvex thoracic vertebral bodies and "donkey back and belly" indicate spondyloepiphyseal dysplasia

Further malformation conditions with biconvex or pear-shaped vertebral bodies include the following:
- Spondyloepiphyseal dysplasia—congenital
- Dysostosis multiplex (especially Hurler syndrome)
  - Fibrochondrogenesis
  - Beta-glucuronidase deficiency
  - Cockayne syndrome

Malformations

Table 4.79   Vertebral fusion

Diagnosis	Findings	Comments
Isolated block vertebra	Predilection for C2-C3 (see subsequent discussion of 22q11.2 deletion), rare in the lumbar region. The anterior aspect of congenital block vertebrae is smooth, usually with a triangular indentation anteriorly. Block of only the most anterior part of the bodies will result in kyphosis.	Can also involve the neural arches. If neural foramina are small or absent, nerve roots or rootlets need other pathways (level above or level below) to exit the spinal canal.
Klippel-Feil syndrome	By definition: fused cervical vertebral bodies; hemivertebrae and fusion of neural arches may be some of the associated segmentation abnormalities.	Neck appears short. Occasionally associated with Sprengel deformity (failure of scapular descent), deafness, or fetal alcohol syndrome.
22q11.2 deletion ▷ Fig. 4.235	Most subjects with this genetic abnormality have changes in the cervical column, including C2-C3 fusion, upswept "swoosh" C2 posterior arch, open posterior C1 arch, platybasia, and dens variations.	The clinical syndromes include DiGeorge, Shprintzen, and Sedlačkova syndromes.
Elsahy-Waters syndrome	Fusion of C2 and C3, mandibular cysts.	Other anomalies: midface hypoplasia, brachycephaly, and hypospadias.

Vertebral fusion (**Table 4.79**) also occurs in the following syndromes:
- Trisomy 18
- Robinow syndrome
- Wildervanck syndrome
- Goltz focal dermal hypoplasia, in which anterior fusion of vertebral bodies may occur.

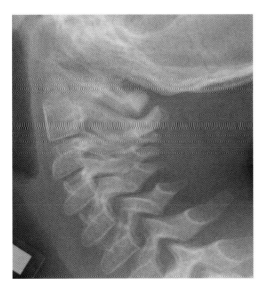

Fig. 4.235   22q11.2 deletion with some characteristic associated cervical vertebral findings, including the upward swoosh (think Nike logo) of the posterior arch of C2 and the lack of ossification of the anterior arch of C1.

Table 4.80 Acquired fusion

Diagnosis	Findings	Comments
JIA	Body and vertebral arch fusions in cervical spine. Apophyseal joint fusions are perhaps the most common. The anterior margins of fused bodies are straight rather than indented. Associated erosion of back of dens and tapering of spinous processes as well as tendency to atlantoaxial subluxation may occur.	Formerly juvenile rheumatoid arthritis (in United States) or juvenile chronic arthritis (in Europe).
Disk destruction from spondylitis-diskitis and other processes	Block vertebra (bodies) formation. If only anterior, will result in local kyphosis.	Fusion can be left/right asymmetric, leading to local scoliosis.
Scheuermann "disease"	Rarely, secondary fusion of affected vertebral bodies.	Both a result and a cause of kyphosis.

Hemivertebrae

Table 4.81 Hemivertebrae

Diagnosis	Findings	Comments
Lateral hemivertebra ▷ Fig. 4.236	Usually has its own rib or transverse process.	In the absence of balancing contralateral hemivertebra (such as butterfly vertebra), scoliosis will result.
Unilateral pulmonary agenesis, neurenteric cyst, anterolateral meningocele	Frequently associated with hemivertebrae or other thoracic vertebral segmentation anomalies.	
VATER and VACTERL associations	Hemivertebrae or combination of hemivertebra with fusion, resulting in 1.5 fused vertebrae, are two manifestations.	VACTERL is vertebral, anal, cardiac, tracheoesophageal, radial or renal, limb.
Posterior hemivertebra ▷ Fig. 4.237	Short, triangular, or trapezoidal vertebral bodies on the lateral image, with diminution of the most anterior body. Retrolisthesis often also present.	Results in acutely angled local kyphosis.
Jarcho-Levin syndrome, spondylocostal dysostosis	Hemivertebrae among many segmentation anomalies possible.	Associated rib deformities.

Hemivertebrae are encountered in Klippel Feil syndrome, diastomatomyelia, and other conditions.
Complex vertebral malformations with hemivertebra, fusions, and other anomalies also in Goldenhar syndrome, mesomelic dysplasias, and Robinow syndrome.

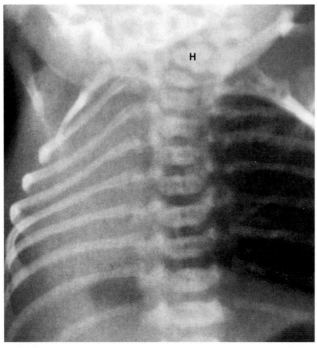

Fig. 4.236 Lateral hemivertebra (H) with associated right pulmonary agenesis. Incidental finding: pseudarthrosis of the left clavicle (newborn).

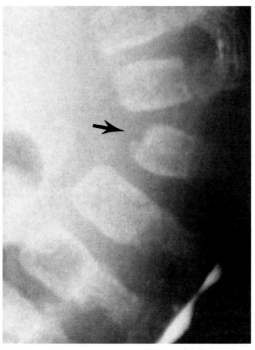

Fig. 4.237 Posterior hemivertebra with sharply angled kyphosis in an 8-month-old boy. Note the typical triangular shape (arrow).

Table 4.82   Absent vertebrae

Diagnosis	Findings	Comments
Caudal regression ▷ *Fig. 4.238*	Associated with sacral agenesis. Absence of variable number of caudal lumbar vertebrae or even distal thoracic.	Association with maternal diabetes in some cases.
Surgical removal	Due to tumor, trauma, or as part of surgical repair of severe kyphosis (kyphectomy) or scoliosis.	Typically stabilized with orthopedic instrumentation.
Achondrogenesis type I Parenti-Faccaro, type II Langer-Saldino	Decrease or absent ossification of vertebrae at birth (and in utero), more pronounced in type I. Decreased ossification also in other skeletal elements (absent ossification of the skull in type I).	Lethal dysplasias with significant micromelia, fetal hydrops.
Dyssegmental dysplasia	Variable size and shape of vertebral ossification; some vertebrae may be absent.	Early demise usually.
Spondylocostal and spondylothoracic dysplasia	Complex vertebral malformations as well as absence of single vertebrae.	Associated rib deformities.

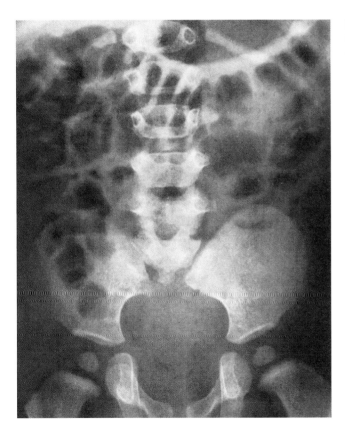

Fig. 4.238   Sacral agenesis/caudal regression. Only one hypoplastic sacral vertebra is present; the medial upper iliac bones approach each other more than normally.

Anomalies of the Spinal Canal and Neural Arches

■ Narrowing of the Spinal Canal (Spinal Stenosis)

Narrowing of the spinal canal may be generalized and thus is an indication of slowed enchondral bone formation in bone dysplasias (**Fig. 4.239**).

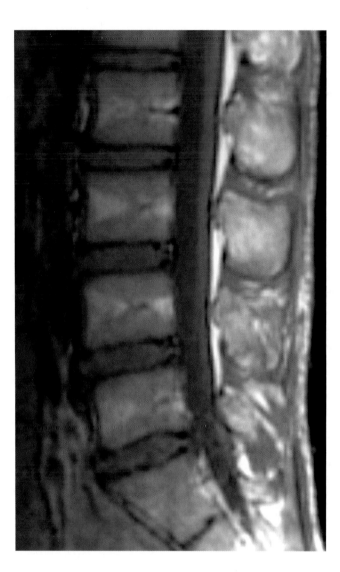

Fig. 4.239 MRI of lumbar spinal stenosis. Sagittal T1-weighted MRI in a 16-year-old with Ehlers-Danlos syndrome. The canal is narrowed in association with shorter than normal lumbar pedicles; the disks bulge somewhat. Note the reduced amount of canal fat, especially compared to **Fig. 4.234**.

Table 4.83   Narrowing of the spinal canal

Diagnosis	Findings	Comments
Achondroplasia ▷ *Fig. 4.240a, b*	Narrowing of the lumbar canal both coronally (progressive narrowing of the space between pedicles at each lumbar level as one goes inferiorly). Posterior margin of lumbar bodies are notably concave. Cervical and thoracic canal also narrow; occasionally severe in upper cervical region.	Minimal lumbar disk herniation can cause severe symptoms. Occasionally, the cervical canal narrowing may cause respiratory difficulty. Narrowed jugular foramina may cause dilated ventricles; foramen magnum also relatively small.
Hypochondroplasia	Less pronounced changes than achondroplasia. The decrease downward in distance between pedicles is less evident or distance may be constant downward.	Allelic to achondroplasia. Head circumference at least fiftieth percentile.
Idiopathic lumbar spinal stenosis	Isolated variation. Perhaps just the lower range of the bell-shaped curve of spinal canal area.	May be associated with back pain from minor disk protrusions.
Metatropic dysplasia	Cervical spinal stenosis frequent.	Develop kyphoscoliosis during childhood. May have dens hypoplasia.
Consequence of fractures of bodies or arches	Oblique plain images may help define, but CT and MRI are definitive.	Associated cord damage.
Intraspinal exostosis	A rare and unfortunate localization in multiple cartilaginous exostoses.	CT and MRI to define.
Hurler syndrome and other heteroglycanoses	Thickened meninges narrow the intraspinal space.	
Hypertrophied ligamentum flavum	CT or MRI to define.	
Sirenomelia	Single midline lower extremity with one or two sets of limb bones in it.	

Other skeletal conditions with narrowing of the spinal canal include the following:
- Atlantoaxial subluxation
- Down syndrome
- Cartilage hair hypoplasia
- Kniest disease
- Alagille syndrome
  -Multiple stippled epiphyses
  -Dyssegmental dysplasia
- Diastrophic dysplasia
- Acrodysostosis
- Gordon syndrome (with narrowed disk spaces)
- Acromesomelic dysplasia

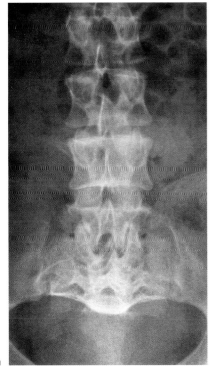 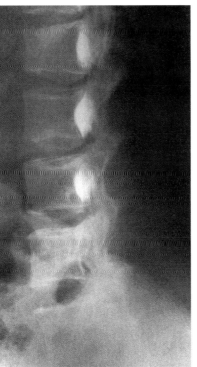

Fig. 4.240a, b   Achondroplasia in a 14-year-old girl. (**a**) Caudally decreasing lumbar transverse interpedicle distance. (**b**) Classic myelogram: marked spinal stenosis with posteriorly concave bodies.

■ Widening of the Spinal Canal

Table 4.84 Widening of the spinal canal

Diagnosis	Findings	Comments
Normal	The interpedicle distance at T11 often wider than T12. Relative widening of cervical or lumbosacral canal on AP projection may be without any association.	Apparent cervical canal widening is striking on infant frontal chest images.
Meningomyelocele and other rachischisis ▷ *Fig. 4.241*	Predominantly lumbosacral. The interpedicle distance wide at involved levels.	Cord examination with US in first months of life, then MRI. Possible association with tethered cord.
Syringomyelia or hydromyelia	Canal widening in involved cervical or thoracic region. MRI to image cord and its roots.	If neurologic symptoms, say in scoliosis, progress rapidly, think of these diagnoses.
Chiari type I or II malformation ▷ *Fig. 4.242a, b*	Wide cervical spinal canal and foramen magnum.	Downward protrusion of cerebellum on CT or MRI.
Diastematomyelia ▷ *Fig. 4.241*	Bony or uncalcified spur in canal, local narrow disk spaces, fusion of laminae craniocaudally at the involved level. Local widened interpedicle distance.	MRI to confirm and evaluate the associated split cord.
Intraspinal space-occupying process	Tumors, vascular malformations, NF1, for example.	MRI to evaluate.
Dural ectasia	NF1, MPS, among other associations. Posterior concavity of vertebral bodies.	Widening of the dural sac at L5 only is a normal variant.
Marfan syndrome ▷ *Fig. 4.243a, b*	Wide lumbar canal associated with relatively long pedicles and laminae.	Dolichostenomelia.

(continues on page 446)

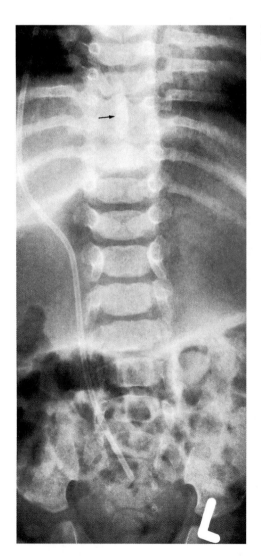

Fig. 4.241 Rachischisis associated with meningomyelocele; diastematomyelia. Widened transverse interpedicle distance is most marked at L3 and L4. Diastematomyelia ossified spur (arrow). VP shunt is also seen.

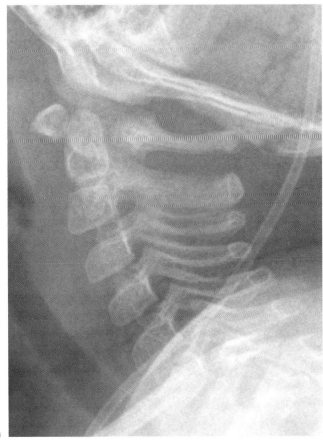

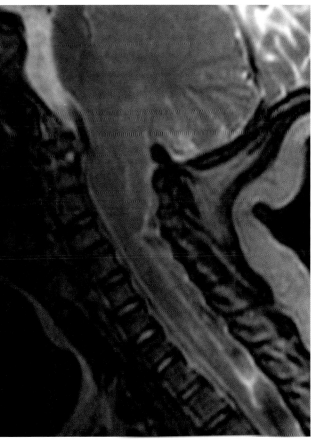

a   b

Fig. 4.242a, b   Chiari type II malformation. (a) On the plain image, the spinal canal behind the upper cervical spine is wider than normal, as may be seen in Chiari types I or II. **(b)** T2 MRI shows the downward protrusion of brainstem into the upper cervical canal. An incidental syrinx is noted in the upper thoracic cord.

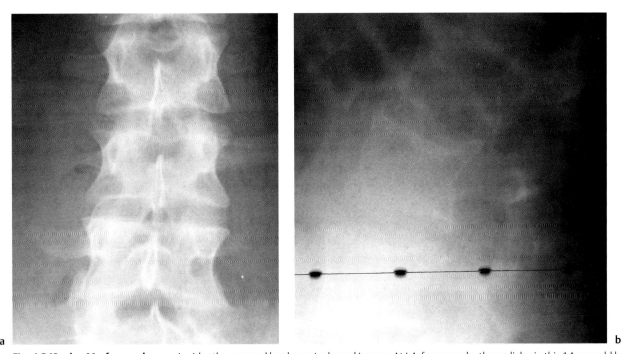

a   b

Fig. 4.243a, b   Marfan syndrome. A wider than normal lumbar spinal canal is seen. At L4, for example, the pedicles in this 14-year-old boy have a distance of 35 mm. According to standards quoted in Lusted and Keats, 33 mm is two standard deviations above the mean at that level at that age. On the lateral, there is some concavity of the posterior margins of the bodies.

Table 4.84   (Cont.) Widening of the spinal canal

Diagnosis	Findings	Comments
Homocystinuria	Wide lumbar canal associated with relatively long pedicles and laminae.	Dolichostenomelia; trunk osteoporosis.
Neurenteric cyst	Associated separation of pedicles.	
Epidural lipomatosis	Wide midthoracic canal.	MRI.
Otopalatodigital syndrome, Taybi syndrome	Widening of the thoracic and lumbar spinal canal.	
Arthrogryposis syndrome of the Eskimos (Kuskokwim)	Increasing displacement of the neural arch at L5 leads to spondylolisthesis. Hypoplastic dens and body of C2.	Joint contractures.

Anomalies of the Intervertebral Foramina

Table 4.85   Enlarged intervertebral foramen

Diagnosis	Findings	Comments
Normal	The widest cervical vertebral foramina are usually at C2-C3 level.	
Congenital absence of a pedicle ▷ *Fig. 4.244a, b*	Two adjacent foramina form one large common foramen. Hypoplasia of the anterior transverse process associated. On frontal radiographs, the pedicle is missing.	In the cervical column, neurologic or vascular symptoms in upper extremity common ("absent cervical pedicle syndrome"), MRI will demonstrate the courses of the involved nerve roots. Thoracic and lumbar are most often asymptomatic variations.

(continues on page 447)

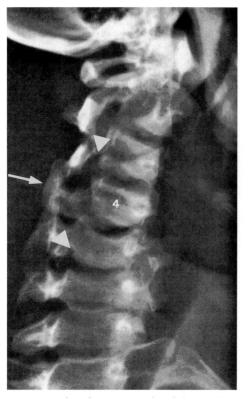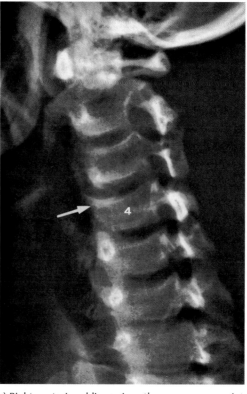

Fig. 4.244a, b   Absent cervical pedicle at right C4. (**a**) Right posterior oblique view: there are common intervertebral foramina from C3–C5 (arrowheads). Through it is seen a hypoplastic C4 transverse process. Arrow shows the right lamina, which is displaced outward and is no longer in line with its fellow laminae. (**b**) Left posterior oblique, the C4 pedicle is lacking (arrow).

Table 4.85   (Cont.) Enlarged intervertebral foramen

Diagnosis	Findings	Comments
"Dumbbell" or "hourglass" tumor ▷ *Fig. 4.245*	Smooth-bordered widening on the lateral image; wide foramen on the oblique images. MRI for full examination.	Commonly neurofibromas or neuroblastoma, ganglioneuroma, or schwannoma. Others: teratoma, lipoma, LCH, hemangioma, vascular malformation, spinal epidural cyst.
Serpiginous vertebral artery	Simulates the dumbbell tumor configuration.	Delineation of vessel by MRA.
NF1 lateral meningocele	Widened dural sac. Soft-tissue density mass along the spine.	Café-au-lait spots on skin.
Nerve root diverticulum	Traumatic in origin.	CT or MRI.
Hypertrophic interstitial polyneuritis	Thickening of the nerves causes erosion of the neural arches with flattening of the upper edges. May have concave posterior vertebral bodies; wide interpedicle distance.	Déjerine-Sottas syndrome. Onset usually in childhood. MRI for definition.

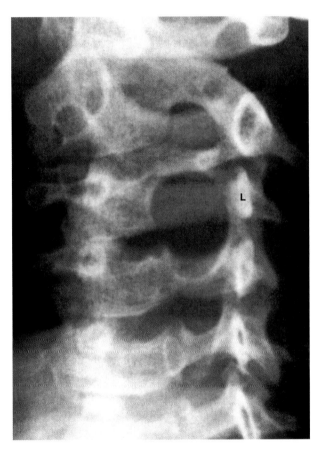

Fig. 4.245   "Hourglass/dumbbell" tumor (neurofibroma). Widening of the intervertebral foramen caused by intraspinal and extraspinal "hourglass" or "dumbbell" tumor (neurofibroma). However, unlike the case of absent pedicle (see **Fig. 4.240**), the consecutive laminae en face maintain a smooth alignment.
L Thinning and deformity of the lamina

Table 4.86   Small intervertebral foramen

Diagnosis	Findings	Comments
Congenital anomaly	Fewer nerve rootlets exit through it than a usual foramen.	Often associated with other anomalies: Klippel-Feil syndrome, vertebral fusions, diastematomyelia, and meningomyelocele, for examples.
Posttraumatic	Bony fragments.	CT for bone; MRI for cord and nerve roots.
Osteoarthrosis	Less common in children unless predisposing condition or repeated activity (e.g., cervical area in wrestlers).	Bone laid down into neural canal as part of the degenerative process.

Table 4.87 Fusion of neural arch elements

Diagnosis	Findings	Comments
JIA ▷ *Fig. 4.246a, b*	Acquired fusion of vertebral bodies, arches, and apophyseal joints.	Especially in cervical spine area. Formerly juvenile rheumatoid arthritis and juvenile chronic arthritis.
Anomalies at the craniocervical junction		Hox gene effects.
Iatrogenic fusion of the neural arch with bone chips	A possible late complication is pseudarthrosis at the level of the fusion.	Fusion also after surgical stabilization of high-grade scoliosis.
22q11.2 deletion	One finding is occipital assimilation of C1 elements.	
Diastematomyelia	Fusion of one lamina to a subjacent lamina.	
Unilateral congenital fusion	May lead to progressive scoliosis, especially unilateral vertical pedicle bar.	Close follow-up for progressive curves.

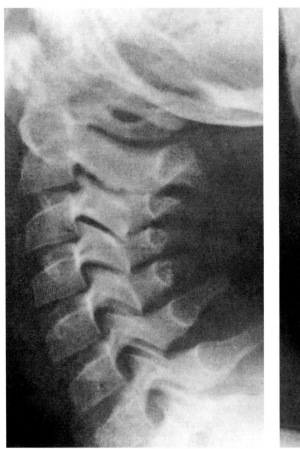 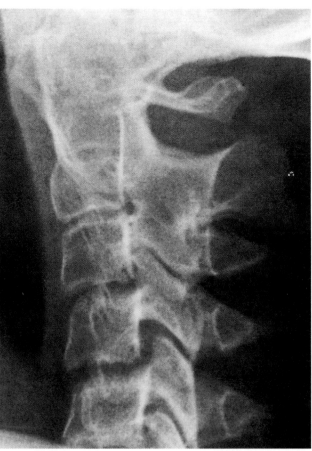

Fig. 4.246a, b Juvenile idiopathic arthritis (JIA). (a) At age 6 years, there are no abnormal fusions. **(b)** At age 16 years, there is bony fusion of C1 arch and C2, the neural arches of C2 and C3, as well as the dens with the occiput.

Table 4.88   Disruption of the contour of the neural arch (clefts, defects, and fractures)

Diagnosis	Findings	Comments
Normal finding	The neurocentral synchondrosis between the neural arches and the body ossifies between 3 and 6 y of age, but remains patent in approximately 2% of individuals. Midline clefts of the thoracic posterior arches fuse sequentially caudocranially in the first 2 y of life; they can remain visible in some children after age 7 y, and then fuse in adulthood. Isolated defects in the neural arch can occur in the cervical and thoracic vertebrae (and be available for forensic identification if known).	Defects in the posterior neural arch can be associated with cleft palate. Median clefts in the neural arch are common in cleidocranial dysplasia, with delayed closure of the neurocentral synchondrosis.
Spina bifida occulta ▷ Fig. 4.247a–c	Narrow midline cleft represents delayed or absent posterior bony union of the laminae. L5 may normally remain ununited until age 10 y, or even later.	No clinical significance unless associated with a dysraphism (skin changes, dermal sinus, progressive foot deformities, for example).
Spina bifida aperta	Associated meningomyelocele or other neural posterior deformities.	MRI for definition. Ultrasound in infancy for associated tethered cord.

(continues on page 450)

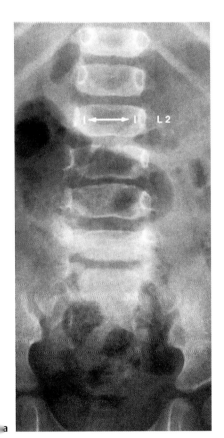
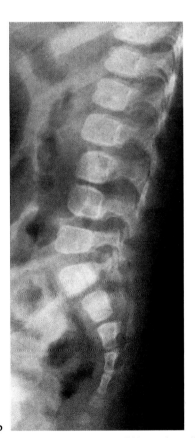
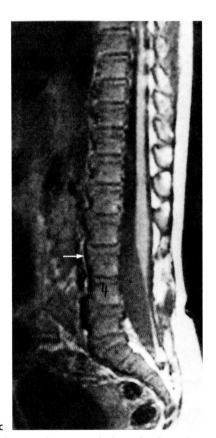

Fig. 4.247a–c   Spina bifida with externally visible finding in a 1 year old boy. Clinically, hypertrichosis over the lower lumbar spine, neurologically intact. (**a**) Widened lumbar spinal canal, interpedicle distance (double arrow) of 25 mm at L2, 29 mm at L3 and L4, and 30 mm at L5. Some pedicles narrow. Disk space is narrowed at L3–L4. (**b**) Lateral view, hypoplastic bodies L3 and L4 with narrow disk space between. (**c**) MRI: the posteriorly tethered spinal cord has conus at L3-L4 (arrow).

Table 4.88   (Cont.) Disruption of the contour of the neural arch (clefts, defects, and fractures)

Diagnosis	Findings	Comments
Dermal sinus ▷ *Fig. 4.248*	In lumbosacral midline, rarely occipital. US in infants to confirm or exclude a fistulous connection to the spinal canal. MRI provides the best delineation.	Skin dimple; may be noticed because of a hairy patch or pigmentation. A true fistula may have recurrent meningitis. The fistula can be demonstrated with sterile contrast injection.
Cleft in the cervical vertebrae ▷ *Fig. 4.249*	Midline cleft common in the posterior arch of C1. Also, lateral clefts (neurocentral synchondroses). The absence of displacement of the anterior lucent fat stripe differentiates C1 anterior clefts from fracture.	Asymptomatic. No specific history of trauma.
Fractures	Uncommon in the neural arches and transverse processes. Oblique images may show; CT is more specific.	Child abuse a possible cause in infants.
Cervical vertebral fractures	Uncommon in the neural arch prior to age 15 y. Hangman fracture through the pedicles of C2, anterior displacement of the vertebral body. Jefferson fracture of C1: burst fracture with lateral displacement of the lateral masses > 3 mm on axial CT.	Associated widening of the prevertebral soft-tissue space. Caution: a pseudo-Jefferson fracture in many children up to age 4 y; widening of the atlas < 3 mm in the absence of a fracture, the synchondrosis still patent.
Spondylolysis ▷ *Fig. 4.250a, b* ▷ *Fig. 4.251a, b* ▷ *Fig. 4.252a, b, p. 452*	Cleft in the interarticular portion of L5. Less often L4. On plain images, suggested on the lateral image; shown on obliques.	Can be bilateral. In unilateral lysis: hyperdensity of contralateral pedicle with increased uptake on bone scan. May lead to spondylolisthesis.
Osteomyelitis	Lysis or sclerosis in the neural arch and in the transverse process.	Not common.
LCH	Rarely affects the neural arches.	
Tumors	Hodgkin disease, leukemia, metastatic neuroblastoma. Primary bone tumors are rare.	
Pseudarthrosis after spinal fusion for scoliosis or kyphosis repair	A break in the fusion mass. Consider when abnormal curvature recurs.	Bone scintigraphy more than 6 months after surgery may be confirmatory.
Multiple stippled epiphyses	Coronal cleft in spinous processes.	Also known as chondrodysplasia punctata.

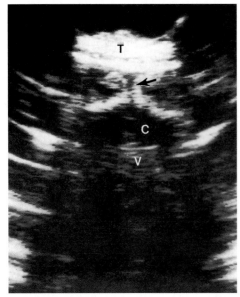

Fig. 4.248   Neural canal-cutaneus fistula. Historic sonographic examination in a neonate. Arrow points to a fistula.
C   Spinal canal
T   Subcutaneous tissue
V   L3 vertebral body

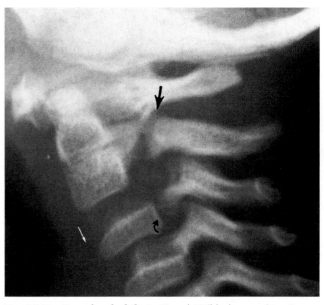

Fig. 4.249   Neural arch clefts in C2 and C3 (black arrows) in a 2-year-old girl. The anterior fat stripe (white arrow) is not displaced. Apposing bone surfaces are smooth. There is no recent remarkable trauma. Appearance is also unchanged from a prior study, so they are not believed to be fractures.

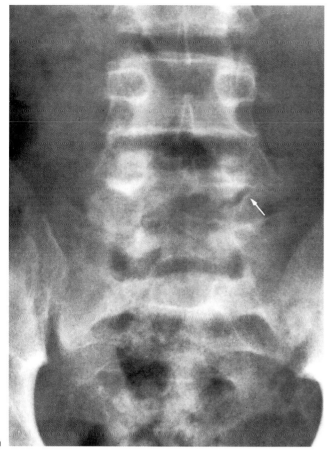

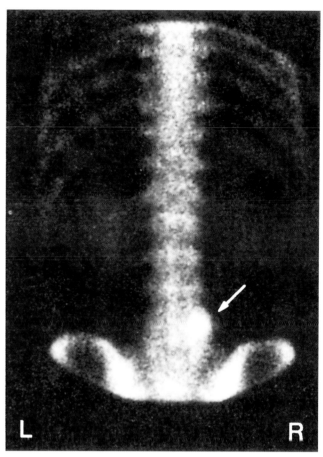

b

Fig. 4.250a, b   Spondylolysis. (a) Interruption of the interarticular pars of L5 (arrow), a hypoplastic left pedicle, and a somewhat dense right pedicle. Clinically, the patient complains of back pain. **(b)** Classic bone scintigram: increased activity in the right pedicle (arrow) due to stress related to the left spondylolysis.

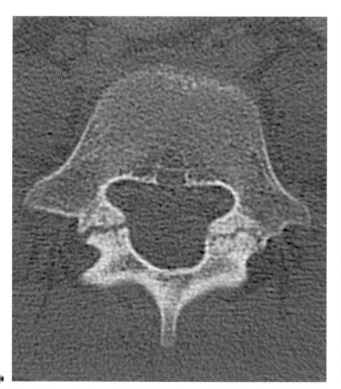

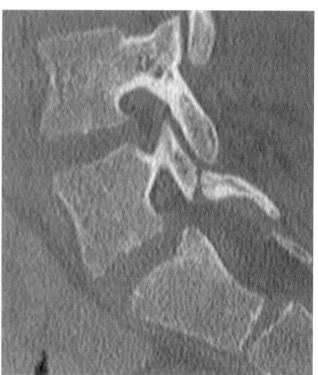

b

Fig. 4.251a, b   Spondylolysis and spondylolisthesis. (a) Axial CT image on this 14-year-old boy shows bilateral irregular lucencies across the pars of the arch of L5, with some sclerosis to either side of the gap. **(b)** Sagittal reconstruction of the CT shows one-sided L5 spondylolysis and the associated grade 1 spondylolisthesis of L5 on S1.

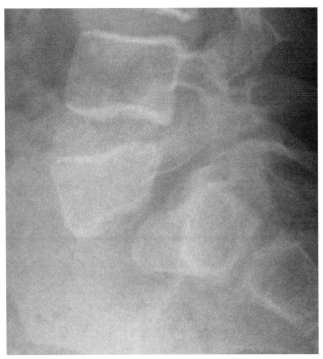

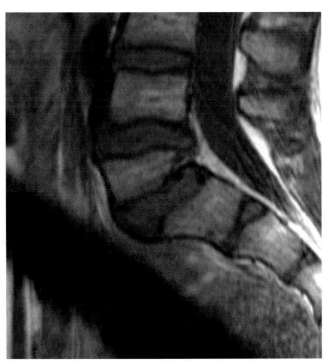

a

Fig. 4.252a, b   Spondylolysis and spondylolisthesis. This is more severe than in **Fig. 4.251a, b**. (**a**) The more severe spondylolisthesis of L5 on S1 on the plain image is considered grade 3 of 4 (over 50% relative displacement). (**b**) T1 MRI reveals the effects on disks and canal contents in this 12-year-old boy with back pain.

Table 4.89   Enlargement of the neural arches

Diagnosis	Findings	Comments
Normal variants	Tendency for development of a large anterior arch of C1 in conjunction with a small posterior arch, and vice versa.	
Bone tumors	Expansion of the neural arch together with simultaneous destruction. May narrow the adjacent intervertebral foramen.	Osteoblastoma, aneurysmal bone cyst, giant cell tumor, osteochondroma, hemangioma, and lymphangioma, for example.
Generalized bone disease	Generalized enlargement in involved skeletal elements in, for example, FD or hyperphosphatasemia	Associated changes in the limb bones.
Unilateral enlargement of a pedicle	The contralateral pedicle undergoes hypertrophy in contralateral unilateral spondylolysis or in congenital absence of contralateral pedicle.	Also may occur as an isolated anomaly.
Congenital hyperplasia of anterior tubercle of transverse process	Typically occurs at C5 and C6.	Neurologic symptoms can accompany. Clarification with CT; MRI for evaluation of the cord and nerve roots.

Table 4.90   Abnormal shape of pedicles

Diagnosis	Findings	Comments
Normal variant	Flattening of the usually ovoid shape on front projection, mainly in the upper lumbar spine. The medial boundaries are not quite concave.	If necessary, MRI to exclude an intraspinal process.
Intraspinal mass	Flattening or concavity of the medial border; possible destruction or total obliteration of the neural arch.	MRI for evaluation.
Dysplastic or small pedicle	In various anomalies of vertebral column, especially rachischisis, postirradiation, and in NF1.	
Achondroplasia	Short pedicles (and laminae).	Slowing of enchondral growth.
Hypochondroplasia	Less severely short than achondroplasia.	Less severely slowed than achondroplasia.
Melnick-Needles syndrome	May have very small pedicles, especially in the lumbar region. The arches are intact, however.	Osteodysplasty. Thin irregularly marginated ribs.
Postirradiation	Abnormally small pedicles may be part of the acquired growth disturbance.	Associated scoliosis if radiation fields were not symmetrically balanced.

Table 4.91   Destruction, sclerosis, and absent pedicles

Diagnosis	Findings	Comments
Congenital absence ▷ *Fig. 4.244, p. 446*	Aplasia, hypoplasia, or absence of one or more pedicles.	Nerve roots rearrange according to the hox gene structure abnormalities.
Osteolysis from tumors, metastases, infection ▷ *Fig. 4.253a, b, p. 254* ▷ *Fig. 4.254, p. 254*	CT shows abnormal bone structure. MRI for better definition of soft tissues and any intraspinal canal pathology.	Metastases, leukemia, Hodgkin disease, LCH, osteoblastoma, Ewing sarcoma, osteogenic sarcoma, among others. Among infections, be on the lookout for community-acquired methicillin-resistant *Staphylococcus aureus*.
Osteoid osteoma	Sclerosis of one pedicle and nearby.	CT, bone scintigraphy. Night pain relieved by aspirin. Secondary scoliosis eventually.
Engelmann disease	Pedicle periosteal reaction leads to dense pedicles.	Progressive diaphyseal dysplasia.
Sclerotic tumors	Sometimes seen in Ewing sarcoma, Hodgkin sarcoma, osteogenic sarcoma, and some metastases.	

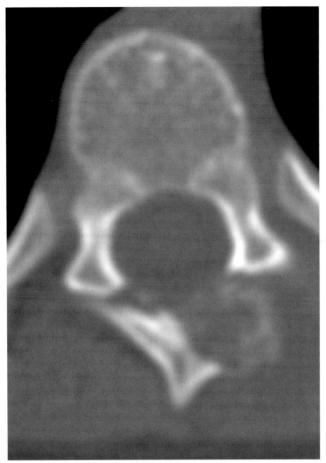

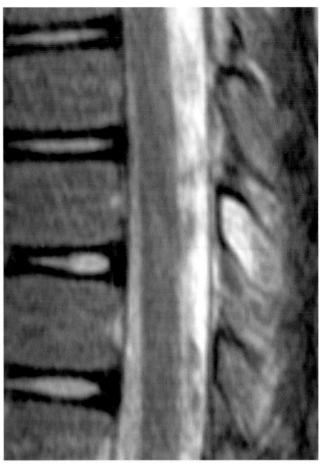

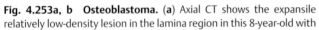
a

b

Fig. 4.253a, b   Osteoblastoma. (a) Axial CT shows the expansile relatively low-density lesion in the lamina region in this 8-year-old with localized pain. **(b)** On sagittal T2 MRI to the left of midline, note the high intensity associated with the osteoblastoma.

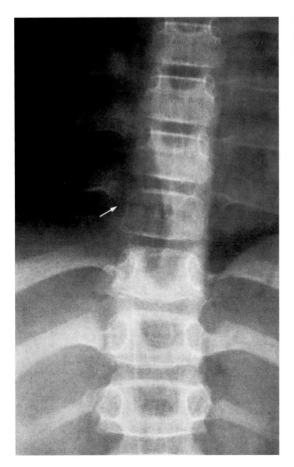

Fig. 4.254   Osteoblastoma obliterating visualization of pedicle. Osteoblastoma replaced the pedicle bony substance (arrow) and caused obstruction of the CSF flow at that level.

■ Abnormalities in Alignment and Position

Abnormalities in alignment and position include scoliosis, kyphosis, lordosis, and dislocation.

Table 4.92   Idiopathic scoliosis

Diagnosis	Findings	Comments
Idiopathic scoliosis ▷ *Fig. 4.255*	Rotation of vertebrae around the long axis is a key element in lateral curvature. Cobb technique for measuring the angle of the scoliosis (**Fig. 4.255**). As scoliosis and rotation of bodies progresses, wedging of the body shape occurs. S-shaped deformity, convex right in the thoracic region is one classic curve. Erect radiographs in two projections are standard. Functional radiographs (lateral bending or perhaps longitudinal stretching) to evaluate the flexibility of curves.	Mostly becoming apparent after the age of 2 y, and especially in second decade. Tendency to progress during growth spurts. Girls much more common than boys. Underlying causes must be excluded, such as NF1, congenital hemivertebra, and intraspinal pathology.
Infantile idiopathic scoliosis	Compensatory, mild (Cobb angle below 15°). Rule out segmentation abnormality such as hemivertebra). Spontaneous regression in first or second year of life.	Believed not uncommonly to be caused by intra-uterine position of the fetus; may have concomitant asymmetry of skull, thorax, or pelvis. Other simulator: active infant during imaging.

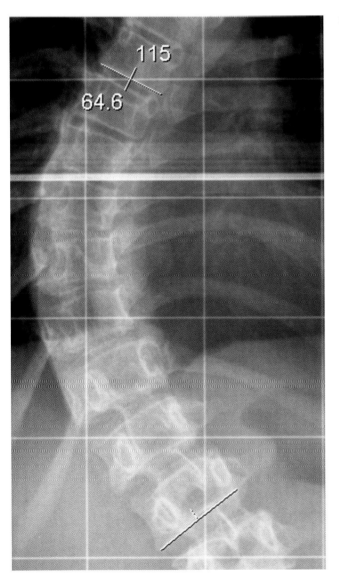

Fig. 4.255   Cobb method of angle measurements, using end plates most tilted from the horizontal. The severe thoracolumbar curve measures 65°.

Table 4.93 Scoliosis arising from bony abnormalities

Diagnosis	Findings	Comments
Vertebral malformations (hemivertebrae, etc.)	Fixed scoliosis. A single lateral hemivertebra will result in a locally angulated scoliosis.	May be a part of VATER association.
Asymmetric lumbosacral transitional vertebra	Frontal view: unilateral fusion of a wide transverse process of L5 with S1.	May also occur without scoliosis. Role in any back pain not established.
Anomalies with hemihypertrophy	Asymmetric vertebral development possible. Upright images to show associated pelvic tilt from leg-length discrepancy.	For example, Klippel-Trénaunay syndrome, Weber syndrome, and Proteus syndrome.
Following vertebral fractures	Scoliosis convex to fractured lumbar transverse processes.	Similar possible scoliosis after unilateral rib resection.
Postirradiation	Scoliosis may be due to underdevelopment of the muscles on unilaterally irradiated side (e.g., after treatment of Wilms tumor).	Can occur after doses of 30 Gy, regularly occurs after 40 Gy; latent period up to 10 y.
Spondylolysis, spondylolisthesis	May coincidentally accompany scoliosis or cause the scoliosis.	Oblique plain images or CT to image.
One hypoplastic lower extremity	Following polio; embryologic reduction deformities in lower extremity sclerotomes. Pelvic tilt on upright images.	Asymmetric thalidomide effect, for example. Any cause of unilaterally shortened lower extremity will lead to functional scoliosis.
Bones weakened from demineralization	Asymmetric compression fractures.	Osteoporosis vs. hyperparathyroidism.
Osteoid osteoma ▷ Fig. 4.256	Painful scoliosis, not fully flexible in severe cases; the circumscribed increased density may be elusive on plain images.	Bone scintigraphy is most useful way to detect. CT and MRI may also be subtle.
Osteoblastoma	Tumor in body or arch.	Larger than osteoid osteoma.
Lateral block vertebra or vertical pedicle bar	The old conventional tomography showed the fusions well; now may need CT with coronal reconstruction.	Pedicle bar: rapidly progressive scoliosis. Therapy: fusion of the other side.
Spondylocostal dysplasia	Multiple rib and vertebral anomalies.	Also known as Jarcho-Levin syndrome.

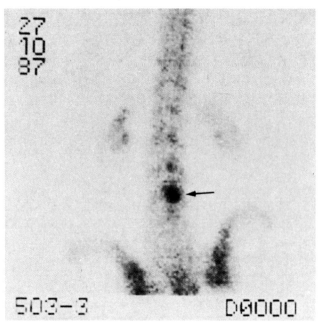

Fig. 4.256 Scoliosis associated with osteoid osteoma in an 11-year-old boy. Bone scintigram: Circumscribed increased uptake in the neural arch of L4 (arrow). Clinically presents as painful fixed scoliosis. CT and MRI had initially been considered unremarkable.

Table 4.94   Spinal and neuromuscular scoliosis causes

Diagnosis	Findings	Comments
Meningomyelocele and related conditions	Often associated with progressive scoliosis.	
Other neuromuscular conditions	Often especially long curves (many vertebral levels).	Seated or standing images helpful.
Syringomyelia, hydromyelia	Diagnosed with MRI.	Consider if rapid worsening of scoliosis after surgery or trauma.
Diastematomyelia	A spur is often present (but frequently overlooked) on a frontal radiograph. Scoliosis may result from associated vertebral anomalies. Wide interpedicle distance; vertical fusion of laminae on one side.	Definitive diagnosis with MRI, although CT good for bony spur. Occasionally accompanied by Sprengel deformity of scapula.
Space-occupying lesion in the spinal canal	May show local canal widening on plain images; diagnosis with MRI.	Painful scoliosis with neurologic manifestations. Among tumors, astocytoma is relatively common.

Kyphosis

Kyphosis occurs frequently as a part of kyphoscoliosis in neuro-muscular diseases and in several skeletal dysplasias.

Other kyphosis arises from malformation syndromes with anterior wedging of vertebral bodies, such as Morquio disease.

Kyphosis may be associated with intraspinal abnormalities (**Fig. 4.257**).

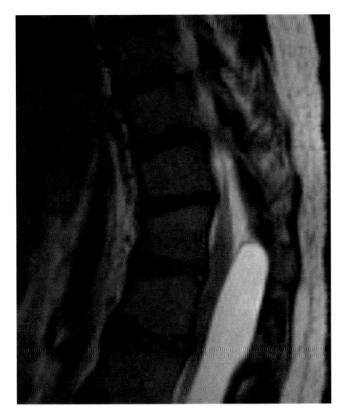

Fig. 4.257   Kyphosis associated with arachnoid cyst. Back pain and worsening kyphosis in a 13-year-old girl. Arachnoid cyst just below the apex of the kyphos shows high intensity on T2 MRI. Did the arachnoid cyst cause the kyphosis, or is it the other way around?

Table 4.95 Kyphosis

Diagnosis	Findings	Comments
Scheuermann "disease," adolescent kyphosis	Anterior wedging in thoracic vertebrae, classically at least three adjacent levels; irregular end plates.	May lead to early degenerative disk disease (in the fourth decade). Often at least one parent also has Scheuermann kyphosis.
Vertebral body fractures	Anterior wedging as loss of height.	MRI for associated cord damage.
Late sequela of spondylitis (pyogenic or tuberculous)	Wedged kyphosis due to vertebral body destruction and loss of height with possible disk destruction.	Gibbus formation, particularly in tuberculosis, in which case it is known as Pott disease.
Following cervical spine laminectomy ▷ Fig. 4.258	Especially laminectomy at several levels.	For example, because of cervical column neurofibroma surgery.
Achondroplasia	Kyphosis increases with age, independent of the lumbar lordosis.	One more reason for short stature in achondroplasia.
LCH	Kyphosis may precede frank vertebra plana.	Eosinophilic granuloma.
Obesity	In overweight children, a tendency to cervical kyphosis.	
Chronic lung disease	Develop barrel-shaped thorax.	As examples, asthma and cystic fibrosis.
Severe cervical kyphosis in diastrophic dysplasia, camptomelic dysplasia, and other dysplasias	Images of chest or cervical spine should include laterals at least once.	Diastrophic dysplasia: hitchhiker thumbs; camptomelic: congenital bent limbs.
Posterior hemivertebra	May be partially compensated for in alignment by anterior overgrowth of adjacent vertebral bodies.	Hox gene effect.
Larsen syndrome	Many vertebral anomalies, which may cause cervical or thoracic kyphosis and other deformities of the region.	Multiple dislocations of joints in the extremities at birth. Overabundant carpal and tarsal bones.

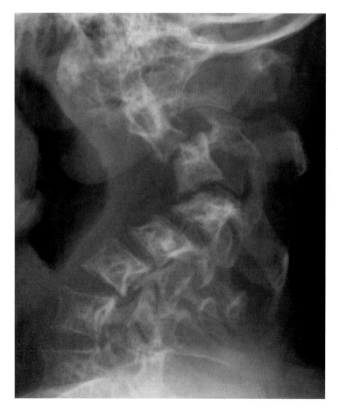

Fig. 4.258 Kyphosis following cervical laminectomy (NF1). Lateral plain image of a 10-year-old who had had a cervical neuroblastoma in the spinal canal.

Table 4.96   Hyperlordosis

Diagnosis	Findings	Comments
Achondroplasia	Increased lordosis at lumbosacral junction.	Sacrum may be seen en face on frontal images.
Idiopathic scoliosis	Curvature changes in all three dimensions in scoliosis.	
Associated with thoracic kyphosis	As an attempt to balance in the sagittal plane.	
Cerebral palsy	Less common than scoliosis; coxa valga.	Abnormal brain MRI.
Pseudoachondroplastic dysplasia and other dysplasias	May show hyperlordosis	

Table 4.97   Abnormally straight vertebral column (on lateral view)

Diagnosis	Findings	Comments
Straight back configuration; straight back syndrome ▷ *Fig. 4.259*	Absence of normal physiologic thoracic kyphosis in conjunction with decreased sagittal diameter of the thorax. Heart and great vessels may appear enlarged on the front view, with heart displaced to the left. Pectus excavatum accentuates the changes even more.	This configuration, or else pectus excavatum alone, is seen in about half of teenagers receiving chest radiographs for chest pain (thus straight back "syndrome"). Many persons with this configuration or with pectus excavatum can be shown to have mitral valve prolapse on sonogram.
Absence of cervical lordosis	Not a rare but a presumably normal finding in childhood.	Also common: pseudosubluxation between C2 and C3, and less often between C3 and C4.
Reflex pain, induced stiff back	Loss of cervical or lumbar lordosis due to pain-induced muscle spasm.	

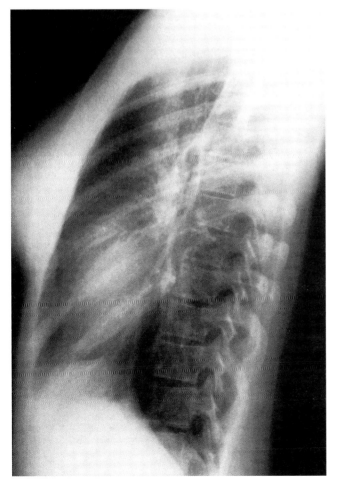

Fig. 4.259   Straight back configuration (syndrome, if associated with chest pain) in a 14-year-old girl. Total absence of thoracic kyphosis, yielding a narrowed thorax in midline.

■ Causes Extrinsic to the Vertebral Bodies

Muscular causes include torticollis (US of the sternocleidomastoid [SCM] muscle), reflex muscle spasm with intra-abdominal or retroperitoneal processes, ophthalmologically induced wryneck, chronic pleural empyema and pleural rind, congenital cardiac disease (atrial septal defect, tetralogy of Fallot), cystic fibrosis, and psychogenic malpositioning.

Table 4.98   Limb and gastroesophageal causes

Diagnosis	Findings	Comments
Leg-length discrepancy	Scoliosis may be seen only on standing images; should be repeated once the discrepancy has been equalized by blocks under the foot, or else by supine image to check flexibility.	Pelvic tilt from idiopathic scoliosis may simulate leg-length discrepancy.
Unilateral upper limb hypoplasia or hyperplasia	Scoliosis may be associated. Observe humerus on scoliosis images.	Today, polio has become a less common occurrence.
Vigorous archery or javelin throwing	Muscular hypertrophy of arm, with cortical thickening of humerus.	Other athletic activities also possibilities (e.g., perhaps discus throwing).
Sandifer syndrome	Torsion spasms, abnormal positioning, and movements of the head, neck, and thorax during or after feeding in a child with a sliding hiatus hernia.	Occasionally only gastroesophageal reflux without a hernia.

Table 4.99   Malformation syndromes, skeletal dysplasia

Diagnosis	Findings	Comments
NF1	The typical scoliosis is short and more angulated than bowed. Thinned ribs.	Idiopathic scoliosis more common in NF1 than the characteristic short curve.
Marfan syndrome	Mild scoliosis may accompany the more common pectus excavatum or carinatum.	Dolichostenomelia and arachnodactyly.
Achondroplasia	Mild scoliosis may occur with the typical lumbar lordosis and frequent thoracolumbar kyphosis.	Rhizomelia including somewhat short ribs.
Fibrous dysplasia	Disturbed local density and contour of involved bones.	Café-au-lait spots. Advanced bone age.
Ehlers-Danlos syndrome[a]	Kyphoscoliosis. Occasional spondylolisthesis.	Hyperextensible joints, cutis laxis.

[a]Because other rare syndromes and dysplasias have associated scoliosis or kyphoscoliosis, this finding is usually not itself a major deciding factor in the differential diagnosis.

Abnormal Position (Dislocation)

Atlantoaxial Subluxation

The atlantoaxial complex normally prevents sagittal dislocation between C1 and C2; this complex consists of the dens that is attached to the body of C2, the transverse ligament of C1 posterior to the dens, and the anterior arch of C1, along with ligaments from the upper tip of the dens to the occiput and to the C1–C2 articular surfaces. The distance between the anterior border of the dens and the posterior margin of the anterior arch of C1 should not exceed 5 mm in flexion or extension in childhood and in most cases is limited to 2 to 3 mm.

The distance between the C1 arch and the dens can only be determined on a well-positioned lateral radiographic image of the cervical spine (or else cross-sectional imaging); subluxation or instability is best visualized in flexion (see **Fig. 4.260**). Rotational injury is to be suspected from the frontal view, then examined with special views or CT. The open mouth view is the best method to assess the dens and the atlantoaxial articulations (supplemented as needed with CT).

Ossification of the anterior arch of C1 usually begins by the end of the first year of life, but some children may already have ossification by birth.

Instability or subluxability is a potential finding; subluxation is the actual event.

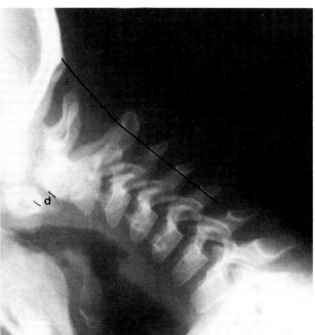

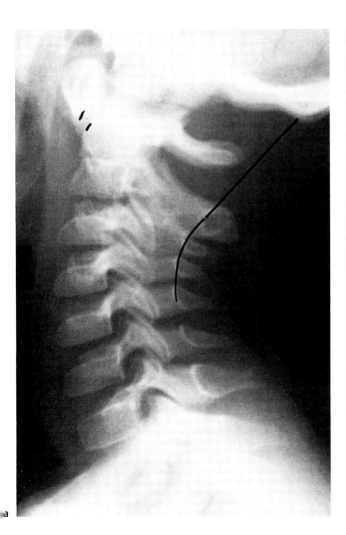

Fig. 4.260a, b   Atlantoaxial subluxation in a 3-year-old girl. Increasing distance (d) in flexion (**b**) between the dens and the anterior arch of C1, compared to neutral position (**a**). Incidental nonossification of the most posterior arch of C1.

Table 4.100　Atlantoaxial subluxation

Diagnosis	Findings	Comments
Down syndrome (trisomy 21) ▷ *Fig. 4.261*	Subluxation possible in severe cases, even in the neutral sagittal position. Some children with Down syndrome have narrow spinal canal behind C1 without subluxability,	About 17% of children with Down syndrome have subluxability; of these, about one-sixth have associated neurologic symptoms.
Retropharyngeal abscess and similar inflammatory processes	Subluxation caused by laxity of the transverse ligament.	Known as Grisel syndrome.
JIA and other arthridites	Subluxation caused by laxity of the ligaments. Dens may have a concave dorsal impression from the transverse ligament.	Tapering of the spinous processes posteriorly. Body- or arch-acquired fusions.
Dens fracture, or epiphyseolysis, with sagittal dislocation	Retropharyngeal soft-tissue swelling with anterior displacement of the cervical fat stripe from hematoma.	Upper cervical spine fractures are uncommon in children below 12 y of age.
Short dens (hypoplasia or even aplasia) ▷ *Fig. 4.262a–c*	Predisposes to subluxation because of lack of dens in front of the transverse ligament. Caution when intubating.	Always rule out in children with generalized platyspondyly. Subluxation is a common danger in Morquio disease, but may happen in other dysplasias. May also be isolated in otherwise normal children.
Marfan syndrome	C1-C2 instability may be present. Fortunately, spinal canal is often wider than average.	
Os odontoideum ▷ *Fig. 4.223, p. 431*	An ossicle in place of the upper dens will not protect from subluxation if free to move from lowest dens and the body of C2.	Os odontoideum may also represent the end result of an unhealed dens base fracture. Os terminale, however, is a normal ossification at the upper tip of the dens and is unlikely to be associated with subluxation.
Dorsal tilt of the dens ▷ *Fig. 4.263, p. 464*	Although this variation may look unusual, subluxation is not likely.	
Congenital anomaly in the atlantoaxialoccipital region ▷ *Fig. 4.264, p. 464*	Partial or full incorporation of the posterior arch of atlas into the skull base is one manifestation.	Variations controlled by hox genes.
Rotary subluxation	Mostly due to trauma. C1 is rotated in axial plane relative to C2 (or vice versa).	The spinous process is displaced on the open mouth plain image; CT is more accurate.
Ehlers Danlos syndrome (and other hyperlaxity conditions)		Especially Ehlers Danlos syndrome type IV.

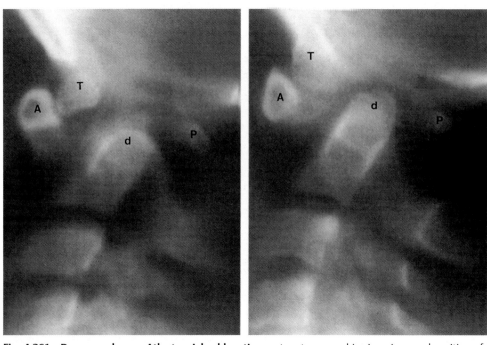

Fig. 4.261　Down syndrome. Atlantoaxial subluxation on two tomographic views in neural position of the cervical spine. The distance between the dens (d) and the anterior arch of C1 is considerably greater than 5 mm and the distance between the dens and the posterior arch (P) of C1 is markedly less than normal.
A　Anterior arch of the atlas
T　Third condyle (condylus tertius), an additional finding in this subject

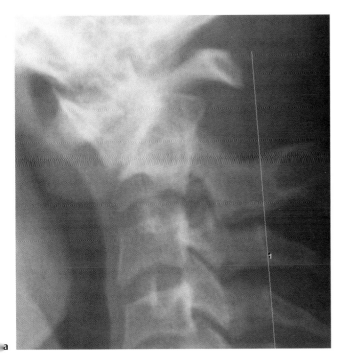

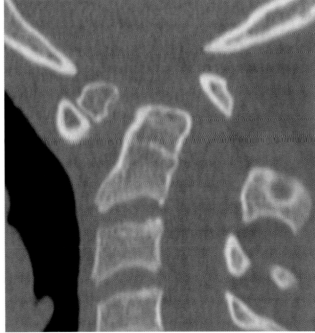

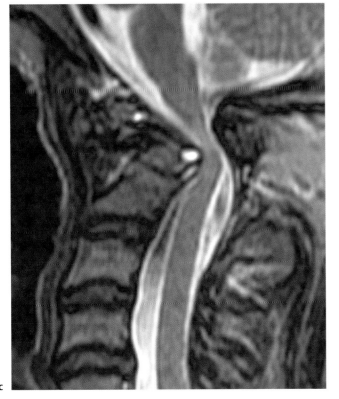

Fig. 4.262a–c   Atlantoaxial subluxation on cross-sectional imaging in 14-year-old girl who may have a spondyloepiphyseal dysplasia. (**a**) Plain image shows severe posterior displacement of the dens, nearly at the same level as the spinolaminal junction of C1. (**b**) CT sagittal reconstruction shows the bony relationships in greater detail, including a likely condylus tertius of the occiput above the anterior arch of C1. (**c**) Sagittal T2 MRI demonstrates the plight of the cord and other canal contents.

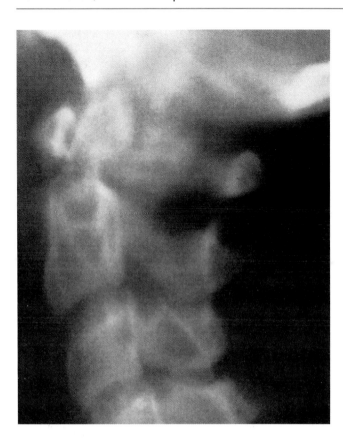

Fig. 4.263   Posterior concavity of the upper dens (tomography) in a 7-year-old girl. Appearance on the plain lateral image had suggested suspicion of a fracture of dens.

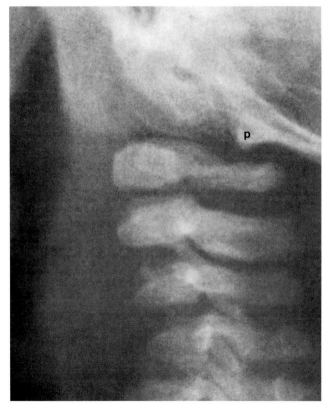

Fig. 4.264   Anomalous craniocervical junction (Hox gene anomaly). The posterior arch of the atlas (p) is incorporated into the occiput. The dens and the anterior arch of the atlas are not (yet) ossified. Midcervical spine kyphosis is also present.

Table 4.101 Other types of dislocation

Diagnosis	Findings	Comments
Normal: C2-C3 pseudosubluxation ▷ *Fig. 4.265a, b*	The spinolaminar line remains intact (posterior border of the spinal canal).	Anterior subluxation of C2 up to 2 mm quite normal, 3–4 mm may also be normal. Similar findings at C3-C4 and even C4-C5.
Atlanto-occipital dislocation	The clival line will no longer touch the posterior surface of the dens.	Severe trauma, including birth trauma. Cord transection; fatal in most cases.
Basilar impression ▷ *Fig. 4.266, p. 466*	Primary or secondary protrusion of the upper vertebrae (dens) through the foramen magnum. Ascending clivus in severe cases.	In osteogenesis imperfecta and in hyperparathyroidism. Also after infectious or neoplastic destruction in the region. Results in tam o'shanter skull configuration.
Trauma ▷ *Fig. 4.267, p. 466*	Displacement with fracture of neural arch; disruption of the spinolaminar line.	
Inflammatory processes or tumors	Dislocation can occur as a relatively late complication.	
Spondylolisthesis	Mainly at L5-S1. The upside-down Napoleon hat sign on frontal radiograph in grade IV.	Four grades per 25% anterior displacement increments.

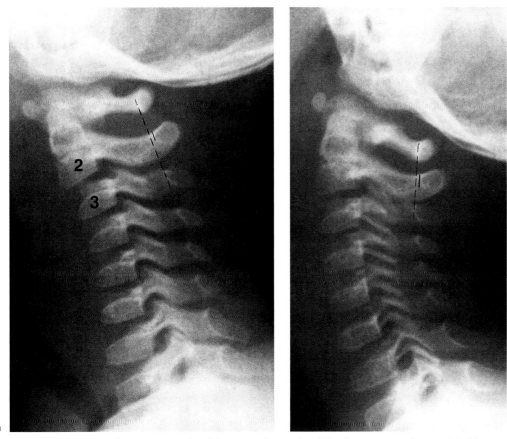

Fig. 4.265a, b   Normal anterior pseudosubluxation of C2 with mild kyphosis on partial flexion (**a**). (**b**) Normal relationships in extension. The posterior borders of the vertebral canal (spinolaminar line) remain unchanged during the position change.

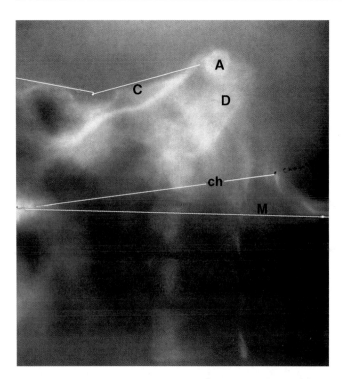

Fig. 4.266   Basilar impression ("protrusio occipital") in **osteogenesis imperfecta** in a 16-year-old patient.
A   Anterior arch of C1
C   Ascending clivus
ch Chamberlain line
D   Dens
M   McGregor line

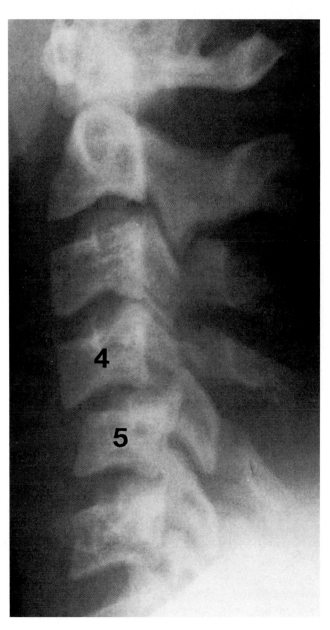

Fig. 4.267   Locked facet joints between C4 and C5 **from trauma**, with displacement of a small fragment to the inferior articular surface of C4.

Alterations in Bone Structure

■ Increased Density

Generalized Increased Density

Please note that humans are not densitometers; we are only recognizers of interfaces. Plain image recognition of increased or decreased density is only possible in relation to adjacent objects.

Sclerosis of the vertebrae can occur in all diseases in which generalized sclerosis of all bones occurs.

Table 4.102   Generalized increased density

Diagnosis	Findings	Comments
Physiologic "bony sclerosis of the neonate"	Apparent increased density of multiple bones, decreasing in the first weeks of life. One explanation is the difference from prenatal bone and the metaphyseal less dense bone created in the first weeks of life. See below for bone-in-bone appearance.	Can closely mimic osteopetrosis. True increased density is in relation to neighboring structures, such as zones of provisional calcification or tooth buds. Bones can be made more or less dense on picture archiving and communication system (PACS) with maneuvering.
Osteopetrosis ▷ *Fig. 4.268, p. 468*	Diffuse sclerosis systematically of all or part of the vertebral bodies and entire skeleton. "Rugger jersey" spine in some older children.	Anemia occurs when too much bone is involved. Increase bone fragility, even in vertebrae. Occasionally has multiple wormian bones. May have jaw osteomyelitis. Osteocytic osteolysis impairment may be a cause.
Bone marrow hyperplasia	Dense trabeculation. If severe, could show extramedullary hematopoiesis.	Chronic iron deficiency and hemolytic anemias, and particularly thalassemia major, MRI shows well the abnormal pattern vs. expected fat in marrow.
Pyknodysostosis	Generalized sclerosis.	Bone fragility. Multiple wormian bones. Short stature. Toulouse-Lautrec's syndrome is a possible example.
Fluorosis	Generalized sclerosis is systematically laid down in bone during exposure.	Osteoporosis can also occur in chronic fluoride intoxication.
Engelmann disease, progressive diaphyseal dysplasia ▷ *Fig. 4.269, p. 468*	Diaphyseal vigorous periosteal reaction leads to sclerotic appearance. In vertebrae, mainly seen in the neural arch.	Also know as Camurati-Engelmann disease. Increased uptake in bone scintigraphy in active stage. Similar pattern in mother-of-pearl industrial exposure.
Osteomesopyknosis	Density similar to osteopetrosis, but limited to trunk and the most proximal limbs.	May have back pain.

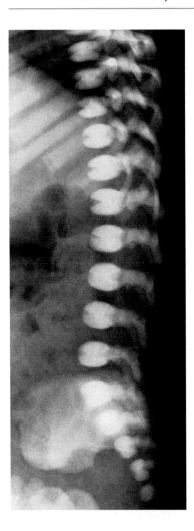

Fig. 4.268 Osteopetrosis in a neonate (compare to **Fig. 4.192**). Denser than normal bones and prominent vascular clefts are noted.

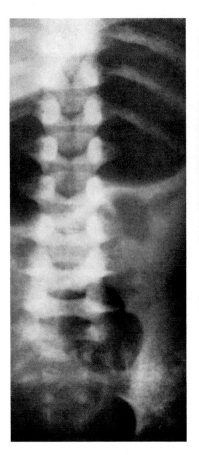
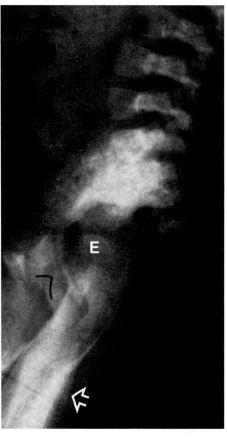

Fig. 4.269 Camurati-Engelmann disease. The neural arches are dense compared to the bodies, as are regions in the ilium. These are analogous to the periosteal reaction of the dense femoral shafts (arrow). The density remains normal in femoral epiphysis (E) and metaphysis, as well as the vertebral bodies. All but the most posterior parts of the posterior ribs also dense.

Table 4.103   Bandlike sclerosis

Diagnosis	Findings	Comments
Bone-in-bone appearance	Normal growth pattern in the very young.	Normal in neonates and prematures in the first 2–8 wk. Evolves to normal spontaneously.
Healing osteoporosis	Newest normal density bone interfaces with osteoporotic bone.	
Growth resumption lines after illness or injury ▷ *Fig. 4.270*	Dense lines parallel to growth plates in vertebral column are less conspicuous than in long bones.	Also known as Harris lines, Park lines, growth arrest lines, or growth recovery lines.
"Rugger jersey" vertebrae ▷ *Fig. 4.271, p. 470*	Denser bone along end plates than centrally.	A characteristic of osteopetrosis and osteomesopyknosis.
Healing renal osteodystrophy	Band of normal bone looks denser than earlier demineralized bone.	
Chronic lead poisoning	Dense bands less conspicuous than those of long bones.	Also in bismuth poisoning.
Idiopathic hypercalcemia and hypervitaminosis D	Bands of increased density during the metabolically active period of the conditions.	Occasionally, hypervitaminosis D leads to less than normal density instead.

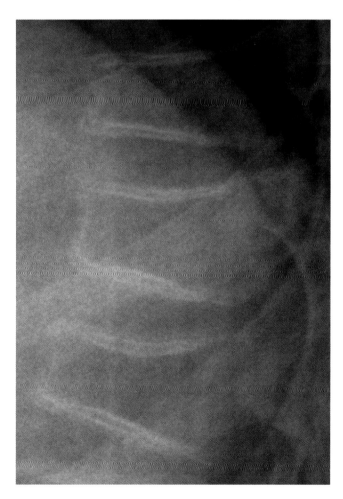

Fig. 4.270   Harris lines. Osteoporotic vertebral bodies show dense thin lines (growth arrest/recovery lines of Harris or Park) paralleling the end plates. This teenager with Duchenne muscular dystrophy has had a heart transplant and thus receives periodic metabolic jolts from immune therapy, resulting in the lines.

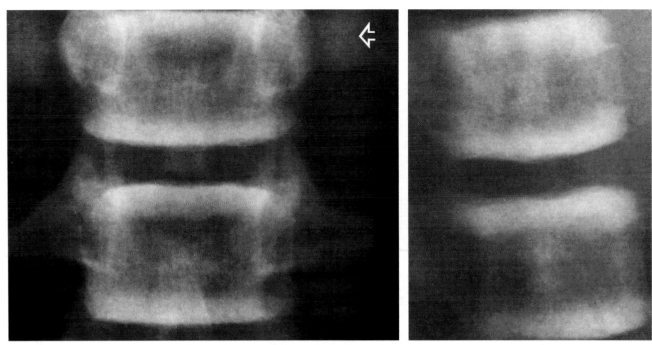

Fig. 4.271   "Rugger jersey" in osteopetrosis in a 1-year-old girl. The metaphyseal equivalents adjacent to the end plates are denser than the central (older) portions of the vertebral bodies. A dense 12th rib is noted (arrow).

Table 4.104   Localized sclerosis

Diagnosis	Findings	Comments
Bone island(s)	Homogeneous, often round, sclerotic, with hazy borders.	Also called osteomas. Of no clinical significance, except diagnostically if part of Gardner syndrome.
Sclerotic pedicle	Contralateral to spondylolysis. Possibly metastasis.	See the subsequent discussion of osteoid osteoma.
Osteoid osteoma ▷ *Fig. 4.272* ▷ *Fig. 4.273*	Sclerotic region with sharp borders; has a predilection for pedicles. Reflex scoliosis common.	Often difficult to demonstrate. Skeletal scintigraphy or CT are best diagnostic methods (rather than MRI).
Compression fracture	Areas of increased density from significant vertebral body compression. Especially when callus occurs during healing phase.	Anterior compression best seen on lateral image; lateral compression best seen on frontal.
Healing phase of spondylitis-diskitis	Increased density at margins of disk material that intrudes through end plate.	Associated disk space narrowing.
Schmorl node margins	Increased density at margins of disk material that intrudes through end plate.	
Healing phase of other lytic and steopenic processes	For example, LCH or rickets.	In healing rickets, the end plates (which are zones of provisional calcification) reappear first.
Melorheostosis	Could involve vertebral elements.	Endosteal in childhood.
Percutaneous vertebroplasty	Dense material injected into treated vertebral body.	After traumatic collapse or in eosinophic granuloma.
Sclerotic neoplasms		
Hodgkin and non-Hodgkin lymphoma ▷ *Fig. 4.274a–d, p. 472*	Predominantly increased density of the affected vertebral bodies.	Marrow replacement on MRI.
Ewing sarcoma	Mostly sclerotic, arch or body.	
Hemangioma	Dense and coarse trabeculae.	Often asymptomatic. Nicely shown on thin-section CT.
Metastases from medulloblastoma		Or retinoblastoma.
Osteogenic sarcoma		Unusual in vertebral location.
Chordoma		Mainly in clivus or sacrum.
Endosteal hyperostosis	Cortex of pedicles and other arch elements is thick at expense of medullary cavity; sclerotic calvarium and jaw.	Worth type is AD; van Buchem type is autosomal recessive.

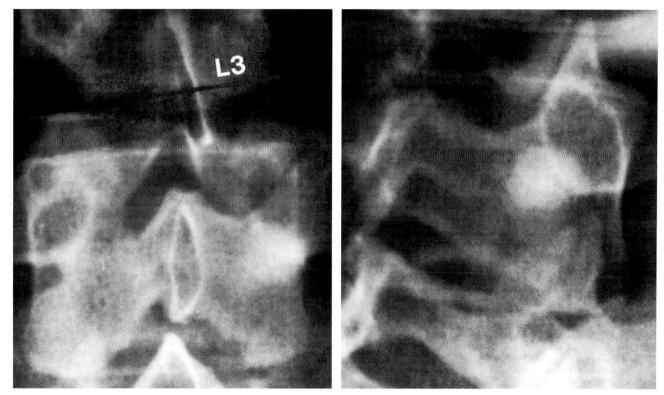

Fig. 4.272   Osteoid osteoma in the pars articularis of L4. A 14-year-old girl with back pain and scoliosis (note tilt of L3).

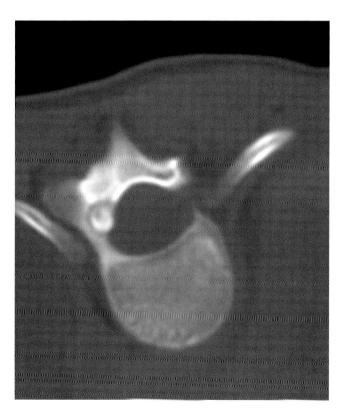

Fig. 4.273   Osteoid osteoma seen on axial CT at the medial right pedicle (on bone scan the lesion was hot). Moderately severe associated scoliosis is reflected by the rotation of the vertebra in the axial plane.

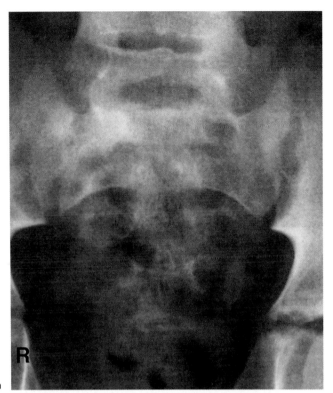

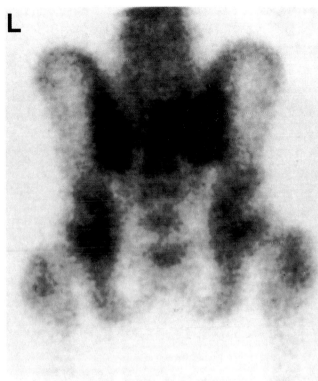

a

b

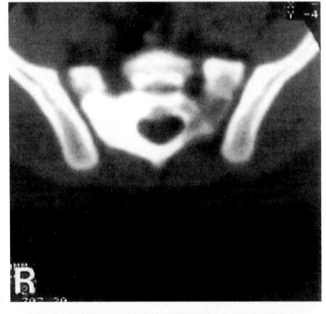

c

Fig. 4.274a–d Non-Hodgkin lymphoma. (**a**) Radiograph with increased density of S2 on the right. (**b**) Classic bone scintigram with increased uptake in the right sacrum, view as from behind. (**c, d**) CT of the sacrum with sclerosis on the right.

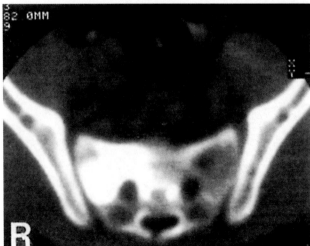

d

■ Decreased Density

Table 4.105   Generalized decreased density

Diagnosis	Findings	Comments
Osteopenia of prematurity	Particularly in very premature infants. Affects the entire skeleton.	Especially after prolonged hospitalization. May relate to insufficient vitamin D.
Osteoporosis	The end plates (zones of provisional calcification) more conspicuous than normal.	May have wedged or codfish vertebra.
Osteogenesis imperfecta	Osteoporosis, tendency to fracture.	Multiple wormian bones in the skull. May have protrusio occipiti.
Rickets, hyperparathyroidism, and renal osteodystrophy	The end plates of the bodies are poorly defined, unlike osteoporosis.	Hand radiograph may help radiologic diagnosis.
Chronic malnutrition		
Untreated hypothyroidism		Inferior anterior breaking of approximately L1 body.
Scurvy	Osteoporosis, with striking periosteal reaction at fractures.	May be a complication of thalassemia therapy.
Leukemia	May present with osteoporosis.	MRI may show bone marrow replacement.
JIA	May have osteoporosis prior to steroid therapy.	Cervical spine fusions and erosions. Formerly juvenile rheumatoid arthritis or juvenile chronic arthritis.
Turner syndrome	Some osteoporosis. Prominently wide finger tufts.	Gonadal dysgenesis. XO genetically. Delayed bone age in second decade.
Fibrous dysplasia	Involved vertebral elements may be of decreased density.	
Homocystinuria	Truncal osteoporosis.	Dolichostenomelia similar to Marfan syndrome.
Glycogenosis and other congenital metabolic diseases		Hepatomegaly in type I (von Gierke syndrome).
Menkes kinky hair syndrome (congenital copper deficiency)	Resembles scurvy at metaphyses. Osteoporosis. Multiple wormian bones.	Decreased copper in hair, blood, and urine. Can be mistaken for child abuse. Very fragile arteries.
Hypophosphatasia	Ricketslike changes involving only a portion of each metaphysis.	Phosphoethanolamine in urine; loose teeth.
I-cell disease	At birth, changes of hyperparathyroidism, plus dysostosis multiplex.	Mucolipidosis II.
Chronic fluoride intoxication	Osteoporosis rather than sclerosis seen in some endemic area cases.	

Table 4.106   Localized decreased density (defect, destruction, and osteolysis)

Diagnosis	Findings	Comments
Spondylitis-diskitis	End plate defects with initially ill-defined margins. Disk space narrowing.	
Central spondylitis	Central defect in body without disk space narrowing.	
Osteolytic malignancies	Initial destruction and later collapse of the vertebral body. Neural arch may also be involved.	CT defines bony change but MRI is preferred to show marrow and soft-tissue components and involvement of cord and nerve roots.
Aneurysmal bone cyst ▷ *Fig. 4.275*	Destruction with ballooning out of the bone structure. Preservation of some cortex in those bony elements with cortex.	May involve sacrum as well.
Fracture ▷ *Fig. 4.276a–c* ▷ *Fig. 4.277, p. 476*	May be subtle on plain images.	Be alert that a fracture may not be alone.
LCH	One or more bodies, not necessarily contiguous.	Eosinophilic granuloma. Common in vertebral body; less common in arch. Often initially painless.
Echinococcal cyst	Soap bubble expansion.	Caution: biopsy with large needle may induce anaphylactic shock.

Metastases: Neuroblastoma (the most common); Wilms tumor (considerably less common); also rhabdomyosarcoma, retinoblastoma, pheochromocytoma (rare).
Hodgkin and non-Hodgkin lymphoma can cause sclerosis as well as destruction.

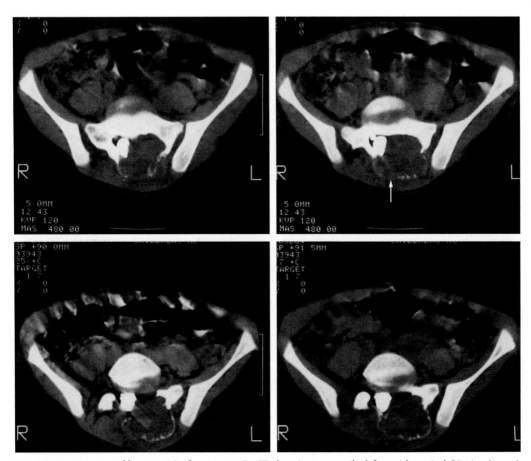

Fig. 4.275   Aneurysmal bone cyst in the sacrum. On CT, there is an expansile defect with cortical thinning (arrow).

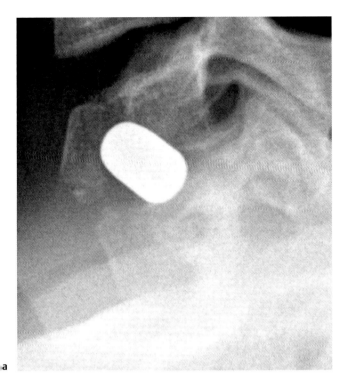

a

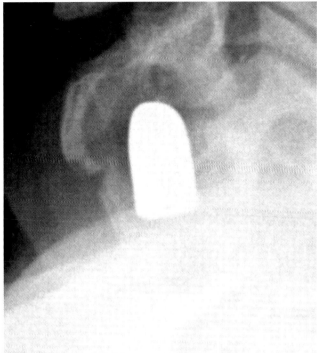

b

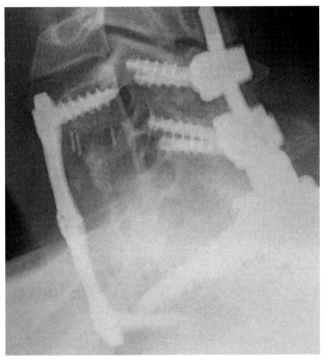

c

Fig. 4.276a–c   **Bullet** from gunshot wound to a 10-year-old lodges in C7 and upper T1 bodies. In August (**a**), one sees the break through the superior end plate of C7. In December (**b**), the bullet has rotated and lies within a wider area of lucency (reaction or infection). (**c**) An image showing the postoperative status.

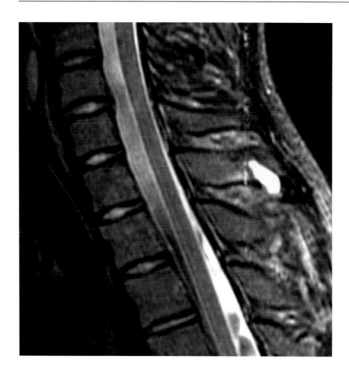

Fig. 4.277 Clay shoveler fracture. On the plain images of this child with neck pain and finger numbness, no fracture was detected initially. The T2 MRI shows the localized posterior spinous process high signal (C7 or T1) which correlates with a so-called clay-shoveler fracture.

The Spinal Canal and Its Contents

■ Localized Spinal Stenosis Caused by Bony Changes

See page 442 for generalized stenosis. Standard investigation includes radiographs in at least two projections and additional work-up with CT. MRI is the method of choice for evaluating the contents of the canal (as well as the medullary portions of bony elements).

Table 4.107 Localized spinal stenosis caused by bony changes

Diagnosis	Findings	Comments
Spondylolisthesis	Posterior displacement of the lower involved level. Mostly L5-S1; less often L4-L5.	Narrowing more pronounced in grades III and IV. Associated spondylolysis.
Displaced fracture fragments	CT for bony detail; MRI for cord involvement and damage.	
Posterior hemivertebra	Often protrudes back into the spinal canal.	Retrolisthesis and kyphosis at that level.
Malformations	For example, Klippel-Feil syndrome.	
Disk prolapse ▷ *Fig. 4.278a, b*	MRI to define.	Causes include spondylodiskitis, calcified nucleus pulposus, and trauma.
Severe scoliosis	Curvature in any direction can narrow the spinal canal and compress nerve roots.	MRI prior to surgery.
Tumors of the vertebral body or arch		
Gibbus	Sharp, severe kyphosis.	Classically, in tuberculosis—may increase rapidly.
Achondroplasia	Short pedicles and laminae in cervical column.	May happen in other dysplasias with enchondral slowing, or even from isolated shortened arch elements.

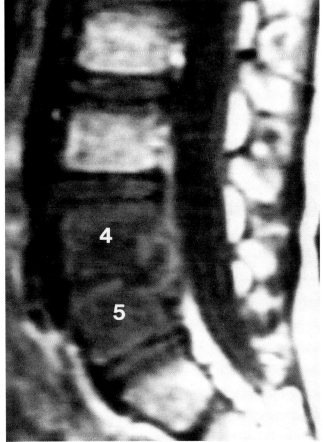

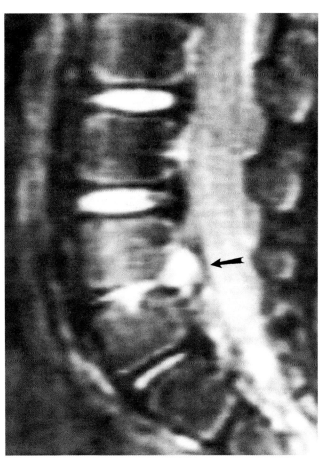

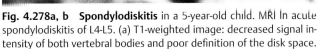

Fig. 4.278a, b   Spondylodiskitis in a 5-year-old child. MRI in acute spondylodiskitis of L4-L5. (a) T1-weighted image: decreased signal intensity of both vertebral bodies and poor definition of the disk space.

(b) T2-weighted image: increased signal intensity of the minimal disk space with posterior prolapse and compression of the dural sac (arrow), as well as protrusion into the body of T5.

■ Masses Within the Spinal Canal

The cervical and lumbosacral canal are normally relatively wide; according to Petersson and Harwood-Nash, the dural sac is significantly wider in approximately 4% of myelograms in children. CT and especially MRI are the diagnostic modalities of choice for those cases that require further diagnostic work-up, whether an intraspinal mass is suspected or if neurologic symptoms occur without bony changes on conventional radiography.

Table 4.108   Masses within the spinal canal

Diagnosis	Findings	Comments
Tumors: extradural and intradural, extramedullary, and intramedullary ▷ *Fig. 4.279, p. 478*	MRI: low signal on T1 and high on T2 (except fat- or cartilage-containing tumors).	Drop metastases result from astrocytoma and cerebellar tumors such as medulloblastoma.
Lipoma ▷ *Fig. 4.280a, b, p. 478*	MRI: high signal intensity on T1.	
Hematoma	MRI: can appear as high signal in the early phase.	Other sequelae of trauma: necrosis, atrophy, syringomyelia, edema.
Edema of cord	MRI: high signal on T2, low on T1.	Narrowing of surrounding spaces.
CSF after failed lumbar puncture	Evident on US and MRI (and CT) around cord.	Typically regresses in a few days. Usually not blood.
Arachnoiditis	MRI: irregular structures of soft tissue within the dural sac (soft-tissue density on CT).	This was relatively common after administration of oily myelographic contrast medium. This is no longer the case.
Meningeal thickening in MPS	Soft-tissue thickening between the dural sac and the bony vertebral structures.	Compression of the cervical cord has been described in MPS I, I-H/S, I-S, II, IV, and VI.
NF1	Posterior scalloping of vertebral bodies.	
Vascular malformations	MRI: signal dropout on T1 and T2, except in small vessels with low-flow velocity.	MRA: artery of Adamkiewicz may be a feeder.
Increased fat deposition in steroid therapy	MRI characteristics the same as lipoma.	Can cause neurologic symptoms.

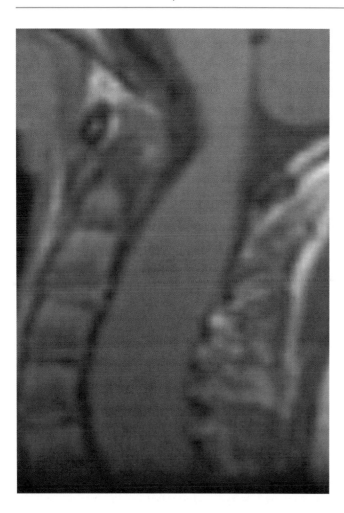

Fig. 4.279 Astrocytoma expanding spinal canal in 6-year-old boy. The mass at the C1–C6 is seen to expand the spinal canal on T1 sagittal MRI.

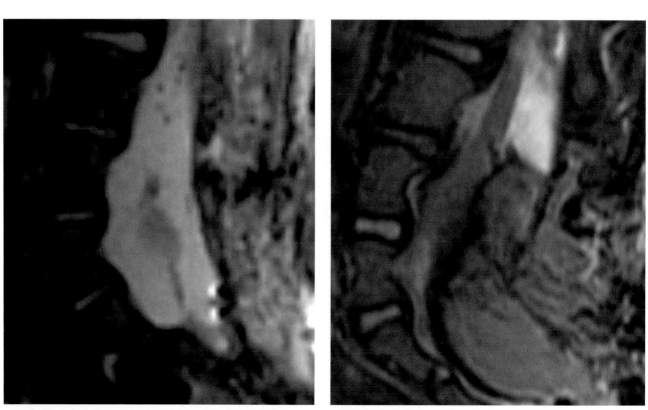

a

b

Fig. 4.280a, b Intraspinal lipoma, part of lipomeningocele. This 4-year-old child has had release of tethered cord and portions of the lipomeningocele. Note the extension of the fatty elements forward to indent and narrow the lowest lumbar bodies.

■ Anomalies of the Spinal Cord With or Without Bony Abnormality

Decreased motion, usually associated with cord tethering, can be determined with US in infants. It is best seen in the first few months of life. Thereafter, MRI shows cord location in sagittal and cranial caudal directions. The conus medullaris does not normally terminate below L3 at any age. Spinal cord tumors are best shown on MRI.

Table 4.109   Anomalies of the spinal cord with or without bony abnormality

Diagnosis	Findings	Comments
Tethered cord	Common in spinal dysraphism. The conus attachment is abnormally low and the cord lacks the normal pulsating motion. Association with meningomyelocele and/or lipoma.	Clinical signs: skin changes, neurologic symptoms, orthopedic abnormalities in the lower limbs such as pes cavus, bladder dysfunction, kyphoscoliosis.
MMC, meningocele, myelocele, lipo-MMC	Spinal dysraphism. MRI: frequently tethered cord with lipoma and high signal of T1.	Severe neurologic deficits. Associated with Chiari type II malformation.
Diastematomyelia ▷ *Fig. 4.281a, b* ▷ *Fig. 4.241, p. 444*	Often a bony spur on radiography or CT. Split cord, conus, and/or filum terminale.	May be associated with hydromyelia, scoliosis, Sprengel deformity. Neurologic symptoms are often minimal.
Syringomyelia, hydromyelia	On radiograph may be widening of the spinal canal. The syrinx is positioned centrally and has low T1 signal.	Occurs after trauma and surgery as well as dysraphism, particularly following shunting of a MMC and with Chiari type II malformation.
Spinal cord *injury* without radiologic *abnormality* (known as SCIWORA)	After trauma, damage to the cord (shown on MRI) without abnormality of bone on plain radiographs.	Neurologic examination is important to suspect it, but also consider depending on mechanism of injury.

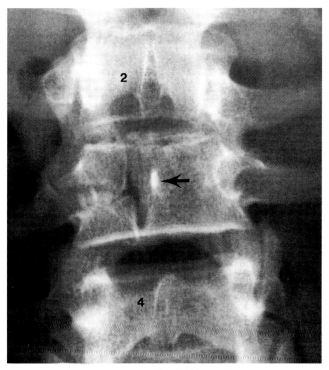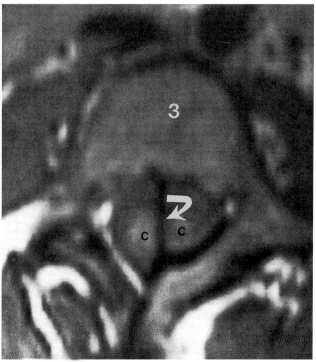

b

Fig. 4.281a, b   Diastematomyelia. (a) Vertical bone spur at L3 level (arrow) and right-sided fused neural arch laminae of L2 and L3. **(b)** Axial MRI: split cord (C) at the level of C3. The arrow indicates the low signal bone spur.

■ Changes in the Disk Spaces

Table 4.110   Narrowed disk spaces

Diagnosis	Findings	Comments
Forme fruste of vertebral body fusion	A step along the way to vertebral body fusion is a narrower than normal disk space.	A possible part of VATER association. A hox gene effect.
Spondylitis-diskitis	Disk narrowing may be the first radiographic finding (but not seen in osteomyelitis limited to the body).	Early scintigraphic diagnosis: increased activity in the adjacent vertebral bodies. Well demonstrated with MRI. Disk material may occasionally protrude through the end plates or posteriorly into the spinal canal.
Scheuermann "disease"	Thoracic kyphosis, narrowed disk spaces, irregular end plates, Schmorl nodes.	May have similar configuration in anterior disk prolapse.
Acute Schmorl nodes	Ill-defined margin of the end plate defect. Later sclerosis of the rim.	MRI (or CT) if needed to confirm.
Trauma	Acute traumatic prolapse of disk into spongiosa uncommon in children.	Demonstrated by CT. Sclerosis of edges later.
JIA	Disk space narrowing precedes full fusion.	Associated arch fusions and areas of erosion in cervical spine.
Spondyloepiphyseal dysplasias, Morquio disease, Kniest disease, Cockayne syndrome	Narrowed disk spaces with irregular end plates may be seen in many syndromes.	

Table 4.111   Widened disk spaces

Diagnosis	Findings	Comments
Normal variant	The normally flat disk may be centrally biconvex.	Also may occur after hyperextension injury.
Platyspondyly	Lower than normal height of vertebral bodies often is associated with taller than normal disks.	See **Tables 4.64** and **4.65**.
Osteoporosis	Weaker than normal end plates allow disks to approach a more spherical shape.	Codfish vertebra configuration.
Other acquired causes of decreased vertebral body height	Sometimes, the disks become taller and sometimes they maintain normal height.	

Table 4.112   Disk calcification

Diagnosis	Findings	Comments
Calcification in the nucleus pulposus, solitary or multiple ▷ *Fig. 4.282*	Most common in the cervical spine, where most commonly associated with pain. Adjacent end plates may be irregular. May prolapse anteriorly or posteriorly.	Persists or resolves spontaneously. Increased incidence in hyperparathyroidism, hypervitaminosis D, homocystinuria, and spondyloepiphyseal dysplasia tarda.
Ochronosis	Disk calcification or ossification; narrows disks.	Onset usually in adulthood. Especially frequent in Czech Republic.

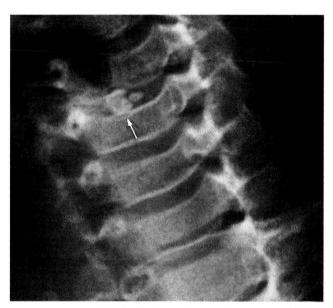 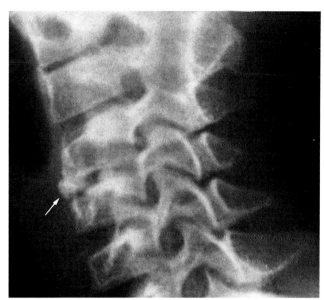

Fig. 4.282   Cervical disk calcification (arrows) in an 8-year-old boy. Intermittent pain and anterior prolapse.

Table 4.113   The vacuum phenomenon

Diagnosis	Findings	Comments
Vacuum phenomenon	In general, air or vacuum with a disk is associated with degenerative disease.	Rare in children. Occurs after trauma. Flexion extension series may reveal a vacuum.

■ Magnetic Resonance Imaging of the Vertebral Column

Table 4.114 Vertebral MRI

Diagnosis	Findings	Comments
Normal bone marrow ▷ *Fig. 4.283a, b*	High signal on T1 because of fat content, relatively low T2 signal intensity. However, the fat distribution changes during normal (or abnormal) development.	In first year of life, signal is similar or less than adjacent disk in most; between 5 and 15 y, it is usually higher.
Bone marrow infiltration or replacement	T1 signal deceases when normal fatty marrow is replaced: Exceptions are hematoma and postradiation change.	Tumors, leukemia, osteomyelitis, and other processes such as Gaucher disease or FD.
Sclerosis	Dense osseous tissue lacks signal on T1 or T2.	For example, bone islands, osteopetrosis.
Diskitis-spondylitis	Decreased T1 signal. May be same intensity between involved body and its disk. On T2, the signal is increased in the disks, bodies, and paravertebral inflammation.	Early diagnosis with scintigraphy or MRI.
Compression fracture	Decreased T1, increased T2 because of associated hematoma.	
Iron deposition	Markedly increased T1.	For example, hemosiderosis; or thalassemia under therapy.
Postirradiation	Increased T1 signal.	
LCH	Low T1, high T2 during active stage. MRI also shows any loss of height.	Whole body MRI may reveal additional lesions.

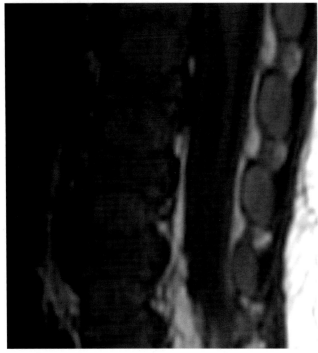
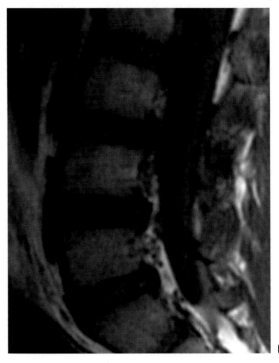

a

b

Fig. 4.283a, b Marrow distribution of red marrow and fat changes during childhood. (**a**) A 6-month-old with sacral dimple. (**b**) A 9-year-old 6 years after release of tethered cord. Sagittal fast spin echo T1 images. In (**a**), body red marrow results in similar low signal in bodies and adjacent disks. In (**b**), the body fat has replaced marrow, yielding a higher intensity in bodies compared to the disks.

■ Sacrum and Soft Tissues

Table 4.115   The sacrum and sacroiliac joint

Diagnosis	Findings	Comments
Sacral agenesis and hypoplasia ▷ Fig. 4.238, p. 441	A spectrum of severity from absence of part of a single sacral vertebra to total absence of the sacrum. The iliac bones are closely approximated medially in the latter case.	Caudal regression. Most have neuropathic bladder and fecal incontinence. Associated anomalies include anal atresia, anterior meningomyelocele, renal and bladder anomalies, hip dysplasia, and Dandy-Walker cyst. Predisposition in infants of diabetic mothers.
Asymmetric sacral defects ▷ Fig. 4.284a, b, p. 484	Associated with anterior of lateral meningocele.	Currarino triad: sacral malformation, presacral mass, and anorectal anomaly (rectal narrowing).
Lumbosacral transitional vertebrae	Asymmetric or symmetric transitional level with lateral elements somewhere between lumbar transverse process and lateral sacral mass in character.	Hox gene variation. If asymmetric side to side, often is thoracolumbar junction asymmetric as well.
Osteomyelitis adjacent to sacroiliac joints	Plain image findings often delayed. Bone scintigraphy, MRI, or CECT for early detection. A widened joint space later gets sclerotic margins.	
Juvenile ankylosing spondylitis	Variety of findings: erosions, widened joint, subchondral sclerosis of spongiosa, and eventually ankylosis. Early diagnosis on scintigraphy or MRI.	Bechterew disease. Look for associated parasyndesmophytes higher in the spinal column. Findings similar in Reiter syndrome, psoriatic arthritis, and colitis-associated arthritis. Somewhat similar changes in paraplegia may occur.
Coccygeal fracture	Difficult to confirm on plain (lateral) images without preinjury comparison.	Sacrococcygeal kyphosis may occur without traumatic episode.
Osteitis condensans ilii	Denser than normal medial iliac bone(s).	Also called hyperostosis condensans ilii. Association with pelvic area inflammation or with pregnancy.
Sacroiliac joints		
Normal	The joint space is normally relatively wide appearing in teenagers, and the apposing bony surfaces are hazy.	
Pelvic fracture complex	Widened sacroiliac joint.	Often additional fractures of the pelvic ring.
Tumors and tumorlike conditions	Destruction in LCH, metastatic disease and primary malignancy, aneurysmal bone cyst (expansion), giant cell tumor, presacral tumors (e.g., teratoma, neuroblastoma, or chordoma). May also be sclerotic, as in some lymphoma.	CT and MRI. Detection elusive on plain images.
Sacrum fractures	Elusive on plain images—check the normal lines carefully. Lateral images and CT images may assist.	
Changes in the paravertebral and presacral soft tissues		
Normal anterior cervical fat stripe	Lateral radiograph of cervical spine: a lucent line parallel to the anterior margin of C2–C5.	Can be simulated by dissecting gas from a retropharyngeal foreign body. The stripe is not displaced forward in expiration the way soft tissue in front of it may be.
Hematoma from fracture, spondylitis; retropharyngeal abscess; vertebral body tumor	Forward displacement (of effacement) of the prevertebral fat stripe.	
Hematoma from fracture, spondylitis; retropharyngeal abscess; vertebral body tumor	Forward displacement (of effacement) of the prevertebral fat stripe.	
Widened thoracic or lumbar paravertebral soft tissue ▷ Fig. 4.285, p. 484	Many causes: most common are neuroblastoma, but also hiatal hernia and round pneumonia or atelectasis (see **Table 4.116**).	Look forward for associated rib and pedicle destruction. Work-up with CT and MRI.
Extramedullary hematopoiesis	Soft-tissue masses along vertebral column and expanded posterior ribs. Same MRI intensities as normal marrow hematopoeitic material.	Severe anemias. Occasionally may displace or compress the spinal cord.
Alterations in presacral soft tissue	Sacral osteomyelitis with abscess; hematoma from sacral fracture; tumor expansion; anterior meningocele.	Look for Currarino triad. Do not confuse stool-distended rectal ampulla for a mass.
Myositis ossificans progressiva congenita	Kyphosis and scoliosis can be a consequence of ossification of the paravertebral musculature; another consequence can be limitation of rib movement.	Also known as fibrositis ossificans progressiva. Associated thumb and great toe abnormalities.

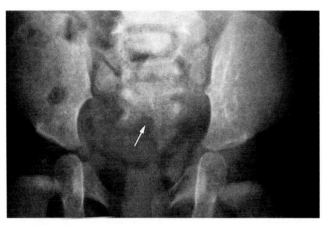

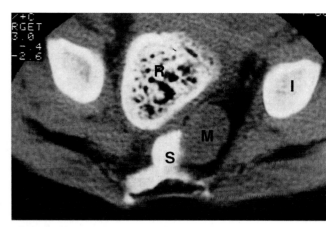

a   b

Fig. 4.284a, b   Currarino triad. (a) Comma-shaped sacrum with lower right lack of bone (arrow). **(b)** Axial CT.
I Iliac bone
M Presacral teratoma
R Rectum, dilated
S Sacrum

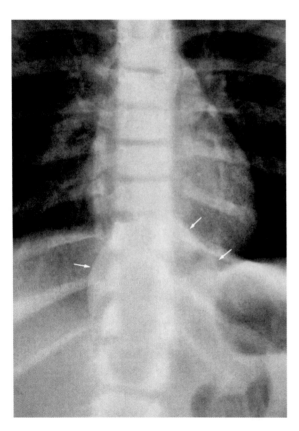

Fig. 4.285   Neuroblastoma in a 5-year-old girl. Bilateral widening of the paravertebral soft tissue (arrows).

Table 4.116 Differential diagnosis for widening of the paravertebral soft space on the frontal radiograph	
Tumors and metastases—many with vertebral changes	Neuroblastoma and other neurogenic tumors (the most common cause, occasionally bilateral): rhabdomyosarcoma; leukemia, lymphoma; LCH.
Inflammatory changes	Spondylitis, tuberculosis, lymphadenopathy.
Other	Scoliosis: abnormal soft-tissue planes. Hiatal and other diaphragmatic hernias, may contain air, may mimic cysts. Pneumonia, pulmonary sequestration, bronchogenic cyst. The left atrium (to right of the vertebral column). Esophagus, particularly in achalasia. • Ectopic, thoracic kidney • Dural ectasia, idiopathic or in NF1 • Lateral meningocele (vertebral anomalies) • Extramedullary hematopoiesis • Chloroma of acute myeloid leukemia

■ References

Barkovich AJ. Diagnostic imaging: pediatric neuroradiology. Salt Lake City: Amirys, 2007

Barkovich AJ. Pediatric neuroimaging. 4th ed. Philadelphia: Lippincott Williams & Wilkins, 2005

Bonneville F, Savatovsky J, Chiras J. Imaging of cerebellopontine angle lesions: an update. Part 2: intraaxial lesions, skull base lesions that may invade the CPA region, and non-enhancing extra-axial lesions. Eur Radiol 2007;17:2908–2920

Brill PW, Baker DH, Ewing ML. "Bone-within-bone" in the neonatal spine: stress change or normal development. Radiology 1973;108: 363–366

Chadwell JB, Halsted MJ, Choo DI, Greinwald JH, Corning Benton C. The cochlear cleft. AJNR Am J Neuroradiol 2004;25:21–24

Chapman S, Nakielny R. Radiological differential diagnosis. Philadelphia: W.B. Saunders, 1992

Dahnert WJ. Radiology review manual. 2nd ed. Philadelphia: Williams and Wilkins, 1993

De Foer B, Vercruysse JP, Bernaerts A, et al. The value of single-shot turbo spin-echo diffusion-weighted MR imaging in the detection of middle ear cholesteatoma. Neuroradiology 2007;49:841

Donnelly L. Diagnostic imaging pediatrics. Salt Lake City: Amirys, 2005

Fielding JW, Hensinger RN, Hawkins RJ. Os odontoideum. J Bone Joint Surg Am 1980;62:376–383

Fernández-Latorre F, Menor-Serrano F, Alonso-Charterina S, Arenas-Jiménez J. Langerhans' cell histiocytosis of the temporal bone in pediatric patients. Imaging and follow-Up. AJR 2000;174: 217–221

Gonzalez BE, Martinez-Aguilar G, Hulten KG, et al. Severe Staphylococcal sepsis in adolescents in the era of community-acquired methicillin-resistant Staphylococcus aureus. Pediatrics 2005;115(3):642–648

Harnsberger HR. Diagnostic imaging head and neck. Salt Lake City: Amirys, 2007

Keats TE. Atlas of roentgenographic measurement. 6th ed. St. Louis: Mosby Year Book, 1990:208–213

Kilborn T, Goodman TR, Teh J. Paediatric manifestations of Langerhans cell histiocytosis: a clinical and radiological review. Clinical Radiology 2003;58:269–278

King SJ, Boothroyd AE. Pediatric ENT radiology. New York: Springer, 2003

Kirks DJ. Practical pediatric imaging: diagnostic radiology of infants and children. Philadelphia: Lippincott Williams & Wilkins, 1998

Koch BL, Moosbrugger EA, Egelhoff JC. Symptomatic spinal epidural collections after lumbar puncture in children. Am J Neuroradiol 2007;28(9):1811–1816

Lachman R. Taybi and Lachman's radiology of syndromes, metabolic disorders and skeletal dysplasias. St. Louis: Mosby, 2006

Larsen WJ. Anatomy: development function clinical correlations. Philadelphia: W.B. Saunders, 2002

Legeais M, Haguenoer K, Cottier JP, Sirinelli D. Can fixed measure serve as a pertinent diagnostic criterion for large vestibular aqueduct in children? Pediatr Radiol 2006;36:1037–1042

Lemmerling MM, Mancuso AA, Antonelli PJ, Kubilis PS. Normal modiolus: CT appearance in patients with a large vestibular aqueduct. Radiology 1997;204:213–219

Mampaey S, Vanhoenacker F, Boven K, et al. Progressive pseudorheumatoid dysplasia. Eur Radiol 2000;10(11):1832–1835

Martin N, Sterkers O, Mompoint D, Julien N, Nahum H. Cholesterol granulomas of the middle ear: MR imaging. Radiology 1989;172: 521–525

McCredie J. Beyond thalidomide: birth defects explained. London: Royal Society of Medicine Press, 2007

Mukherji S. Neuroimaging clinics of North America: pediatric head and neck imaging. Philadelphia: W.B. Saunders, 2000

Nackos JS, Wiggins RH 3rd, Harnsberger HR. CT and MR imaging of giant cell granuloma of the facial bones. AJNR 2006;27(8): 1651–1653

Pettersson H, Harwood-Nash DCF. CT and myelography of the spine and cord, techniques, anatomy and pathology in children. Berlin: Springer, 1982

Sebag GH, Dubois J, Tabet M, Bonato A, Lallemand D. Pediatric spinal bone marrow: assessment of normal age-related changes in the MRI appearance. Pediatr Radiol 1993;23(7):515–518

Siegel MJ. Pediatric sonography. Philadelphia: Lippincott Williams & Wilkins, 2002

Som P, Curtin H. Head and neck imaging. 3rd ed. St. Louis: Mosby, 1996

Soto G. Ultrasound of the salivary glands. In Syllabus 28th Postgraduate Course 7-11; ESPR 2005

Taybi H, Lachman R. Radiology of syndromes: metabolic disorders and skeletal dysplasias. 4th ed. St. Louis: Mosby, 1996

Treves ST, ed. Pediatric nuclear medicine/PET. 3rd ed. New York: Springer, 2007

Vandekerckhove K, Van Den Abeele K, Van Den Broecke C, Verstraete K, Meire F. Psammomatoid ossifying fibroma of the ethmoid. Bull Soc belge Ophtalmol 2003;287:9–14

Wieselthaler N, Kilborn T, Grier D. Prepontine haematoma on CT brain post trauma: an indication for urgent cervical spine MRI. Pediatric Radiology 2006;136:72

5 The Skeleton and Soft Tissues

→

Metaphysis

Diaphysis (Long Bones)

Terminology of Limb Alteration

Dysmelia

Alterations in Shaft Width

Bowing

Hands and Feet

→

Brachydactyly

Osseous Alterations

Soft-Tissue Alterations

Tumors and Focal Bone, Joint, and Soft-Tissue Lesions

Periosteal Reaction

→

Bone Marrow Patterns

Changes in Bone Density

Increased

Decreased

Skeletal Maturation

Lethal Dysplasias

Fracture Dating

Child Abuse

Chest Wall (Including the Scapula and Clavicle)

The Sternum

Table 5.1 Sternum: congenital, genetic, and syndromic diseases that may alter the sternum[1]

Diagnosis	Findings	Comments
Variations in normal anatomy[2]	Sternal foramen, sclerotic bands, manubriosternal, and sternoxiphoidal fusions.	Cortical irregularity, expansion, and soft tissue mass help distinguish a pathologic process from normal variations in anatomy.
Pectus excavatum	Concave posterior depression of the sternum often with rotation along the transverse plane results in a reduction of the prevertebral space, leftward displacement and axial rotation of the heart, and reduction in the space occupied by the lungs (usually the left lung).[3]	Most common congenital deformity of the sternum. The pectus (Haller) index, derived by dividing the transverse diameter of the chest by the anteroposterior (AP) diameter, obtained on axial computed tomography (CT) or magnetic resonance imaging (MRI). A pectus index greater than 3.25 necessitates surgical correction.
Trisomy 21	Multiple manubrial ossification centers (hypersegmentation).	Probability of trisomy 21 increases with the number of anomalies present on the chest radiograph (11 rib pairs and a bell-shaped chest).[4]
Sickle cell ▷ Fig. 5.1	Sternal cupping at the ends of the segments.[5]	Similar appearance as end plate depressions in vertebral bodies. May be seen in up to 8% of patients.
Turner syndrome	Short, premature fusion of manubriosternal junction or mesosternum, decreased ratio of sternal body to manubrium, two ossification centers, bowing, mild pectus excavatum.[6]	(see Table 5.30)
Poland syndrome	Deformity of the sternum associated with absence of muscles and clavicle.	(see Table 5.15)
Chronic recurrent multifocal osteomyelitis (CRMO)	Hyperostosis and osteomyelitis.	Chronic inflammatory condition of unknown etiology. Usually multifocal. Children 5–15 y old. Accompanied by synovitis, acne, pustulosis. Adult form is SAPHO (synovitis, acne, pustulosis, hyperostosis, and osteitis).[7]

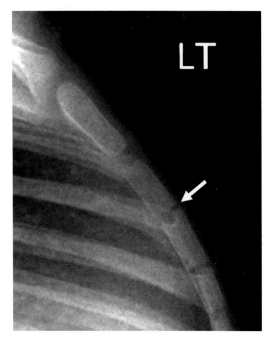

Fig. 5.1 Sickle cell disease with sternal infarcts at the ends of the ossification centers (arrow shows an example of one area of involvement).

Table 5.2   Sternum: masses

Diagnosis	Findings	Comments
Pectus carinatum	Anterior displacement of sternum.	May be confused with malignancy on physical examination. Also known as pigeon breast and is less common (1:1500 births) than pectus excavatum.
Malignant	(see **Table 5.74**)	Rare. Chondrosarcoma, lymphoma, Ewing sarcoma, osteosarcoma.
Benign		Rare. Enchondroma, osteochondroma, hemangioma, hemangiopericytoma, osteoid osteoma, osteoblastoma, fibrous dysplasia, Langerhans cell histiocytosis, brown tumor.

The Ribs

Short ribs do not extend as far anteriorly as the sternum; they lead to a decreased chest volume that may cause respiratory insuffi- ciency. The more widely know dysplasias and syndromes with short ribs as a feature are discussed in **Tables 5.3** through **5.10**.

Table 5.3   Ribs: short ribs

Diagnosis	Findings	Comments
Achondroplasia	Short and wide ribs with concavity at the rib end.	Narrowing of the intrapedicular distance (as apposed to normal widening) from L1 to L5 on AP projection. Rhizomelic shortening of the humeri, macrocephaly, depression of the nasion, scalloping of the posterior aspects of the vertebral bodies, square iliac bones, and a champagne glass–shaped pelvic inlet. DD: hypochondroplasia.
Thanatophoric dysplasia	Very short ribs that do not extend beyond the anterior axillary line.	Most common form of skeletal dysplasia that is lethal in the neonatal period. "H-" or "U-"shaped vertebral bodies, short and curved humeri, cloverleaf skull deformity, polydactyly, and hypoplastic iliac bones. DD: thanatophoric variants, asphyxiating thoracic dysplasia, homozygous achondroplasia, and achondrogenesis.
Asphyxiating thoracic dysplasia (Jeune) ▷ *Fig. 5.2*	Short ribs with a horizontal course. The chest diameter is smaller in comparison to the abdomen.	Long bones are shortened, the iliac wings are small, and the acetabula may have spurs. The proximal humeral and femoral epiphyses may be ossified at birth. ± polydactyly. Adults have a high prevalence of medullary cystic renal disease. DD: Ellis-van Creveld dysplasia.

(continues on page 494)

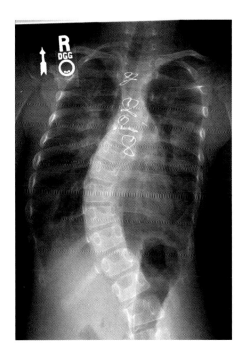

Fig. 5.2   Asphyxiating thoracic dysplasia. Jeune syndrome. Short ribs and scoliosis.

Table 5.3 (Cont.) Ribs: short ribs

Diagnosis	Findings	Comments
Chondroectodermal dysplasia (Ellis-van Creveld syndrome) ▷ *Fig. 5.3*	Small chest accentuates the size of the cardiomegaly.	Congenital heart disease (atrial septal defects) with cardiomegaly. Severe respiratory insufficiency results in high neonatal mortality (~50%). High prevalence among the Amish. Appearance of pelvis is similar to Jeune dysplasia. DD: Jeune dysplasia and short rib–polydactyly syndromes.
Other dysplasias and syndromes		For example, atelosteogenesis, Barnes syndrome, campomelic dysplasia, metatropic dysplasia, otopalatodigital syndrome, Schneckenbecken dysplasia.

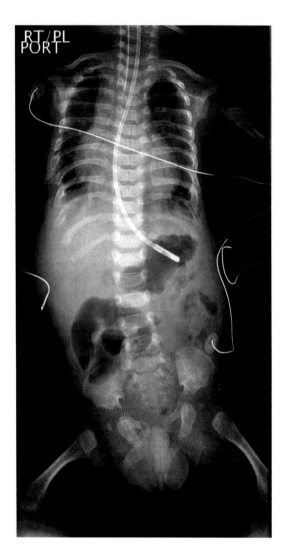

Fig. 5.3 Chondroectodermal dysplasia. Ellis-van Creveld syndrome with a narrow chest, small iliac bones, and iliac spurs.

Table 5.4 Ribs: slender ribs

Diagnosis	Findings	Comments
Trisomies 8, 13, 18, and 21	Hypoplastic and thin ribs. 11 rib pairs.	In trisomy 18, a short sternum produces a shield deformity of the chest. Acute iliac angle is diagnostic. Ulnar deviation and flexion deformity of the fingers with curled thumb grasped by the fingers.
Neurofibromatosis	Slender, twisted, and/or deformed ribs that may be separated by neurofibromas.	
Chondrodysplasia punctata	(see **Table 5.35**)	
Other dysplasias and syndromes		For example, achondrogenesis, campomelic dysplasia, progeria, and Cockayne, Gorlin, Larsen, and Turner syndromes.

Table 5.5   Ribs: wide ribs

Diagnosis	Findings	Comments
Thalassemia major	Undertubulated and broad ribs with heterogeneous ossification.	The rib findings as well as widened dipole, hypoplasia of paranasal sinuses, paraspinal extramedullary foci, and hepatosplenomegaly are rarely seen with aggressive marrow replacement and chelation therapy. DD: other chronic anemias, storage disease, and fibrous dysplasia.
Fibrous dysplasia	Affected ribs are widened.	
Sickle cell anemia and thalassemia		
Mucopolysaccharidosis	Ribs are thin proximally near the costovertebral junction and then wider distally.	External flaring of the iliac bones, vertebral body flattening and beaking, atlantoaxial instability, and brachydactyly. DD: Gaucher and Niemann-Pick diseases.
Gorlin (basal cell nevus) syndrome	Bifid, fused, or markedly splayed ribs.	Sprengel and pectus deformities, syndactyly, calcified falx cerebri, flame-shaped lucencies of the hands and feet. Radiologic findings contribute to the list of clinical criteria used to diagnose the syndrome.[8]
Other dysplasias and syndromes		For example, achondroplasia, Erdheim-Chester disease, Niemann-Pick disease, osteopetrosis, pacman dysplasia, tuberous sclerosis.

Table 5.6   Ribs: miscellaneous rib anomalies[9]

Diagnosis	Findings	Comments
Cervical ribs	Unilateral or bilateral, arise from the seventh cervical vertebra, and resemble hypoplastic first thoracic ribs.	Incidental finding (0.2% to 8% prevalence) or are associated with Klippel-Feil anomaly. Can compress adjacent nerves supplying the brachial plexus and vessels (thoracic outlet syndrome or aneurysm formation).
Eleven paired ribs		Occurs in 5%–8% of normal individuals and in one-third of patients with trisomy 21. Associated with several skeletal dysplasias including cleidocranial and campomelic dysplasia.
Pectus excavatum	Posterior ribs are horizontal, whereas the anterior ribs have a more vertical course.	(see **Table 5.1**)
Bifid rib	A portion of the rib splits into two separate ribs.	May be incidental and discovered as a palpable mass. DD: Gorlin (or basal cell nevus) syndrome (fourth rib most commonly bifid).
Supernumerary ribs		Trisomy 21 syndrome (although 11 paired ribs is more common) and with VATER (*v*ertebral defects, *a*nal atresia, *t*racheoesophageal fistula with *e*sophageal atresia, *r*adial or *r*enal dysplasia, and *l*imb anomalies) association. Rarely seen as a variation of normal.
Rickets ▷ *Fig. 5.4a, b, p. 496*	Cupping and enlargement at the rib ends of the costochondral junctions (rachitic rosary).	
Rib notching ▷ *Fig. 5.5, p. 496*	Concave notches found on the inferior rib surface.	Most commonly found as a variation of normal anatomy. Pressure erosion (saucerization) from enlarged vascular or neural structures. Notching associated with aortic coarctation usually affects ribs 4–8 (costal arteries are enlarged above the aortic stenosis) and is rare before the age of 8 y. DD: coarctation of the aorta, neurofibromatosis, thalassemia, and postoperative Blalock-Taussig shunt (right-sided notching).
Cerebrocostomandibular syndrome	Ribs have abnormal costovertebral articulations and posterior ossification gaps that resemble fractures.	Gaps will eventually ossify. Usually 11 pairs of ribs. Microcephaly, micrognathia, and congenital heart disease. DD: multiple rib fractures.

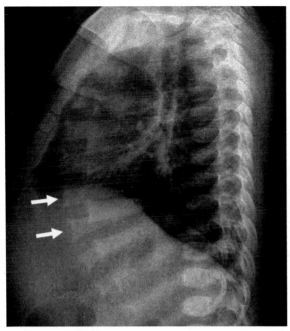
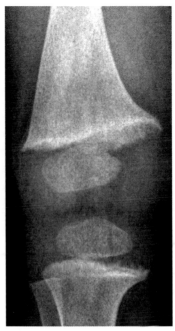

a   b

Fig. 5.4a, b   **Rickets** with cupping at the rib ends (arrows in **a**) and metaphyses about the knee (**b**).

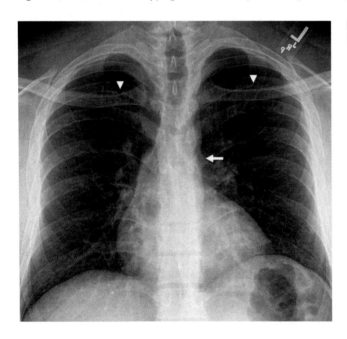

Fig. 5.5   Rib notching. Coarctation of the aorta. Rib notching (arrowheads) and the figure-three sign (arrow).

Table 5.7   Ribs: expansile rib deformity

Diagnosis	Findings	Comments
Fibrous dysplasia	Expansile mixed lucent and sclerotic non-aggressive lesion with a ground-glass matrix, cortical thinning, and modeling deformity.	Most common cause of a benign expansile rib lesion. DD: simple bone cyst, enchondroma, and brown tumor of hyperparathyroidism.
Brown tumor of hyperparathyroidism	Lucent lesion.	(see **Table 5.75**)
Other benign tumors		DD: enchondromatosis, osteochondroma, xanthogranuloma.
Malignant tumors ▷ *Fig. 5.6* ▷ *Fig. 5.7*	Bone destruction and attempt at remodeling usually with associated soft-tissue mass (see **Table 5.74**).	DD: Ewing sarcoma, primitive neuroectodermal tumor.
Langerhans cell histiocytosis ▷ *Fig. 5.8*	Expansile and well-defined lucent lesion.	Skeletal survey may be useful to detect multiple lesions.
Lymphangiomatosis (Gorham disease)	Well-defined areas of lucency that may coalesce and replace large portions of bone. Osteolytic with a thin sclerotic rim. Osteolysis may be massive.	Thought to be due to malformation/proliferation of lymphatic vessels in bone.

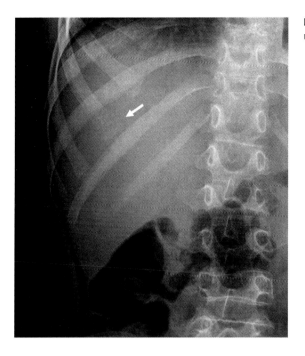

Fig. 5.6   Malignant tumors. Rib expansion and destruction from metastatic rhabdomyosarcoma (arrow).

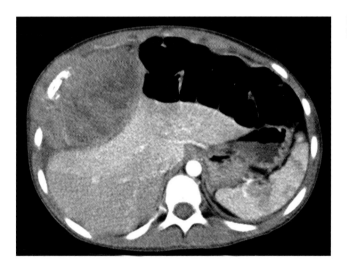

Fig. 5.7   Malignant tumors. Chest wall mass with rib destruction from Ewing sarcoma.

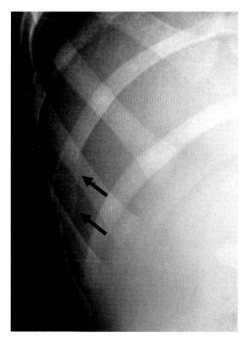

Fig. 5.8   Langerhans cell histiocytosis. Lucent and expansile rib lesion produced by Langerhans cell histiocytosis (arrows).

Table 5.8 Ribs: rib absence

Diagnosis	Findings	Comments
Eleven paired ribs		(see **Table 5.6**)
Unilateral absent rib		Postsurgical resection, tumor, osteomyelitis.

Table 5.9 Ribs: supernumerary ribs

Diagnosis	Findings	Comments
Turner syndrome	Cervical ribs.	(see **Table 5.30**)
Trisomy 8	Eleven or thirteen ribs. Rib abnormalities (wide, sloping, or rib gap).	Vertebral segmentation anomalies. Large and small joint contractures. Congenital heart disease and corneal opacities
Cornelia de Lange syndrome	Thirteen ribs	(see **Table 5.50**)

Table 5.10 Ribs: increased sclerosis

Diagnosis	Findings	Comments
Tuberous sclerosis	Patchy regions of bone expansion and sclerosis.	May be confined to a single rib.
Osteopetrosis (Albers-Schönberg disease)	Generalized increase in bone density.	
Melorheostosis ▷ *Fig. 5.9*	Intramedullary sclerosis with the appearance of dripping candle wax.	Follows dermatomes.
See Table 5.91		

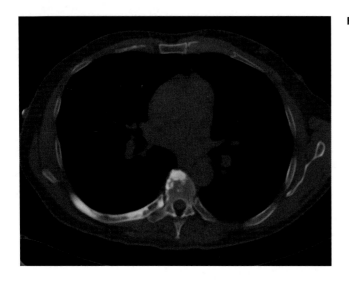

Fig. 5.9 Melorheostosis.

Clavicle[10]

Table 5.11   Clavicle: erosions and contour irregularities of the sternoclavicular and acromioclavicular joints

Diagnosis	Findings	Comments
Pseudofracture	False appearance of midshaft fracture due to rotation or projection, especially in children.	A vascular channel in the bone may simulate a fracture.
Conoid tubercle	Bump on posteroinferior distal one-third of clavicle.	Attachment for the conoid portion of the coracoclavicular ligament. Ligament between conoid tubercle and coracoid process may undergo ossification, usually secondary to trauma.
Posttraumatic osteolysis ▷ *Fig. 5.10* ▷ *Fig. 5.11a, b*	Resorption of the distal or proximal ends of the clavicle. Acromioclavicular (AC) joint appears widened with erosions at the distal end.	May follow 6–8 wk after trauma at the AC joint.
Osteomyelitis	Destruction and periosteal reaction.	Primary infection of bone (spread from trauma or blood) or secondary spread from sternoclavicular or AC joints.

(continues on page 500)

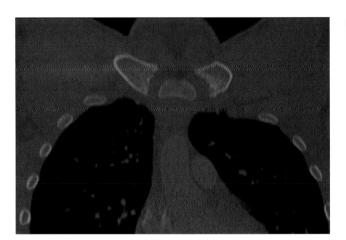

Fig. 5.10   Posttraumatic osteolysis. Osteolysis of the sternoclavicular joint in a 17-year-old weightlifter, likely secondary to overuse.

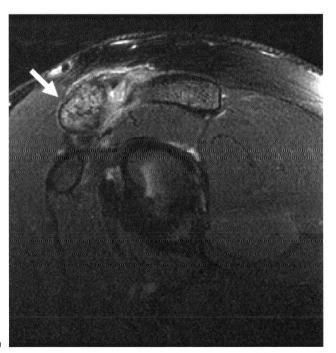 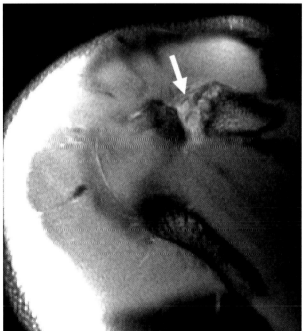

a   b

Fig. 5.11a, b   Posttraumatic osteolysis. Osteolysis of the AC joint from overuse in a football player (arrow in **a**). Bone marrow edema is seen on sagittal oblique MRI in the acromion with subchondral cysts and fluid in the AC joint (arrow in **b**) on axial imaging.

Table 5.11 (Cont.) Clavicle: erosions and contour irregularities of the sternoclavicular and acromioclavicular joints

Diagnosis	Findings	Comments
Hyperparathyroidism	Generalized bone demineralization, erosion of the distal ends of the clavicles, and bone resorption along the inferior border of the distal clavicle at the attachment of the coracoclavicular ligament.	Brown tumor may be seen in primary hyperparathyroidism (see **Table 5.75**). Pseudofractures (Looser zones).
Osteonecrosis	Aseptic necrosis of the medial end of the clavicle (Friedrich disease).	Sclerosis of the medial end of the clavicle may persist.
Juvenile idiopathic arthritis (JIA)	Erosions at the ends of the clavicles with widening of AC joint.	Sternoclavicular joint involvement may be difficult to appreciate on radiographs and may require cross-sectional imaging for detection of inflammatory changes.
Ankylosing spondylitis	Enthesopathy at the coracoclavicular and costoclavicular ligaments with bone proliferation and ligamentous calcification on radiographs and bone marrow edema on MRI.	
Tumor ▷ *Fig. 5.12*		Langerhans cell histiocytosis, aneurismal bone cyst, hemangioma. Clavicle is rare site of involvement for fibrous dysplasia, metastasis, osteosarcoma, Ewing sarcoma, leukemia, and lymphoma.
Radiation necrosis	Spectrum of findings from localized bone demineralization to frank bone destruction.	An osteochondroma may arise at the medial end of the clavicle following irradiation of the bone during childhood. Pathologic fractures often fail to heal (pseudarthrosis). Secondary osteosarcoma may develop as a late complication.
Neurofibromatosis	Pressure erosions. Tapering of the clavicle ("pencil pointing," distal > proximal).	
Infantile cortical hyperostosis (Caffey disease)	Cortical hyperostosis. Clavicle appears thick and wide and is surrounded by exuberant periosteal reaction.	Infants less than 5 mo of age. Clavicles, ribs, and mandible are most common sites. DD: vitamin A toxicity.
CRMO	Bone destruction, extensive sclerosis, and bone enlargement.	(see **Table 5.1**)
Melorheostosis	Marked cortical thickening and characteristic dripping candle wax appearance.	Localized painful swelling and growth disturbances. Follows distribution of dermatomes.

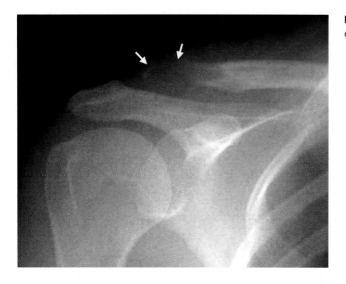

Fig. 5.12 Clavicle tumor. Aneurysmal bone cyst expanding the distal end of the clavicle (arrows).

Table 5.12 Clavicle: handlebar deformity or lateral clavicle hook—angulated clavicle or superior inclination of the clavicles (Fig. 5.13)[11]

Diagnosis	Findings	Comments
Brachial plexus injury		Handlebar deformity is acquired presumably from neuromuscular weakness.
VACTERL (vertebral defects, anal atresia, cardiac malformations, tracheoesophageal fistula with esophageal atresia, radial or renal dysplasia, and limb anomalies) association		(see **Table 5.50**)
Radial ray defects (Holt-Oram syndrome, thrombocytopenia absent radius syndrome, Fanconi pancytopenia)	In addition to handlebar, clavicles may be hypoplastic with bulbous ends.	
Pierre Robin syndrome	Radiohumeral synostosis, hypoplasia of the mandible, congenital amputations, syndactyly.	Overlap with other syndromes/anomalies: amniotic band syndrome, Beckwith-Wiedemann syndrome, CHARGE syndrome.
Campomelic dysplasia ▷ *Fig. 5.14a, b*	Hypoplastic tibia, scapula, and vertebral bodies. Pear-shaped iliac bones, long femora that are anteriorly bowed, and deficient ossification of the pubis.	Lethal skeletal dysplasia. Pulmonary hypoplasia and laryngeal and tracheal stenosis. Ureteral stenosis. Thoracic platyspondyly and kyphosis. Multiple cutaneous dimples in the arms and legs.
Osteogenesis imperfecta		Handlebar deformity is acquired.
Cornelia de Lange syndrome		(see **Table 5.50**)
Schneckenbecken dysplasia	Snail-shaped ilia, flat acetabular roofs, handlebar clavicles, hypoplastic scapula, dumbbell-shaped very short long bones, wide fibula, and round vertebral bodies.[12]	Hypoplastic vertebral bodies with relatively well-preserved posterior arches.[13]

Fig. 5.13 Handlebar deformity of the clavicles.

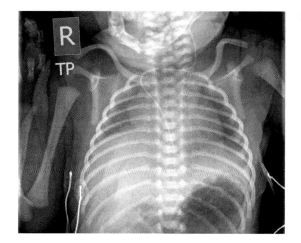

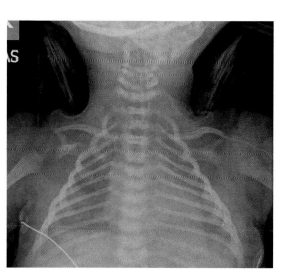
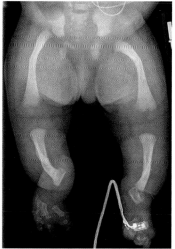

a   b

Fig. 5.14a, b Campomelic dysplasia with hypoplastic scapulae and cervical vertebral bodies (**a**) and bowing of the extremities, dislocated hips, deficient ossification of the pubis, and hypoplastic fibulae and tibiae (**b**).

Table 5.13 Clavicle: pseudarthrosis

Diagnosis	Findings	Comments
Posttraumatic pseudarthrosis	Continued lucency through the fracture with smooth fracture margins and adjacent sclerosis beyond when healing with union is expected. Exuberant callus formation without bridging.	Nonunion common in fractures that occur distal to the coracoclavicular ligament attachment.
Congenital	Defect in the middle clavicle with no callus formation. Ends may be sclerotic and tapered.	Usually seen within 2 wk after birth. Right clavicle involved. Left clavicle if dextrocardia.
Cleidocranial dysplasia ▷ *Fig. 5.15a–d*	Hypoplastic or absent clavicles: often central portion of the clavicle is absent with rudimentary medial and lateral portions remaining.	Clavicle findings may be confused with congenital pseudarthrosis.

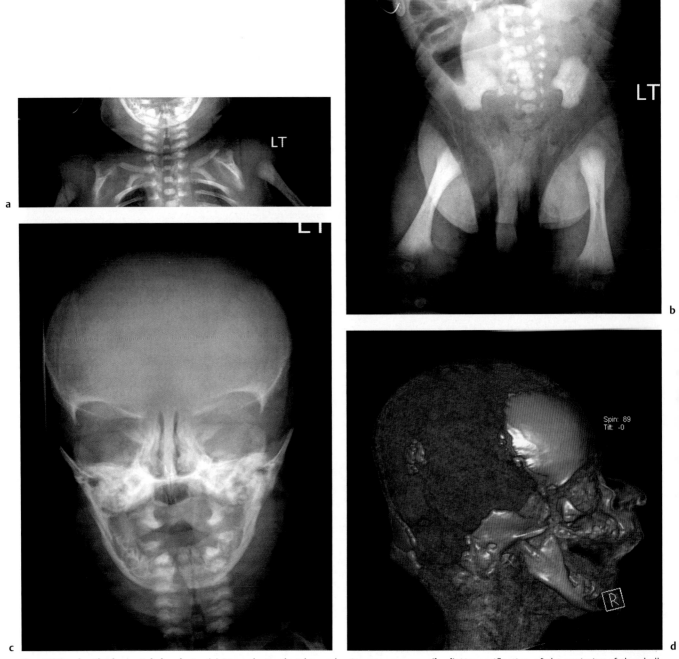

Fig. 5.15a–d Cleidocranial dysplasia. (**a**) Hypoplastic clavicles and spinous processes. (**b–d**) Nonossification of the majority of the skull, pubic, and ischial bones.

Table 5.14   Clavicle: hypoplasia or absence

Diagnosis	Findings	Comments
Posttraumatic osteolysis ▷ *Fig. 5.10, p. 499* ▷ *Fig. 5.11, p. 499*		(see **Table 5.11**)
Postsurgical resection ▷ *Fig. 5.16*		
Destructive process		Tumor, infection.
Trisomy 13 and 18		
Osteogenesis imperfecta	Slender, osteoporotic, and hypoplastic clavicles.	± Fracture with exuberant callus formation.
Cleidocranial dysplasia ▷ *Fig. 5.15a–d*	(see **Table 5.13**)	
Cardiomelic syndrome **(Holt-Oram syndrome)**	Hypoplastic clavicles with bulbous ends (handlebar).	
Otopalatodigital spectrum **(e.g., Melnick-Needles syndrome)**	(see **Table 5.26**)	Scoliosis, joint subluxations, long fingers and toes.
Focal dermal hypoplasia **(Goltz syndrome)**		Syndactyly, polydactyly, camptodactyly, and skeletal absence deformities.
Pycnodysostosis	Generalized bone sclerosis and mild modeling deformity of the bones.	Short-limbed dwarfism with generalized increase in bone density. Acroosteolysis. Brittle bones.
Progeria	Usually distal portion of clavicle affected.	Absent due to fibrosis. Rare: 1 in 8 million. Infant with an "old man appearance." Generalized skeletal hypoplasia. Small mandible and face.

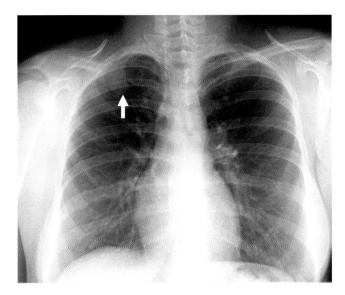

Fig. 5.16   Postsurgical resection. Postsurgical appearance of the medial right clavicle (arrow) after resection of Ewing sarcoma.

Table 5.15   Clavicle: congenital, genetic, and syndromic diseases that may alter the clavicle

Diagnosis	Findings	Comments
Thalassemia	Generalized osteopenia and coarse trabecular pattern in the intramedullary cavity.	Myeloid hyperplasia produces the radiographic findings that commonly involve the clavicle.
Turner syndrome	Short, premature fusion of manubriosternal junction or mesosternum, decreased ratio of sternal body to manubrium, two ossification centers, bowing, mild pectus excavatum.[6]	(see **Table 5.30**)
Poland syndrome	Absence of the pectoralis major muscle and syndactyly.	Other associated chest wall abnormalities: deformity of the sternum, absence or atrophy of the second to fifth ipsilateral ribs and other chest wall muscles, aplasia of the ipsilateral breast or nipple, and simian crease of the affected extremity.
Cleidocranial dysplasia ▷ *Fig. 5.15a–d, p. 502*	Hypoplastic or absent clavicles: often central portion of the clavicle is absent with rudimentary medial and lateral portions remaining.	Delayed ossification of the pubic bones. Increased shoulder joint mobility. Delayed closure of the anterior fontanelle.
Primary hyperoxaluria (oxalosis)	Sclerosis and bulbous deformity of the medial ends (drumstick clavicles). Osteoporosis in the early phase and diffuse bone sclerosis in the advanced stage. Subchondral sclerosis in the long bones. Metaphyseal sclerosis, dense epiphyses.	Growing ends of bones show bulbous enlargement. Pathologic fractures are common. Growth disturbance and increased incidence of urinary calculi due to hyperoxaluria.

Scapula

Table 5.16   Scapula: hypoplasia

Diagnosis	Findings	Comments
Brachial plexus palsy (Erb palsy) ▷ *Fig. 5.17a, b*	Variable degrees of hypoplasia of the inferior glenoid with posterior subluxation of the humeral head.	Severity may be placed into various categories with cross-sectional imaging.[14]
Recurrent shoulder dislocations ▷ *Fig. 5.18*	Osseous Bankart and Hill-Sachs lesions.	Recurrent impaction and wear on the anteroinferior glenoid (most commonly) by the humeral head.
Osteonecrosis	Subchondral collapse leads to joint destruction.	DD: sickle cell disease, steroids, radiation and chemotherapy treatments, pancreatitis, etc.
Sprengel deformity ▷ *Fig. 5.19a–c, p. 506*	Small elevated and rotated scapula ± omocervical (or omovertebral) bone that joins scapula to C5 or C6.	Most common congenital anomaly of the shoulder girdle. Complex anomaly that is associated with malposition and dysplasia of the scapula, regional muscle hypoplasia/atrophy. Associated with Klippel-Feil syndrome.
Dysplasias and syndromes		Achondroplasia, hypochondroplasia, achondrogenesis, campomelic dysplasia, cleidocranial dysplasia, Alpert syndrome.
Glenoid hypoplasia	Hypoplasia of the scapular neck, widened glenohumeral joint space. Bilateral.	± Hypoplasia of other regional structures (humeral head, acromion, clavicle).

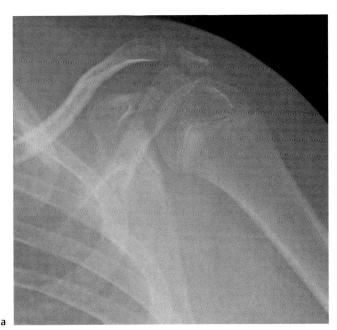

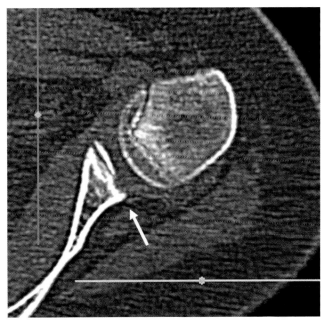

a   b

Fig. 5.17a, b   Brachial plexus palsy in an 8-year-old. Although the humeral head appears relatively normal, the glenoid is hypoplastic (**a**) and sloped posteriorly (arrow in **b**).

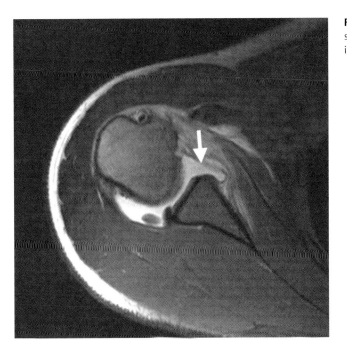

Fig. 5.18   Recurrent shoulder dislocations. Osseous Bankart lesion from recurrent shoulder dislocation (arrow) and accompanying intraarticular body in the posterior joint.

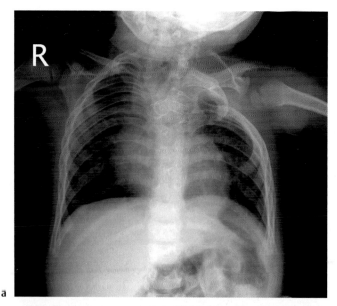

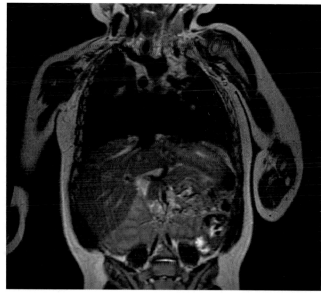

Fig. 5.19a–c   Sprengel deformity. Klippel-Feil syndrome with small left ribs (**a**) and a hypoplastic and superiorly located left scapula (Sprengel deformity) that articulates with the neck (**b, c**).

Table 5.17   Scapula: expansion and destruction

Diagnosis	Findings	Comments
Osteomyelitis	Permeative or moth-eaten pattern of bone destruction.	DD: round blue cell tumors.
Tumors or metastases	Permeative or moth-eaten pattern of bone destruction.	DD: osteosarcoma (new bone formation) and Ewing sarcoma.
Infantile cortical hyperostosis (Caffey disease)	(see **Table 5.11**)	
Langerhans cell histiocytosis	Lytic lesion or expansile hyperplastic lesion.	May be indistinguishable from osteomyelitis and tumors (round blue cell).

Pelvis

Acetabulum

Table 5.18   Pelvis: increased acetabular angle

Diagnosis	Findings	Comments
Developmental dysplasia of the hip ▷ *Fig. 5.20a–c* ▷ *Fig. 5.21, p. 508*	Hypoplastic acetabular roof with later development of increasing sclerosis. Posterosuperior dislocation of the femoral head ± flattening of the femoral head.	Ultrasound (US) is the screening modality of choice before ossification excludes visualization of the hip structures (below the age of 6 mo).
Secondary hip dysplasia	Increased acetabular angle. Shallow acetabulum. Coxa valga, ± femoral head dislocation and flattening.	Generally occurs in neuromuscular diseases with spasticity of the lower extremities. May develop in a previously normal hip.
Arthrogryposis	Very thin diaphyses, osteopenia, dislocation and subluxation of large joints.	Joint contractures and decreased muscle bulk.
Ehlers-Danlos syndrome types III and VII	Hip dislocation with an otherwise normal appearing skeleton.	Calcified round areas of subcutaneous fat necrosis.
Campomelic dysplasia ▷ *Fig. 5.14, p. 501*	(see **Table 5.12**)	
Larsen syndrome	Accessory carpal ossification centers, double calcaneal ossification center. Dislocation of large joints.	Flat facies. Clinical DD: Marfan syndrome, arthrogryposis, and Ehlers-Danlos syndrome.

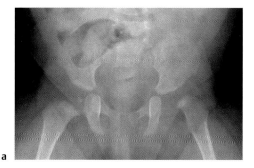

a

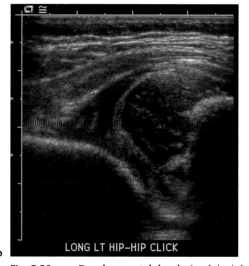

b LONG LT HIP-HIP CLICK

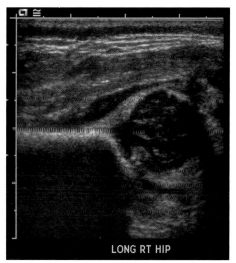

c LONG RT HIP

Fig. 5.20a–c   Developmental dysplasia of the left hip with dislocation and delayed ossification of the proximal femoral epiphysis (**a**). (**b**) US shows dislocation. (**c**) Normal side for comparison.

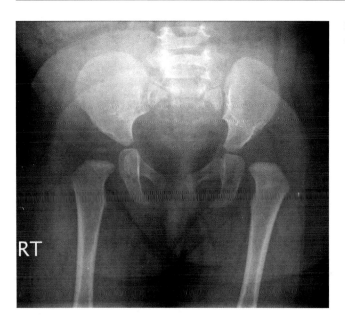

Fig. 5.21 Developmental dysplasia of the left hip with a shallow acetabulum.

■ Lateral and Medial Spurs of the Acetabulum (Trident Acetabulum)

Spurs are seen in skeletal dysplasias when the base of the iliac bone is small and the entire iliac bone is decreased in size. The spur is visible in neonates and young infants and disappears as the skeleton matures.

■ Acetabular Protrusio

Acetabular protrusio is likely the result of remodeling of weak, medial acetabular bone and may also result after multiple, recurring microstress fractures. Protrusio is present when the femoral head is medial to Kohler line (line drawn tangential to the lateral margin of the pelvic brim and the obturator foramen).[15]

Table 5.19 Pelvis: acetabular protrusio

Diagnosis	Findings	Comments
Septic arthritis ▷ *Fig. 5.22a–d*	Uniform joint space narrowing and possible disorganized remodeling of bone at sites of prior infection.	May occur 1 mo or later after the acute joint infection.
Trauma	Remodeling after fracture through the acetabulum.	
Connective tissue disorder		DD: Ehlers-Danlos and Marfan syndromes.
Inflammatory arthropathy (e.g., JIA)	Protrusion with uniform joint space narrowing.	Late finding in inflammatory arthritis at the hip.
Complication of hip arthroplasty	Medial position of the acetabular cup.	May be due to osteolysis from particle wear and foreign body granuloma formation or chronic infection.
Renal osteodystrophy	Medial migration of the acetabulum with intact cartilage joint space.	Long-standing disease may result in protrusion.

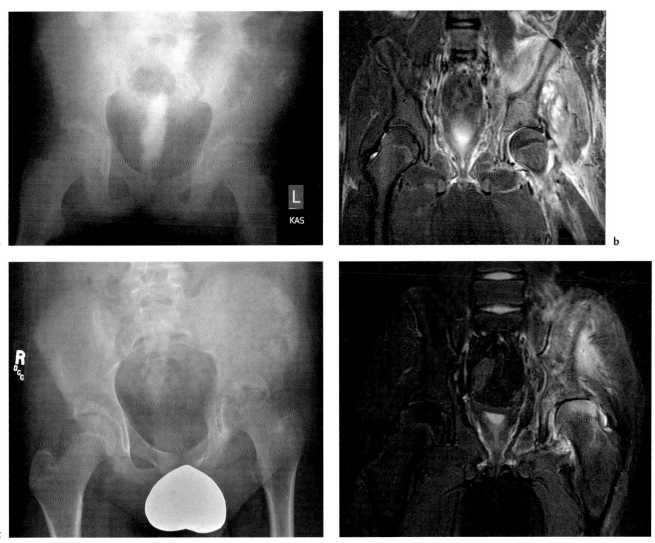

Fig. 5.22a–d Septic arthritis with interval joint space narrowing. (**a**) On presentation, the radiograph shows mild joint space narrowing and adjacent soft-tissue swelling about the left hip. (**b**) MRI shows mild cartilage loss, joint effusion, osteomyelitis, myositis, and an adjacent soft-tissue abscess. (**c, d**) One month later, the joint space has further narrowed from diffuse cartilage loss, osteomyelitis has enveloped more of the bones about the acetabulum, and acetabular protrusio has developed.

Iliac Bone

Almost every lethal bone dysplasia is characterized by a small iliac bone and horizontal acetabular roofs or flat acetabular angle, acetabular spurs, and a narrow sacrosciatic notch.

Table 5.20 Pelvis: small iliac bone

Diagnosis	Findings
Achondroplasia	Champagne-glass appearance of the inner margins of the pelvis, squared iliac wings (elephant ears), short and narrow sciatic notch, flat acetabular roof, short and narrow sciatic notch, and flat acetabular roof. Large skull, canal stenosis at the foramen magnum, narrowing (rather than widening) of the interpediculate distance from upper to lower lumbar spine, short vertebral pedicles with spinal canal stenosis, scalloped vertebral bodies.
Pseudoachondroplasia	Poorly formed, irregular acetabulum and round ilium. Spinal, metaphyseal, and epiphyseal changes.
Thanatophoric dysplasia	Short and small iliac bones, horizontal acetabular roofs, small sacroiliac notches, bowed femurs (French telephone receiver), "H"-shaped appearance of vertebral bodies, very short ribs, small scapula.
Campomelic dysplasia	Narrow and tall iliac wings, incomplete ossification of pubis and ala of sacrum, narrow vertical ischia. Hip dislocation.[12]
Chromosome disorders (particularly 13 and 18)	
Achondrogenesis types I and II	Poor osseous mineralization. Deformed and short iliac wings, absent ossification of pubis and sacrum. Often lethal.
Asphyxiating thoracic dysplasia (Jeune syndrome)	(see **Table 5.3**)
Chondroectodermal dysplasia (Ellis-van Creveld syndrome)	Flared hypoplastic iliac wing, horizontal acetabulum with medial and lateral spurs (trident pelvis), small sacroiliac notch. Short limbs, short ribs, postaxial polydactyly, and dysplastic nails and teeth. Sixty percent have congenital heart disease.[13] Ninth carpal bone (after the age of 5 y).
Dyggve-Melchior-Clausen dysplasia and Smith-McCort syndrome	Lacy appearance of iliac crest, wide sacroiliac joints, small sacrosciatic notches, wide pubic symphysis, and ischiopubic synchondrosis.[12] Smith-McCort syndrome similar to Dyggve-Melchior-Clausen dysplasia but without mental retardation.
Metatropic dysplasia	Flat irregular acetabular roof, short squared iliac wings, narrow sacrosciatic notches, and accessory ossification centers of the ischia. Tail (small appendage or cutaneous fold in coccygeal region).[12]
Short rib-polydactyly syndrome (types I and III)	Small iliac bones and flattened acetabular roofs. Types range from lethal to more mild forms. Types II and IV have near normal pelvis.
Barnes syndrome	Small bell-shaped thorax, small iliac wings and pelvis, small sacroiliac notch. Laryngeal stenosis.
Schneckenbecken dysplasia	Snail-shaped ilia, flat acetabular roofs, handlebar clavicles, hypoplastic scapula, dumbbell-shaped very short long bones, wide fibula, and round vertebral bodies.[12]
Schwartz-Jampel syndrome	Triangular deformity of the pelvis, flared iliac wings, femoral head dysplasia.[12]
Kniest dysplasia ▷ *Fig. 5.23a–c*	Trefoil-shaped pelvis and coxa vara. Spondyloepiphyseal dysplasia associated with deafness or myopia. Large epiphyses at the knees, large flattened proximal femoral epiphyses with broad metaphyses.

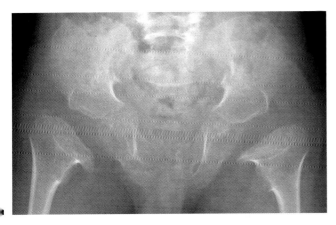

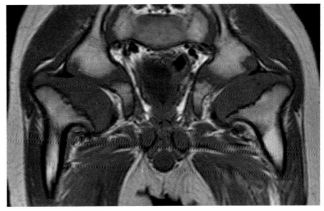

b

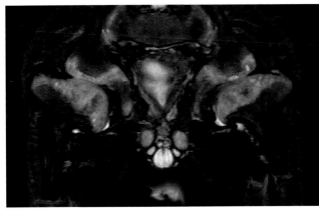

c

Fig. 5.23a–c   Kniest dysplasia. (a) Frontal view of the pelvis shows hip dysplasia, small sacrosciatic notches, and spurs at the proximal femurs. Corresponding T1-weighted (**b**) and coronal short time-inversion recovery (STIR; **c**) images show the contribution of epiphyseal cartilage.

Ischium and Pubic Bones

Table 5.21   Pelvis: widening (diastasis) of the pubic symphysis

Diagnosis	Findings	Comments
Trauma	Separation of the medial ends of the pubic bones.	A second pelvic fracture is usually present to complete a break through the pelvic ring.
Osteitis pubis	Lysis of the pubic symphysis and marginal sclerosis during healing phase. Bone marrow edema in the pubis about the pubic symphysis. Increased uptake on bone scan.	Typically occurs in athletes.[16]
Bladder exstrophy ▷ *Fig. 5.24, p. 512*	Tilted iliac bone with horizontal acetabular roof. True widening of the symphysis.	DD: variants of exstrophy (cloacal, superior vesicle fissure, duplicated exstrophy), epispadias, anorectal anomalies, and urogenital anomalies.[17]
Metabolic ▷ *Fig. 5.25, p. 512* ▷ *Fig. 5.26, p. 512*	Margins may appear eroded.	Hyperparathyroidism/renal osteodystrophy.
Infection/Inflammation	Lysis and erosions. Widening may be asymmetric.	DD: bacterial, tuberculosis, JIA, reactive arthritis.
Connective tissue disorders		Marfan and Ehlers-Danlos syndromes, for example.
Campomelic dysplasia ▷ *Fig. 5.14, p. 501*	(see **Table 5.12**)	
Prune belly syndrome (Eagle-Barrett syndrome)	Flared iliac wings and wide interpubic distance.	Spectrum of congenital anomalies of the gastrointestinal and genitourinary systems. Associated with other syndromes.
Cleidocranial dysplasia ▷ *Fig. 5.15a–d, p. 502*	Delayed ossification of the pubis.	(see **Table 5.15**)
Spondyloepiphyseal dysplasia ▷ *Fig. 5.27, p. 512*	Absent ossification of the pubis during infancy.	Bone dysplasia with premature osteoarthritis (OA) of the hips. Platyspondyly, short stature. No ossification of the epiphyses of the knees, talus, and calcaneus. Ovoid pear-shaped vertebra in infancy progressing to platyspondyly.

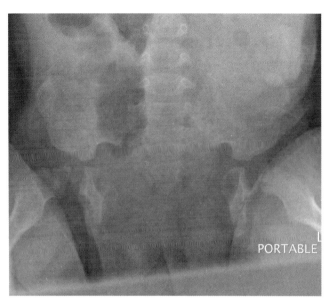

Fig. 5.24 **Bladder exstrophy.** A 5-month-old with diastasis of the pubic bones from bladder exstrophy.

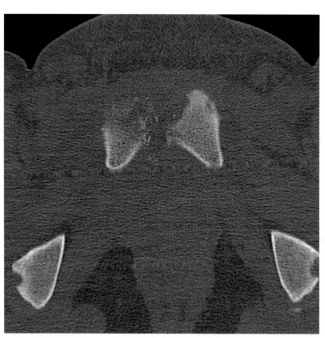

Fig. 5.25 **Metabolic.** Widening of the pubic symphysis with lysis in a patient with renal osteodystrophy. Note the erosions in the ischia.

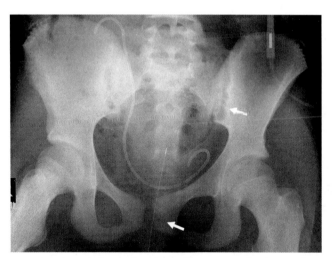

Fig. 5.26 **Metabolic.** Widened sacroiliac joints and pubic synchondrosis from renal osteodystrophy (arrows).

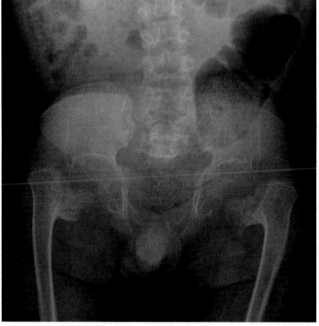

Fig. 5.27 **Spondylometaphyseal dysplasia** with changes at the hips and iliac bones and widening of the inferior portion of the pubic symphysis.

Table 5.22 Pelvis: flat and rotated iliac bone

Diagnosis	Findings	Comments
Trisomy 21 ▷ *Fig. 5.28*	Flattened, broad pelvis with flared iliac wings, and decreased acetabular and iliac angles.	An enlarged iliac angle may be seen by fetal US in the second trimester of fetal life.[18]
Exstrophy-epispadias complex	Wide pubic symphysis.	Spectrum of anomalies of the lower abdominal wall, bladder, anterior bony pelvis, and external genitalia.
Sacral agenesis and hypoplasia		Associated abnormalities include deformities of the lower extremities and anomalies of the genitourinary tract, lower gastrointestinal tract, and spine.

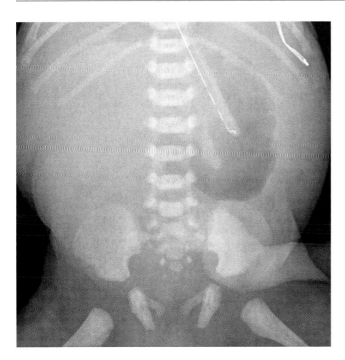

Fig. 5.28 **Trisomy 21** with flattened broad pelvis (flared iliac wings), six non–rib-bearing lumbar vertebral bodies (11 pairs of ribs not shown), and double bubble of duodenal atresia.

Table 5.23 Pelvis: narrow sacrosciatic notch

Diagnosis	Comments
Achondroplasia	(see **Table 5.20**)
Pseudoachondroplasia	(see **Table 5.20**)
Thanatophoric dysplasia and variants	(see **Table 5.20**)
Short rib-polydactyly syndrome, type I (Saldino-Noonan type)	(see **Table 5.20**)
Chondroectodermal dysplasia (Ellis-van Creveld syndrome)	Short limbs, short ribs, postaxial polydactyly, and dysplastic nails and teeth. Sixty percent have congenital heart disease.[13]
Spondyloepimetaphyseal dysplasia	▷ *Fig. 5.29a, b*

A narrow sacrosciatic notch may be seen in almost all the bone dysplasias with a small iliac bone (see **Fig. 5.23**).

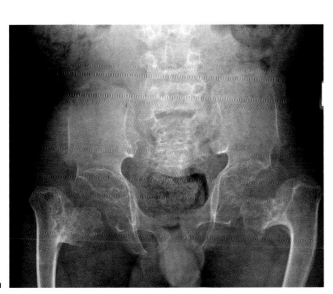
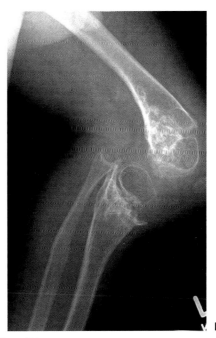

a   b

Fig. 5.29a, b **Spondyloepimetaphyseal dysplasia** at the hips (**a**) and knee (**b**).

Joints

Widened Joint Space

Table 5.24 Joints: joint effusion

Diagnosis	Findings	Comments
Toxic synovitis ▷ *Fig. 5.30a, b*	Sterile hip aspiration.	Patients tend to have less painful hip symptoms than those with bacterial synovitis.
Septic arthritis ▷ *Fig. 5.31a–d*	Pus or bacteria found on hip aspiration.	Other clinical parameters that increase the likelihood of bacterial infection prior to aspiration when US shows an effusion are increases in temperature, leukocyte count, and erythrocyte sedimentation rate.[19]
Renal osteodystrophy (primary and secondary hyperparathyroidism) ▷ *Fig. 5.26, p. 512*	Widened sacroiliac joints.	
JIA		Mono- and polyarticular forms. Likely to have more chronic symptoms.
Pigmented villonodular synovitis (PVNS) ▷ *Fig. 5.32a–d, p. 516*	Synovium is dark on T1 and T2-weighted MRI.	Masses of PVNS may appear similar to hypertrophied synovium of JIA on MRI and US.
Rheumatic fever		Symptoms change more rapidly in rheumatic fever than JIA.
Hemarthrosis (trauma, hemophilia) ▷ *Fig. 5.33a, b, p. 517*	Uniform joint space narrowing. Hemosiderin in the synovium (dark on T1- and T2-weighted MRI).	Tends to affect large joints. Patients usually already have a diagnosis of trauma or a bleeding disorder.

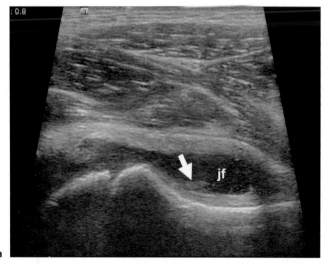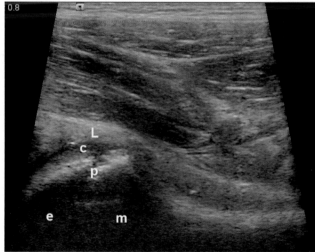

Fig. 5.30a, b Toxic synovitis left hip. (**a**) US of the left hip shows a joint effusion and synovial thickening (arrow) when compared to the unaffected right hip (**b**).

c Cartilage
e Epiphysis
jf Joint fluid
L Labrum
m Metaphysis
p Physis

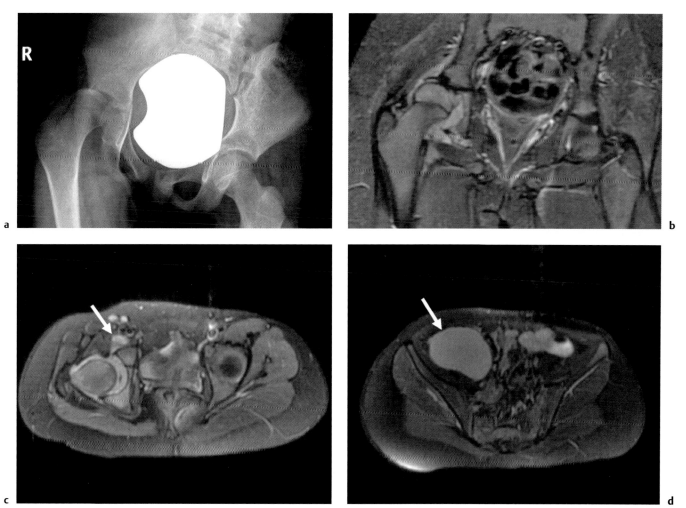

a

b

c

d

Fig. 5.31a–d Septic arthritis in an 8-year-old with hip subluxation from a large joint effusion (**a, b**) that extends into a pus-filled iliopsoas bursa (arrows in **c** and **d**).

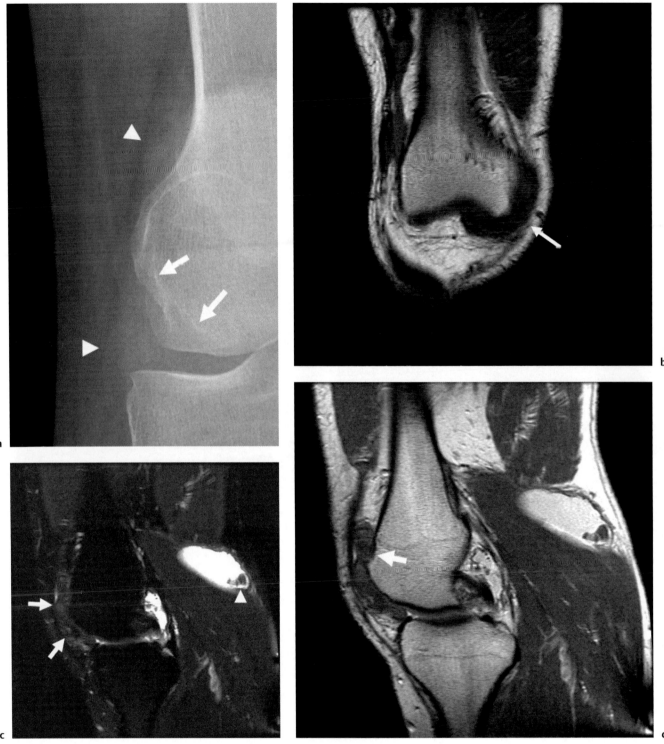

Fig. 5.32a–d Pigmented villonodular synovitis. (a) Radiography shows erosions (arrows) with adjacent soft-tissue masses (arrowheads). The PVNS is intermediate to low in signal intensity on T1 (arrow in **b**) and T2 fat-saturated (arrows in **c**) imaging. Erosions (arrow in **d**) adjacent to PVNS are better demonstrated on proton-density imaging.

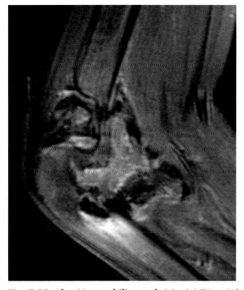
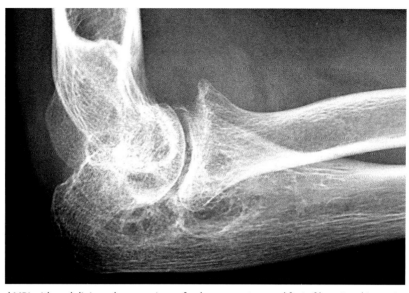

a   b

Fig. 5.33a, b Hemophiliac arthritis. (a) T1-weighted MRI with gadolinium shows regions of enhancement around foci of low signal intensity from chronic deposition of blood products in the elbow joint. **(b)** Four years later, advanced stages of arthritis have manifested with joint space narrowing and bone remodeling.

Table 5.25 Joints: widened and/or dislocated joint space—traumatic and congenital

Diagnosis	Findings	Comments
Traumatic: transient dislocation of the patella ▷ *Fig. 5.34a–c, p. 518*	Lateral subluxation of the patella.	May be associated with patellofemoral dysplasia. Secondary findings of impaction fractures at the medial pole of patella and lateral femoral condyle, tears of medial retinaculum and vastus medialis.
Traumatic: radial head dislocation ▷ *Fig. 5.35, p. 518*	Forearm held in pronation on tangential views of the elbow.	Caused by a sudden pull on the extended pronated forearm.
Brachial plexus palsy ▷ *Fig. 5.17, p. 505*	Widened joint space in the affected shoulder. ± Flattened epiphysis proximal humerus, ± glenoid dysplasia.	Muscular hypotonia from the brachial plexus paresis causes joint instability and dysplasia as the child grows.
Developmental dysplasia of the hip ▷ *Fig. 5.20, p. 507*		Pulvinar may produce widening of the hip joint and complicate adequate relocation.
Legg-Calvé-Perthes disease ▷ *Fig. 5.36a–d, p. 519*	Findings depend on the phase of the disease.	
Traumatic epiphyseal separation	Widening of the physis ± subluxation of the epiphysis.	Restricted to unossified epiphyses. Humerus (proximal and distal) is commonly affected.
JIA ▷ *Fig. 5.37a, b, p. 519*	Joint space may be widened from erosions.	Early findings of bone marrow edema on MRI may herald later erosions.
Radial head dislocation	Long axis of the radius does not bisect the capitellum.	Progressive radial head deformity is common.
Potter sequence	Dislocated knees, bell-shaped thorax.	Oligohydramnios due to renal agenesis leads to fetal malposition with dislocation of large joints, club feet, typical facies, and pulmonary hypoplasia.
Osteochondromas	Joint space may be widened by an osteochondroma.	Typically between the radioulnar or tibiofibular joints (proximal or distal).
Arthrogryposis	Contractures.	
Collagen vascular disorders	Joint space widening, subluxations, and dislocations.	DD: Marfan and Ehlers-Danlos syndromes.
Diastrophic dysplasia	Micromelic dysplasia with wide metaphyses, dislocations, subluxated elbows, hips, patellae.	Classic hand radiograph with subluxated thumb joints, oval phalanges, joint contractures, scoliosis.
Larsen syndrome	Dislocation of large joints (knees, hips, and elbows).	

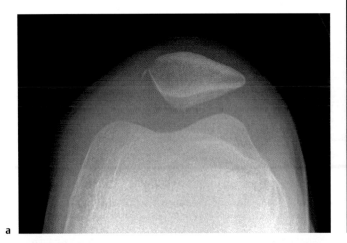

a

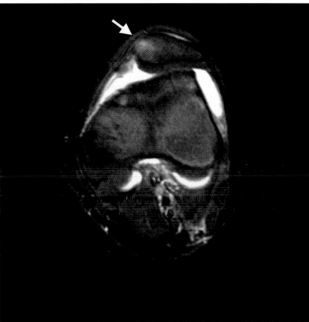

b

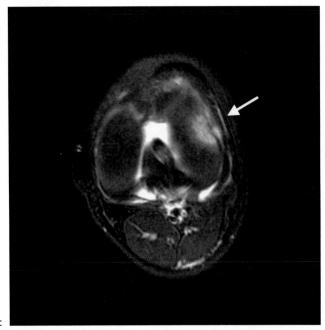

c

Fig. 5.34a–c Transient dislocation of the patella. (a) Lateral sub-luxation of the patella with an avulsion fraction off the medial pole. Bone contusions in the medial pole of the patella (arrow in **b**) and on the lateral condyle of the distal femur (arrow in **c**) from impaction by the patella.

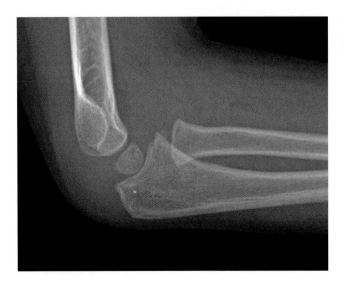

Fig. 5.35 Radial head dislocation. A line drawn through the center of the long axis of the proximal radius does not bisect the center of the capitellum.

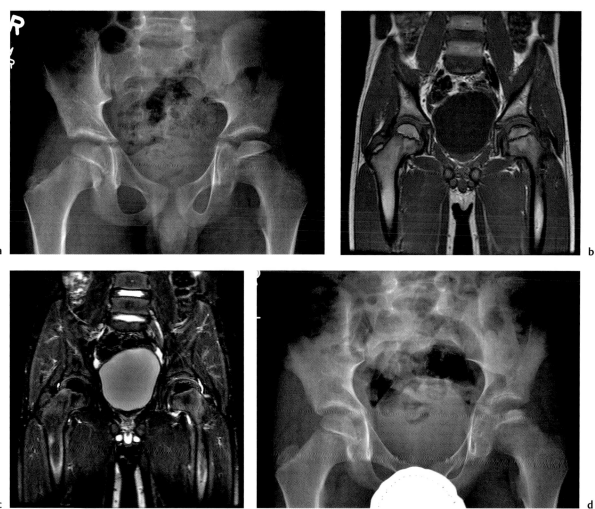

Fig. 5.36a–d   Legg-Calvé-Perthes disease. Avascular necrosis (AVN) at the proximal epiphysis of the left femur in a patient with Legg-Calvé-Perthes disease. Mild increased sclerosis on presentation (**a**) with de-creased T1-weighted signal intensity (**b**) and increased T2-weighted signal intensity on MRI (**c**), as well as increased sclerosis 6 months later (**d**).

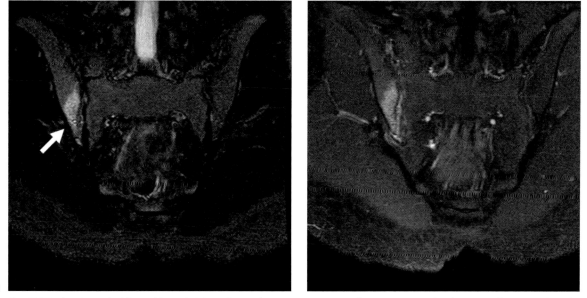

Fig. 5.37a, b   Juvenile idiopathic arthritis and sacroiliitis. Bone marrow edema on T2-weighted imaging (arrow in **a**) at the right sacroiliac joint with enhancement on T1-weighted imaging (**b**).

Table 5.26   Joints: congenital radial head dislocation

Diagnosis	Comments
Noonan syndrome	Male Turner syndrome. Multisystem involvement. Anterior bowing of the sternum, genu valgum, finger anomalies, scoliosis, vertebral anomalies, Klippel-Feil syndrome.
Holt-Oram syndrome	Radial ray anomalies, hypoplastic clavicle and/or glenoid, Sprengel deformity, pectus deformities, rib anomalies.
Ulnar hypoplasia	Isolated ulnar hypoplasia or associated with other anomalies.
Campomelic dysplasia	(see **Table 5.96**)
Osteoonychodysplasia (nail–patella syndrome)	Hypoplastic or absent patella, iliac horn arising off the central outer surface of the ilium, flared iliac wing, and small iliac angle.
Multiple epiphyseal dysplasia, Fairbank type	Small irregular epiphyses. Flattened and multicentric epiphyses at the femoral head.
Léri-Weill dyschondrosteosis	Most common form of mesomelic dwarfism. Madelung deformity, shortening of both tibias.
Russell-Silver syndrome	Finger anomalies, asymmetric skeletal maturation (left vs. right), urinary system anomalies.
Cornelia de Lange syndrome	(see **Table 5.50**)
Acromesomelic dysplasia	Short tubular bones particularly at the forearms, cone-shaped epiphyses of the phalanges and metacarpals, premature epiphyseal fusion of hands and feet, large great toes.
Auriculoosteodysplasia	Dysplasia of the radiocapitellar joint, ± radial head dislocation. Characteristic ear shape and short stature.
Larsen syndrome	(see **Table 5.34**)
Mesomelic dysplasia, Nievergelt type	(see **Table 5.51**)
Otopalatodigital syndrome I (Taybi syndrome)	Hypoplastic clavicle, scoliosis, joint subluxations, long fingers and toes. Dense skull base, under-pneumatization of skull, short thumbs and great toes.
Trichorhinophalangeal dysplasia, types I and II	(see **Table 5.33**)

Narrowed Joint Space and Ankylosis

Table 5.27   Joints: ankylosis

Diagnosis	Findings	Comments
Postsurgical	Bone bridges prior to joint	Ankylosis correlates with the locations of fusion; surgical defects and hardware may be present.
Sequelae of septic arthritis	Frank destruction of joint leads to eventual ankylosis.	
JIA	Joint space narrowing from cartilage loss leads to ankylosis.	Locations correspond to sites of inflammation.
Infantile cortical hyperostosis (Caffey syndrome)	Smooth interosseous bridging and cortical thickening between long bones (e.g., radius and ulna). Involves diaphysis and spares epiphysis.	Synostosis may occur between two adjacent long bones after resolution of the acute phase.
Radioulnar synostosis ▷ Fig. 5.38 Isolated ▷ Fig. 5.39a, b	Proximal radius and ulna are fused by a bone bridge.	The trabecular bone between the proximal radius and ulna is continuous.
Fibrodysplasia ossificans progressiva	Soft-tissue ossification bridging joints.	Intermittent progressive heterotopic bone replaces skeletal muscle and connective tissues.

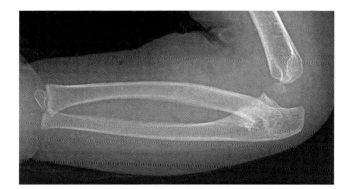

Fig. 5.38 Radioulnar synostosis.

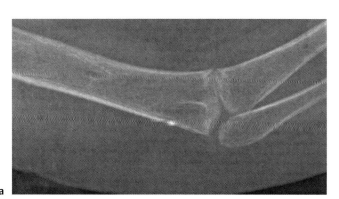

a

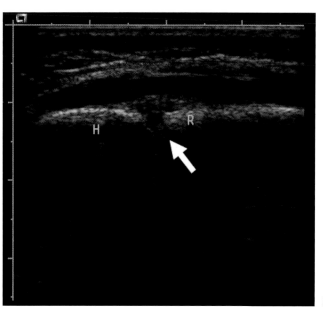

b

Fig. 5.39a, b Isolated ankylosis. (a) Radiohumeral synostosis. **(b)** US shows a synchondrosis (arrow) where the joint should be located.
H Humerus
R Radius

Table 5.28 Joints: narrow joint space

Diagnosis	Findings	Comments
OA ▷ *Fig. 5.40, p. 522*	Cartilage loss, marginal osteophytes, subchondral bone marrow edema, sclerosis, and cysts.	Although typically seen in adults, secondary OA may complicate JIA or the later stages of AVN. Any disorder that causes abnormal mechanics may lead to OA: posttraumatic, after repair of anterior cruciate ligament.
Sequela of septic arthritis ▷ *Fig. 5.22, p. 509*		Presumably, pyarthrosis increases intracapsular pressure and compromises epiphyseal blood flow. Inflammation contributes to acute cartilage loss.
JIA ▷ *Fig. 5.41a, h, p. 522*	Joint space narrowing at sites of inflammation. May have imaging findings of synovial thickening and hyperemia, bone marrow edema (MRI), and erosions.	Inflammation contributes to acute cartilage loss.
Hemophilia	Resembles JIA. Epiphyses of affected joints are often enlarged.	

Narrowing of the joint space usually results from diseases that cause cartilage loss. A narrowed joint space may be a precursor to ankylosis.

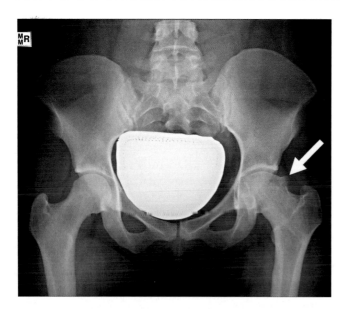

Fig. 5.40   Osteoarthritis. Advanced joint degeneration from slipped capital femoral epiphysis of the left hip with joint space narrowing and osteophyte formation limiting abduction (arrow).

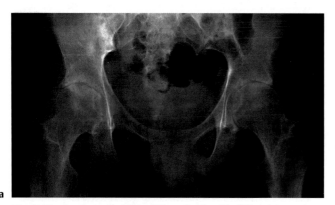

a

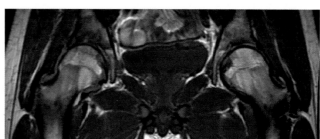

b

Fig. 5.41a, b   Juvenile idiopathic arthritis with diffuse joint space narrowing at both hips (**a**) that is greater on the right. (**b**) Corresponding coronal T1-weighted image.

Table 5.29   Joints: proximal radioulnar synostosis

Diagnosis	Comments
Congenital	Autosomal dominant and sporadic forms.
Associated skeletal anomalies	Developmental dysplasia of the hip, club feet, missing or diminutive thumb, coalescence of carpal bones, symphalangism, and dislocation of radius.
Associated syndromes	Multiple exostoses, acrocephalopolysyndactyly, Holt-Oram, mandibulofacial dysostosis, Nievergelt dysplasia and Apert, Williams, Klinefelter (and other variants of Klinefelter syndrome with extra sex chromosomes), Nievergelt-Pearlman, and fetal alcohol syndromes.

Proximal radioulnar synostosis may arise from a defect in longitudinal segmentation at the seventh week of development and is bilateral in 60% of cases. Surgery is rarely indicated (because bridge regrows) except for severe pronation deformities.[20]

Epiphysis

Overgrowth

Solitary overgrowth is most commonly associated with chronic inflammation or chronically increased blood flow.

Table 5.30 Epiphyses: solitary overgrowth

Diagnosis	Findings	Comments
JIA ▷ *Fig. 5.42a–c*	Periarticular osteopenia, erosions at the margins of joints, synovial hypertrophy, subchondral cysts and sclerosis, joint space narrowing.	The knee is the most commonly affected large joint.
Septic arthritis	Pus or organisms on arthrocentesis.	Although acute bacterial infections are usually rapidly destructive and thus tend not to alter epiphyseal growth, infantile osteomyelitis may accelerate development of the affected epiphysis.

(continues on page 524)

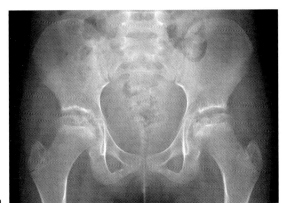

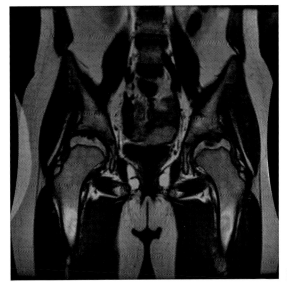

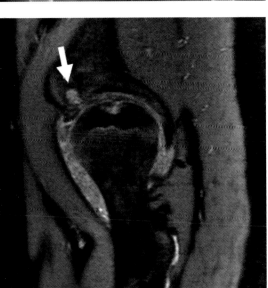

Fig. 5.42a–c Juvenile idiopathic arthritis. Epiphyseal overgrowth at the proximal femur in a child with JIA. (**a**) Enlarged epiphysis of the proximal femurs with erosions on T1-weighted imaging (**b**) and erosions (arrow in **c**) and rice bodies on proton density fat-saturated imaging.

Table 5.30 (Cont.) Epiphyses: solitary overgrowth

Diagnosis	Findings	Comments
Legg-Calvé-Perthes disease	The femoral head is enlarged (coxa magna) and the epiphysis is flattened and deformed from AVN.	Coxa magna develops during the reparative stage.
Status post hip dislocation	Coxa magna with normal architecture.	Accelerated growth of the affected side occurs after successful relocation of a previously small proximal femoral epiphysis. Necrosis of the femoral head is more common than coxa magna.
Hemophilia	Soft-tissue swelling, periarticular osteopenia, epiphyseal overgrowth. Later stages progress to joint space narrowing, marginal osteophyte formation. Synovium is decreased in T1- and T2-weighted signal intensity on MRI.	
Turner syndrome	Small medial tibial plateau with hypertrophy of the medial femoral condyle (Kosovicz sign).	Short stature, shortening of the fourth metacarpals, radiocarpal angulation, cervical ribs, Scheuermann disease, Madelung deformity.
Hypochondroplasia	Large proximal femoral epiphyses with broad metaphyses and short femoral neck.	Mild form of short-limbed dwarfism. Between the spectrum of achondroplasia to normal. Spinal stenosis.
Hemihypertrophy	Unilateral hypertrophy.	Increased incidence of embryonal tumors, Wilms tumor, neuroblastoma, and hepatoblastoma.
Klippel-Trenaunay syndrome	Uneven enlargement of the parts of the affected limb, including the epiphysis.	Triad of unilateral capillary hemangioma, varices, and localized gigantism with overgrowth of the skeleton and soft tissues.
Tibia vara (Blount disease) ▷ Fig. 5.43a, b	Unilateral enlargement of the distal femoral epiphysis (medal or lateral condyle).	Overgrowth in distal femur may be in response to changes in the proximal tibia.
Neurofibromatosis and other phakomatoses		
Macrodystrophia lipomatosa ▷ Fig. 5.44 ▷ Fig. 5.45a, b	Digits > other parts of the extremities.	
Metaphyseal chondrodysplasia, Schmid type	Affects proximal femoral epiphyses in 75% of patients. Irregular metaphyses resemble rickets.	Short-limbed dwarfism with a large degree of genu valgum from the age of 2 y.
Dysplasia epiphysealis hemimelica (Trevor disease) ▷ Fig. 5.46a–c, p. 526	(see Table 5.68)	

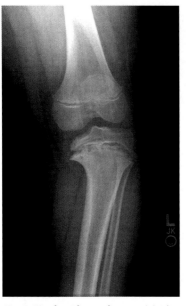

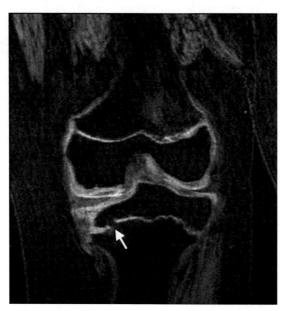

a   b

Fig. 5.43a, b   Blount disease. (a) Tibia vara. **(b)** Double echo steady state (DESS) MRI shows bone bridge (arrow) on the medial side of the tibia and reactive changes in the lateral physis of the distal femur.

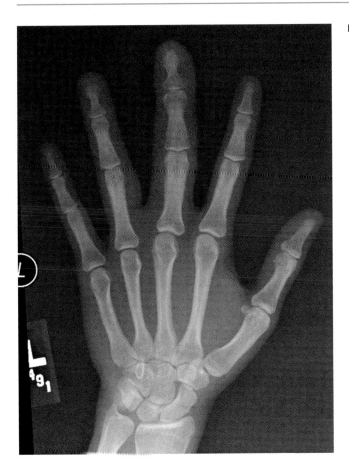

Fig. 5.44   Macrodystrophia lipomatosa of the middle finger.

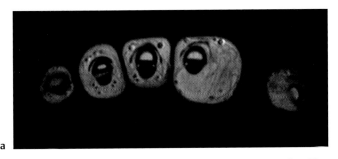

a

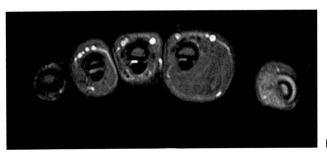

b

Fig. 5.45a, b   Macrodystrophia lipomatosa with hypertrophy of fat around the index finger and thumb on T1-weighted (**a**) and fat-suppressed T2-weighted (**b**) MRI.

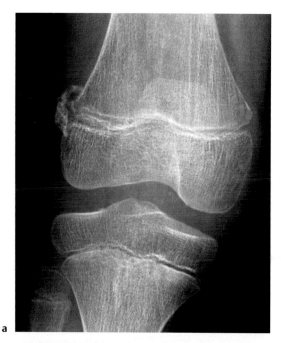

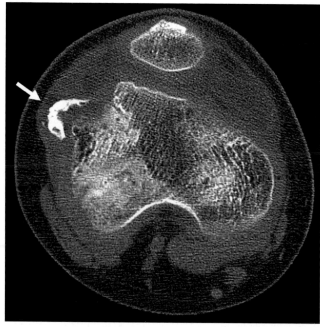

a

b

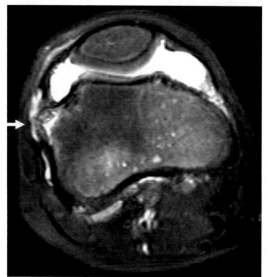

Fig. 5.46a–c   Dysplasia epiphysealis hemimelica (Trevor disease). Radiograph (**a**) and CT (arrow in **b**) show ossific excrescence projecting off the lateral aspect of the distal femoral epiphysis in an 8-year-old. (**c**) T2-weighted MRI shows cartilage cap (arrow).

c

Table 5.31   Epiphyses: generalized overgrowth

Diagnosis	Findings	Comments
Hyperthyroidism	Cone-shaped epiphyses.	Advanced skeletal maturation. Premature closure of cranial sutures. Brachydactyly.
Acromegaly	Epiphyses are enlarged but normal in shape.	Accelerated skeletal growth with delay in closure of growth plates. Widened joint spaces from increased amount of cartilage. Spadelike appearance of hands and feet.
Polyostotic fibrous dysplasia with precocious puberty (McCune-Albright syndrome)	Multifocal fibrous dysplasia. Advanced bone age, pathologic fractures, and pseudarthrosis.	Triad of fibrous dysplasia, precocious puberty in girls, skin pigmentation mainly in the trunk and proximal limbs. Two to three percent of patients with fibrous dysplasia. Bone involvement tends to be asymmetric.
Kniest dysplasia ▷ Fig. 5.47 ▷ Fig. 5.23, p. 511	Large epiphyses at the knees, large flattened proximal femoral epiphyses with broad metaphyses.	Spondyloepiphyseal dysplasia associated with deafness or myopia.

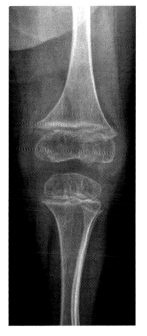

Fig. 5.47   Kniest dysplasia. AP view of the knee in a 4.5-year-old shows large epiphyses and broad metaphyses.

Small Epiphysis

Table 5.32   Epiphyses: solitary small epiphysis

Diagnosis	Findings	Comments
AVN		Several different staging systems of AVN illustrate the imaging features of early vs. advanced disease.[21] DD: Legg-Calvé-Perthes disease (idiopathic), slipped capital femoral epiphysis, sequelae of infection or inflammation, sequelae of trauma.
Joint dislocation/ subluxation ▷ *Fig. 5.48a, b*	Epiphysis is small and irregular in contour.	Proximal femoral epiphysis is the most common site (developmental dysplasia of the hip). The epiphysis of the affected side may be smaller.
Osteochondrosis (e.g., osteochondritis dissecans)		Focal disruption of endochondral ossification.
Postirradiation	Proportionally decreased growth, osteopenia, coarse trabeculae in area of field.	Disruption in cell growth from high-dose irradiation.
Meyer dysplasia ▷ *Fig. 5.49a, b, p. 528*	Delayed or smaller multiple ossification centers of the femoral head. No collapse or metaphyseal abnormality.	Symptomless developmental disorder of the hip. Forty to sixty percent are bilateral. Heals completely. May be mistaken for Legg-Calvé-Perthes disease.

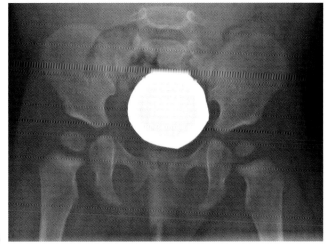

a

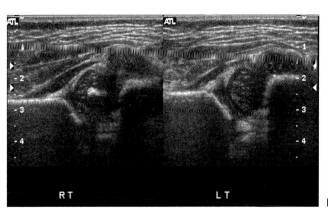

b

Fig. 5.48a, b   Joint dislocation/subluxation. Developmental dysplasia of the left hip with asymmetric epiphyses. (**a**) Delayed epiphyseal growth on radiography. (**b**) US shows the developmental dysplasia of the left hip with mild acetabular changes, uncovering of the femoral head, and lack of a secondary ossification center (no echogenic focus) in the epiphysis.

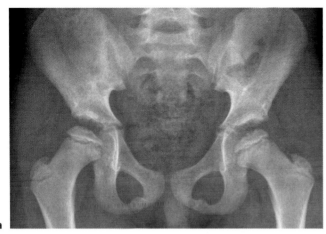
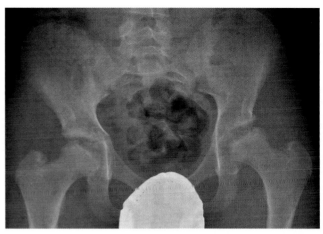

a   b

Fig. 5.49a, b   Meyer dysplasia. On presentation at 7 years of age (**a**) and then progression to joint degeneration 6 years later (**b**).

Table 5.33   Epiphyses: generalized small epiphyses

Diagnosis	Findings	Comments
Hypothyroidism	Multiple ossification centers may be present in the epiphyses.	Proximal femoral epiphyses may resemble Legg-Calvé-Perthes: the growth plates are widened and the epiphyses are prone to slippage due to mechanical instability of the physis.
Multiple epiphyseal dysplasia, Fairbank and Ribbing types	Small irregular epiphyses. Flattened and multicentric epiphyses at the femoral head.	Most commonly affected locations include the hip, knee, hand, and ankles.
Multiple epiphyseal dysplasia ▷ *Fig. 5.27, p. 512*	Delay in the appearance of the secondary ossification centers of the long bones, hands, and feet.	May have small, flattened, and fragmented epiphyses. Femoral head epiphyses may develop AVN.
Pseudoachondroplasia	Delayed small and irregular secondary ossification centers.	Premature OA.
Hereditary arthro-ophthalmopathy (Stickler syndrome)	All epiphyses are small. Classically, the distal epiphyses are flattened.	Thoracic platyspondyly. Premature OA. Severe myopia and retinal detachment.
Mucopolysaccharidosis	Small and irregular epiphyses.	
Conorenal syndrome	Somewhat flattened and small femoral heads.	Cone epiphyses in the hands and nephronophthisis (medullary cystic kidney disease).
Trichorhinophalangeal syndromes, types I and II ▷ *Fig. 5.50* ▷ *Fig. 5.51*	Small flattened proximal femoral epiphyses.	Type II has multiple osteochondromas. Premature OA. Brachyphalangy with deformation of the fingers and wedge-shaped epiphyses.

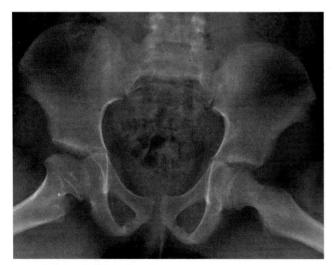

Fig. 5.50   Trichorhinophalangeal syndrome with small flattened proximal right femoral epiphysis.

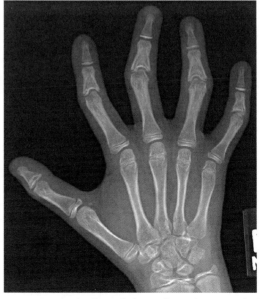

Fig. 5.51   Trichorhinophalangeal syndrome with brachydactyly and wedge-shaped epiphyses.

Supernumerary Epiphyseal Ossification Centers

Supernumerary epiphyseal ossification centers are often seen
in diseases with greatly delayed bone growth.

Table 5.34   Epiphysis: supernumerary epiphyseal ossification centers

Diagnosis	Findings	Comments
Normal epiphyseal maturation	Bipartite ossifications centers eventually fuse during development	Bipartite often seen at the proximal femoral epiphysis.
Hypothyroidism		
Multiple epiphyseal dysplasia		Knees and hips.
Larsen syndrome	Multicentric epiphyseal ossification centers.	Bilateral dislocation of the knees (anterior dislocation of the tibia), pes cavus, cylindrically shaped fingers, and characteristic facies. Cervical kyphosis due to vertebral body hypoplasia (usually C4 and/or C5).

Table 5.35   Epiphysis: punctate and irregularly shaped epiphysis or apophysis

Diagnosis	Findings	Comments
Normal variation in skeletal maturation ▷ *Fig. 5.52*	Irregular ossification at the border between the epiphyseal ossification center and epiphyseal cartilage.	Classically described at the medial condyle of the distal femur, medial aspect of the proximal tibia, and distal fibula.
Osteochondrosis ▷ *Fig. 5.53* ▷ *Fig. 5.54a–c, p. 530* ▷ *Fig. 5.55a–c, p. 531* ▷ *Fig. 5.56a–d, p. 532*	Focal lucency and sclerosis of the secondary ossification centers and apophyses.	Common sites are distal femoral condyle and olecranon of the elbow. Other sites are shown in **Fig. 5.53**.

(continues on page 533)

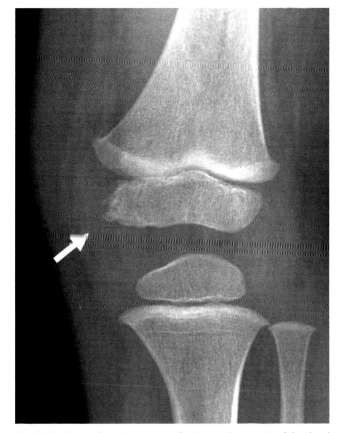

Fig. 5.52   Normal variation in ossification at the margin of the distal epiphysis of the femur (arrow) in a 2-year-old. Also note the normal cone-shaped appearance of the femur epiphysis.

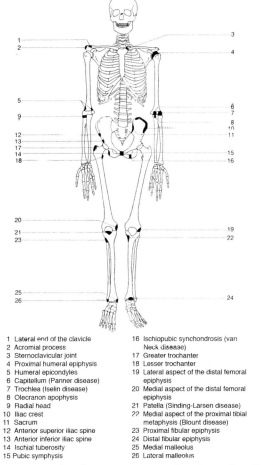

1 Lateral end of the clavicle
2 Acromial process
3 Sternoclavicular joint
4 Proximal humeral epiphysis
5 Humeral epicondyles
6 Capitellum (Panner disease)
7 Trochlea (Iselin disease)
8 Olecranon apophysis
9 Radial head
10 Iliac crest
11 Sacrum
12 Anterior superior iliac spine
13 Anterior inferior iliac spine
14 Ischial tuberosity
15 Pubic symphysis
16 Ischiopubic synchondrosis (van Neck disease)
17 Greater trochanter
18 Lesser trochanter
19 Lateral aspect of the distal femoral epiphysis
20 Medial aspect of the distal femoral epiphysis
21 Patella (Sinding-Larsen disease)
22 Medial aspect of the proximal tibial metaphysis (Blount disease)
23 Proximal fibular epiphysis
24 Distal fibular epiphysis
25 Medial malleolus
26 Lateral malleolus

Fig. 5.53   Osteochondrosis. Uncommon locations of pediatric osteochondritis.

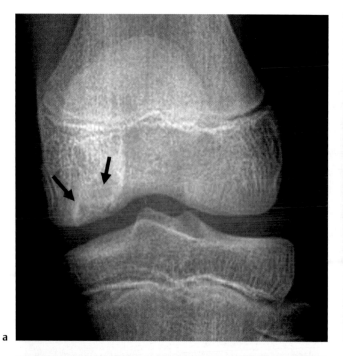

a

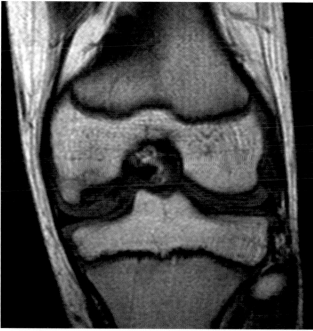

b

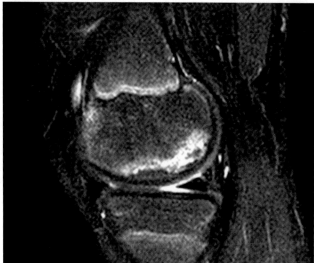

c

Fig. 5.54a–c   Osteochondritis dissecans at the medial femoral condyle (stable lesion). (**a**) Lucent lesion surrounded by sclerosis (arrows). Low signal intensity on T1 (**b**) and subchondral bone marrow edema with intact overlying cartilage on fluid-sensitive MRI (**c**).

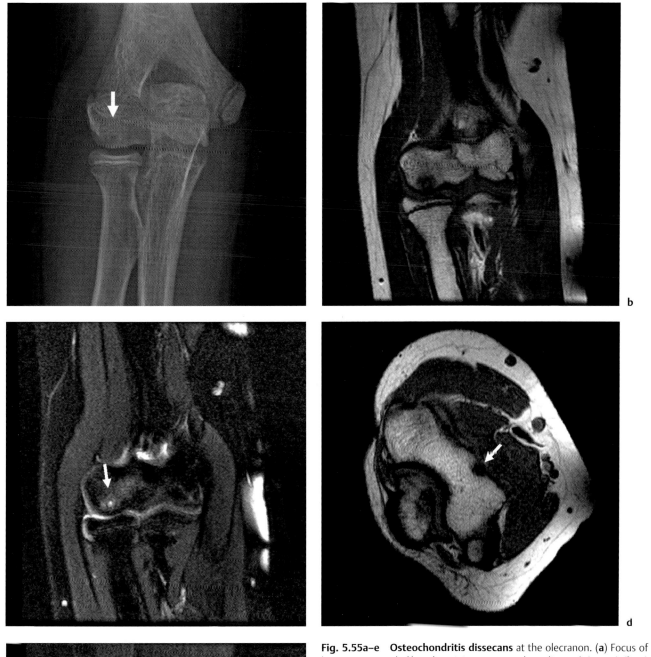

Fig. 5.55a–e   Osteochondritis dissecans at the olecranon. (**a**) Focus of lucency surrounded by sclerosis is present on the radiograph (arrow). (**b–e**) MRI further characterizes the size and stability of the lesion (arrows, **c–e**) on fluid-sensitive and T1 imaging in axial, coronal, and sagittal planes.

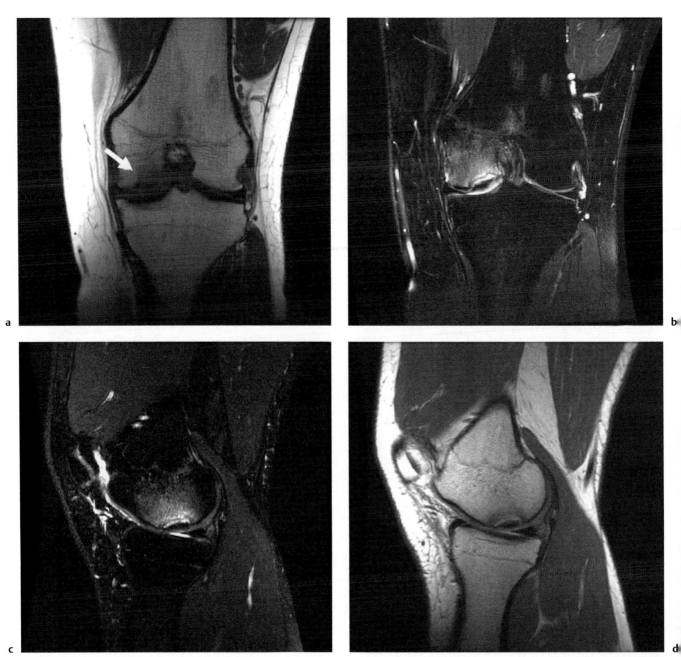

Fig. 5.56a–d **Osteochondritis dissecans** at the lateral femoral condyle (unstable lesion). (**a**) Bone marrow edema suppresses the fat around the lesion (arrow) on T1-weighted imaging. (**b, c**) Fluid undercuts the fragment on T2-weighted fat-saturated imaging. (**d**) The fragment is low in signal intensity on all pulse sequences, including proton-density imaging.

Table 5.35 (Cont.) Epiphysis: punctate and irregularly shaped epiphysis or apophysis

Diagnosis	Findings	Comments
Steroid therapy	Generalized osteopenia with bone infarcts.	MRI usually shows much more extent of involvement than radiographs alone.
Physiologic epiphyseal defect (femoral notch) ▷ *Fig. 5.57a–d*	Characteristic focus of lucency and sclerosis at the boundary of the secondary ossification center and epiphyseal cartilage. Heterogeneously increased T2-weighted signal intensity at characteristic location at distal femur.	Younger patients than with osteochondritis dissecans. Controversial whether it is a result of normal maturation or region of ischemia.[22]
Sickle cell anemia	Bone infarct due to AVN.	
Maternal ingestion of certain anticoagulants	Stippled epiphyses.	Dicoumarol or warfarin taken in early pregnancy.

(continues on page 534)

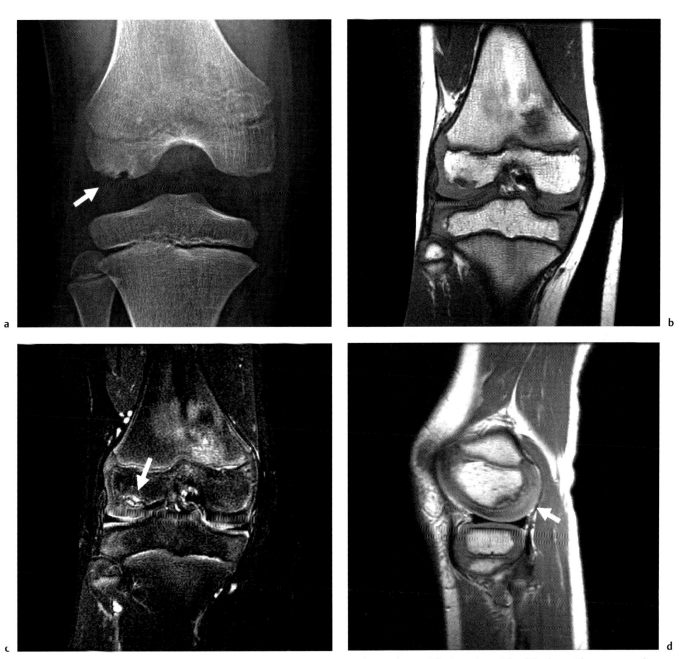

a

b

c

d

Fig. 5.57a–d Condylar notch. Radiograph shows a defect (arrow in **a**) in the epiphysis of the lateral condyle of the knee. The corresponding coronal T1 (**b**), coronal T2 fat-saturated (arrow in **c**), and sagittal proton-density (arrow in **d**) MRI suggests a diagnosis of normal variation of skeletal maturation rather than osteochondritis dissecans.

Table 5.35 (Cont.) Epiphysis: punctate and irregularly shaped epiphysis or apophysis

Diagnosis	Findings	Comments
Meyer dysplasia of the hip ▷ *Fig. 5.49, p. 528*	Delayed or smaller multiple ossification centers of the femoral head. No collapse or metaphyseal abnormality.	Symptomless developmental disorder of the hip. Forty to sixty percent are bilateral. Heals completely. May be mistaken for Legg-Calvé-Perthes disease.
Chondrodysplasia punctata ▷ *Fig. 5.58a, b*	Punctate calcifications in cartilage.	Multiple genetic forms. Type I: stippled foci of calcification in hyaline cartilage, coronal vertebral clefts, dwarfism, and joint contractures. X-linked: hypoplasia of the distal phalanges of the fingers
Mucopolysaccharidosis		
Dysplasia epiphysealis hemimelica (Trevor disease) ▷ *Fig. 5.46, p. 526*	Irregular ossification at sites of epiphyseal enchondromas. Cartilage may be seen capping the stalks of the enchondromas on MRI.	Osteochondromas of the epiphyses usually restricted to one side of the body.
Kniest dysplasia ▷ *Fig. 5.23, p. 514* ▷ *Fig. 5.47, p. 527*	Large epiphyses at the knees, large flattened proximal femoral epiphyses with broad metaphyses.	Spondyloepiphyseal dysplasia associated with deafness or myopia.

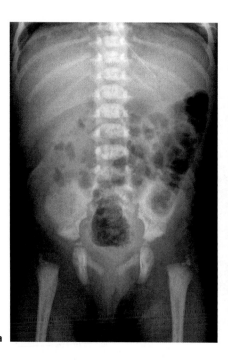
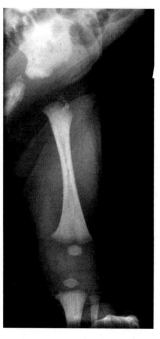

a   b

Fig. 5.58a, b Chondrodysplasia punctata. (a, b) Punctate calcifications involve the epiphyses of the proximal femurs and cartilage centers of the triradiate cartilage and transverse processes of the spine.

Cone-shaped epiphyses may be seen in the phalanges of the hand in many syndromes and bone dysplasias and after local epi-/metaphyseal trauma (osteomyelitis, hemorrhagic disruption in scurvy, bone infarction in sickle cell anemia, as well as after long-term ischemia of an extremity). A cone-shaped epiphysis in the foot is a normal variant (**Fig. 5.59**).

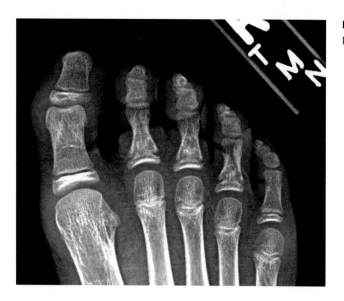

Fig. 5.59 Cone-shaped epiphysis of the second to fourth proximal phalanges. A normal variant of the foot.

Table 5.36   Epiphysis: cone-shaped epiphyses

Diagnosis	Findings	Comments
Physiologic cone shape of the distal epiphysis of the femur ▷ *Fig. 5.52, p. 529*	Slightly cone-shaped without central fusion of the physis.	Common normal variant in young children.
Acquired ▷ *Fig. 5.60a–c*	Bone bar formation after trauma.	Causes of disruption include prior trauma, infection, and scurvy (Trümmerfeld zones; see **Table 5.43**).
Vitamin A toxicity	Usually greatest in the distal epiphyses. Often symmetric premature closure of the physes.	Seen after chronic overdose. Thickened cortex after the first year of life in the long bones (ulna and metatarsals).
Syndrome-associated ▷ *Fig. 5.51, p. 528*		Acrodysostosis, asphyxiating thoracic dystrophy, cleidocranial dysplasia, trichorhinophalangeal syndrome, etc.

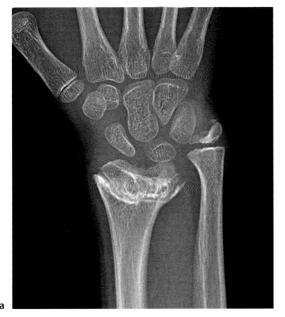

a

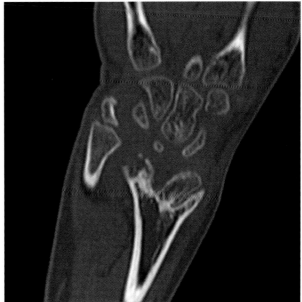

b

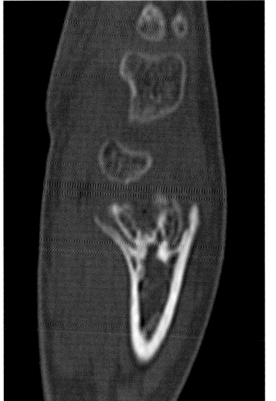

c

Fig. 5.60a–c   Acquired cone-shaped epiphysis. Bone bridge after meningococcemia produces cupping (**a**) at the metaphysis of the distal radius on radiography and coronal (**b**) and sagittal (**c**) CT.

Table 5.37   Epiphysis: focal defects[23]

Diagnosis	Findings	Comments
Physiologic epiphyseal defect ▷ *Fig. 5.57, p. 533*	Characteristic focus of lucency and sclerosis at the boundary of the secondary ossification center and epiphyseal cartilage. Heterogeneously increased T2-weighted signal intensity at characteristic location at distal femur.	Younger patients than with osteochondritis dissecans. Controversial whether it is a result of normal maturation or region of ischemia.[24]
Osteochondritis dissecans ▷ *Fig. 5.53, p. 529* ▷ *Fig. 5.54, p. 530* ▷ *Fig. 5.55, p. 531* ▷ *Fig. 5.56, p. 532*	Focal lucency in the subchondral bone with a rim of sclerosis	Characteristic locations include the medial aspect of the lateral femoral condyle, capitellum, and tibiotalar joint. MRI can stage the lesion as stable or unstable
AVN including Legg-Calvé-Perthes disease ▷ *Fig. 5.61a, b* ▷ *Fig. 5.36, p. 519*	Segmental defects usually in the large epiphyses of the limbs. The appearance of the epiphyseal defect will depend on the stage of the disease.	Early disease will show bone marrow edema on MRI or increased activity on bone scan with normal radiographs. Focal lucencies and/or sclerosis; intact joint space progresses to collapse of the subchondral bone.
Dorsal defect of the patella	Round and lytic lesion with well-defined margins located in the superolateral aspect of the patella adjacent to the subchondral bone.	Controversy over whether this is an incidental finding or a cause of anterior knee pain.
Osteomyelitis	(see **Table 5.68**)	
JIA	Cortical epiphyseal erosions and subchondral osteolysis.	Erosions in juvenile forms of inflammatory arthropathies are less common than in adults. New disease-modifying antirheumatic drug (e.g., tumor necrosis factor inhibitors) also have decreased the severity and number of erosions.
Osteoid osteoma	Well-defined lucency with a dense central calcification of the nidus.	
Chondroblastoma	(see **Table 5.68**)	
Langerhans cell histiocytosis	(see **Table 5.68**)	

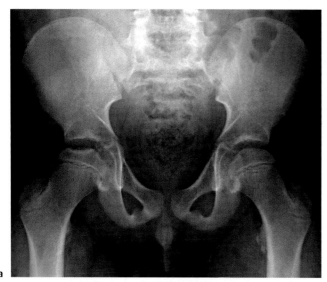
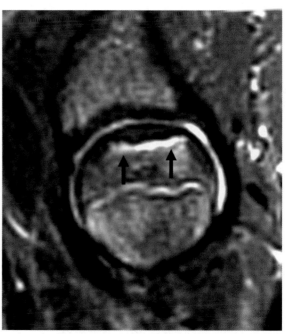

Fig. 5.61a, b   Legg-Calvé-Perthes disease. Focal epiphyseal lucency produced by AVN at the right hip (**a**) and corresponding subchondral signal abnormality on sagittal STIR MRI (arrows in **b**).

A ring epiphysis may develop when ossification is either decreased centrally or osteoblasts are active in the provisional zone of ossification. Increased bone formation in the provisional zone of ossification may be seen in the healing phase of diseases such as hyperparathyroidism and renal osteodystrophy.

Table 5.38 Ring epiphysis

Diagnosis	Findings	Comments
Osteopenia	Decreased bone demineralization that highlights the edge of the epiphysis.	
Healing rickets ▷ *Fig. 5.62*	Widened area of density in the epiphysis caused by calcium deposition in the provisional zone of ossification.	Visible approximately 3 wk after commencing therapy.
Scurvy	Well-delineated cortex of the epiphysis (Wimberger ring).	Metaphyseal changes (Trümmerfeld zones) are nearly always associated with the thickened zone of provisional calcification with osteopenia in the epiphysis (see **Table 5.43**).
Osteogenesis imperfecta		Osteopenia is due to insufficient synthesis of collagen matrix. Thin gracile long bones, wormian bones in the lambdoid sutures, fractures, and nonunion.

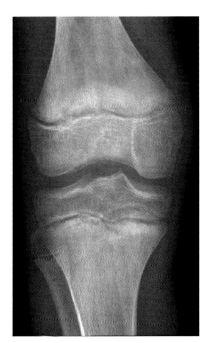

Fig. 5.62 Healing rickets. Vitamin D–resistant rickets with metaphyseal widening, irregularity, and sclerosis.

Growth Plate

Table 5.39 Physis: widened growth plate

Diagnosis	Findings	Comments
Rickets ▷ Fig. 5.63	Blurring and widening of the margins of the physis. Osteopenia with resorption of trabeculae.	Deficient ossification of the zone of provisional calcification. Etiology is vitamin D deficiency, either acquired or congenital (malabsorption, failure of conversion to active form of vitamin D, renal osteodystrophy, etc.).
Legg-Calvé-Perthes disease ▷ Fig. 5.64	Widening of the physis of the proximal femur.	Early sign of Legg-Calvé-Perthes disease may be widening of physis with intact epiphysis.
Epiphyseal fracture and slipped capital femoral epiphysis	Although the physis is typically narrowed, widening of the physis may occur in association with slippage of the epiphysis.	
Slipped capital femoral epiphysis ▷ Fig. 5.65a, b	The epiphysis is separated and sometimes displaced from the metaphysis.	Distal humerus in infants and young children. Although the physis is typically narrowed in slipped capital femoral epiphysis, widening of the physis may occur in association with slippage of the epiphysis.
Metaphyseal chondrodysplasia		Several different types, some with known genetic deficiencies in either parathyroid hormone or collagen function.

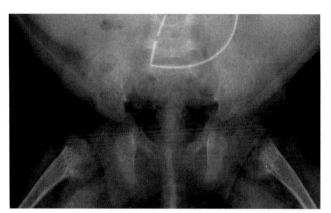

Fig. 5.63 Rickets. Renal osteodystrophy with diffuse bone demineralization and resorption.

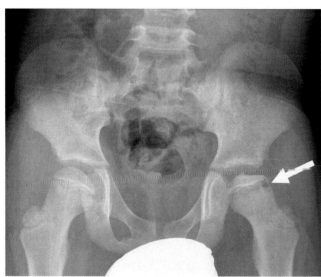

Fig. 5.64 Legg-Calvé-Perthes disease. In addition to the epiphyseal sclerosis the physis is widened (arrow).

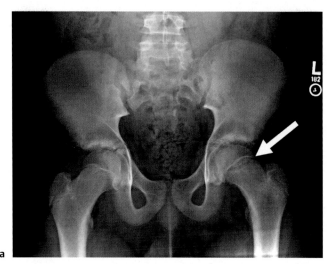

a

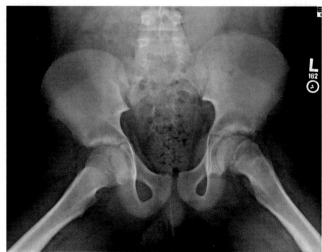

b

Fig. 5.65a, b Slipped capital femoral epiphysis (SCFI). The left physis is widened on the frontal projection (**a**) and SCFI is confirmed on the frog-leg view (**b**).

Table 5.40   Physis: narrowing and premature closure of the growth plate

Diagnosis	Findings	Comments
Posttraumatic ▷ *Fig. 5.66a–d* ▷ *Fig. 5.60, p. 535*	Usually focal bone bridge (bar) with limb-length discrepancy ± angular deformity.	Frank destruction or local ischemia results in bridging after fracture or infection. Recruitment of osteoprogenitor cells via blood vessels that cross the physis may promote bone bridge formation.[25] MRI may help quantify amount of bone bridge and direct treatment.
Advanced bone age	Normal architecture and mineralization.	All growth plates are affected similarly. A child's current height and bone age can be used to predict adult height. DD: prolonged elevation of sex steroid levels (precocious puberty or congenital adrenal hyperplasia), premature adrenarche, obesity from a young age, lipodystrophy, genetic overgrowth syndromes (Sotos, Beckwith-Wiedemann, and Marshall-Smith syndromes).

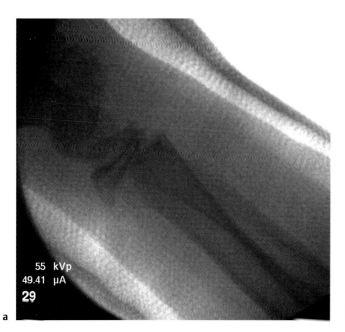

55 kVp
49.41 µA
29

a

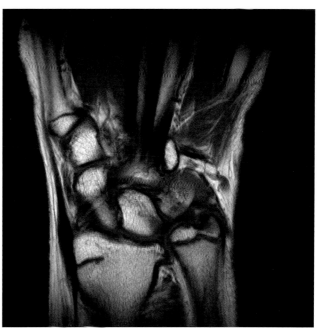

b

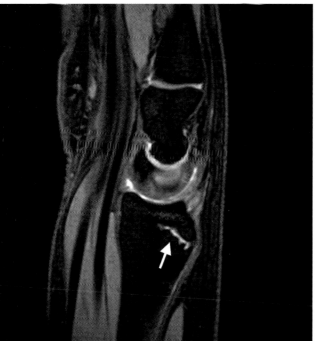

c

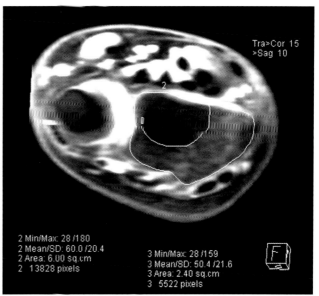

2 Min/Max: 28 /180
2 Mean/SD: 60.0 /20.4
2 Area: 6.00 sq.cm
2 13828 pixels

3 Min/Max: 28 /159
3 Mean/SD: 50.4 /21.6
3 Area: 2.40 sq.cm
3 5522 pixels

d

Fig. 5.66a–d   Bone bridge formation after physeal injury. Acute Salter-Harris fracture (**a**) followed 1 year later by premature physeal closure on T1 (**b**) and DESS MRI (arrow in **c**). (**d**) Maximum intensity projection imaging from the DESS data quantifies the amount of bridging (area 3).

Metaphysis

The Erlenmeyer flask shape describes the distal femur when the metaphysis is broad and the transition zone of the diaphysis is wide (**Fig. 5.67**). The Erlenmeyer flask shape is always the result of a pathologic process: either failure of remodeling (bone dysplasia) or expansion of the marrow space (infiltrative processes).

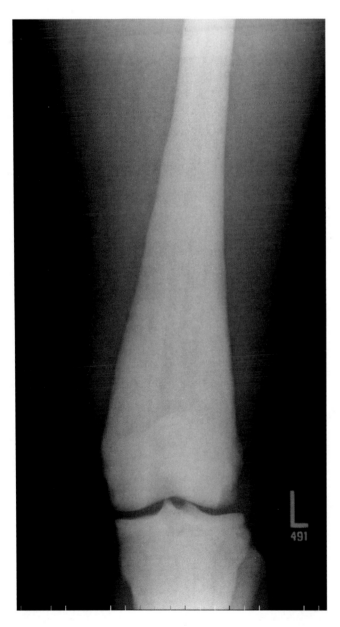

Fig. 5.67 Osteopetrosis. Erlenmeyer flask deformity in a patient with osteopetrosis.

Table 5.41 Metaphysis: broad metaphysis without cupping (Erlenmeyer flask)

Diagnosis	Findings	Comments
Fibrous dysplasia	Well-demarked lucent lesion with ground-glass matrix and cortical thinning in areas of expansion.	Bowing of the affected bones is common (shepherd's crook in the proximal femur). Most lesions are located in the diaphysis. McCune-Albright syndrome: polyostotic fibrous dysplasia, skin pigmentation, and endocrinopathies (precocious puberty).
Thalassemia major	Coarse trabecular pattern. The medulla is expanded, causing cortical thinning.	Marrow infiltration from increased red marrow.
Sickle cell anemia (homozygous)	Similar appearance as thalassemia except for bone infarcts and AVN.	The marrow hyperplasia is milder in the heterozygous form, thus without the Erlenmeyer flask deformity.
Healing rickets	Erlenmeyer flask deformity seen during the healing phase.	
Posttraumatic ▷ *Fig. 5.68a, b*	Healing with periosteal new bone formation may extend into the diaphysis.	Normal width of the native metaphysis may sometimes be discerned within the periosteal new bone of the healing fracture. Follows metaphyseal fracture of infancy (child abuse, osteogenesis imperfecta).
Chronic lead and bismuth toxicity	Dense transverse metaphyseal band.	
Gaucher disease	Symmetric and marked widening of the distal femoral metaphyses with bone infarcts.	
Osteopetrosis (Albers-Schönberg disease) ▷ *Fig. 5.67* ▷ *Fig. 5.80, p. 549*		
Congenital erythropoietic porphyria (Günther disease)	Diffuse osteopenia. Thin and porous cancellous bone.	Hemolytic anemia due to enzymatic defects in heme synthesis, which results in the accumulation and increased excretion of porphyrins or porphyrin precursors. Light sensitization and severe damage to skin. Acroosteolysis, soft-tissue atrophy, skin calcifications, osteopenia, pathologic fractures.[26]
Other rare disorders		Metaphyseal dysplasia (Pyle disease), Léri-Weill dyschondrosteosis, Melnick-Needles syndrome (including frontometaphyseal dysplasia and otopalatodigital syndromes 1 and 2), craniometaphyseal dysplasia, osteopetrosis, pycnodysostosis.

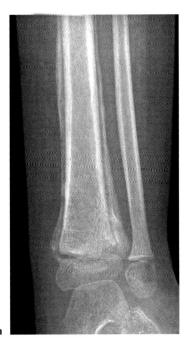
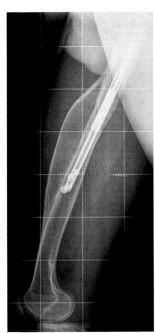

a   b

Fig. 5.68a, b Posttraumatic periosteal reaction. Subacute subperiosteal hemorrhage with periosteal cloaking (**a**) and, in another patient, chronic subperiosteal hemorrhage with large subperiosteal lucency and mature remodeling (**b**).

Table 5.42   Metaphysis: broad metaphysis with cupping and irregular cortical outline

Diagnosis	Findings	Comments
Physiologic	The ulna in infants and young children.	The distal radial metaphysis is normal with no osteopenia.
Vitamin D–deficiency rickets ▷ *Fig. 5.69a–c* ▷ *Fig. 5.70* ▷ *Fig. 5.4, p. 496*	Cupping is greatest in the early healing phase. The zone of provisional ossification is obliterated. Osteopenia and coarsened trabeculae are the result of secondary hyperparathyroidism. Cortices are thinned.	Metaphyses about the knees and wrists, distal tibia and fibula, and costochondral junctions (rachitic rosary) are most severely affected.
Vitamin D–resistant rickets	Similar findings as vitamin D–deficiency rickets.	DD: chronic renal failure with secondary hyperparathyroidism, intestinal malabsorption, premature infants on long-term parenteral nutrition, Menkes syndrome with copper deficiency, infantile, hypophosphatasia, and long-term anticonvulsant therapy (barbiturates and hydantoin).
Scurvy	(see **Table 5.43**)	
Other disorders ▷ *Fig. 5.71*		Ischemic infarct, achondroplasia, chronic vitamin A toxicity, hypophosphatasia, bone dysplasias.

a,b
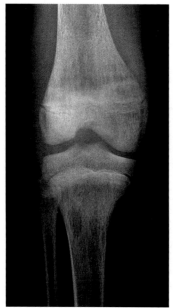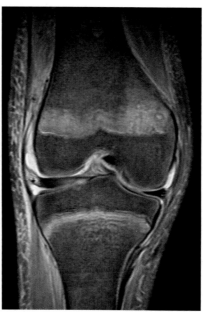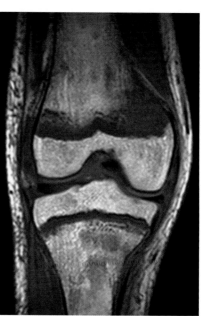
c

Fig. 5.69a–c   Vitamin D–deficiency rickets. Rickets and renal osteodystrophy. (**a**) Coarse trabeculae, increased bone density, and physeal irregularity on radiographs. Widened growth plate on proton-density fat-saturated (**b**) and T1-weighted (**c**) MRI.

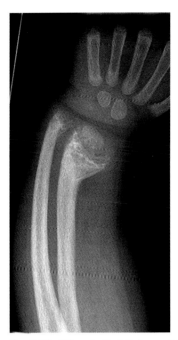

Fig. 5.70   **Vitamin D–deficiency rickets.** Healing rickets.

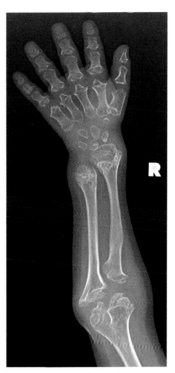

Fig. 5.71   **Metaphyseal epiphyseal dysplasia,** unknown type.

Table 5.43   Metaphysis: metaphyseal lucent bands

Diagnosis	Findings	Comments
Premature infants and neonates ▷ *Fig. 5.72, p. 544*	Variable width of lucency from 0.5 mm to several millimeters.	Occurs due to calcium mobilization from the bones.
Leukemia ▷ *Fig. 5.73a, b, p. 544*	Metaphyseal bands may be solitary or multiple. MRI will show marrow replacement.	Decreased endochondral bone formation is most visible in the most rapidly growing bones. Bone pain.
Healing rickets	Irregular bands.	Irregular bands help differentiate rickets from other diseases.
Scurvy	Trümmerfeld zone. Increased signal intensity in the metaphysis on T7-weighted MRI.	Trümmerfeld zone or scurvy line is the lucent band in metaphysis more proximal to the diaphysis than the white line of Frankel at the zone of provision calcification. Metaphyseal irregularities with spurring (Pelkan sign). White lines surrounding the epiphyses. Rare in industrialized countries and widespread in areas of the world dependent on external food aid.
Congenital syphilis	Single or multiple metaphyseal lucent bands.	Periosteal reaction. Lucent lesion in the proximal medial tibial metaphysis (Wimberger sign). Epiphyses are usually spared.
Congenital rubella infection	Longitudinal striation of sclerotic and radiolucent areas (celery stalk appearance) at the metaphyses.	May also appear similar to other TORCH (*toxoplasmosis, other infections, rubella, cytomegalovirus, and herpes simplex virus*) infections with a more irregular pattern of sclerosis and lucency at the metaphysis.
Other TORCH Infections	Nonspecific appearance seen after birth with irregular sclerosis and lucency at the metaphysis.	
Hypervitaminosis D	Wide submetaphyseal lucent bands.	After long term ingestion of high doses of vitamin D.

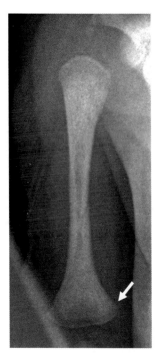

Fig. 5.72   Lucent metaphyseal line (arrow) in an infant with long-term care in the intensive care unit.

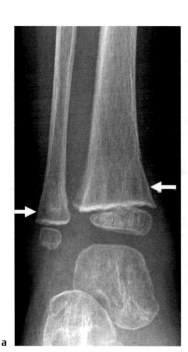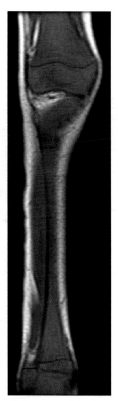

a

b

Fig. 5.73a, b   Metaphyseal lucent bands (arrows in **a**) in a 3-year-old boy with pre-B cell acute lymphoblastic leukemia infiltrating the bone marrow. (**b**) Diffuse bone marrow infiltration is seen on the T1-weighted MRI with suppression of fat in all visualized bone marrow.

Although metaphyseal corner fractures have a strong association with child abuse, imaging findings at the corners of the metaphyses may also arise from normal variation during skeletal maturation and a wide array of syndromes, dysplasias, and metabolic conditions.[27]

Table 5.44   Metaphysis: corner fractures and spurs (see Table 5.98)

Diagnosis	Findings	Comments
Subperiosteal bone collar (normal variation)	Discrete mineralized spur at the periphery of the physis or an abrupt step-off of the metaphyseal cortex as it approaches the physis.	Osseous ring that surrounds the primary spongiosa of the metaphysis and, to a variable extent, the physis. The collar has a variety of imaging appearances that may simulate metaphyseal fractures. Most common at the knees and wrists. A follow-up radiograph may be necessary to exclude healing from trauma.
Child abuse ▷ *Fig. 5.74a, b* ▷ *Fig. 5.75a, b*	Classic metaphyseal lesion.	(see **Table 5.98**)
Metabolic ▷ *Fig. 5.76a–c, p. 546* ▷ *Fig. 5.180, p. 622*		DD: neonatal rickets with hyperparathyroidism, congenital hyperparathyroidism
Obstetric injury		Extraction from a breech or armling presentation may produce traction and torsion similar to the forces occurring in child abuse.
Bone dysplasias	Follow-up radiograph will show no change in appearance, unlike the healing that would occur after trauma.	Although the underlying dysplasia is often clinically evident, several dysplasias may manifest only with modest osseous changes in early infancy (e.g., Metaphyseal chondrodysplasia, Schmid type).
Iatrogenic		Children with underlying neuromuscular disorders (myelodysplasia) may sustain metaphyseal injuries during physical therapy.[28] Infants after orthopedic manipulation.[29]
Osteogenesis imperfecta		In rare cases, blue sclera are absent (type IV), and osteopenia may be difficult to detect to establish a diagnosis of osteogenesis imperfecta before the incorrect diagnosis of child abuse is entertained.

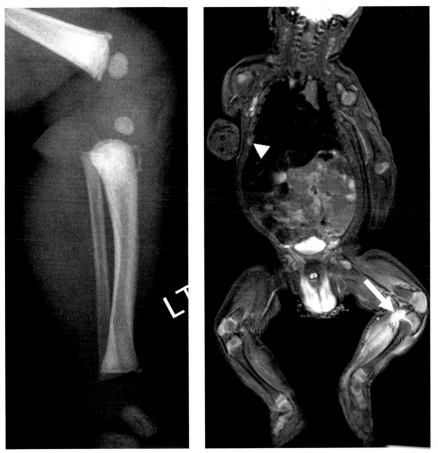

a b

Fig. 5.74a, b Child abuse with metaphyseal corner fractures at the distal femur and proximal and distal tibia (**a**). (**b**) Whole-body STIR MRI shows the corner fractures, epiphyseal separation at the left tibia (arrow), and rib fracture (arrowhead). Note the lymph nodes in the right axilla.

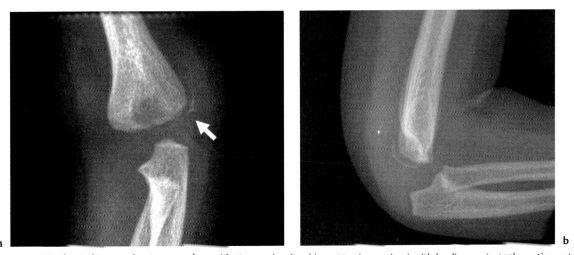

a b

Fig. 5.75a, b Subacute classic metaphyseal lesion at the distal humerus (arrow in **a**) with healing periosteal reaction extending proximally along the diaphysis (**b**).

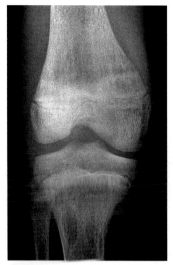
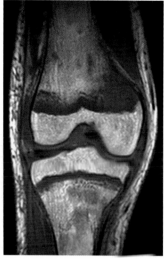
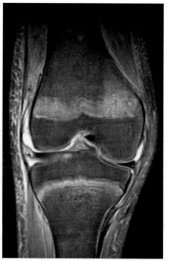

a,b

c

Fig. 5.76a–c Metabolic metaphysis. Renal osteodystrophy with metaphyseal widening on radiography (**a**) and edema on T1- and T2-weighted MRI (**b, c**).

Table 5.45 Metaphysis: metaphyseal dense bands

Diagnosis	Findings	Comments
Physiologic growth recovery lines ▷ *Fig. 5.77a, b*	Symmetric distribution of very fine lines perpendicular to the physis.	Evidence of variable rates of bone growth similar to rings on a tree. Usually less dense and numerous than after a severe systemic disease (see subsequent discussion).
Healing rickets	Increased metaphyseal density.	Asymmetric ossification immediately adjacent to the zone of provisional ossification.
After severe systemic disease ▷ *Fig. 5.78a–c*	Similar to physiologic growth recovery lines but often more thick and more numerous.	
Insufficiency or stress fracture ▷ *Fig. 5.79, p. 548*	Horizontal sclerosis located ~1–3 cm from the physis.	
Neuroblastoma	Mixed lytic and sclerotic lesion(s).	May affect metaphysis or diaphysis.
Scurvy	Normal or increased mineralization of the zone of provisional calcification on the metaphyseal side of the growth plates and surrounding the epiphyses.	(see **Table 5.43**)
Postirradiation	Additionally, increased trabecular thickening and fine periosteal reaction.	

(continues on page 548)

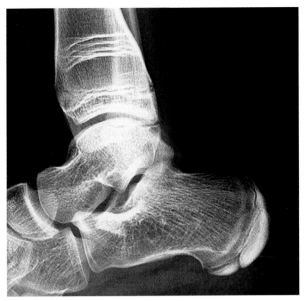

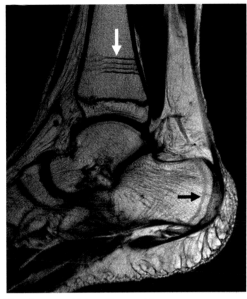

a

b

Fig. 5.77a, b   Growth recovery lines about the ankle (**a**) and hind foot (arrow in **b**) in a 12-year-old.

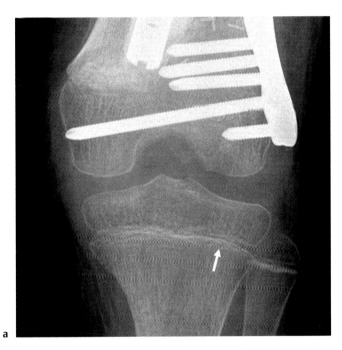

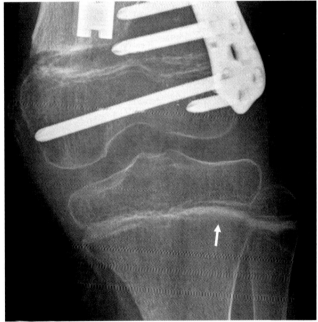

a

b

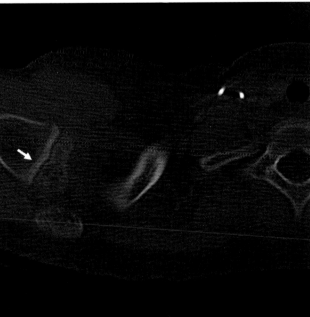

c

Fig. 5.78a–c   Dense horizontal metaphyseal bands. Five months time had passed between the initial (**a**) and follow-up (**b, c**) imaging when the dense bands (arrows) developed in this child recovering from tumor therapy.

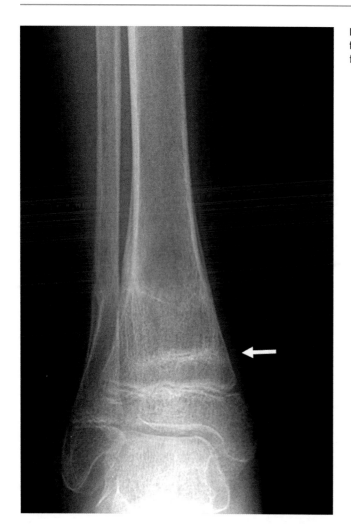

Fig. 5.79 Dense metaphyseal line (arrow) from an insufficiency fracture. The insufficiency fracture has developed near old healing fractures in the fibula and tibia.

Table 5.45 (Cont.) Metaphysis: metaphyseal dense bands

Diagnosis	Findings	Comments
Chronic lead poisoning	Very dense broad metaphyseal bands.	Similar changes in other types of heavy metal poisoning. Density does not represent deposition of metal but rather inhibition of osteoclasts with subsequent preferential activity of osteoblasts.
Hypoparathyroidism	Irregular zones of density in the long bones, atypical growth lines.	
TORCH	(see **Table 5.43**)	
Hypothyroidism	Similar to rickets but without cupping.	Delayed skeletal maturation. Small and irregular ossified femoral capital epiphyses.
Osteopetrosis (Albers-Schönberg disease) ▷ *Fig. 5.80* ▷ *Fig. 5.67, p. 540*	Broad transverse metaphyseal bands in the late disease.	Generalized bone sclerosis.
Williams-Beuren syndrome (Williams syndrome) ▷ *Fig. 5.81*	Metaphyseal density with generalized osteosclerosis.	Infantile hypercalcemia, supravalvular aortic stenosis, elfin face, multiple peripheral pulmonary arterial stenoses, mental retardation, and other defects.
Homocystinuria	Metaphyseal spicules.	Osteoporosis, flattening of the vertebral bodies (codfish vertebrae), scoliosis and kyphosis, bowed radius and ulna.

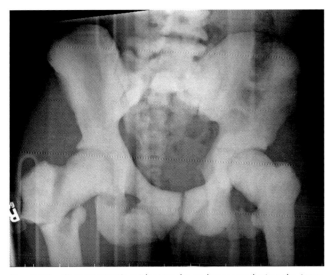

Fig. 5.80   Osteopetrosis with very dense bones replacing the intramedullary space and a pathologic fracture.

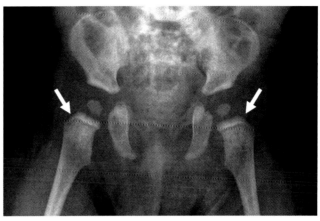

Fig. 5.81   Williams-Beuren syndrome. Dense femoral metaphyses (arrows) in a child with Williams syndrome.

Table 5.46   Metaphysis: perpendicular linear bands of metaphyseal lucency and sclerosis

Diagnosis	Findings	Comments
Normal variant ▷ *Fig. 5.82*	Almost always restricted to the distal femoral metaphyses.	Increased thickening of the longitudinal trabeculae.
Osteomyelitis and CRMO ▷ *Fig. 5.83a–c, p. 550* ▷ *Fig. 5.84, p. 550*	Brodie abscess or focal lysis marginated by sclerosis.	Usually seen in the chronic course of osteomyelitis.
Bone metastasis	Punctate and linear areas of lucency with surrounding sclerosis.	May resemble osteomyelitis.
Rubella and cytomegalovirus	(see **Table 5.43**)	
Enchondromatosis (including Ollier disease and Maffucci syndrome) ▷ *Fig. 5.126, p. 580* ▷ *Fig. 5.127, p. 581*	Arcs and whirls of sclerosis.	
Exostosis	Two parallel lines of cortex en face.	The perpendicular view will usually reveal the exostosis.
Hypophosphatasia, infantile	Long bone bowing and characteristic Bowdler transverse spurs of the long bones.[30]	Symmetrical central defects in the distal femoral metaphyses.
Osteopathia striata	Fine longitudinal lines in the metaphyses of long bones.	Little consequence in the long bones, but osteosclerosis in the cranial and facial bones leads to disfigurement and to disability due to pressure on cranial nerves.

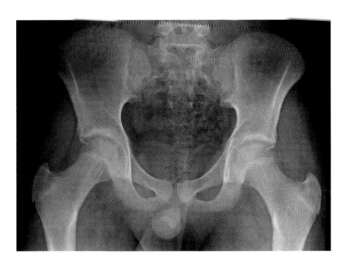

Fig. 5.82   Variation of normal. Perpendicular linear bands in the proximal femurs to be distinguished from osteopathia striata.

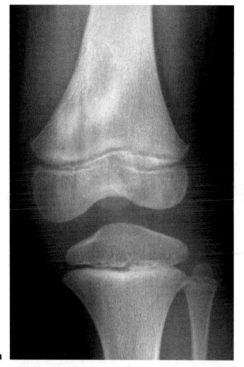

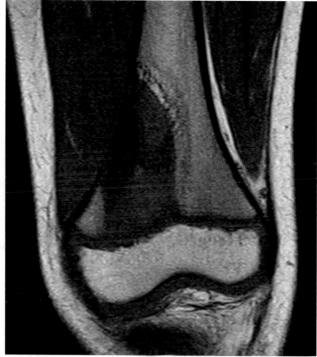

a

b

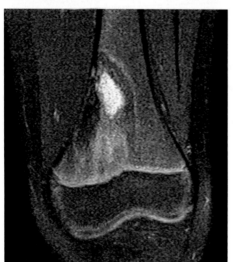

Fig. 5.83a–c Chronic recurrent multifocal osteomyelitis. (a) AP view of the knee shows a mixed lucent and sclerotic lesion in the distal femur in a 6-year-old. **(b)** Coronal T1-weighted image shows replacement of fat and extension to the physis. **(c)** Coronal proton-density–weighted fat-suppressed image shows central increased signal intensity.

c

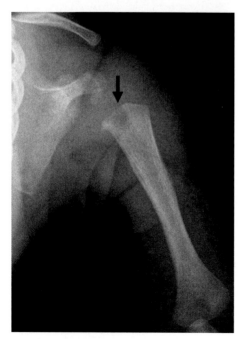

Fig. 5.84 Osteomyelitis in a 1-year-old. The infection has produced a focal lucency in the proximal metaphysis of the humerus (arrow).

Diaphysis (Long Bones)

Terminology of Limb Alteration

Dysmelia is the malformation of a limb due to disturbance in embryonic development and may range from mild hypoplasia of a single bone to aplasia of the entire limb. The radius and fibula are the most commonly affected, followed by the femur, ulna, humerus, and tibia. Abnormalities may be categorized into the following groups of defects:

- Fingers (see **Table 5.59**)
- Hands and feet (acromelia)
- Calf and forearm (mesomelia)
- Thigh and arm (rhizomelia)
- Complex (phocomelia)
- Amniotic band syndrome

Table 5.47 Types of limb shortening

Diagnosis	Findings	Comments
Acromelia	Hypoplastic hands or feet.	A spectrum of genetic syndromes may have acromelia as one of the skeletal findings.[13] Acromelic dysplasia includes three rare disorders: Weill-Marchesani syndrome, geleophysic dysplasiaa, and acromicric dysplasia.[32]
Mesomelia	Shortening of the middle limb segments (calf or forearm), often more pronounced in one limb.	Heterogeneous group of bone dysplasias[12] including but not limited to mesomelic dysplasia (many forms/types such as Langer, lethal, upper limbs), chondroectodermal dysplasia, chondrodysplasia punctata, dyschondrosteosis.
Rhizomelia	Shortening of the proximal limb segments (thigh or arm).	Heterogeneous group of bone dysplasias[12] including but not limited to achondroplasia, chondrodysplasia punctata, femoral dysplasia, multiple epiphyseal dysplasia, rhizomelic bone dysplasia (several types).
Phocomelia	Absence or underdevelopment of the proximal portion of the limb with the hand or foot attached to the body by a short flipperlike stump.	Patients have severe but unclassifiable extremity deformities. The deformity may be drug- or toxin-induced (see **Table 5.48**) or genetic. Traditionally, phocomelia has been described as a transverse, intercalary segmental defect; however, genetic and developmental biological research has provided further insight into the complexity of the possible derangements in development, and alternative approaches to classification are under development.[31]

Dysmelia

Table 5.48 Dysmelia: general syndromes

Diagnosis	Findings	Comments
Amniotic band syndrome ▷ **Fig. 5.85a, b, p. 552**	The skeleton proximal to the deformity is characteristically normal.	The most common cause of congenital amputation. May be the following etiologies: (1) a true amniotic band constricting the limb and (2) focal and circumferential apoptosis of the soft tissues.
Hypoplasia isolated to a single bone	(see **Tables 5.49, 5.50, 5.51, 5.52, 5.53, 5.54**)	
Drug- or toxin-induced	Proximal phocomelia combined with incomplete formation of the distal skeletal segment.	Variable spectrum of limb anomalies arising from maternal ingestion of a drug or toxin that disrupts early fetal skeletal development. Drugs include thalidomide and retinoic acid.

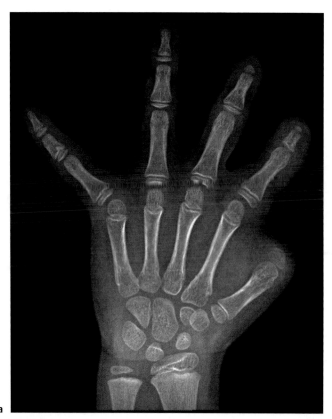 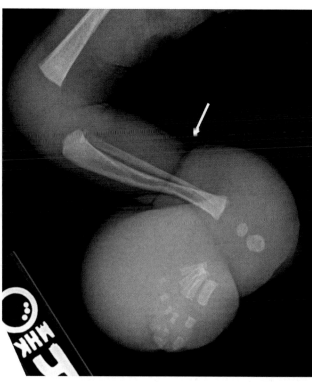

a   b

Fig. 5.85a, b   Amniotic band syndrome. (a) Amputation of the fingers. **(b)** A second child with soft-tissue swelling from a constricting band about the tibia (arrow).

Table 5.49   Dysmelia: humeral hypoplasia

Diagnosis	Findings	Comments
Rhizomelia	(see **Table 5.48**)	
Omodysplasia	Short humerus, dysplastic distally; the femora may also be shortened with resultant rhizomelic dwarfism.	Two forms (isolated to upper limbs or upper and lower with severe dwarfism)

Table 5.50   Dysmelia: radial hypoplasia and aplasia

Diagnosis	Comments
VATER/VACTERL association	The nonrandom association of vertebral defects, anal atresia, cardiac malformations, tracheoesophageal fistula with esophageal atresia, radial or renal dysplasia, and limb anomalies.
Trisomies 13 (Patan syndrome) and 18 (Edward syndrome)	
Mesomelia	(see **Table 5.48**)
Cornelia de Lange syndrome	Characteristic facies, maxillary prognathism, long philtrum, ("carp" mouth), prenatal and postnatal growth retardation, mental retardation, ± upper limb anomalies. Marked variability in presentation.
Poland syndrome	Unilateral absence of hypoplasia of the pectoralis muscle (usually sternocostal portion of the muscle) and a variable degree of ipsilateral hand and digit anomalies.
Oculoauriculovertebral dysplasia (Goldenhar syndrome)	Sporadic, unilateral malformation syndrome of the first and second brachial arches (hypoplastic mandible and maxilla), vertebral anomalies.
Cardiomelic syndrome (Holt-Oram syndrome) ▷ *Fig. 5.86*	Congenital heart disease, hand anomalies (triphalangeal thumbs, os centrale), radioulnar synostosis.
Mesomelic dysplasia	Several associated anomalies exist. Langer type is considered to be the homozygote form of the Leri-Weill dyschondrosteosis.
Léri-Weill dyschondrosteosis	Mesomelic dwarfism.
Fanconi anemia, thrombocytopenia-absent radius	Autosomal recessive disorder affecting all bone marrow elements (decrease in one or several hematopoietic cell lines) and associated with cardiac, renal, and limb malformations, and changes in dermal pigmentation.

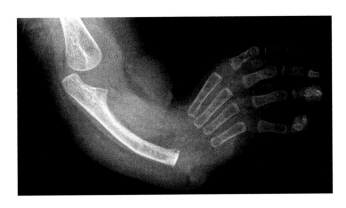

Fig. 5.86 Cardiomelic syndrome (Holt-Oram syndrome). Absent radius in a patient with Holt-Oram syndrome.

Table 5.51 Dysmelia: ulnar aplasia and hypoplasia

Diagnosis	Findings
Mesomelic skeletal dysplasias	Heterogeneous group of bone dysplasias with disproportionate shortening of the middle segments of the limbs (ulna/radius and/or fibula/tibia). DD: Langer, Nievergelt, Ellis-van Creveld, Maroteaux, Campailla-Martinelli, Reinhart-Pfeiffer, and Robinow syndromes.[12]
Ulnar hypoplasia	May be isolated or associated with other deficiencies (brachydactyly, lobster-claw deformity of feet, mental retardation).[13]
Cornelia de Lange syndrome	Micromelia, phocomelia, hemimelia[12] (see **Table 5.50**).
Nievergelt mesomelic dysplasia	Hypoplasia of the radius and ulna as well as the tibia and fibula. Radioulnar synostosis and a typical rhomboid shape of the tibia and fibula. Mesomelic type dwarfism.

Table 5.52 Dysmelia: femoral hypoplasia

Diagnosis	Findings	Comments
Rhizomelia	(see **Table 5.48**)	
Congenital short femur ▷ **Fig. 5.87**	Relatively small (short) femur with near normal morphology.	May be a separate entity from mild proximal focal femoral deficiency (PFFD).
PFFD ▷ **Fig. 5.88a–c, p. 554** ▷ **Fig. 5.89, p. 555**	The proximal femur is partially absent, and the entire limb is overall shortened.	The proximal deficiency is a misnomer, as PFFD is often accompanied by aplasia or hypoplasia of the fibula and/or knee (e.g., absence of one or both cruciate ligaments).

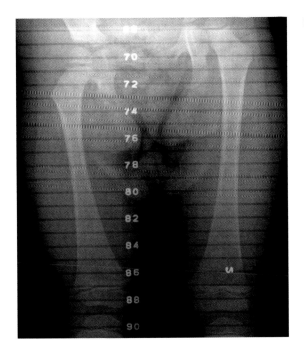

Fig. 5.87 Congenitally short femur.

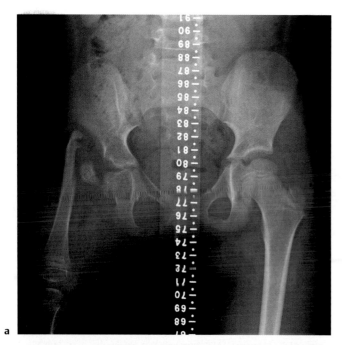

a

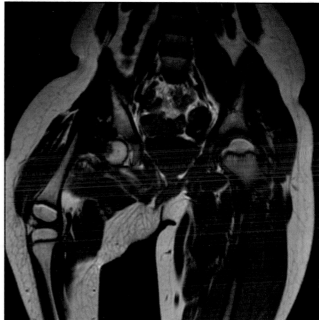

b

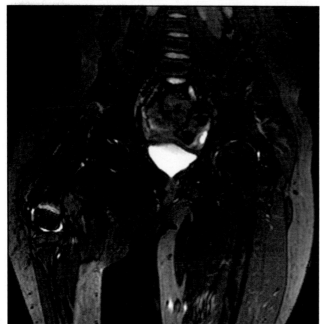

c

Fig. 5.88a–c Proximal focal femoral deficiency. (a) Radiograph shows the short and malformed proximal femur. T1-weighted (**b**) and STIR (**c**) imaging show the relative amount of cartilage in the proximal femur.

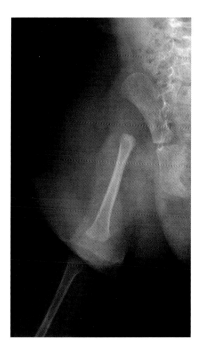

Fig. 5.89   Proximal focal femoral deficiency with fibular aplasia.

Table 5.53   Dysmelia: tibial aplasia and hypoplasia

Diagnosis	Findings
Mesomelia	(see **Table 5.48**)
Tibial aplasia associated with hand and foot anomalies	Tibial aplasia is associated with clefts, polydactyly, triphalangeal thumbs, and congenital deafness.
Nievergelt types of mesomelic dysplasia	Hypoplastic tibia. Radioulnar synostosis and a typical rhomboid shape of the tibia and fibula.
Werner mesomelic dysplasia	Bilateral hypoplasia of the tibia with polydactyly in the feet and hands.

Table 5.54   Dysmelia: fibular hypoplasia and aplasia

Diagnosis	Findings	Comments
VATER/VACTERL association		The nonrandom association of vertebral defects, anal atresia, cardiac malformations, tracheoesophageal fistula with esophageal atresia, radial or renal dysplasia, and limb anomalies.
PFFD ▷ **Fig. 5.88** ▷ **Fig. 5.89**	Hypoplastic or aplastic fibula may accompany dysmelia at the proximal femur.	(see **Table 5.52**)
Chondroectodermal dysplasia (Ellis-van Creveld syndrome)	Short fibula.	Short limbs, short ribs, postaxial polydactyly, and dysplastic nails and teeth. Sixty percent have congenital heart disease.[13]
Seckel syndrome	Fibular hypoplasia.	Growth retardation, microcephaly with mental retardation, and a characteristic "bird-headed" facial appearance.
Campomelic dysplasia	(see **Table 5.12**)	
Mesomelia	(see **Table 5.49**)	
Fibular hypoplasia and complex brachydactyly (Du Pan syndrome)	Fibular aplasia → hypoplasia, short-limbed dwarfism, and complex brachydactyly.	

Alterations in Shaft Width

■ Slender Diaphysis

Neuromuscular and soft-tissue diseases lead to skeletal atrophy with osteopenia.

Table 5.55   Diaphysis—overtubulation: slender, thin, and gracile bones

Diagnosis	Findings	Comments
Arthrogryposis	Bones are not dysplastic. Bone demineralization and dislocation of large joints.	Heterogeneous group of diseases that are all characterized clinically by joint contractures already evident at birth. Muscle weakness and fibrosis.
Spinal muscular atrophy	Slender long bones, increased height of vertebral bodies, and bell-shaped chest.	Cardinal feature is proximal muscle weakness due to degeneration of motor neurons. Childhood and adult onset forms. Molecular characterization has led to subtypes (e.g., 1–4).
Osteogenesis imperfecta	Slender long bones and osteopenia with frequent fractures.	Defect in connective tissue usually due to deficiency of type-1 collagen. Types I through VIII have different age of onset and severity. Type II = fatal, type IV = normal color of sclera.
Marfan syndrome	Scoliosis is common. Ascending aortic aneurysm and dissection are major findings	Long fingers and toes (arachnodactyly).
Caudal regression sequence	Aplasia-hypoplasia of the sacrum with hypoplasia of the lower extremities, at the extreme sirenomelia.	
Homocystinuria		Autosomal recessive trait; cystathionine beta synthase deficiency.
Schwartz-Jampel syndrome		Short stature, myotonic myopathy, and dystrophy of epiphyseal cartilage.
Cockayne syndrome	Decreased intramedullary space of the long bones, vertebrae, skull, and pelvis. Disproportionately long limbs and joint contractures.	Short stature, mental retardation, retinal atrophy, cataracts, and hearing loss. Shows overlap with xeroderma pigmentosum, another disorder caused by defective deoxyribonucleic acid repair.
Hallermann-Streiff syndrome		Birdlike facies with hypoplastic mandible and beaked nose, proportionate dwarfism, hypotrichosis, microphthalmia, and congenital cataracts.
Diaphyseal tubular narrowing (Kenny-Caffey syndrome)	Characteristic cortical thickening and intramedullary stenosis of the long bones.	Hypocalcemia and hypoparathyroidism.

■ Broad Diaphysis

Bone dysplasias with short stature will display some change in the proportions of the bone length and diaphyseal width, and the vast majority have an increase in the diaphyseal width. The metaphysis may also be affected (see **Tables 5.41** and **5.42**). The exceptions to this rule are included in **Table 5.55**. Infiltrative disorders of the bone marrow may also cause a diffuse increase the width of the diaphysis. Benign and malignant tumors may produce more focal increases in the width of the diaphysis.

Table 5.56   Diaphysis: widened diaphysis or undertubulation (short and squat [wide] bones)

Diagnosis	Findings	Comments
Achondroplasia	(see **Table 5.3**)	
Storage disorders		
Osteogenesis imperfecta type II	Short wide bones with fractures.	
Other skeletal dysplasias		Many skeletal dysplasias have this finding in the diaphyses. For exceptions, see **Table 5.55**.
Diaphyseal dysplasia (Camurati-Engelmann disease)	Increased bone density. Spindle-shaped bone expansion limited to diaphysis (spares the metaphyses).	Thickening of the cortex along the diaphysis. Bone expansion caused by endosteal new bone formation. Periosteal new bone may be laid down in layers.
Primary hypertrophic osteoarthropathy	Subperiosteal new bone formation produces widening of diaphyses. Increased bone density.	Digital clubbing and osteoarthropathy, variable features of pachydermia, delayed closure of the fontanels, and congenital heart disease.[33]
Endosteal hyperostosis (van Buchem and Worth types)	Cortical thickening with thinning of the intramedullary space and dense metaphyseal bone. Increased bone density.	Onset in puberty. Elevated alkaline phosphatase. Cranial nerve palsies. Worth type is benign form.

Bowing

Bowing may be congenital or acquired. The direction of bowing of the tibia may suggest the etiology. Anterolateral bowing of the tibia is associated with neurofibromatosis, tibial fractures, and congenital pseudarthrosis of the tibia. Posteromedial tibial bowing is an isolated finding not associated with other conditions.

Table 5.57   Diaphysis: bowing[34]

Diagnosis	Findings	Comments
Physiologic bowling of toddlers	Femur and tibia are mildly bowed.	Predilection for the first 2 y of life. Corrected within 6 mo of walking. Reaches adult pattern of mild valgus by 6–7 y.
Plastic/bowing fracture	Bowing of radius or ulna are the most common sites.	If the radius is fractured, the accompanying bone (ulna) may be fractured (and vice versa).
Rickets ▷ *Fig. 5.90*	(see **Table 5.42**)	Widening of the medial aspect of the growth plate in older children with an ossified distal femoral epiphysis. The weight-bearing part is always the widest.
Recurrent fracture with malposition	Bowing of fragile bones after repeated fractures.	Occurs in all bone disorders with increased bone fragility (e.g., osteogenesis imperfecta and other intrinsic sclerotic bone dysplasias).
Fibrous dysplasia ▷ *Fig 5.91a, b, p. 558*	Expansile and lucent lesion with a ground-glass matrix.	Typically restricted to the polyostotic variety. Medial bowing of the proximal femur (Shepherd crook deformity).
Intrauterine malposition/ congenital bowing of the tibia	Unilateral bowing, mostly involving the tibial diaphysis. Lateral and posterior bowing. Fibula is also bowed.	Believed to result from an abnormal intrauterine position. Usually heals in the neonatal period.
Neurofibromatosis ▷ *Fig. 5.92a, b, p. 558*	Anterolateral bowing.	Ten percent of patients with neurofibromatosis will have pseudarthrosis of the tibia.
Tibia vara (Blount disease) ▷ *Fig. 5.43, p. 524*	Varus angulation of the proximal tibia.	Changes in the posteromedial proximal tibial epiphysis that lead to growth suppression. Any varus angulation at the knee in children > 2 y is considered abnormal.
Pseudarthrosis of the tibia	Anterolateral bowing.	Almost always unilateral. Associated with neurofibromatosis (40%–50% of pseudarthroses of the tibia).
Other syndromes and dysplasias ▷ *Fig. 5.93, p. 559* ▷ *Fig. 5.94, p. 559* ▷ *Fig. 5.95a, b, p. 559*		Osteogenesis imperfecta, achondroplasia, and campomelic dysplasia, for example.

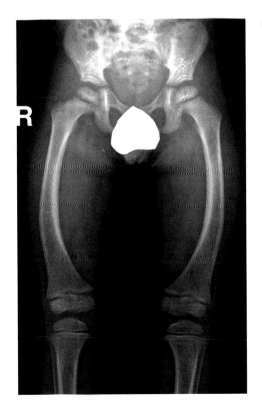

Fig. 5.90   Rickets. Hypophosphatemic rickets and bowing of both femurs.

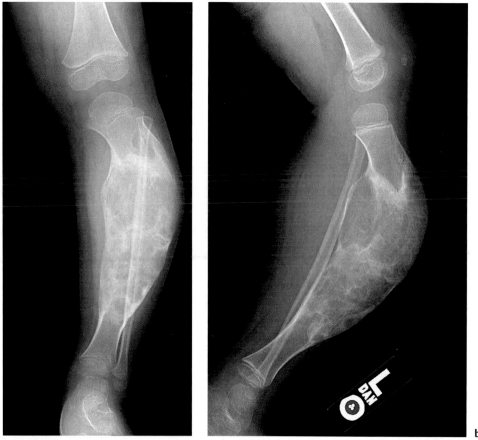

a
b

Fig. 5.91a, b   Fibrous dysplasia with ground-glass matrix producing anterolateral bowing of the tibia.

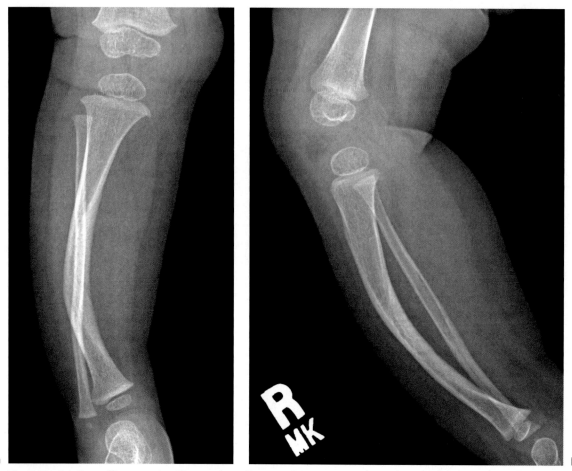

a
b

Fig. 5.92a, b   Neurofibromatosis with anterolateral bowing of the tibia.

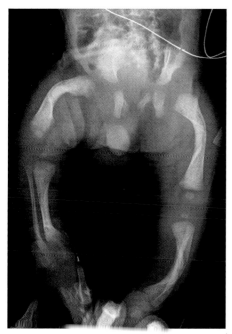

Fig. 5.93   Unknown congenital syndrome with congenitally bowed femurs and dislocated hips.

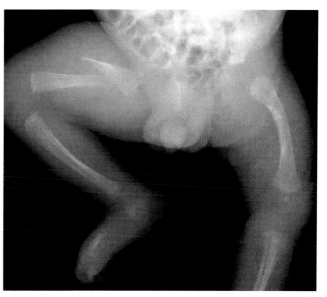

Fig. 5.94   Osteogenesis imperfecta with a bowed left femur and a contralateral fracture.

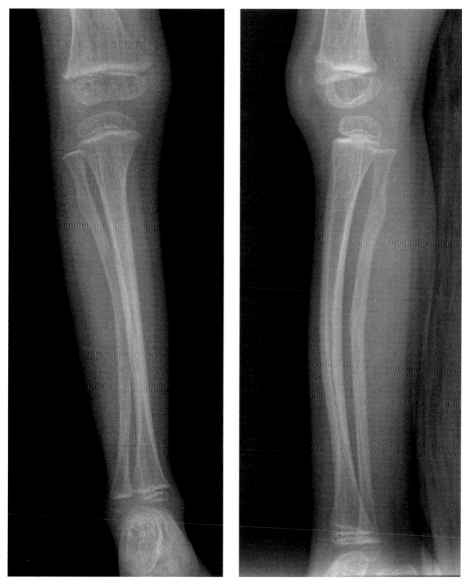

a   b

Fig. 5.95a, b   Osteogenesis imperfecta. Anteromedial bowing of the tibia in a 4-year-old with osteogenesis imperfecta.

Hands and Feet

Vocabulary to Describe Deformities of Hands and Feet

Table 5.58 Vocabulary to describe deformities of hands and feet[35]

Diagnosis	Findings	Comments
Adactyly ▷ *Fig. 5.96*	Absence of metacarpal or metatarsal.	DD: sporatic, Kniest dysplasia, aplasia cutis congenita, Adams-Oliver syndrome.
Brachydactyly[36]	Shortness of the digits.	Often an isolated finding. Associated with many inherited disorders[13] (see **Table 5.59**).
Camptodactyly	Flexion deformity of one or more fingers or toes.	Inherited as an autosomal dominant trait with variable penetrance. Seventy percent are bilateral. Generally affects the interphalangeal joints, mainly the little finger. Although most often an isolated anomaly, it may be occasionally seen with congenital disorders.[13]
Clinodactyly ▷ *Fig. 5.97*	Radial bowing of the little finger.	Most often a sporadic incidental finding. DD: trisomy 21, Klinefelter, Russell-Silver, Feingold, Robinow, and Cornelia de Lange syndromes.
Macrodactyly	Enlarged digit.	DD: progressive macrodystrophia lipomatosa, vascular malformation, congenital lymphangioma. Associated conditions: neurofibromatosis type I, lipofibromatosis, hemihypertrophy, tumors, macrodactyly simplex congenital, macromelia, proteus syndrome.
Perodactyly	Congenitally deformed fingers or toes.	Hypoglossia-hypodactylia syndrome, Cornelia de Lange syndrome, thalidomide embryopathy, amniotic band syndrome.
Polydactyly	Ranges from total duplication to a rudimentary appendage.	Most commonly affects the little finger or toe.
Preaxial = radial	Usually unilateral, mainly duplication of the thumb. Total duplication generally the same size on both sides (e.g., entire thumb or just a small appendage).	Total: Fanconi anemia, thrombocytopenia absent radius syndrome, Holt-Oram, Greig cephalopolysyndactyly, Alpert, Carpenter, Pfeiffer, trichorhinophalangeal (type II), and other syndromes.
Postaxial = ulnar ▷ *Fig. 5.98*	Mainly left-sided, frequently short metacarpal or phalanx. The carpals are rarely affected.	Asphyxiating thoracic dysplasia and Ellis-van Creveld, Greig cephalopolysyndactyly, Bardet-Biedl, short rib-polydactyly syndromes type I and II (Saldino-Noonan and Majewski), and other syndromes.
Symphalangism	Congenital ankylosis of one or more phalangeal joints.	Not always recognizable at birth because ossification has not yet occurred. May coincide with carpal and tarsal fusion. DD: hereditary absence of the proximal or distal interphalangeal joints, Apert syndrome, diastrophic dysplasia.
Syndactyly ▷ *Fig. 5.99*	Incomplete separation of the soft tissues and bones of one or more digits.	Failure of differentiation. Greig cephalopolysyndactyly syndrome.

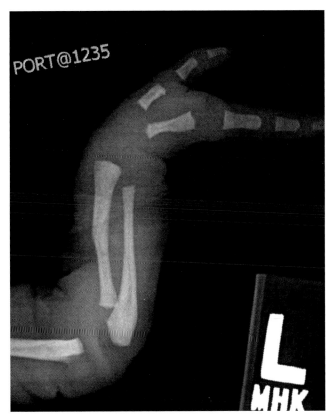

Fig. 5.96   Adactyly.

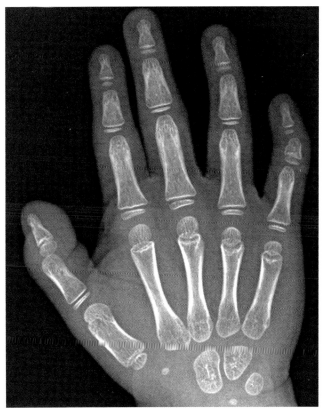

Fig. 5.97   Clinodactyly. Radial bowing of the little finger.

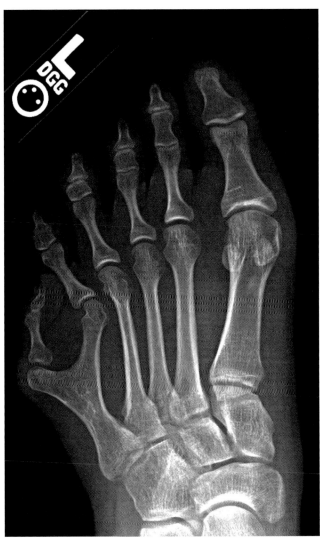

Fig. 5.98   Postaxial polydactyly.

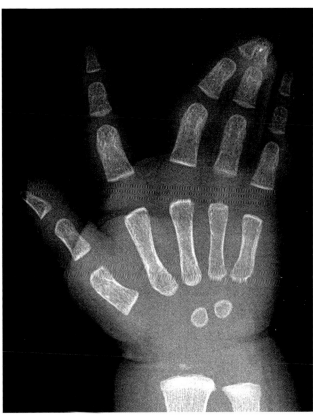

Fig. 5.99   Syndactyly with soft-tissue and bone fusion.

Brachydactyly

Brachydactyly may be isolated or associated with a syndrome. Isolated forms of brachydactyly have been typed A1–5, B, C, D, E, IV, Sugarman brachydactyly, and Kirner deformity as an extension of the original Bell classification system.[36] Isolated brachydactyly is rare except for types A3 (short middle phalanx of the little finger) and D (short distal phalanx of the thumb). Over 260 syndromes and genetic disorders have brachydactyly as a feature[13] and several of them are listed below. Delta phalanx (longitudinally bracketed epiphysis) is a triangular phalanx with continuous epiphyseal cartilage bridging the base and head (**Fig. 5.100**).

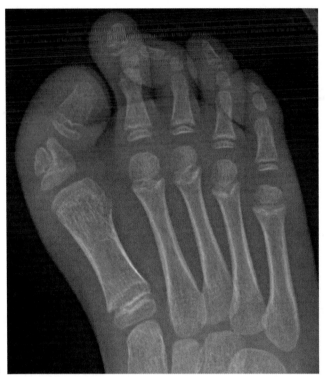
a

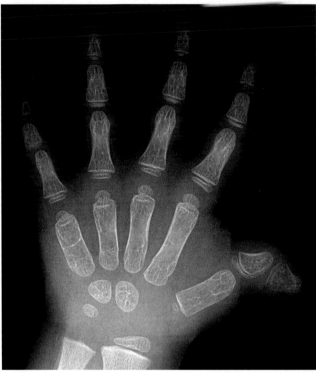
b

Fig. 5.100a, b **Delta phalanx** of the great toe (**a**) and thumb (**b**) in separate children.

Table 5.59 **Classification of isolated brachydactyly**[36]

Type	Findings	Comments
A1	Short middle phalanges: first through fourth.	Acrodysostosis, diastrophic dysplasia, and Larsen, Saldino-Robinow, and brachydactyly-distal symphalangism syndromes.
A2	Short middle phalanx: second.	
A3	Short middle phalanx: fifth.	Trisomy 21 and Aarskog, Noonan, Silver, and Shwachman syndromes.
A4	Short middle phalanges: second and fifth.	
A5	Absent middle phalanges: second through fifth with nail dysplasia.	
B	Absent or hypoplastic distal phalanges: second through fifth. Flattening, splitting, or duplication of the distal phalanx of the thumb. Feet are similarly affected.	Apical dystrophy. Must be distinguished from causes of acroosteolysis (see **Table 5.61**).
C	Brachymesophalangy of the second and third. The ring finger is usually the longest digit.	
D	Short distal phalanx of the thumb.	Rubinstein-Taybi, hand-foot-genital, Carpenter, Pfeiffer, Apert, and Robinow syndromes.
E (brachymetatarsus)	Shortening of metacarpals ± metatarsals. Note: rare as an isolated finding. Usually associated with syndromes.	Beckwith-Wiedemann syndrome, Turner syndrome, pseudohypoparathyroidism, pseudopseudohypoparathyroidism, Albright hereditary osteodystrophy, brachydactyly with hypertension. Acquired: JIA, sickle cell anemia.
Kirner (dystelephalangy)	Radial bowing distal phalanx little finger. Usually bilateral.	Differentiate from camptodactyly (flexure contraction) and type A3.

Osseous Alterations

Table 5.60   Hands and feet: alterations in size, shape, contour, or architecture

Diagnosis	Findings	Comments
Osteosclerosis ▷ Fig. 5.101	Increased focal density with a narrow zone of transition.	DD: enostosis (bone island), terminal phalangeal sclerosis (associated with JIA), melorheostosis.
Enchondroma ▷ Fig. 5.102 ▷ Fig. 5.103, p. 564	(see **Table 5.71**)	
Periostitis	(see **Table 5.81**)	
Elongation, megadactyly	(see **Table 5.95**)	
Slender phalanges, arachnodactyly	Long and slender fingers.	Homocystinuria, Marfan syndrome, congenital arachnodactyly with contractures.

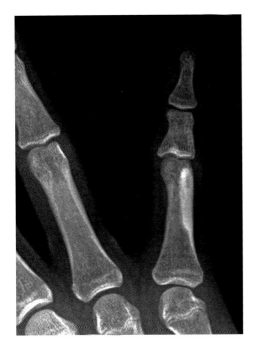

Fig. 5.101   Phalangeal osteosclerosis (differental diagnosis includes enostosis and melorrheostosis).

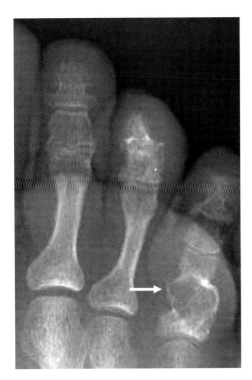

Fig. 5.102   Enchondroma in the proximal phalanx of the fourth toe (arrow).

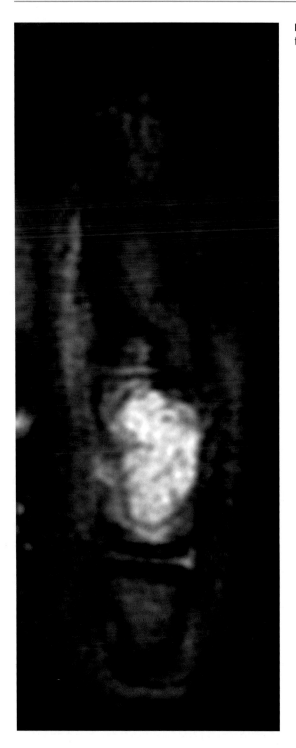

Fig. 5.103 **Enchondroma** of the proximal phalanx of the toe with a pathologic fracture.

Table 5.61 Hands and feet: alterations in distal phalanges

Diagnosis	Findings	Comments
Clubbing	Bulbous thickening of the ends of the fingers. Confined to the soft tissues and spares the bones.	Cyanotic heart disease, chronic lung disease, lung tumors, pachydermoperiostosis, chronic gastrointestinal disease, gigantism.
Hyperplasia	Widening of the tuft with a narrow shaft (drumstick appearance).	Normal variant, Coffin-Lawry (drumstick terminal phalanges), Holt-Oram syndrome (triphalangeal thumb).
Hypoplasia	(see **Table 5.59**)	
Acroosteolysis ▷ *Fig. 5.104*	Resorption or erosions of the distal phalanges, especially the tufts.	Congenital: brachydactyly type B (see **Table 5.59**). DD: trauma, infection, frostbite, leprosy, psoriasis, hyperuricemia, polyvinyl toxicity, insensitivity to pain, epidermolysis bullosa, secondary hyperparathyroidism.

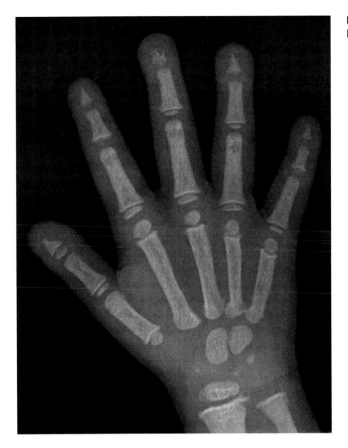

Fig. 5.104   Acroosteolysis. A 3-year-old with resorptive metabolic bone disease of unclear etiology.

Table 5.62   Hands and feet: digit I

Diagnosis	Findings	Comments
Brachydactyly isolated		(see **Table 5.59**)
Radial ray anomalies ▷ *Fig. 5.86, p. 553*		VACTERL, Holt-Oram syndrome, thrombocytopenia absent radius syndrome, Fanconi pancytopenia.
Triphalangeal thumb	Thumb has an extra phalanx.	DD: Blackfan-Diamond syndrome, Holt-Oram syndrome, trisomy 13, Poland syndrome, VATER, Werner mesomelic dysplasia, Juberg-Hayward syndrome, thalidomide and phenytoin embryopathy, and sporadic (rarely). Associated with duplication or absence of the contralateral thumb.
Acrocephalosyndactyly (Apert syndrome) ▷ *Fig. 5.105, p. 566*	Widened, short thumbs. Thumbs and great toes may also be duplicated.	Craniosynostosis, midface hypoplasia, and syndactyly of the hands and feet. Crouzon and Pfeiffer syndromes are allelic disorders with overlapping features.[13]
Rubinstein-Taybi syndrome	Widened, short thumbs. Thumbs and great toes may also be duplicated.	Characterized by mental retardation, broad thumbs and toes, and facial abnormalities.
Other syndromes	Abnormal shape (usually short or broad) thumbs and great toes.	Nonspecific finding seen in oropalatodigital syndrome, frontodigital syndrome, hand-foot-uterus syndrome, progressive myositis ossificans, diastrophic dysplasia (hitchhiker thumb), Larsen syndrome, Leri pleonosteosis, hemifacial microsomia (Goldenhar syndrome), trisomy 13 (polydactyly), Poland syndrome (syndactyly), thalidomide embryopathy, Juberg-Hayward syndrome, etc.

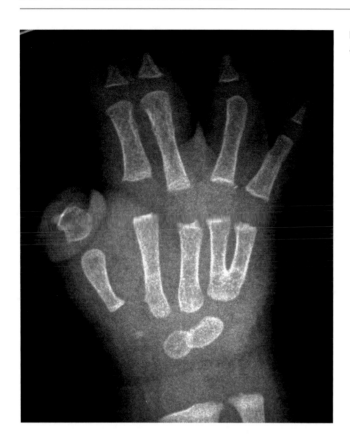

Fig. 5.105   Apert syndrome with syndactyly, fusion of metacarpals, and hypoplasia of the thumb.

Table 5.63   Hands and feet: digit V

Diagnosis	Findings	Comments
Kirner (dystelephalangy)	Radial bowing distal phalanx of the fifth finger. Usually bilateral.	Differentiate from camptodactyly (flexure contraction) and type A3 brachydactyly.
Clinodactyly	Radial bowing of the fifth finger.	Most often a sporadic incidental finding. DD: includes genetic syndromes such as trisomy 21, Russell-Silver, Feingold, Robinow, and Cornelia de Lange syndromes (see **Table 5.59** and brachydactyly type A3).
Senior syndrome	Shortening of middle phalanx of the fifth finger, fusion of middle and distal phalanges of the fifth toe, and absence of middle and distal phalanx of fifth toe.	Short children with tiny toenails.
Coffin-Siris syndrome	Absence of the distal phalanges of the fifth fingers and fifth toes.	Mental retardation with absent nail and terminal phalanx of the fifth finger.

Table 5.64   Hands and feet: metacarpals and metatarsals

Diagnosis	Findings	Comments
Idiopathic	Short fourth and fifth metatarsals.	Seen in 10% of normal population.
Radial ray anomalies	Hypoplastic thumb metacarpal.	The radial ray anomaly may be confined to the first metacarpal.
Turner syndrome	Short fourth and fifth and ± third metacarpals.	
Sickle cell disease		Shortening secondary to infarction.
Pseudohypoparathyroidism, pseudopseudohypoparathyroidism	Short fourth and fifth metacarpals.	Subcutaneous calcifications. Shortening not seen in pseudohypoparathyroidism types 1b and 2.
Homocystinuria	Short fourth metacarpal.	
Other disorders associated with short metacarpals or metatarsals		Over 200 syndromes are associated with short metacarpals or metatarsals.[13]

Table 5.65 Hands and feet: carpal and tarsal bones

Diagnosis	Findings	Comments
Coalition/fusion	Fibrous or osseous union between one or more carpal or tarsal bones.	Sporadic, acquired (trauma, JIA), or associated with syndromes (Holt-Oram, Turner, arthrogryposis, acrocephalosyndactyly).
Pseudocyst, intraosseous lipoma, bone cyst, osteonecrosis	Well-defined region of lucency in the distal calcaneus.	MRI may help with the differential diagnosis.
JIA, infection, pigmented villonodular synovitis ▷ Fig. 5.106a–c	Multiple cystic lucencies.	Spotty carpus.

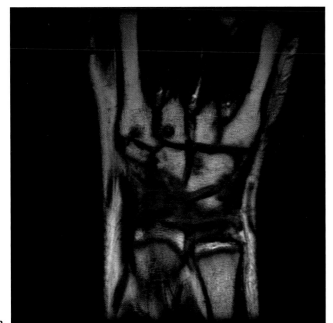

a

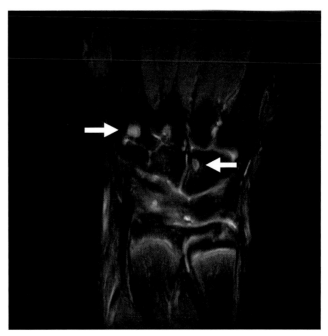

b

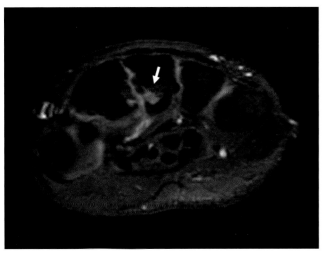

c

Fig. 5.106a–c Juvenile idiopathic arthritis and spotty carpus. T1- (**a**) and T2-weighted (**b**) MRI show osteitis and separate regions of synovium that have eroded into several carpal bones (arrows). (**c**) The intraosseous synovitis enhances with gadolinium (arrow).

Soft-Tissue Alterations

Table 5.66   Hands and feet: soft-tissue calcifications (localized)[37]

Diagnosis

Posttraumatic

Iatrogenic

Myositis ossificans
▷ *Fig. 5.107*
▷ *Fig. 5.108a–c*

Hemangioma
▷ *Fig. 5.109a–c, p. 570*

Lipoma

Subcutaneous fat necrosis

Bone tumor

Progressive systemic sclerosis
(Thibierge-Weissenbach syndrome)

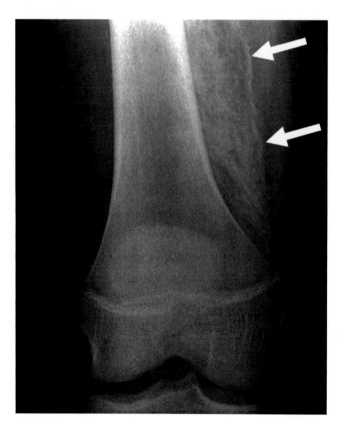

Fig. 5.107   Myositis ossificans in the vastus medialis after trauma (arrows).

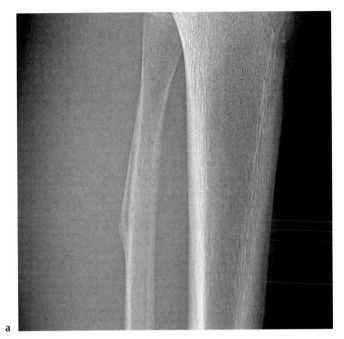

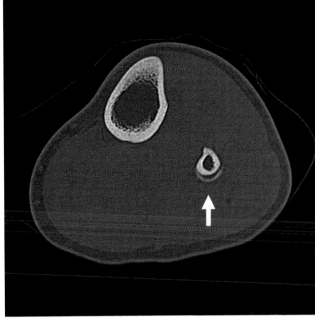

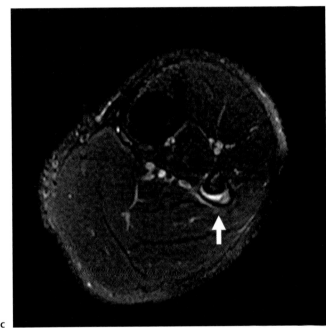

Fig. 5.108a–c   Juxtacortical myositis ossificans. (a, b) One month after trauma, a region of extraskeletal ossification has developed adjacent to the proximal fibula (arrow in **b**). (**c**) Increased fluid signal intensity is seen between the new bone formation and underlying fibula on T2-weighted MRI (arrow).

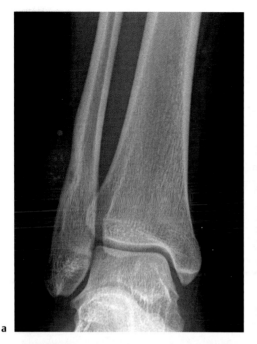

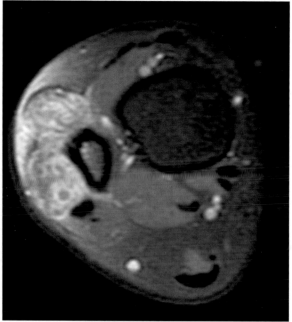

a

b

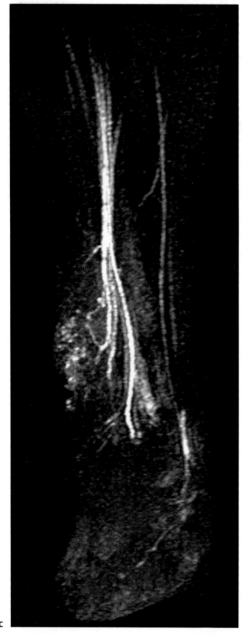

Fig. 5.109a–c Hemangioma with phleboliths (**a**) produces saucerization of the distal fibula. MRI shows avid enhancement and periosteal reaction on T1-weighted fat-suppressed imaging (**b**) after the administration of gadolinium and the contributions of blood vessels on time-resolved imaging with contrast kinetics (**c**).

c

Table 5.67   Hands and feet: soft-tissue calcifications (generalized)[37]

Diagnosis	Findings	Comments
Dermatomyositis ▷ *Fig. 5.110*	Muscle calcifications.	Increased T2-weighted signal intensity and enhancement in muscles on MRI may help direct area for biopsy.
Connective tissue disorders ▷ *Fig. 5.111*	Amorphous and punctuate calcifications in the subcutaneous soft tissues.	
Vitamin D toxicity		
Diastrophic dysplasia	Premature calcification of the cartilage.	Premature costochondral calcification. Scoliosis, clubbed feet, malformed pinnae, cleft palate. Hitchhiker thumb.
Fibrodysplasia ossificans progressiva	Intermittent progressive heterotopic bone replaces skeletal muscle and connective tissues.	Malformations of the great toes.
Progeria	Soft-tissue calcifications.	Precocious senility with early death from coronary artery disease.

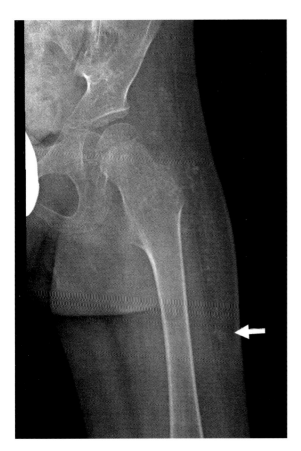

Fig. 5.110   Dermatomyositis with muscle atrophy, diffuse bone demineralization, and soft tissue calcifications (arrow).

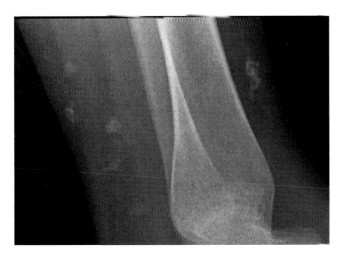

Fig. 5.111   Systemic lupus erythematosus with soft-tissue calcifications.

Tumors and Focal Bone, Joint, and Soft-Tissue Lesions[1–3]

The average annual incidence rate of primary bone sarcomas is approximately 8.7 per million children younger than 20 years of age, and primary bone sarcomas occur 10 times less frequently than soft tissue sarcomas.

Table 5.08   Tumors and focal lesions: epiphyseal lesions before closure of growth plate

Diagnosis	Findings	Comments
Osteomyelitis ▷ *Fig. 5.112a, b*	Erosion in the epiphysis or well-defined lucency from an intraosseous abscess.	Bacterial infections in the epiphyses are not as common as in the metaphyses. Tuberculosis has a predilection for the ends of long bones in children.[38]
Avascular necrosis (AVN) ▷ *Fig. 5.113a, b* ▷ *Fig. 5.36, p. 519*	Mixed sclerosis and lucency ± subchondral collapse.	MRI shows early findings of marrow edema, and bone scan shows increased uptake prior to changes on radiography.
Langerhans cell histiocytosis	Lytic (punched out) defect in the epiphysis.	Uncommon location of Langerhans cell histiocytosis.[39]
Chondroblastoma (Codman tumor) ▷ *Fig. 5.114a–d*	Osteolytic lesion with a fine sclerotic rim, 25%–50% have a stippled matrix ("popcorn" calcifications), ± internal trabeculations.	Common locations: proximal humerus, distal femur, and proximal tibia.
Articular osteocondroma/dysplasia epiphysealis hemimelica (Trevor disease) ▷ *Fig. 5.46, p. 526*	Irregular ossification at sites of epiphyseal enchondromas. Cartilage may be seen capping the stalks of the enchondromas on MRI.	Sixty to seventy percent of patients have enchondromas at multiple epiphyses. Most common sites are the talar dome and distal tibial epiphyses.

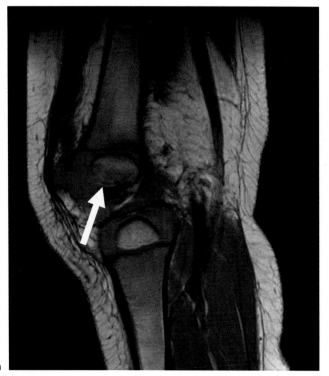
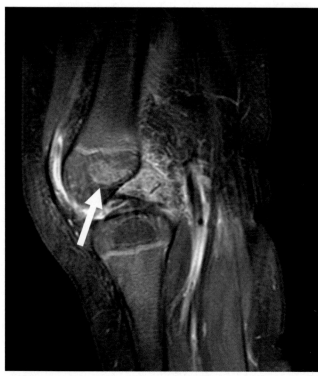

a   b

Fig. 5.112a, b   Osteomyelitis affecting the epiphysis. Decreased T1-weighted signal intensity (**a**) and enhancement in the femoral epiphysis after gadolinium (**b**; arrows; compare with normal ossification center in the tibia).

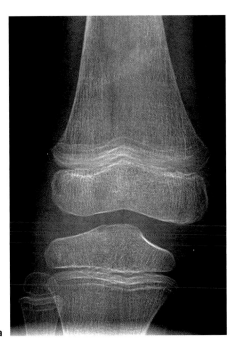

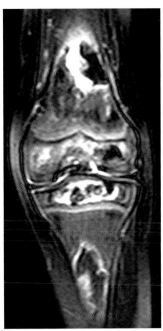

a

b

Fig. 5.113a, b   Avascular necrosis. (**a**) Diffuse bone demineralization, faint sclerosis in the metaphyses, and growth recovery lines around the knee in a 4-year-old with acute lymphoblastic leukemia in remission. (**b**) T2-weighted MRI reveals the underlying AVN and bone infarcts.

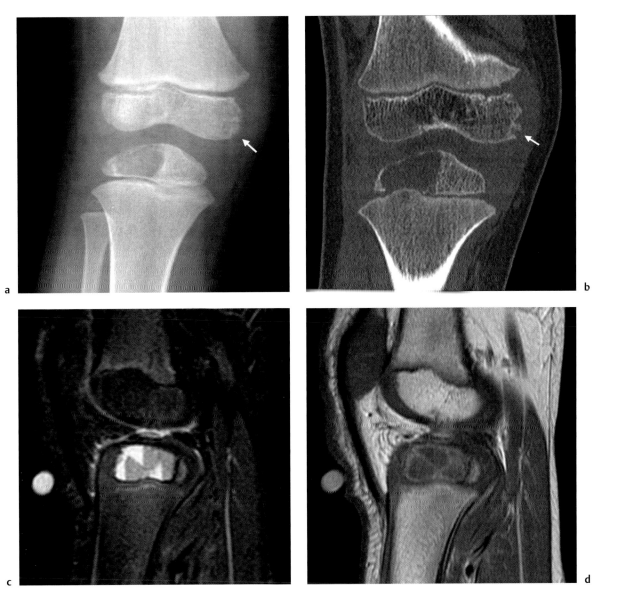

a

b

c

d

Fig. 5.114a–d   Chondroblastoma presenting as a well-marginated lucency in the proximal epiphysis of the tibia on radiography (**a**) and CT (**b**). MRI reveals increased T2-weighted signal intensity with fluid-fluid levels (**c**) and T1-weighted enhancement about the margins of the lesions (**d**). Note the normal appearance of the margins of the distal femoral epiphysis with punctate bone formation (arrow in **a** and **b**).

Table 5.69 Tumors and focal lesions: epiphyseal lesions after closure of growth plate

Diagnosis	Findings	Comments
AVN	Mixed sclerosis and lucency ± subchondral collapse.	MRI shows early findings of marrow edema, and bone scan shows increased uptake prior to changes on radiography.
Giant cell tumor ▷ *Fig. 5.115*	Osteolytic lesion with a geographic type of bone destruction. Lucent expansile lesion eccentrically located without marginal sclerosis, but narrow zone of transition. Internal trabeculations.	Abuts the subchondral bone. Typical locations: ends of the distal femur, proximal tibia, distal radius, and proximal humerus.
Fibrous dysplasia ▷ *Fig. 5.116*	(see **Table 5.71**)	
Subchondral cysts ▷ *Fig. 5.117a, b*	Well-marginated lucency subjacent to the subchondral bone.	May arise from herniation of synovium into the bone (synovial herniation pit).
Clear cell chondrosarcoma	Expansile lytic lesion with thinning of the cortex.	Extensive bone formation may mimic osteosarcoma.[40]

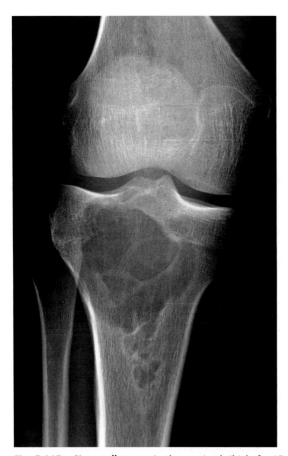

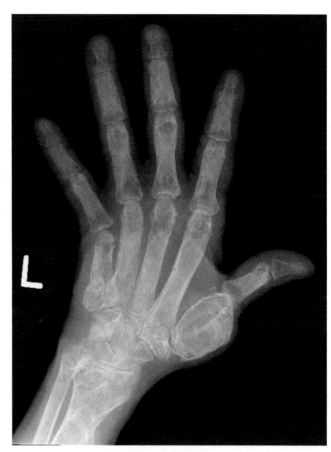

Fig. 5.115 Giant cell tumor in the proximal tibial of a 15-year-old. Bubbly, lucent, and expansile lesion.

Fig. 5.116 Polyostotic fibrous dysplasia.

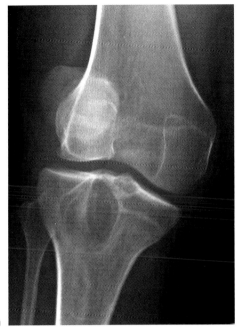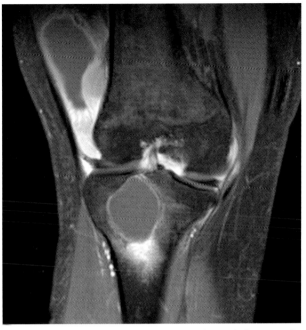

a   b

Fig. 5.117a, b   Large subchondral cyst in a patient with trisomy 21 and inflammatory arthritis. (**a**) Radiograph shows a well-marginated lucent lesion with a narrow zone of transition. (**b**) The wall of the cystic cavity enhances, as does the inflamed and thickened synovium in the suprapatellar pouch.

Table 5.70   Tumors and focal lesions: metaphysis

Diagnosis	Findings	Comments
Fibrous cortical defect (metaphyseal defect) and nonossifying fibroma (NOF; nonosteogenic fibroma) ▷ *Fig. 5.118a, b*	Well-demarcated, eccentric, lucent defect communicating with the cortex and marginated by a thin rim of sclerosis.	Radiography is usually diagnostic. Observed in 30% of normal population < 20 y of age. Proximal and distal tibial and distal femur > proximal humerus and fibula. 1. Large lesions = NOF 2. Small lesions = fibrous cortical defect.
Distal femoral cortical defect (periosteal desmoids, avulsive cortical irregularity, distal metaphyseal femoral defect, cortical desmoid, or medial supracondylar defect) ▷ *Fig. 5.119a–d, p. 576*	Cortically based lesion at posteromedial aspect of distal femur. Similar in appearance to fibrous cortical defect.	May be bilateral. Occurs in 12- to 20-y-olds. Fibrous proliferation of periosteum. Lesions resolve spontaneously. Located at posteromedial aspect of distal femur.[41]

(continues on page 577)

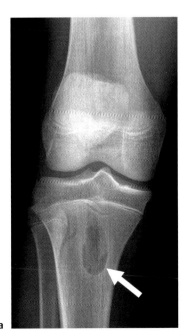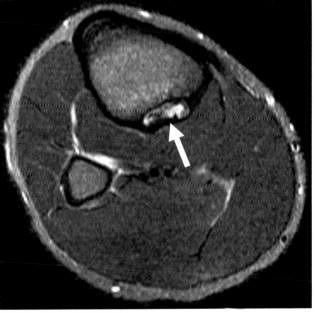

a   b

Fig. 5.118a, b   Fibrous cortical defect (arrows) in the proximal tibia on radiography (**a**) and axial T2 fat-saturated MRI (**b**).

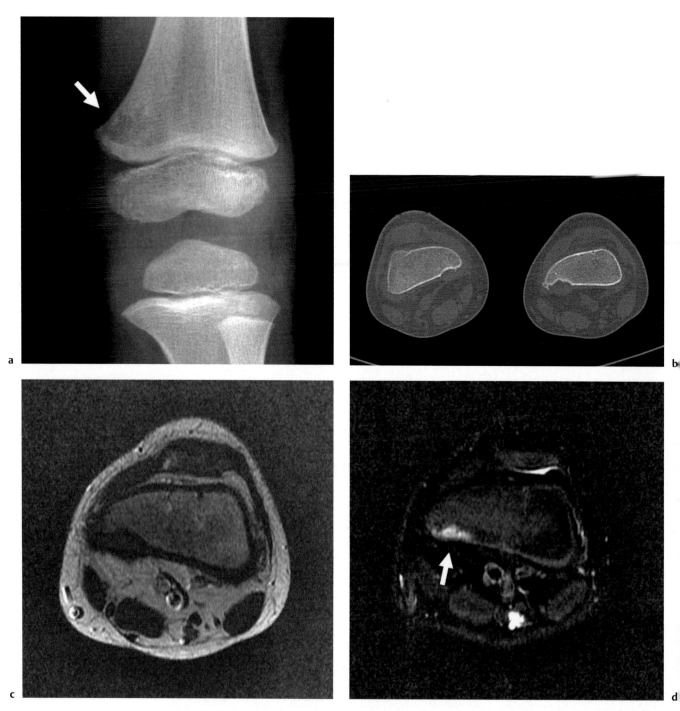

Fig. 5.119a–d Distal femoral cortical defect. (**a**) The defect is lucent with irregular margins on radiography (arrow). (**b**) Because of pain and a limp, additional imaging was performed that showed the classic appearance of the lesion on CT with a smaller cortical defect on the contralateral side. The lesion is associated with the cortex and is dark on T1- (**c**) and bright on T2-weighted (arrow in **d**) MRI.

Table 5.70   (Cont.) Tumors and focal lesions: metaphysis

Diagnosis	Findings	Comments
Osteochondroma (osteocartilaginous exostosis) ▷ *Fig. 5.120a–c* ▷ *Fig. 5.121, p. 578*	Pedunculated: Slender osseous stalk (continuous with the medulla) that projects away from the joint. Capped with hyaline cartilage. Sessile: broad based attached to the cortex.	Very common benign bone lesion. Usually discovered before age 20 y. Knees, hips, shoulders, and ankles. Mass effect on structures. Rarely may transform into chondrosarcoma. Multiple hereditary osteochondromatosis: autosomal dominant. Features of trichorhinophalangeal (Langer-Giedion) and Potocki-Shaffer syndromes.
Aneurysmal bone cyst ▷ *Fig. 5.122a, b, p. 578*	Multicystic and eccentric expansile lesion encased in a thin shell of cortical bone.	May abut the metaphyseal side of the growth plate. Fluid-fluid levels on MRI or CT similar to telangiectatic osteosarcoma. Common sites: proximal tibia and femur, proximal humerus, scapula, and spine.
Unicameral bone cyst ▷ *Fig. 5.123a, b, p. 579*	Centrally located, well-circumscribed, lucent lesion with sclerotic margins. May contain septations. Prior to treatment or pathologic fracture, follows the signal intensity of fluid on MRI pulse sequences.	Tumorlike lesion of unknown cause. May be the result of local disturbance of bone growth. Common locations in patients < 20 y include proximal humerus and femur; > 20 y include scapula, ilium, distal femur, proximal tibia, and calcaneus. May reoccur and reabsorb surgical packing material. Fallen fragment sign: cortical fragment layering in the cyst after pathologic fracture.

(continues on page 579)

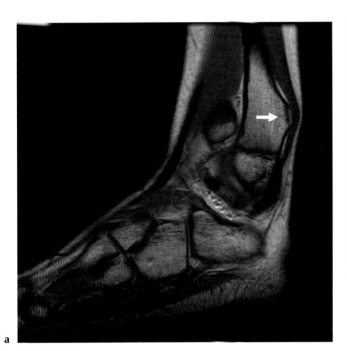

a

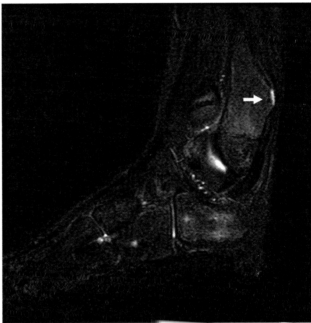

b

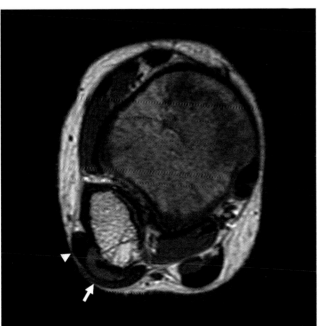

c

Fig. 5.120a–c   Osteochondroma displacing the peroneal tendons. (a) The osteochondroma (arrow) projects off the posterior aspect of the distal fibula and displaces the peroneal tendons posteriorly. (b) The cartilage cap has increased T2-weighted signal intensity (arrow). (c) The tendons are also displaced laterally (arrowhead) by the cartilage cap (arrow).

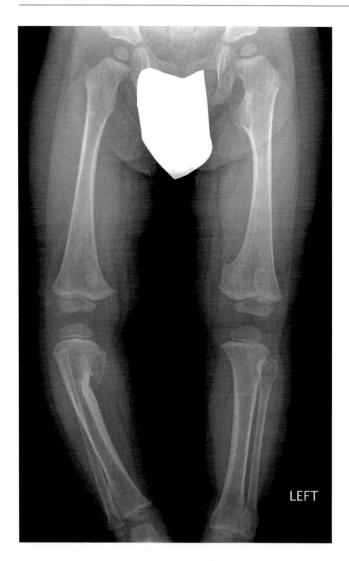

Fig. 5.121   Osteochondroma. Multiple hereditary exostoses.

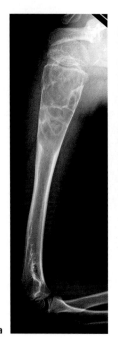

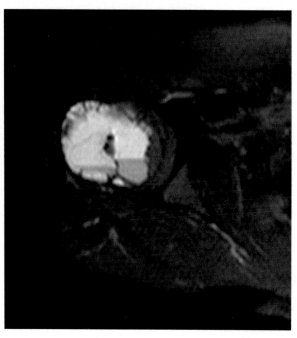

Fig. 5.122a, b   Aneurysmal bone cyst arising from the metaphysis. Bubbly lucent and expansile lesion (**a**) with fluid-fluid levels on MRI (**b**).

a

b

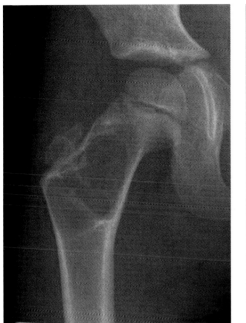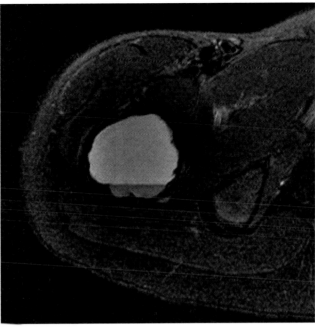

Fig. 5.123a, b   Unicameral bone cyst at the proximal femur. Expansile lucent lesion on radiography (**a**) with a fluid-fluid level on fat-saturated T2-weighted MRI (**b**).

Table 5.70   (Cont.) Tumors and focal lesions: metaphysis

Diagnosis	Findings	Comments
Osteosarcoma ▷*Fig. 5.124a, b* ▷*Fig. 5.125a–c, p. 580*	(see **Table 5.76**)	
Enchondromatosis (including Ollier disease and Maffucci syndrome) ▷*Fig. 5.126a, b, p. 580* ▷*Fig. 5.127a–c, p. 581*	(see **Table 5.75**)	

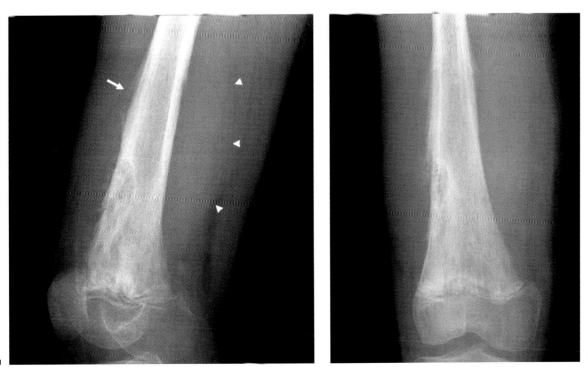

Fig. 5.124a, b   Osteosarcoma arising from the distal femur with a Codman triangle (arrow), soft-tissue mass (arrowheads), and exuberant bone formation (**a, b**).

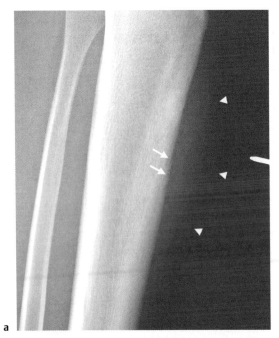

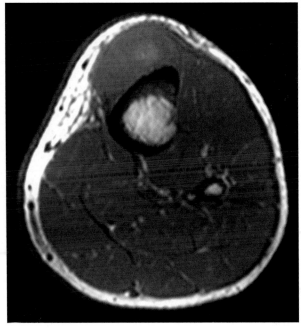

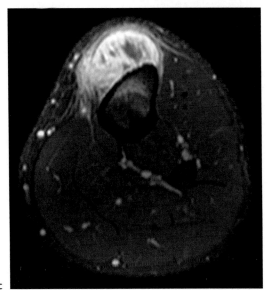

Fig. 5.125a–c   Periosteal osteosarcoma arising from the proximal tibia. (**a**) Patient presented with swelling (arrowheads) after minor trauma. (**b, c**) Cortical erosion (arrows in **a**) on radiography prompted a subsequent MRI that showed an enhancing mass eroding the underlying bone.

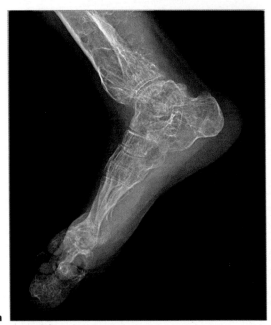

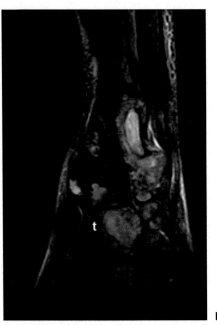

Fig. 5.126a, b   Ollier disease with diffuse enchondromatosis on radiograph (**a**) and STIR MRI (**b**).
t   Talus

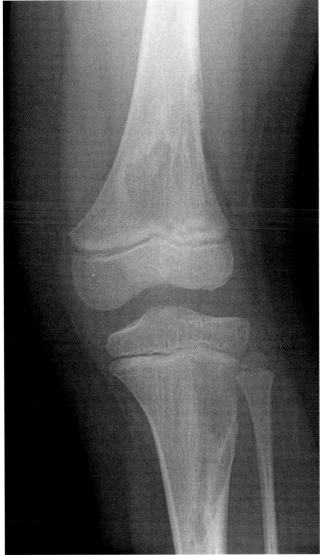

a

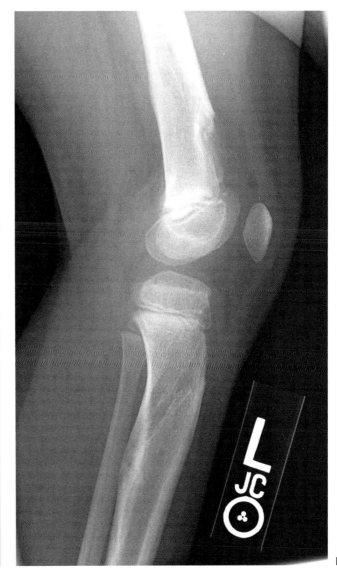

b

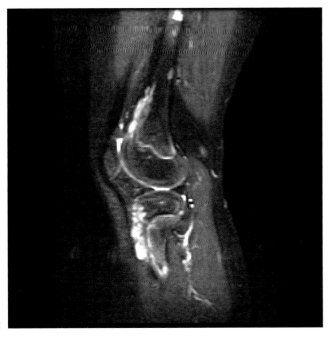

c

Fig. 5.127a–c Enchondromatosis about the knee. (a, b) Radiography shows lucencies in the metaphyses. **(c)** T2-weighted MRI shows cartilage signal intensity.

Table 5.71   Tumors and focal lesions: diaphyseal lesions

Diagnosis	Findings	Comments
Subacute osteomyelitis	Mixed lucent and sclerotic lesion.	
Bone infarct ▷ *Fig. 5.128* ▷ *Fig. 5.113, p. 573*	Coarse sclerotic calcifications confined to the medulla. Serpiginous alternating bands of high and low T2-weighted signal intensity on MRI.	DD: Enchondroma, fibrous dysplasia, NOF, interosseous lipoma. Patients usually have predisposing history for infarcts (sickle cell disease, steroids, etc.). Differentiate from AVN = osteonecrosis of the subchondral bone predisposing to collapse of the joint.
Fibrous dysplasia (monostotic) ▷ *Fig. 5.91, p. 558*	Well-defined geographic lesion with narrow zone of transition. Appearance depends on the relative contribution of fibrous tissue and bone. More fibrous lesions have a cystic or ground-glass matrix. More osseous lesions have scattered calcifications or thick rim (rind sign) of sclerosis. Variable appearance on MRI.	Monostotic 70%–80% of case. Age 10–50 y. Replacement of cancellous bone by fibrous tissue. Common sites: midshaft of tibia, proximal femur, and ribs.
Fibrous dysplasia (polyostotic) ▷ *Fig. 5.116, p. 574*	Multiple lesions. Similar features as monostotic form but may appear more aggressive.	Polyostotic 20%–30% of cases. Tends to involve only one side of body. Similar locations as monostotic form plus: jaw, pelvis, forearm, hands, feet, and fibula. McCune-Albright syndrome is associated with geographic nevi and endocrine abnormality (precocious puberty). Mazabraud syndrome: fibrous dysplasia and intramuscular myxomas.
Unicameral bone cyst	(see **Table 5.70**)	
Osteoid osteoma	(see **Table 5.76**)	
Osteoblastoma	(see **Table 5.76**)	
Langerhans cell histiocytosis	Lesions in diaphysis may have more periosteal reaction than the lytic lesions in other sites.	Variable appearance from a punched out lytic lesion to a mixed lytic and sclerotic lesion.
Ewing sarcoma family of tumors ▷ *Fig. 5.129a–c*	Variable appearance. Poorly marginated lesion with permeative or moth-eaten pattern of bone destruction. Lamellated periosteal new bone formation or sunburst periosteal reaction. Large soft-tissue mass. Soft-tissue mass may cause saucerization.	Age 5–25 y. Second most common bone tumor of childhood. Long bones of lower extremity > pelvis > spine. Femur > ilium > tibia.[42] Varying degrees of neuroectodermal differentiation (Ewing sarcome, Askin sarcoma, primitive neuroectodermal tumor [PNET]). Sclerosis in tumor may resemble osteoid formation of osteosarcoma.
Lymphoma ▷ *Fig. 5.73, p. 544*	Variable appearance. Tends to involve a large portion of bone. Geographic lytic destruction with moth-eaten or permeative pattern. Ivory bone (especially vertebra). Periosteal reaction and soft-tissue masses. Diffuse marrow infiltration on MRI.	Occurs in patients aged 10–70 y. Primary lymphoma of bone is very uncommon. DD: metastatic neuroblastoma, Ewing sarcoma, osteosarcoma.
Enchondroma ▷ *Fig. 5.130, p. 584*	Matrix of coarse sclerotic, punctate, or annular calcifications (arcs and whirls). Homogeneous high signal intensity on T2-weighted MRI with a lobular configuration.	Small lesions may appear similar to bone infarcts. Difficult to distinguish enchondroma from a low-grade chondrosarcoma (localized cortical thickening and lesions > 4 cm in length may indicated chondrosarcoma). Occurs in patients aged 15–40 y.
Benign fibrous histiocytoma (xanthofibroma or fibrous xanthoma)	Similar features as NOF but often develops at an atypical location or appears more aggressive.	Occurs in patients aged 15–60 y. Located in diaphysis or, in contrast to NOF, the articular end of a long bone, ribs, and pelvis. Locally aggressive with recurrence after resection.
Adamantinoma	Well-demarcated, elongated osteolytic lesion separated by sclerotic bone ± soap bubble lucencies. Heterogeneous signal intensity on MRI.	Rare malignant tumor mainly arising at the proximal diaphysis of the tibia ≫ middle humerus, proximal radius, and proximal fibula. Occurs in patients aged 10–40 y. May have satellite lesions.
Osteofibrous dysplasia	Similar in appearance to NOF and fibrous dysplasia.	Classically seen at proximal or middle third of the tibia.

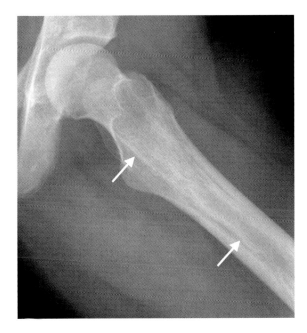

Fig. 5.128 Bone infarct with increased sclerosis in the proximal diaphysis and characteristic bone-within-bone appearance (arrows) in sickle cell disease.

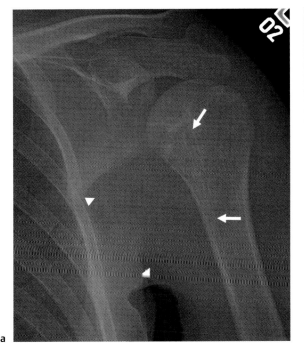

a

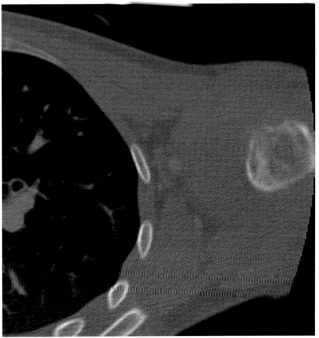

b

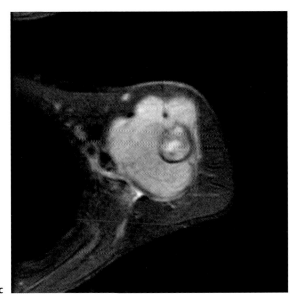

c

Fig. 5.129a–c Ewing sarcoma arising from the proximal humerus with a mottled bone architecture, wide zone of transition (arrows in **a**), and large soft-tissue mass (arrowheads in **a**). (**b**) The cortical destruction is demonstrated on the coned-down image from the screening chest CT. (**c**) The mass enhances and displaces the biceps tendons on MRI.

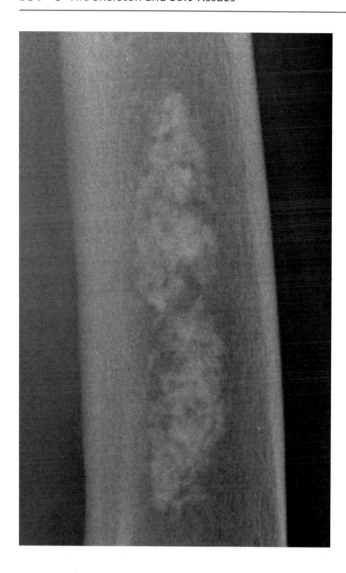

Fig. 5.130   Enchondroma with arcs and rings pattern of mineralized chondroid matrix.

Table 5.72   Tumors and focal lesions: pelvic lesions

Diagnosis	Findings	Comments
Fibrous dysplasia	(see **Table 5.71**)	
Aneurysmal bone cyst ▷ *Fig. 5.131a–c*	(see **Table 5.70**)	Pelvis is less common site.
Ewing sarcoma	(see **Table 5.71**)	
Chondrosarcoma	Similar appearance to an enchondroma but more aggressive.	Rare in children. Occur in children in atypical locations and may have a poorer prognosis.

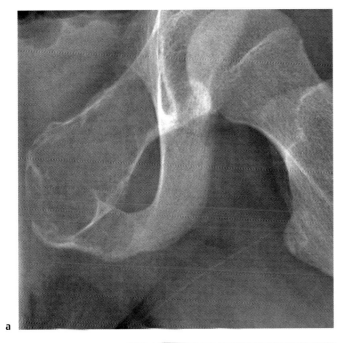

a

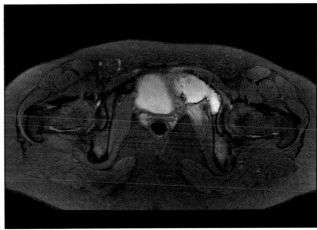

b

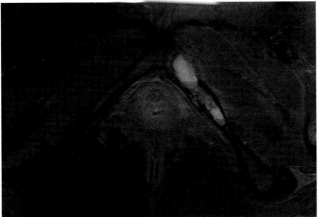

c

Fig. 5.131a–c   Aneurysmal bone cyst arising in the left pubic bone. Expansile and lucent lesion (a) with fluid-fluid levels on MRI (b, c).

Table 5.73   Tumors and focal lesions: scapular lesions

Diagnosis	Findings	Comments
Round blue cell tumors ▷ *Fig. 5.132, p. 586*	Destructive lesion with periosteal reaction and cortical disruption usually extending throughout the entire glenoid.	Ewing sarcoma, Langerhans cell histiocytosis, and osteomyelitis may be indistinguishable on imaging.
Osseous Bankart lesion	Fracture of the anteroinferior glenoid after an anteroinferior dislocation of the humeral head.	
Stress fracture ▷ *Fig. 5.133a–d, p. 586*	Typically occurs at the neck or body.	
Inflamed bursa (snapping scapula syndrome) ▷ *Fig. 5.134, p. 587*	Focal region of soft-tissue thickening/fluid in the chest wall between the chest wall and undersurface of the body of the scapula (usually near the medial tip).	A snapping or clicking may be reproduced on shoulder adduction and abduction.

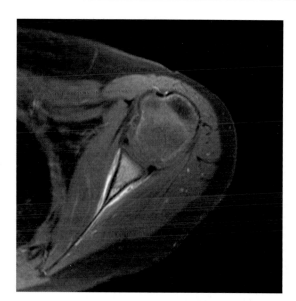

Fig. 5.132　Langerhans cell histiocytosis. Diffuse bone marrow edema and periosteal reaction involve the body and glenoid of the scapula on T2-weighted fat-saturated MRI.

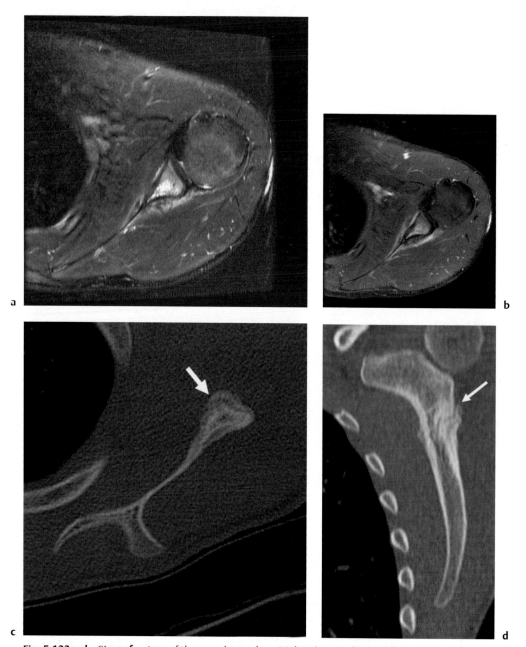

Fig. 5.133a–d　Stress fracture of the scapula may be mistaken (as was this one) for a tumor on MRI. MRI shows increased T2-weighted signal intensity (**a**) and enhancement about the body and glenoid (**b**). Screening chest CT for lung metastases (**c**) shows smooth periosteal reaction and reconstructed coronal images (**d**) confirm a healing fracture line (arrows in **c** and **d**).

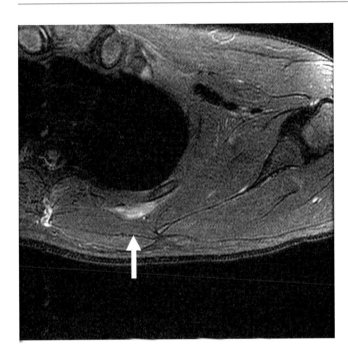

Fig. 5.134 Snapping scapula syndrome with an inflamed bursa between the scapula and chest wall (arrow).

Table 5.74 Tumors and focal lesions: chest wall masses[43,44]

Diagnosis	Findings	Comments
Benign (anatomic variation)	Variation in anatomy of rib, costal cartilage, tilted sternum, bifid rib, breast tissue.	(see **Tables 5.1** and **5.6**)
Lipoma	Fat density on CT and follows the signal intensity of fat on all MRI pulse sequences.	May contain septations.
Ewing sarcoma and PNET ▷ *Fig. 5.7, p. 497*	Chest wall mass with bone destruction ± pleural effusion.	Typically involves one rib at the time of presentation. May invade lung.
Infection ▷ *Fig. 5.135a–c, p. 588*	Large chest wall mass with underlying bone destruction.	DD: Actinomycosis, tuberculosis, blastomycosis, cryptococcosis, nocardiosis. May be misinterpreted as a tumor.
Vascular malformation	(see **Table 5.77**)	May extend from the chest wall into the neck, upper extremity, and/or mediastinum.
Rhabdomyosarcoma	Large soft-tissue mass with variable density due to cystic and solid components.	Rib involvement is uncommon, unlike Ewing sarcoma and PNET. Invasion into adjacent structures.
Chondrosarcoma	Large mass with bone destruction and scattered areas of calcification with a chondroid matrix.	Typically arises from the anterior chest wall (sternum or costochondral arches) or scapula. Rare in children.
Osteosarcoma	(see **Table 5.76**)	Chest is a rare site of involvement. Arises from a rib, scapula, or clavicle. Ossification may not be visible in some patients.
Other sarcomas		Rare: synovial, malignant peripheral nerve sheath tumors (neurofibromatosis type 1), leiomyosarcoma, fibrosarcoma, hemangiopericytoma, etc.
Neuroblastoma	Soft-tissue mass ± bone destruction either a metastasis or extension from paraspinal disease.	Chest wall is an uncommon site for neuroblastoma.
Lipoblastoma	Fat containing.	Locally invasive.
Desmoid tumor	Heterogeneously enhancing mass with destruction of the ribs.	

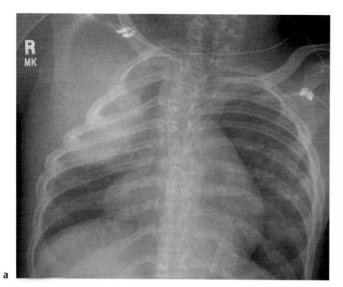

a

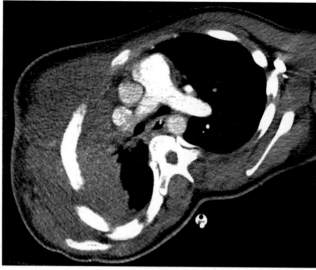

b

c

Fig. 5.135a–c   Actinomycosis mass arising from the right chest wall displaces the scapula on radiography (**a**). The soft-tissue mass encases the upper chest wall (**b**) and causes periosteal reaction in the ribs (**c**).

Table 5.75   Tumors and focal lesions: multiple lesions

Diagnosis	Findings	Comments
Metastasis ▷ *Fig. 5.136a–c* ▷ *Fig. 5.137a, b, p. 590*	Multiple lytic or blastic lesions on radiography. Altered bone marrow signal intensity on MRI. Pathologic fractures. Bone demineralization.	Neuroblastoma, leukemia, Langerhans cell histiocytosis, rhabdomyosarcoma.
Fibrous dysplasia ▷ *Fig. 5.116, p. 574*	(see **Table 5.71**)	
Brown tumor	Well-circumscribed lucent regions in bone. May be accompanied by other findings of hyperparathyroidism: erosions, granular (salt-and-pepper) skull, etc.	Hyperparathyroidism presents as "stones, bones, and groans." Both primary and secondary forms of hyperparathyroidism may lead to lytic lesions in bone. Tumors in the primary form are usually seen in adults. The secondary form is most often the result of chronic renal failure and lytic lesions have an increased incidence with age.[45]
Langerhans cell histiocytosis ▷ *Fig. 5.8, p. 497*	Expansile and well-defined lucent lesion.	Skeletal survey may be useful to detect multiple lesions.
Multiple hereditary exostoses	(see **Table 5.70**)	Growth of multiple osteochondromas around areas of active bone growth. May lead to shortening and bowing of bones and mass effect on adjacent soft tissues.

(continues on page 591)

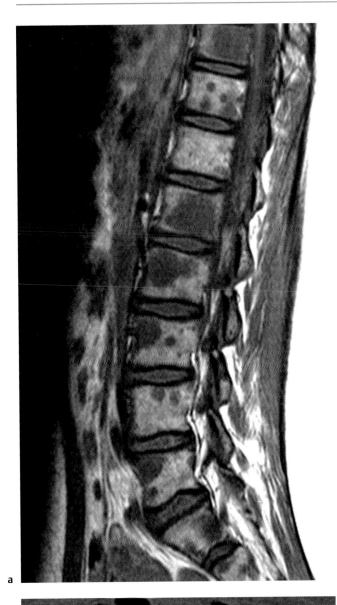

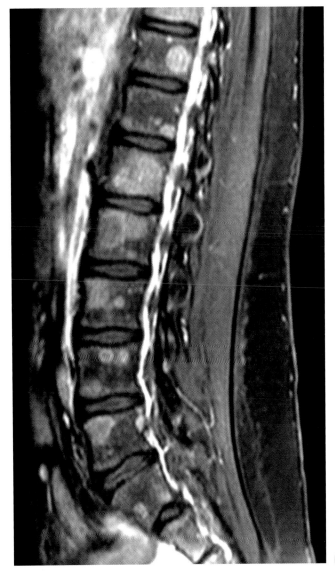

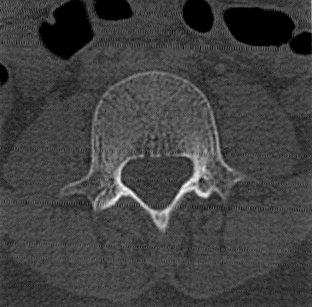

Fig. 5.136a–c   Pre-B cell acute lymphocytic leukemia. Multiple lesions on T1-weighted MRI (**a, b**) enhance after gadolinium administration were occult on CT imaging (**c**).

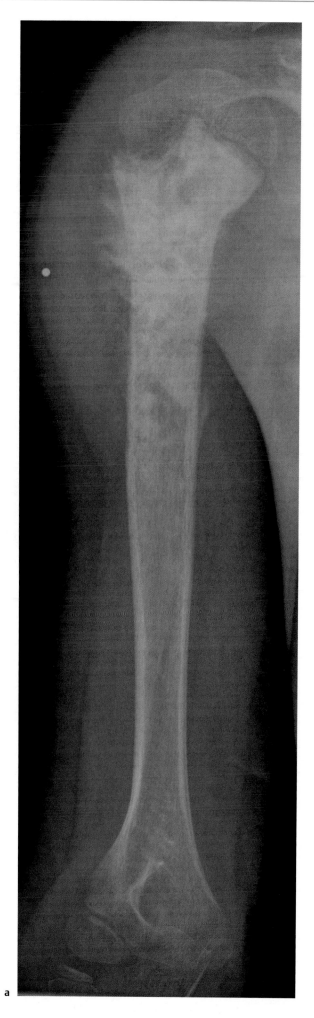

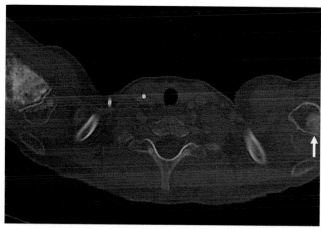

Fig. 5.137a, b   Blastic metastasis. The primary osteosarcoma in the proximal right humerus (**a**) and blastic metastatis (arrow in **b**).

Table 5.75 (Cont.) Tumors and focal lesions: multiple lesions

Diagnosis	Findings	Comments
Enchondromatosis (including Ollier disease and Maffucci syndrome) ▷ *Fig. 5.126, p. 580* ▷ *Fig. 5.127, p. 581*	Multiple enchondromas (see **Table 5.71** for description of an enchondroma).	Ollier: extensive involvement of enchondromas usually unilateral and distributed in metaphyses and diaphyses most commonly in the hands. Maffucci: similar distribution of enchondromas as Ollier plus soft-tissue hemangiomas.
Angiomatosis (hemangiomatosis and lymphangiomatosis) ▷ *Fig. 5.138a–c* ▷ *Fig. 5.139, p. 592*	Osteolytic lesion rimmed by sclerosis or with a narrow zone of transition. May have a honeycomb appearance.	Occurs in patients aged 8–30 y. Diaphyses of long bones, pelvis, and spine. May rarely appear sclerotic. Gorham disease (congenital with massive destruction of bone).
Angiosarcoma	Nonspecific imaging appearance. Aggressive lytic lesion with wide zone of transition. May have a honeycomb appearance similar to angiomatosis.	Occurs in patients aged 10–60 y. More common in skin and soft tissues than bone (~6%). Long bones > pelvis.

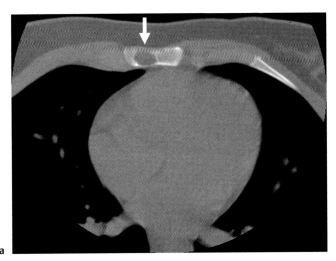

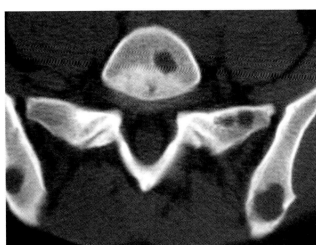

a

c

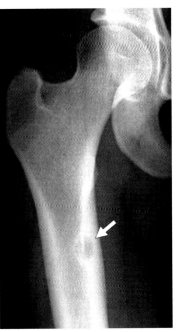

b

Fig. 5.138a–c **Lymphangiomatosis** with lytic lesions involving the sternum (arrow in **a**), femur (arrow in **b**), and pelvis (**c**).

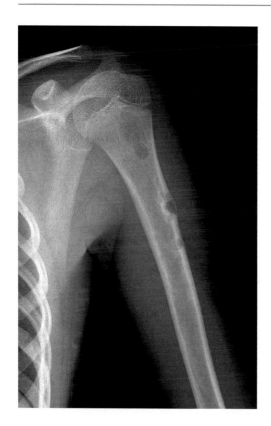

Fig. 5.139 Lymphangiomatosis with bone involvement (Gorham disease).

Table 5.76   Tumors and focal lesions: bone- or cartilage-forming

Diagnosis	Findings	Comments
Benign		
Enostosis (bone island) ▷ *Fig. 5.101, p. 563*	Well-marginated focus of cortical bone within cancellous (trabecular) bone.	Endosteal equivalent of an osteoma.
Osteoma ▷ *Fig. 5.140*	Dense ivorylike sclerotic mass with sharply demarcated boarder attached to the bone.	Slow-growing solid lesion after 10 y of age. Skull and jaw > long bones.
Enchondroma	Calcifications in the intramedullary space. Calcifications range from punctuate to rings. ± Endosteal scalloping and expansion.	May be difficult to distinguish between enchondroma and low-grade chondrosarcoma.
Osteoid osteoma ▷ *Fig. 5.141a, b* ▷ *Fig. 5.142a–c, p. 594*	Very thick smooth cortical thickening and a lucent center (nidus). DD: chronic osteomyelitis and cortical stress fracture.	Fifty percent have typical clinical presentation of night pain relieved with anti-inflammatory medications. Two-y delay from onset of symptoms until diagnosis.
Osteoblastoma ▷ *Fig. 5.142a–c, p. 594* ▷ *Fig. 5.143a, b, p. 595*	Spherical or slightly oval lucent lesions marginated by sclerosis.	Four distinct types: (1) almost identical to osteoid osteoma but larger (> 2 cm diameter), (2) expansive lesion, (3) simulating an aggressive neoplasm, (4) periosteal (juxtacortical).[46]
Heterotopic bone formation ▷ *Fig. 5.144, p. 595*	Soft-tissue ossification near joints.	May lead to bridging and ankylosis of the joint.
Juxtacortical myositis ossificans ▷ *Fig. 5.108, p. 569*	Ossified lesion abutting the cortex.	History of trauma may be difficult to elicit from a child.
Tuberous sclerosis ▷ *Fig. 5.145, p. 595*	Dense sclerotic lesions.	Not to be confused with an osteoblastic lesion in a patient with tuberous sclerosis.
Melorheostosis ▷ *Fig. 5.9, p. 498*	Intramedullary sclerosis with the appearance of dripping candle wax.	Follows dermatomes.
Malignant		
Osteosarcoma primary ▷ *Fig. 5.146a–c, p. 596* ▷ *Fig. 5.124, p. 579*	Aggressive mixed lucent and sclerotic lesion: permeative or moth-eaten bone destruction, wide zone of transition, cloudlike opacities of new bone formation, aggressive periosteal reaction (Codman triangle), soft-tissue mass.	Variable amount of bone formation. May be classified into subtypes based on World Health Organization.[46]

(continues on page 597)

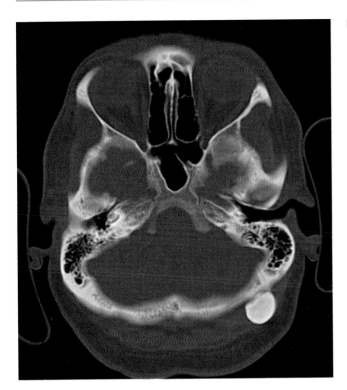

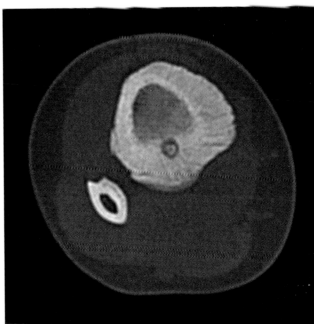

Fig. 5.140   Osteoma arising off the posterior skull.

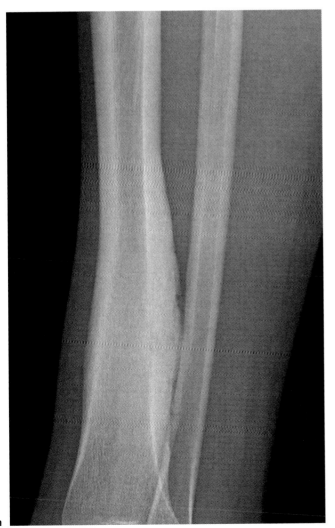

a

b

Fig. 5.141a, b   Osteoid osteoma. Thick periosteal reaction from osteoid osteoma on radiography (**a**). (**b**) The periosteal reaction surrounds the central nidus on CT.

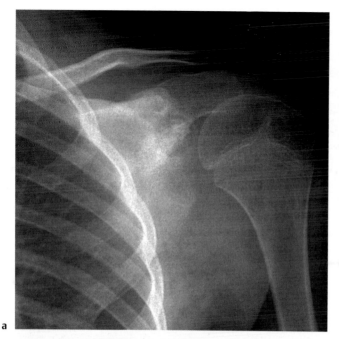

a

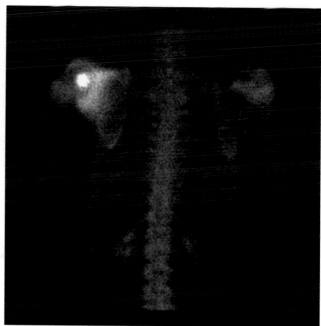

b

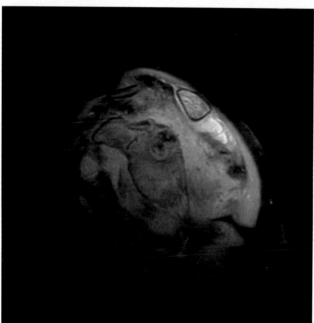

c

Fig. 5.142a–c   **Osteoblastoma** with a mixed lucent and sclerotic lesion in the left scapula (**a**). (**b**) Intense activity is seen in the nidus on bone scan. (**c**) A large region of bone marrow edema surrounds the nidus on the sagittal proton-density fat-saturated MRI.

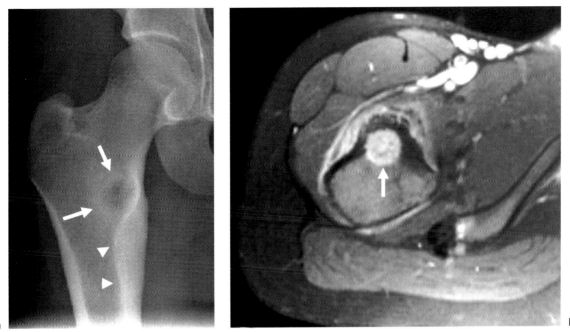

a

b

Fig. 5.143a, b   Osteoblastoma in the proximal femur of a 15-year-old (**a**) with lucent nidus (arrows) and thick periosteal reaction (arrowheads). (**b**) T1-weighted MRI shows the periosteal reaction enhancement in the nidus (arrow).

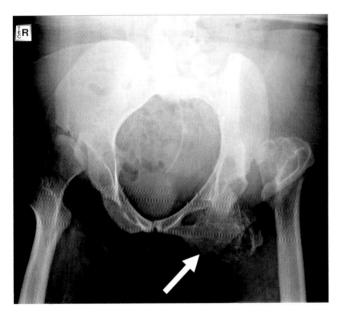

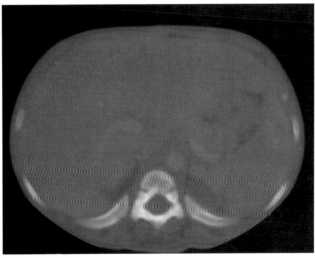

Fig. 5.144   Chronic heterotopic bone formation (arrow) in a 29-year-old with spina bifida and chronic hip dislocations.

Fig. 5.145   Tuberous sclerosis simulating a blastic metastasis.

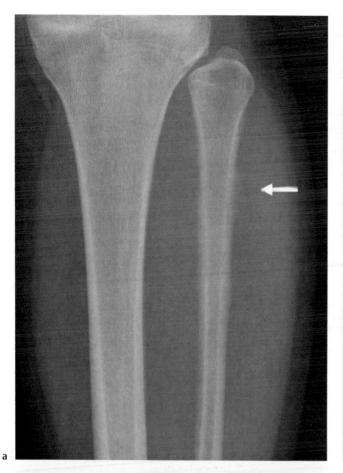

a

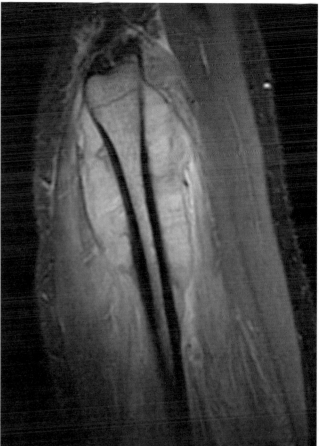

b

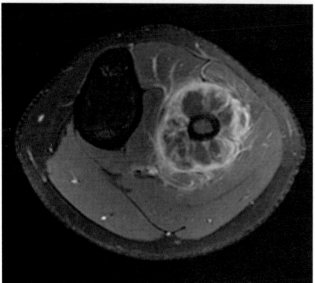

c

Fig. 5.146a–c Osteosarcoma primary. Sunburst pattern of periosteal reaction from chondroblastic osteosarcoma (arrow in **a**) with corresponding appearance on (**b**) STIR and (**c**) T1-weighted post-contrast imaging.

Table 5.76   (Cont.) Tumors and focal lesions: bone- or cartilage-forming

Diagnosis	Findings	Comments
Malignant (cont.)		
Chondrosarcoma	Aggressive mixed lucent and sclerotic lesion. Calcifications range from punctuate to rings.	Clues to differentiate from enchondroma include pain, progressive destruction of the chondroid matrix, large size, and a large unmineralized component.
Secondary sarcoma ▷ *Fig. 5.147a–c*	May arise in area of prior intervention or disturbance.	Following extraskeletal irradiation, chemotherapy, and treatment for retinoblastoma.[47] Malignant transformation within a benign process (Paget disease, fibrous dysplasia, bone infarct) usually occurs in adulthood.

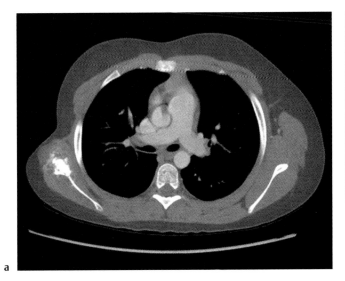
a

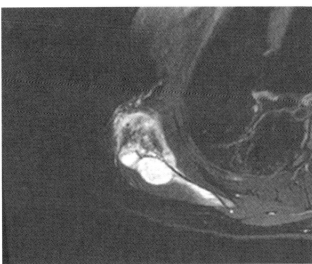
b

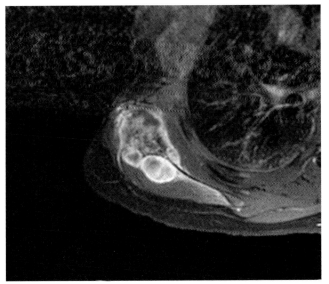
c

Fig. 5.147a–c   Secondary chondrosarcoma arising from the scapula in a patient 7 years after treatment for rhabdomyosarcoma of the axilla. (**a**) CT shows bone destruction and soft-tissue mass. (**b**) MRI shows increased T2-weighted signal intensity and enhancement of the mass (**c**).

Table 5.77 Tumors and focal lesions: soft-tissue masses[48]

Diagnosis	Findings	Comments
Benign		
Cyst or bursa ▷ *Fig. 5.148a, b* ▷ *Fig. 5.31, p. 515*	Fluid-filled cyst (anechoic on US; dark on T1- and bright on T2-weighted MRI sequences).	Rim of cyst may enhance. Examples: synovial cyst, ganglion cyst, popliteal cyst, iliopsoas bursa, etc.
Myositis ossificans ▷ *Fig. 5.107, p. 568* ▷ *Fig. 5.108, p. 569*	Soft-tissue mass rimmed by a peripheral margin of ossification separate from the adjacent bone. May appear aggressive on MRI with increased T2-weighted signal intensity and enhancement.	History of trauma not always elicited from children. Amorphous calcifications may be seen early (1–2 wk) after trauma.
Abscess	Fluid-filled structure with a thick wall that may be hyperemic on US and enhance on MRI or CT.	Clinical signs and symptoms of infection are typically present.
Myositis/cellulitis ▷ *Fig. 5.149*	Soft-tissue swelling on radiography. Increased fluid signal, swelling, and enhancement on MRI.	May be focal or diffuse.
Myonecrosis ▷ *Fig. 5.150*	Soft-tissue mass with central necrosis.	May be seen in patients after trauma or with sickle cell disease.

(continues on page 599)

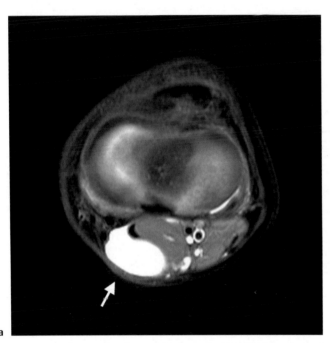
a

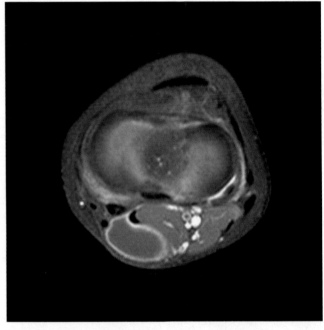
b

Fig. 5.148a, b Popliteal cyst. MRI shows the fluid-filled cyst (arrow in **a**) with rim enhancement (**b**).

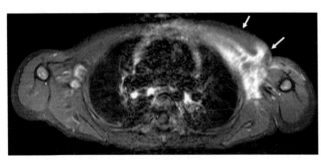

Fig. 5.149 Myositis of the left pectoralis muscles with gadolinium enhancement and swelling on MRI (arrows).

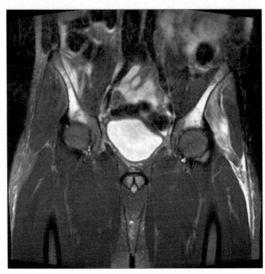

Fig. 5.150 Osteonecrosis and myonecrosis in a child with sickle cell disease.

Table 5.77   (Cont.) Tumors and focal lesions: soft-tissue masses[48]

Diagnosis	Findings	Comments
Benign (cont.)		
Vascular malformation ▷ *Fig. 5.109, p. 570*	May produce periosteal reaction, chronic cortical thickening or remodeling of adjacent bone. High or low flow vascular mass on US or magnetic resonance angiography/magnetic resonance venography.	Venous malformations may contain phleboliths. Classified as capillary, venous, lymphatic, or combined malformations.
Lipoma	Usually well-defined mass that follows signal intensity of fat (T1 bright, T2 fast spin echo bright, and dark on STIR and fat-saturated pulse sequences).	
Giant cell tumor of the tendon sheath	Nodular mass attached to a tendon. Characteristic low to intermediate T1- and low T2-weighted signal intensity on MRI. Variable gadolinium enhancement.	Not really a tumor, but more of a reactive lesion. Seen at tendons that have a synovial-lined tendon sheath. Localized form is usually seen at hands and feet. The diffuse form is rare, affects the lower extremities, and is the counterpart to PVNS affecting joints.
Peripheral nerve tumors ▷ *Fig. 5.151a–d*	Focal mass. Similar or slightly increased in intensity to adjacent muscle on T1- and T2-weighted MRI. Target sign (hyperintense rim with low central T2-weighted signal intensity).	DD: schwannoma, neurofibroma, and neurofibromatosis.

(continues on page 600)

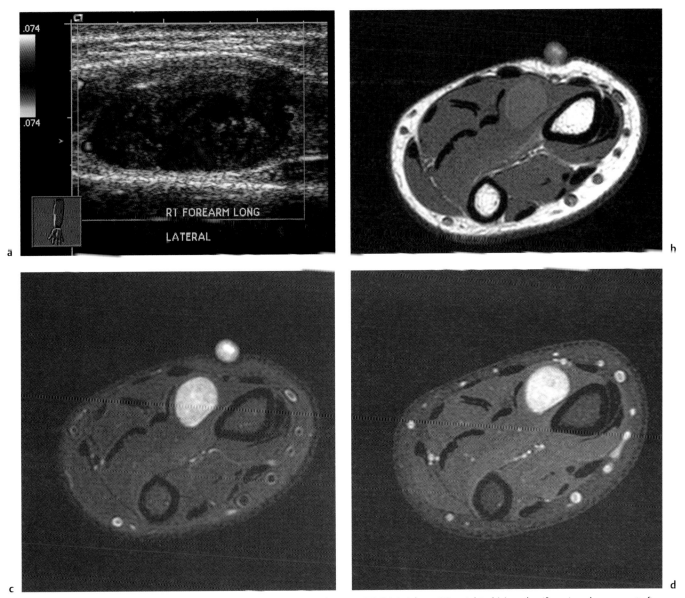

Fig. 5.151a–d   Peripheral nerve tumor. Schwannoma arising in the muscles of the forearm. (**a**) US shows a solid mass with blood flow. MRI shows an encapsulated mass that is intermediate in signal intensity on T1 (**b**), bright on T2-weighted (**c**), and uniform in enhancement after gadolinium administration (**d**).

Table 5.77 (Cont.) Tumors and focal lesions: soft-tissue masses[48]

Diagnosis	Findings	Comments
Benign (cont.)		
Rheumatoid nodules ▷ *Fig. 5.152a–c*	Subcutaneous soft-tissue masses usually 1–4 cm located near joints.	Common locations include the posterior elbow and inferior heal.
Juvenile fibromatosis	Variable appearance on MRI. Focal or infiltrative with enhancement in the cellular portions of the tumor.	Local recurrence.
Nodular fasciitis ▷ *Fig. 5.153a, b*	Soft-tissue mass arising from the fascia.	Rapidly growing benign mass most commonly found in the superficial fascia.
Osteoblastoma	(see **Table 5.76**)	Extraskeletal osteoblastoma is a rare presentation.
Infantile digital fibroma	Enlarging soft-tissue mass ± erosion of a phalanx.	Occurs in patients aged 1–5 y. Recurrent.
Malignant		
Rhabdomyosarcoma ▷ *Fig. 5.154a–c*	Variable appearance of a soft-tissue mass ± bone invasion.[49]	Limb involvement is less common than in the central nervous system and genitourinary system.
Nonrhabdomyosarcoma ▷ *Fig. 5.155a–c, p. 602*	Variable appearance of a soft-tissue mass.	DD: synovial sarcoma, epithelioid sarcoma, liposarcoma, malignant peripheral nerve sheath tumor, clear cell sarcoma, infantile fibrosarcoma, hemangiopericytoma, leiomyosarcoma, alveolar soft part sarcoma, malignant fibrous histiocytoma, angiosarcoma, fibromyxoid sarcoma, extraskeletal myxoid chondrosarcoma, spindle-cell sarcoma, etc.
Lymphoma	Variable appearance of a soft-tissue mass.	May present with symptoms localized to the site of soft-tissue involvement, as an incidental finding on imaging for other reasons, or as part of the staging of the disease.

(continues on page 602)

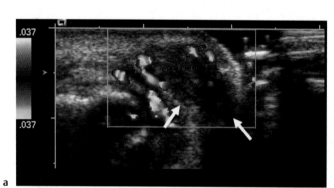

a

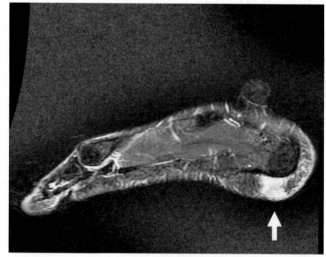

b

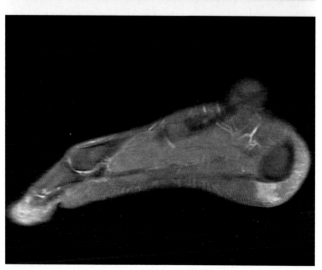

c

Fig. 5.152a–c Rheumatoid nodules (**a–c**) in the superficial soft tissues of the heel (arrows in **a** and **b**) as demonstrated on us (**a**) and T2-weighted fat-saturated MRI (**b**) and T1-weighted postcontrast MRI (**c**).

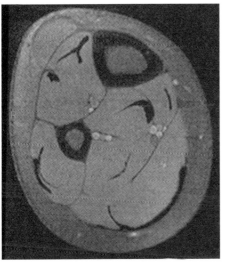
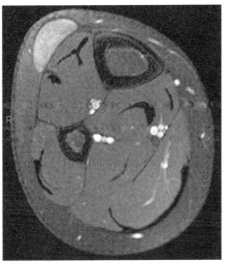

Fig. 5.153a, b   Nodular fasciitis (**a**) arising from the anterior compartment fascia of the proximal calf (**b**) enhances after gadolinium.

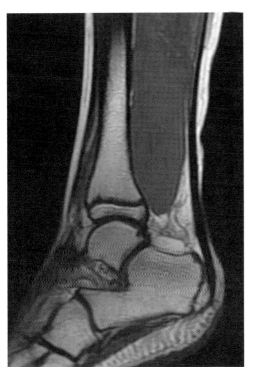
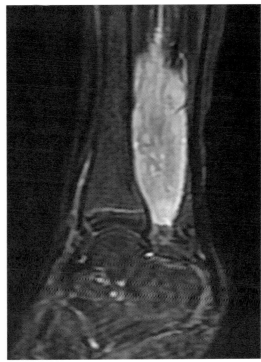

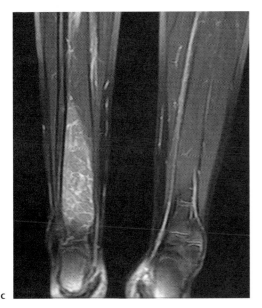

Fig. 5.154a–c   Rhabdomyosarcoma. (a–c) A soft-tissue mass arising in the distal calf.

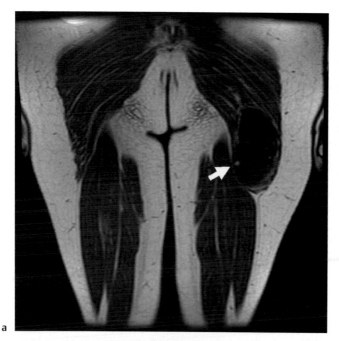

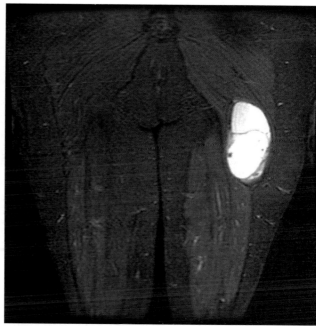

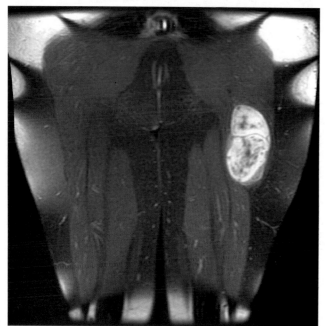

Fig. 5.155a–c   Cystic liposarcoma of the thigh. The signal intensity from a tiny nodule of fat (arrow in **a**) on T1-weighted imaging (**a**) is suppressed on STIR (**b**) and gadolinium-enhanced T1-weighted fat-suppressed (**c**) imaging.

Table 5.77   (Cont.) Tumors and focal lesions: soft-tissue masses[48]

Diagnosis	Findings	Comments
Malignant (cont.)		
Myofibroma ▷ *Fig. 5.156a, b*		
Synovial cell sarcoma ▷ *Fig. 5.157a–c*	Soft-tissue mass typically located in close proximity to a joint.	One of the nonrhabdomyosarcomas most commonly seen adjacent to the knee. Tissue type is unrelated to the synoviocytes that line the joint spaces.
Extraskeletal Ewing sarcoma ▷ *Fig. 5.158, p. 604*	Variable appearance of a soft-tissue mass.	Occurs in patients aged 3–71 y. May develop in the extremities, genitourinary and gastrointestinal tracts and central nervous system.
Extraskeletal osteosarcoma[50]	Ill-defined heterogeneous mineralized tumor mass.	Lower extremity and buttock. May be difficult to distinguish from early myositis ossificans. High rate of metastatic disease. Rare: ~4% of all osteosarcomas. More often seen in adults. DD: calcified hematoma, nodular fasciitis, ossifying lipoma, and myositis ossificans.

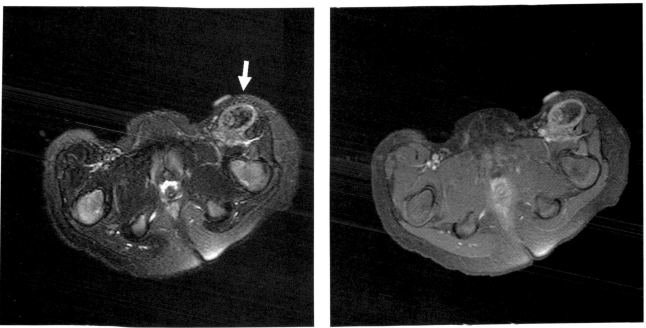

Fig. 5.156a, b **Myofibroma** arising from the proximal thigh (arrow in **a**) on T2-weighted fat-saturated (**a**) and T1-weighted fat-saturated postcontrast–enhanced (**b**) imaging.

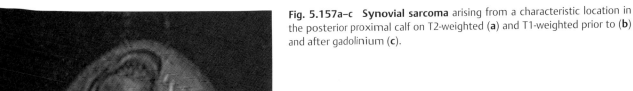

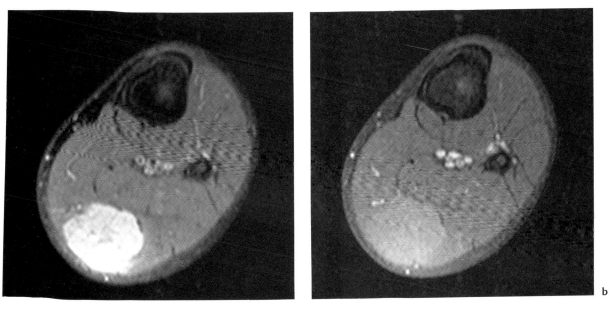

Fig. 5.157a–c **Synovial sarcoma** arising from a characteristic location in the posterior proximal calf on T2-weighted (**a**) and T1-weighted prior to (**b**) and after gadolinium (**c**).

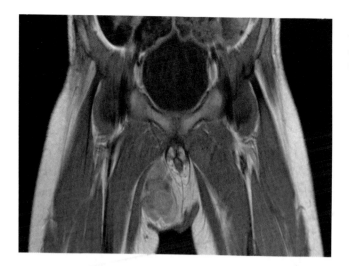

Fig. 5.158 Extraskeletal Ewing sarcoma. A 20-month-old boy with a mass on the medial side of the right upper leg. Gadolinium-enhanced MRI shows a discrete enhancing mass remote from osseous structures; histology showed an extraosseous Ewing sarcoma.

Virtually all palpable, asymptomatic anterior chest wall lesions in children are benign and related to normal variations in the chest wall bone or cartilage.

Table 5.78 Tumors and focal lesions: joints

Diagnosis	Findings	Comments
PVNS ▷ Fig. 5.32, p. 516	Juxta-articular soft-tissue masses with erosive changes in the underlying bone. Masses arising from the synovium have low signal intensity on both T1- and T2-weighted sequences and signal dropout on gradient echo.	Locally destructive proliferative disorder of the synovium. May affect the tendon sheath (giant cell tumor) and bursa (pigmented villonodular bursitis). Adults > children. Vary rarely calcifications may be seen.
Synovial osteochondromatosis ▷ Fig. 5.159a, b	Soft-tissue swelling and joint effusion with many radiopaque bodies, small and uniform in size.	Benign metaplastic proliferation of multiple cartilaginous nodules in the joint, bursa, or tendon sheath. Rarely polyarticular. Differentiate from secondary osteochondromatosis = caused by OA with intra-articular bodies.
JIA ▷ Fig. 5.42, p. 523	Hypertrophied synovium ± enhancement on MRI or increased blood flow on US.	May affect joint or tendon sheaths. Erosions and joint space narrowing are a later finding.
Hemarthrosis (trauma, hemophilia) ▷ Fig. 5.33, p. 517	Uniform joint space narrowing. Hemosiderin in the synovium (dark on T1- and T2-weighted MRI).	Tends to affect large joints. Patients usually already have a diagnosis of trauma or a bleeding disorder.
Synovial hemangioma	Radiographs are often normal. Phleboliths, periosteal thickening, and advanced maturation of the epiphysis may be seen. MRI may characterize the vascular components of the lesion.	Occurs in patients aged 9–49 y. Most commonly affects the knee joint > elbow, wrist, ankle, and tendon sheaths.

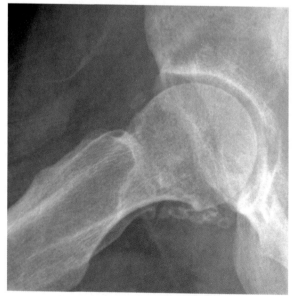

a

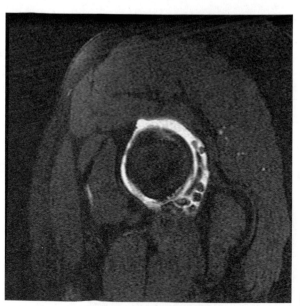

b

Fig. 5.159a, b Synovial osteochondromatosis of the right hip. Ossicles surround the right hip on radiography (**a**) and T1 suppressed magnetic resonance arthrogram (**b**) shows that the osteochondromatosis is located in the joint.

Table 5.79   Tumors and focal lesions: infancy[51]

Diagnosis	Findings	Comments
Vascular malformation	(see **Table 5.77**)	Thrombocytopenia from consumptive coagulopathy.
Congenital fibrosarcoma ▷ *Fig. 5.160*	Radiographically evident soft-tissue mass enveloping, splaying, and resorbing bones without frank bone destruction. Mixed solid and cystic mass with ± areas of necrosis on MRI and ± large draining vein.	Rapidly enlarging soft-tissue mass ± ulceration. More favorable prognosis than adult fibrosarcoma. Thrombocytopenia from disseminated intravascular coagulopathy.
Rhabdomyosarcoma	Soft-tissue mass that usually does not invade bone. Solid or partially cystic on MRI. Well-defined or infiltrative margins.	Approximately 50% arise caudally (buttock, sacrum, bladder, vagina). Approximately 50% have widespread metastatic disease.
Infantile hemangiopericytoma	Large soft-tissue mass ± bone invasion, ± calcific stippling. Vascular mass with feeding vessels but usually no draining vein.	Rapid growth. One-third occur in extremities, one-third the trunk, and one-third head and neck. Rarely metastasize.
Malignant peripheral nerve sheath tumor	Similar appearance as peripheral nerve sheath tumor but more aggressive. May displace or invade bone (see **Table 5.77**).	Rare before the age of 10 y. Associated with neurofibromatosis type 1.
Extrarenal rhabdoid tumor	Variable appearance of a rapidly enlarging soft-tissue mass.[52]	Age < 1 y. Infrequently involves extremities.

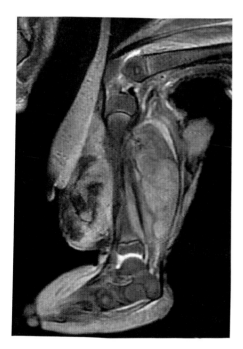

Fig. 5.160   Congenital fibrosarcoma arising from the calf of a neonate on sagittal STIR MRI.

Table 5.80   Soft-tissue alteration without mass

Diagnosis	Findings	Comments
Infection	Increased T2-weighed signal intensity and enhancement in the superficial soft tissues (cellulitis), fascia, or muscles. Soft-tissue swelling and increased echogenicity on US.	Imaging findings that support a clinical diagnosis of necrotizing fasciitis include enhancement and thickening of fascia and gas in the soft tissues.
Muscle or tendon tear	Abnormality confined to the muscle or tendon with increased T2-weighted signal intensity and fluid. Fluid, alterations in the muscle fibers, and a tendon or muscle gap may also be seen on US.	
Dermatomyositis ▷ *Fig. 5.161a–c, p. 606*	Increased T2-weighted signal intensity and enhancement confined to muscles Increased echogenicity and swelling on US.	Usually distributed in muscle groups in the proximal limbs. DD: inclusion body myositis, juvenile myositis, polymyositis.
Fat necrosis ▷ *Fig. 5.162a, b, p. 606*	Linear regions of decreased signal intensity on non–fat-suppressed MRI that have a scarlike appearance.	Although typically localized to sites of prior trauma, patients may not always be able to recall the trauma.

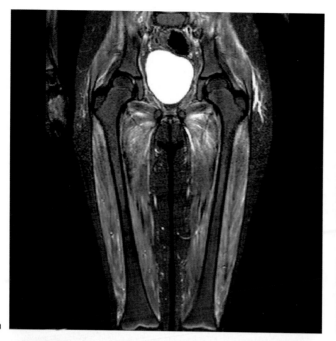

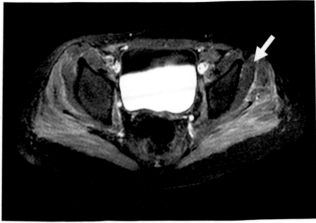

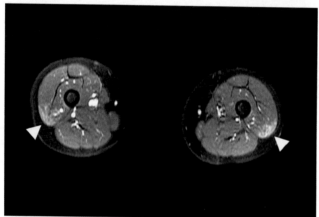

Fig. 5.161a–c Dermatomyositis. Inflammation involves essentially all the muscles of the pelvis and thighs on coronal STIR (**a**) and gadolinium-enhanced T1-weighted fat-suppressed MRI (**b**). Muscle groups around the ilia are less affected (arrow). (**c**) After 6 months of treatment, residual inflammation is seen only in the distal thighs with a small amount of enhancement (arrowheads).

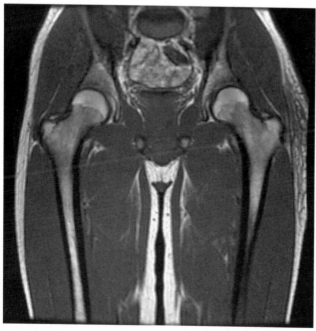

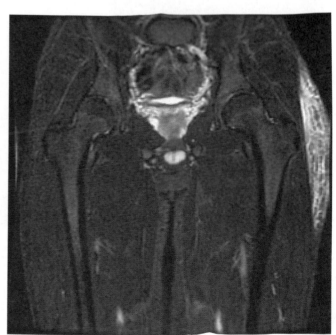

Fig. 5.162a, b Fat necrosis. A 16-year-old with firmness and swelling at the right hip and no clinical signs of cellulitis.

Periosteal Reaction[53]

The periosteum is a membrane that covers the majority of bone except at locations at and near cartilage. How periosteum responds to stimuli (e.g., trauma, infection, metabolic process, and neoplasm) can often give clues to the etiology of the underlying stimulus. An aggressive or destructive process will often greatly alter the periosteum, whereas a nonaggressive process usually gives the periosteum the opportunity to remodel with a more orderly architecture. The distribution of periosteal reaction (focal or diffuse) may give clues to the underlying process.

Periosteal reaction may also be grouped into several patterns: smooth, solid or thick, and aggressive (laminar, sunburst, Codman triangle, and cloaking).

Smooth periosteal reaction consists of one or multiple unbroken layers of ossified periosteum along the cortical surface. Smooth periosteal reaction indicates orderly new bone formation; the bone has had time to heal or remodel toward its original architecture. As a rule, the unbroken lamellar reaction suggests a process that is not very aggressive.

Table 5.81 Periosteal reaction: smooth

Diagnosis	Findings	Comments
Benign periosteal reaction of the newborn ▷ *Fig. 5.163*	Smooth symmetric periosteal reaction of rapidly growing bones.	Typically involves rapidly growing bones: femur, tibia, and humerus. Symmetric distribution and age (newborn) also support this diagnosis.
Healing fracture or infection	Smooth periosteal reaction at and adjacent to the injury.	Often seen in plastic/bowing fractures.
Margins of an aggressive process		The periosteum at margins of an aggressive process may be less affected than at the site of maximal destruction. The lesion should be classified based on the more aggressive features.
Vascular insufficiency	Periostitis of affected limb(s).	Especially venous stasis.
Hypertrophic osteoarthropathy	Symmetric periostitis of the radius and ulna > femur, humerus, metacarpals, and metatarsals.	Associated with underlying cardiopulmonary diseases (e.g., cystic fibrosis), infection, and malignancy. Adults > children. Digital clubbing. May affect a single extremity in arterial infections.
Idiopathic hypertrophic osteoarthropathy (pachydermoperiostosis)	Early stage: symmetric subperiosteal new bone formation along the diaphyses of the extremities, hands, and feet. Advanced stage: diffuse subperiosteal bone formation, ossification of ligaments and tendons, ankylosis, acroosteolysis.	Rare hereditary disorder: Digital clubbing, thickened skin and periostosis. Increased uptake along cortical margins on bone scan.

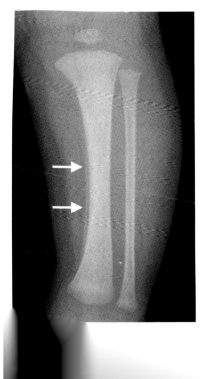

Fig. 5.163 **Benign periosteal reaction of the newborn** (arrows).

Table 5.82   Periosteal reaction: solid or thick new bone formation

Diagnosis	Findings	Comments
Mature fracture healing	Thick bridging callus formation.	
Chronic osteomyelitis ▷ *Fig. 5.164a–c*	Thick periosteal reaction with adjacent mixed lucency and sclerosis.	When thick periosteal reaction is seen on radiographs, CT is useful to distinguish among chronic osteomyelitis, stress fracture, and osteoid osteoma.
Stress fracture	Thick periosteal reaction surrounding a thin fracture line.	Fracture line may only be detectable by CT.
Osteoid osteoma ▷ *Fig. 5.141, p. 593*	Thick periosteal reaction superficial to the nidus.	Periosteal reaction may be related in part to prostaglandin synthesis by the nidus.[54]
Osteoblastoma ▷ *Fig. 5.142, p. 594* ▷ *Fig. 5.143, p. 595*	Similar appearance as osteoid osteoma but larger nidus.	
Chronic sclerosing osteomyelitis (Garré)	Regional periosteal and endosteal new bone formation.	Primarily affects mandible and proximal tibia.
Idiopathic hypertrophic osteoarthropathy (pachydermoperiostosis)	(see **Table 5.81**)	

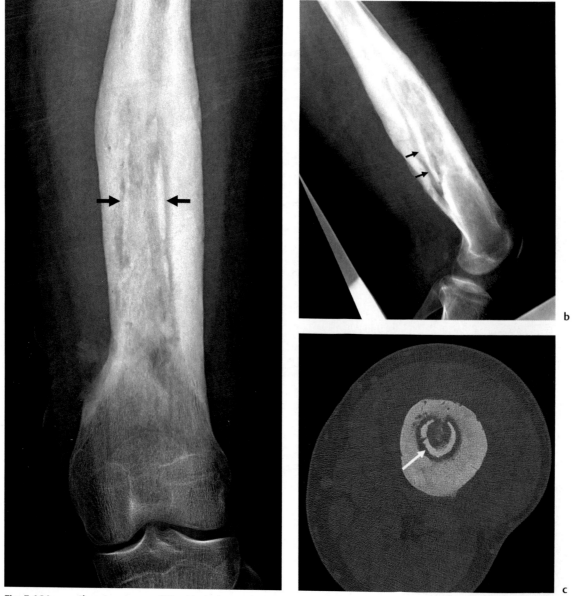

Fig. 5.164a–c   Chronic osteomyelitis with thick irregular periosteal reaction enveloping a sequestrum (arrows) on radiography (**a, b**) and CT (**c**).

Aggressive periosteal reaction is likely the result of disorganized new bone in response to a destructive process. New bone formation cannot keep pace with the accelerated rate of bone destruction. In response to a rapidly destructive process, new bone formation along the periosteum produces several characteristic patterns. Lamellar (onion peel) periosteal reaction appears as successive layers of new bone arising from the periosteal surface. Spiculation is caused by calcification of the periosteal Sharpey fibers, which are oriented perpendicular to the cortical surface. The radial sunburst pattern is a classic sign of osteosarcoma and affects mainly mineralized osteoid. However, the sunburst pattern may also be seen in hemolytic anemias, thalassemia, and sickle cell anemia. The Codman triangle is another sign indicating an aggressive process. The Codman triangle is an acutely-angled triangle of periosteal reaction along the cortex surface and indicates the transition between the periosteum of the aggressive disease process and the uninvolved bone. No tumor cells are found in the Codman triangle. Just as the physis will act as a temporary barrier to the spread of tumor or infection, the periosteal collar will remain intact.

Table 5.83   Periosteal reaction: aggressive (laminar, sunburst, and Codman triangle)

Diagnosis	Findings/Comments
Acute osteomyelitis ▷ *Fig. 5.165a–c*	Bone destruction with varying types of periosteal reaction: Codman triangle, cortical and periosteal destruction, and disorganized periosteal new bone formation.
Thalassemia ▷ *Fig. 5.166, p. 610*	Perpendicular speculation of the long bones and hair-on-end periosteal reaction. Hyperplastic hematopoiesis may extend into the subperiosteal space.
Sickle cell disease ▷ *Fig. 5.167 , p. 610*	Hair-on-end appearance of the skull. Hand-foot syndrome in infancy with dactylitis (periosteal elevation and subperiosteal new bone formation).
Osteosarcoma ▷ *Fig. 5.124 , p. 579* ▷ *Fig. 5.146 , p. 596*	Codman triangle, sunburst pattern, and disorganized periosteal new bone formation.
Ewing sarcoma	Codman triangle and disorganized periosteal new bone formation.
Leukemia	Lamellar periosteal reaction in the long bones. Multiple sites.
Metastasis ▷ *Fig. 5.168 , p. 610*	Cortical destruction. Aggressive periosteal reaction.

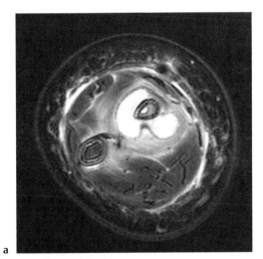

a

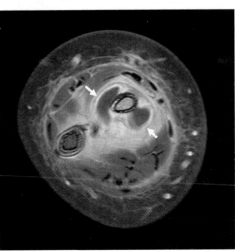

b

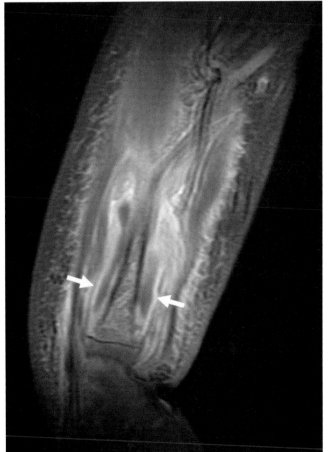

c

Fig. 5.165a–c   Acute osteomyelitis and subperiosteal abscess formation. Fluid has developed deep to the periosteum (arrows in **b** and **c**) around the radius on T2-weighted (**a**) and enhanced T1-weighted (**b, c**) MRI.

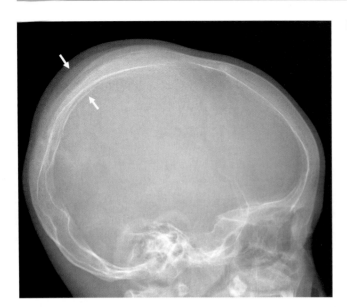

Fig. 5.166 Thalassemia. Hair-on-end appearance of the skull (arrows).

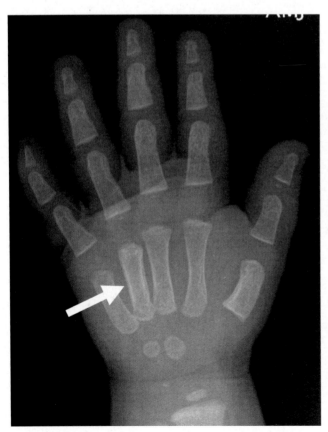

Fig. 5.167 Sickle cell disease with aseptic dactylitis. Periostitis layers along the diaphysis (arrow).

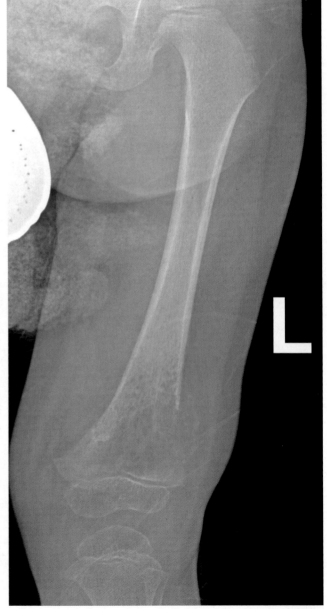

Fig. 5.168 Metastatic neuroblastoma with moth-eaten pattern of lytic bone destruction in the femoral diaphysis and distal metaphysis.

Periosteal cloaking occurs when a long segment of periosteal membrane is altered by disease and results in a long segment of exuberant thickening. Rapidly growing bones appear to be predisposed to producing cloaking in response to injury. Trauma and infection are the most common causes of cloaking.

Table 5.84   Periosteal reaction: cloaking

Diagnosis	Comments
Osteomyelitis	Including syphilis.
Subperiosteal hemorrhage ▷ *Fig. 5.68, p. 541*	Usually after trauma. May be seen in neurofibromatosis type 1 or hemophilia after minor trauma, which leads to chronic dysplastic changes in the bone.
Prostaglandin therapy	Periosteal elevation early in treatment (9–11 d) followed by cloaking.[55] Periosteal elevation is relatively common in infants treated with prostaglandins. After cessation of therapy, the periostitis resolves and the bones normalize.
Rickets	
Metaphyseal fractures in infants	(see **Table 5.98**)
Fractures in neuropathic diseases	
Mucopolysaccharidosis II (Hunter syndrome) ▷ *Fig. 5.169*	Severe osteopenia, widened ribs, and periosteal reaction including cloaking.
Minor trauma in scurvy	Subperiosteal hemorrhage (see **Table 5.43**).
Infantile cortical hyperostosis (Caffey disease)	Subperiosteal cortical hyperostosis. Epiphyses spared. Fever and soft-tissue swelling adjacent to involved bones. Rarely appears after 5 mo and usually resolves spontaneously by 2 y. Imaging appearance will depend on phase of disease.

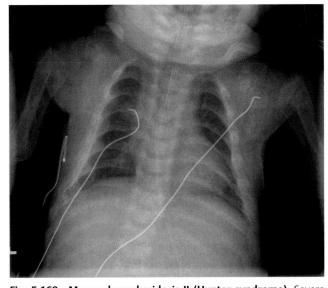

Fig. 5.169   Mucopolysaccharidosis II (Hunter syndrome). Severe osteopenia, widened ribs, and periosteal reaction including cloaking that involves the ribs and humeri.

Table 5.85   Periosteal reaction: fluffy or indistinct

Diagnosis	Comments
Metabolic	Appearance of periosteum will depend on the stage of treatment.
Infantile cortical hyperostosis (Caffey disease)	(see **Table 5.84**)

Table 5.86   Periosteal reaction: focal

Diagnosis	Comments
Trauma	Appearance will vary depending on the stage of healing.
Infection	
Tumor	Langerhans cell histiocytosis, osteoid osteoma, osteosarcoma, Ewing sarcoma.
Vascular	Vascular malformation or venous status.

Table 5.87   Periosteal reaction: diffuse

Diagnosis	Comments
Physiologic ▷ *Fig. 5.163, p. 607*	Benign periosteal reaction of infancy
Infection	Sepsis, chronic granulomatous disease of childhood, syphilis, tuberculosis, fungal
Inflammation	Infantile cortical hyperostosis (Caffey disease)
Hematologic	Sickle cell anemia, thalassemia, hemophilia, leukemia
Metabolic	Rickets, scurvy
Congenital	Pachydermoperiostosis, Camurati-Engelmann disease
Medication/ overdose	Prostaglandin therapy, hypervitaminosis
Tumor	Leukemia, metastases
Miscellaneous	Secondary hypertrophic osteoarthropathy

Bone Marrow Patterns

Table 5.88 Bone marrow: foci of increased T2-weighted signal intensity

Diagnosis	Findings	Comments
Normal variation in residual red marrow and/or vascular channels ▷ *Fig. 5.170a, b* ▷ *Fig. 5.171a, b*	Foci of decreased T1- and increased T2-weighted signal intensity distributed throughout fatty marrow.	The pattern typically seen at the hands and feet usually resolves around 15 y of age, although various patterns may also be seen in adults.[56,57]
Rebound or stimulated hematopoietic marrow ▷ *Fig. 5.172a, b*	Foci of decreased T1- and increased T2-weighted signal intensity distributed throughout fatty marrow.	After initiation of hematopoietic stimulating therapy or on cessation of therapies toxic to red marrow.
Chronic repetitive trauma		Presumably from trabecular microfractures.
Juvenile rheumatoid arthritis ▷ *Fig. 5.106, p. 567*	Foci of bone marrow edema adjacent to joints seen on MRI.	Bone marrow edema (osteitis) has been correlated with future erosions.[58]
Reflex sympathetic dystrophy	Bone marrow edema tends to be larger, more focal, and confluent.	Often accompanied by osteopenia and soft-tissue atrophy in the appropriate clinical setting.
AVN ▷ *Fig. 5.173a, b, p. 614* ▷ *Fig. 5.174, p. 614* ▷ *Fig. 5.175, p. 614*	Early: occult on radiographs with diffuse bone marrow edema on MRI and increased activity on bone scan. Middisease: alternating serpiginous bands of alternating low and high signal intensity on MRI ± characteristic findings of osteonecrosis on radiography.[21]	
Transient osteoporosis	Radiographs may show bone demineralization.	
Osteoid osteoma and osteoblastoma	Intense bone marrow edema on MRI.	The bone marrow edema tends to extend well beyond the nidus.
Metastatic disease ▷ *Fig. 5.132, p. 586* ▷ *Fig. 5.136, p. 589*	More confluent edema ± soft-tissue mass or bone destruction.	

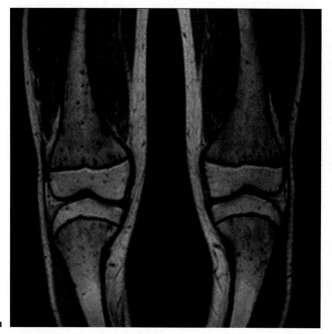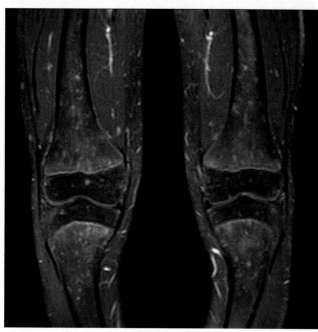

a　　　　　　　　　　　　　　　　　　　　　　　　　　　　　　　　　　　　　　b

Fig. 5.170a, b　Normal variation in red marrow. (a, b) Speckled appearance of biopsy-proven normocellular red marrow on T1 and postgadolinium T1-weighted fat-saturated MRI.

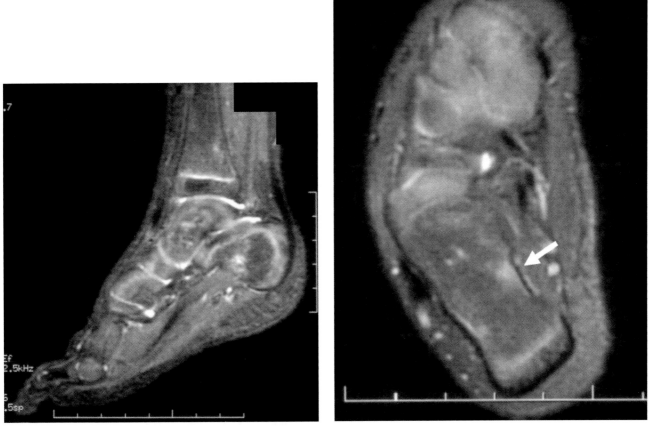

Fig. 5.171a, b   Normal variation in red marrow. (a, b) Speckled increased T2-weighted signal intensity in the marrow of a 3-year-old (arrow in **b**).

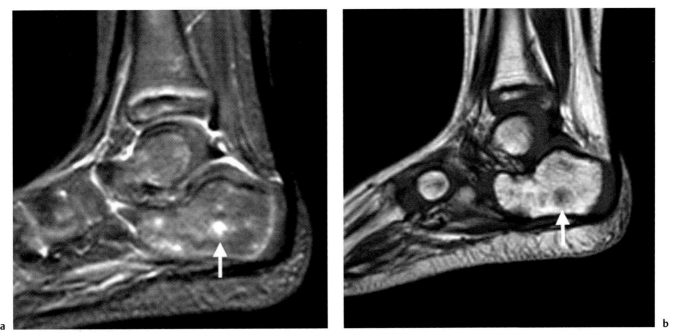

Fig. 5.172a, b   Biopsy-proven red marrow. (a, b) Foci of increased T2-weighted signal intensity (arrows) may mimic a neoplastic process in this patient in remission from acute lymphoblastic leukemia.

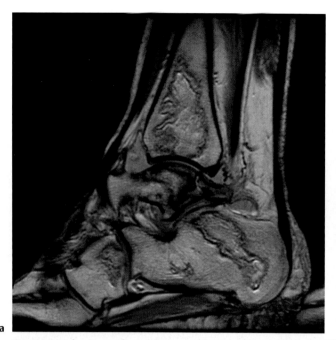

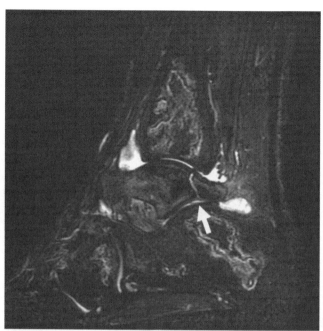

a

b

Fig. 5.173a, b   Avascular necrosis. (a, b) Osteonecrosis of the middle and hind foot on MRI with a vertical fracture through the talus that extends to the posterior facet (arrow in **b**).

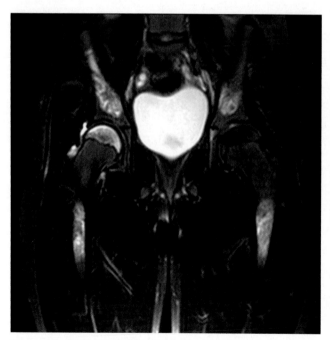

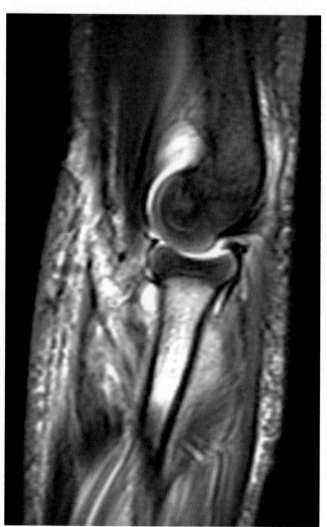

Fig. 5.174   Acute avascular necrosis with bone marrow edema in the right proximal femoral epiphysis. Note the bone infarcts in the ilium and femoral diaphysis. Also, the anemia decreases T2-weighted signal intensity in the regions of the pelvis unaffected by osteonecrosis.

Fig. 5.175   Avascular necrosis. Sickle cell disease with acute bone infarct in the proximal radius with adjacent muscle necrosis on STIR MRI.

Table 5.89 Bone marrow: diffuse alteration in marrow

Diagnosis	Findings	Comments
Overproduction of hematopoietic marrow	Diffusely decreased T1- and increased T2-weighted marrow signal intensity on MRI.	DD: sickle cell disease, thalassemia, and other hemoglobinopathies.
Hematologic malignancy ▷ *Fig. 5.176a, b*	MRI marrow changes may be accompanied by lucent metaphyseal bands on radiographs.	
Inflammation	Diffusely decreased T1- and increased T2-weighted marrow signal intensity on MRI may be accompanied by periosteal reaction.	
Infection	Similar findings as with inflammation.	
Rebound following bone marrow stem cell transplantation		

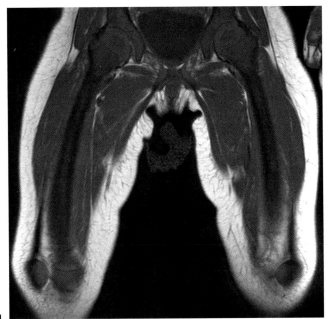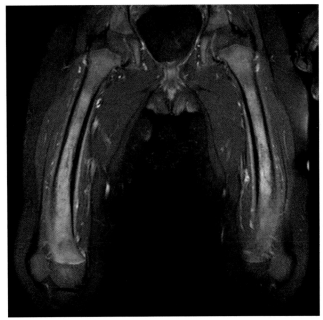

a b

Fig. 5.176a, b Hematological malignancy. Diffuse marrow infiltration from acute megakaryocytic leukemia with replacement of marrow fat in the epiphyses (**a**) and diffuse periosteal reaction and marrow enhancement in the diaphyses (**b**).

Table 5.90 Alterations in the apophysis and sesamoid bones

Diagnosis	Findings	Comments
Apophysitis	Increased fluid signal intensity in the apophysis ± increased fluid signal intensity in the synchondrosis.	Common locations: patella (bipartite patella), ankle (os trigonum), shoulder (os acromiale).
Avulsion	Large gap in the expected location of the synchondrosis suggests avulsion.	
Pseudofracture	Synchondrosis may simulate a fracture.	Bipartite patella.

Changes in Bone Density

Increased

Table 5.91 Bone density: increased density (osteosclerosis)

Diagnosis	Findings	Comments
Osteosclerosis of premature infants and neonates	Generalized increased density of all the bones.	Physiologic variant with no clinical signs. Normalizes within the first 3 mo.
Bone infarcts ▷ Fig. 5.36, p. 519	Patchy regions of increased sclerosis that may coalesce.	Bone infarcts after steroid therapy for inflammatory conditions or tumor treatment. Sickle cell disease.
Renal osteodystrophy with secondary hyperparathyroidism ▷ Fig. 5.69, p. 542	Diffuse sclerosis with trabecular thickening.	
Vitamin D–resistant rickets on vitamin D therapy ▷ Fig. 5.62, p. 537	Increased density of diaphyses and metaphyses.	During therapy, sclerosis develops at sites of prior lucency.
Intrauterine infections	Increased diaphyseal and metaphyseal density.	Celery stalk pattern of the metaphyses. Congenital rubella and cytomegalovirus infections.
Osteopetrosis (Albers-Schönberg disease) ▷ Fig. 5.67, p. 540 ▷ Fig. 5.80, p. 549	Generalized increase in bone density.	Sclerosis obliterates bone marrow preventing hematopoiesis.
Hypervitaminosis D	Increased metaphyseal cortical density, particularly at the diaphyseal junction.	After long-term ingestion of high doses of vitamin D.
Williams-Beuren syndrome (Williams syndrome)	(see Table 5.45)	
Fluorosis	Combined picture of osteomalacia, osteoporosis, and osteosclerosis.	Excessive consumption of fluoride. Bone pain and arthralgias. Calcification of ligaments.
Melorheostosis ▷ Fig. 5.9, p. 498	Marked cortical thickening and characteristic dripping candle wax appearance.	Localized painful swelling and growth disturbances. Follows distribution of dermatomes.
Primary hypertrophic osteoarthropathy	(see Table 5.56)	
Endosteal hyperostosis (van Buchem and Worth types)	(see Table 5.56)	
Pycnodysostosis	Generalized bone sclerosis and mild modeling deformity of the bones.	Short-limbed dwarfism with generalized increase in bone density. Brittle bones. Acroosteolysis.
Diaphyseal dysplasia (Camurati-Engelmann disease)	(see Table 5.56)	
Erdheim-Chester disease (polyostotic sclerosing histiocytosis)		Usually affects adults. Progressive and widespread patchy sclerosis of the intramedullary region of bones with loss of the corticomedullary junction. Coarse trabecular architecture. Focal rib lesions.
Primary hyperoxaluria (oxalosis)	Osteoporosis in the early phase and diffuse bone sclerosis in the advanced stage. Subchondral sclerosis in the long bones. Metaphyseal sclerosis, dense epiphyses.	Growing ends of bones show bulbous enlargement. Pathologic fractures are common. Growth disturbance and increased incidence of urinary calculi due to hyperoxaluria.

Decreased

Several terms are commonly used to describe the decreased density of bones. Osteoporosis is a disease of reduced bone mineral density that leads to fracture and is defined as measured by dual energy X-ray absorptiometry or quantitative CT.[59,60] Osteomalacia describes bone softening due to defective bone mineralization. In children, osteomalacia is known as rickets, and because of this the term osteomalacia is often restricted to the adult form of the disease. Although many of the features of osteoporosis and osteomalacia overlap, they are distinct disorders.

Osteomalacia is a defect in mineralization of osteoid, the protein framework in bones, and is usually the result of low vitamin D levels. *Osteopenia* is a term for low bone mineral density and may be a precursor to osteoporosis.

Table 5.92   Bone density: decreased

Diagnosis	Findings	Comments
Osteopenia from disuse	Regional decreased bone density involving immobilized limbs. Cortex is diffusely thinned and the trabeculae are rarified. Metaphyseal ends may be sharply defined.	Commonly observed during immobilization after trauma/fracture. May accompany soft-tissue atrophy in chronic disuse, arthrogryposis, and other degenerative disorders of muscle and nerves.
Rickets ▷ *Fig. 5.177, p. 618* ▷ *Fig. 5.178, p. 618* ▷ *Fig. 5.4, p. 496* ▷ *Fig. 5.62, p. 537* ▷ *Fig. 5.69, p. 542*	Skeletal changes depend on the patient's age. Wide and hazy growth plates, ill-defined architecture of the trabeculae. Hazy metaphyseal end plates with cupping.	All forms of rickets (vitamin D–deficiency, renal osteodystrophy, vitamin D–resistance, etc). Cortical erosions occur in secondary hyperparathyroidism.
Steroid therapy ▷ *Fig. 5.113, p. 573*	Systemic decrease in bone density. Cortex is diffusely thinned and the trabeculae are rarified.	Decrease in osteoblast activity relative to osteoclasts.
Hematologic disorders	Systemic decrease in bone density may be accompanied by changes characteristic for a particular disorder (e.g., hair-on-end skull in thalassemia major).	Proliferation of cells or deposition of metabolites replaces bone. DD: sickle cell disease, thalassemia major, lysosomal storage disease, leukemia, mastocytosis, mucolipidosis.
Diffuse metastatic disease ▷ *Fig. 5.179, p. 618*	Diffuse bone demineralization may mask lytic lesions.	Pathologic fractures.
JIA	Periarticular bone demineralization.	Demineralization may be accompanied by soft-tissue swelling (synovial hypertrophy), joint space narrowing, and/or periarticular erosions.
Scurvy	(see **Table 5.43**)	
Hyperphosphatasia	Meshed radiolucent bone texture.	Progressive skeletal deformity. Enlargement and thickening of the skull and bowed limbs. High levels of serum alkaline phosphatase.
Congenital hyperparathyroidism	Pronounced bone demineralization, cortical erosions, and Trümmerfeld fractures in the metaphyses.	Coarse bone trabeculae, subperiosteal bone resorption, and metaphyseal cupping.
Osteogenesis imperfecta types I and IV	Diffuse osteopenia	
Idiopathic juvenile osteoporosis	Disseminated osteoporosis and vertebral body collapse.	Presents with bone pain between 8–14 y of age. May spontaneously resolve.
Homocystinuria	(see **Table 5.45**)	
Metaphyseal chondrodysplasia, Jansen type	Osteopenia in 70%. Extensive irregularity in mineralization of markedly expanded and cup-shaped metaphyses.	Relatively preserved epiphyses. The deformity of the metaphyses decreases in adult life.

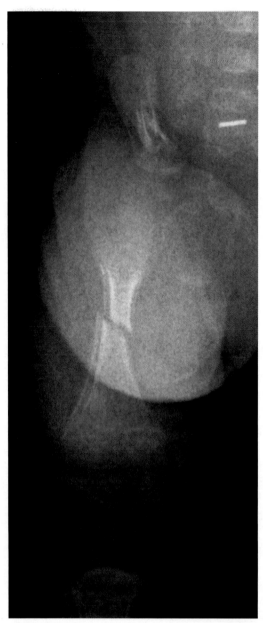

Fig. 5.177 Rickets of prematurity with a pathologic fracture. Cupping at the metaphysis and smooth periosteal reaction along the diaphysis.

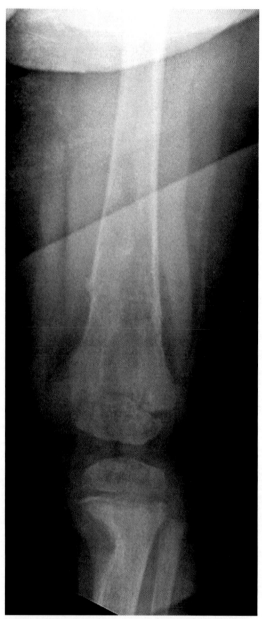

Fig. 5.178 Renal osteodystrophy. Subperiosteal resorption at the proximal tibia and a pathologic fracture at the distal femur.

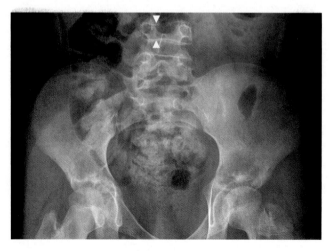

Fig. 5.179 Diffuse metastatic disease. Diffuse bone demineralization and pathologic vertebral body fractures (arrowheads) from metastatic rhabdomyosarcoma.

Skeletal Maturation

Table 5.93   Skeletal maturation: accelerated maturation

Diagnosis	Comments
Endocrine	Comparison with an atlas of normal maturation will show the acceleration. Prolonged elevation in sex steroids. DD: precocious puberty and congenital adrenal hyperplasia, premature adrenarche, obesity, hyperthyroidism, lipodystrophy, gonadotropin-producing tumors.
Idiopathic	
Beckwith-Wiedemann syndrome	Exomphalos, macroglossia, and gigantism in the neonate. Increased risk of developing adrenal carcinoma, nephroblastoma, hepatoblastoma, and rhabdomyosarcoma.
Sotos syndrome	Acromegalic features. Mental retardation. Although growth may be rapid in first years and bone age advanced, final height may not be excessive.
Marshall-Smith syndrome	Failure to thrive, mental retardation, blue sclera, and unusual facies with large forehead, shallow orbits, and depressed nasal bridge.
Polyostotic fibrous dysplasia (McCune-Albright syndrome)	(see **Table 5.31**)

Table 5.94   Skeletal maturation: delayed maturation

Diagnosis	Findings	Comments
Abnormal endocrine function	Comparison with an atlas of normal maturation will show the delay.	Global delay in maturation. DD: growth hormone deficiency, hypothyroidism, Addison disease, Cushing disease, craniopharyngioma, psychosocial dwarfism.
Chronic illness		
Severe malnutrition		
Chromosomal abnormalities		Trisomy 18 and 21, Turner syndrome.
Skeletal dysplasias with epiphyseal involvement	(see **Table 5.33**)	

Table 5.95   Skeletal maturation: classification of asymmetric maturation (hemihypertrophy)[61]

Diagnosis	Comments
Congenital, total	Involvement of all organ systems.
Congenital, limited	Only muscular, vascular, skeletal, or neurologic involvement.
Acquired	Localized hyperemia.
Associated with a syndrome	Neurofibromatosis and Beckwith-Wiedemann (approximately 13% of patients), Klippel-Trénaunay-Weber, Proteus, McCune-Albright, and many other syndromes.
Tumors associated with hemihypertrophy	DD: Wilms tumor, adrenal carcinoma, rhabdomyosarcoma, and hepatoblastoma.[62]
Macrodystrophia lipomatosa ▷ *Fig. 5.44, p. 525* ▷ *Fig. 5.45, p. 525*	Progressive overgrowth of all the mesenchymal elements with a disproportionate increase in the fibroadipose tissues.[63]

Lethal Dysplasias

Lethal skeletal dysplasias have been classified into 11 major categories[64] and the genes responsible are known for several. Several may be diagnosed prenatally. The more common ones are described in **Table 5.96**.

Table 5.96 Lethal bone dysplasias

Diagnosis	Findings	Comments
Campomelic dysplasia ▷ *Fig. 5.14, p. 501*	Hypoplastic tibia, scapula, and vertebral bodies. Pear-shaped iliac bones, long femora that are anteriorly bowed, and deficient ossification of the pubis. Radial head dislocation.	Pulmonary hypoplasia and laryngeal and tracheal stenosis. Ureteral stenosis. Thoracic platyspondyly and kyphosis. Multiple cutaneous dimples in the arms and legs.
Thanatophoric dysplasia	Kleeblattschädel (cloverleaf skull), very short ribs, small scapulae, severe platyspondyly, U- or H-shaped vertebral bodies, small iliac bones, horizontal acetabular roofs, small sacroiliac notches, bowing of long bones (French telephone receiver femurs).	Most common form of skeletal dysplasia that is lethal in the neonatal period.
Achondrogenesis	Poor mineralization of skull, absent or minimal ossification of vertebral bodies, short thin ribs, multiple fractures, deformed and short iliac wings and long bones, absent ossification of pubis.	Micromelic dwarfism. Fetal hydrops and polyhydramnios.
Achondroplasia, homozygous form	Short long bones, flat vertebral bodies, large skull.	Radiographic manifestations lie between thanatophoric dysplasia (see subsequent discussion) and heterozygous achondroplasia (see **Table 5.3**). May be diagnosed in second trimester.[65]
Asphyxiating thoracic dysplasia (Jeune syndrome) ▷ *Fig. 5.2, p. 493*	Small thorax with short bulbous ribs, small pelvis with short flared iliac bones, trident acetabula, infero-lateral spur adjacent to sciatic notch, cone-shaped epiphyses of hands.	Spectrum from lethal to latent forms. Renal, hepatic, and pancreatic dysplasia. Medullary cystic change of the kidneys. Retinal dystrophy.
Osteogenesis imperfecta type II	Very little ossification of skull, wormian bones, beaded ribs, short distorted long bones, multiple fractures, flattened acetabula and iliac wings.	Blue sclera. Types I, III, IV have better prognosis.
Chondrodysplasia punctata (rhizomelic type) ▷ *Fig. 5.58, p. 534*	Symmetric rhizomelic shortening of long bones, punctate calcific deposits in cartilaginous skeleton.	Approximately fifty percent may survive to 6 y. Other types have better prognosis.[12]
Hypophosphatasia, lethal form	Partially ossified skull, no ossification of vertebral pedicles, short abnormal ribs, bent and unusually shaped long bones, spurs in the middle portions of long bones (Bowdler spur).	Blue sclera. Infantile (lethal), childhood, and adult types. Fetal type on prenatal US: failure to observe a fetal head by 16 wk gestation.
Schneckenbecken dysplasia	Snail-shaped ilia, flat acetabular roofs, handlebar clavicles, hypoplastic scapula, dumbbell-shaped very short long bones, wide fibula, and round vertebral bodies.[12]	Hypoplastic vertebral bodies with relatively well-preserved posterior arches.[13]
Short rib-polydactyly syndromes (types I–III)	Dolichocephaly, hypoplastic mandible, short horizontally oriented ribs. Short long bones. Small iliac bones and flattened acetabular roofs.	Types range from lethal to more mild forms. Types II and IV have near normal pelvis. Polydactaly is sometimes absent in types III and IV.[12]

Fracture Dating

Estimation of fracture age should be approached with caution. The current timeline for estimating fracture age (**Table 5.97**) is based on anecdotal experience of seasoned pediatric radiologists and several small series of children.[66] Although fracture dating is not an inexact science, experienced radiologists should be able to differentiate recent from old fractures separated by weeks or months in time.[66,67]

Table 5.97   Fracture dating on conventional radiographs[68]

Feature	Early	Peak	Delayed
Resolution of soft tissues	2–5 d	4–10 d	10–21 d
Subperiosteal new bone formation	4–10 d	10–14 d	14–21 d
Loss of fracture line definition	10–14 d	14–21 d	
Soft callus	10–14 d	14–21 d	
Hard callus	14–21 d	21–42 d	42–90 d
Remodeling	3 mo	1 y	2 y to physeal closure

Table 5.97 reproduced with permission from Kleinman PK. Diagnostic imaging of child abuse. 2nd ed. St. Louis: Mosby, 1989.

Child Abuse

Table 5.98   Child abuse: conditions that masquerade as child abuse and simulate the classic metaphyseal lesion[69] (see Table 5.44)

Diagnosis	Comments
Birth trauma	After low segment cesarean sections.
Iatrogenic	After orthopedic manipulations.
Osteomyelitis	Osteomyelitis has a predilection for the metaphysis in infants. Although systemic signs and symptoms of infection may be lacking in infants and multiple sites of osteomyelitis and different stages of healing may simulate child abuse, the metaphyseal erosions in osteomyelitis tend to be less well-defined than classic metaphyseal lesions (CMLs; see **Table 5.43**).
Rickets and metabolic bone disease ▷ *Fig. 5.180*	Controversy exists as to whether or not osseous fragments resembling CMLs are always accompanied by more obvious changes of rickets such as metaphyseal irregularity and physeal widening.[70,71] Laboratory findings may also help support a diagnosis of rickets.
Bone dysplasias	Skeletal survey will reveal other abnormalities associated with the given skeletal dysplasia. DD: osteogenesis imperfecta, metaphyseal chondrodysplasia (Schmid type), and spondylometaphyseal dysplasia (corner fracture type).
Leukemia	Bone demineralization, osteolytic lesions, and subperiosteal new bone formation. Radiolucent bands at the metaphyses. Imaging findings may be due to a combination of nutritional disturbance and leukemic invasion (see **Table 5.43**).
Scurvy	Subperiosteal hemorrhage and metaphyseal and epiphyseal changes. Characteristic findings of scurvy may help to distinguish from child abuse (see **Table 5.43**).
Vitamin A intoxication	Subperiosteal new bone formation predominantly in the tubular bones.
Lower extremity paralysis	Routine handling of infants with paralysis may cause fractures.
Infantile cortical hyperostosis (Caffey disease)	Subperiosteal new bone formation and cortical thickening. Preference for the mandible, clavicle, and ulna.
Menkes syndrome (kinky hair disease)	Rare genetic disorder resulting in defective gastrointestinal absorption of copper. Metaphysis of the long bones have spurs ± fractures. Subperiosteal new bone formation and bone demineralization. Tortuous and irregular cerebral and abdominal arteries.
Congenital indifference/ insensitivity to pain	Lack of sensation of pain may lead to a delay in diagnosis of both minor and major trauma. Imaging may show metaphyseal injuries, subperiosteal hemorrhage, fractures, and epiphyseal separations in various stages of healing during infancy. Charcot-type joints manifest later in childhood.

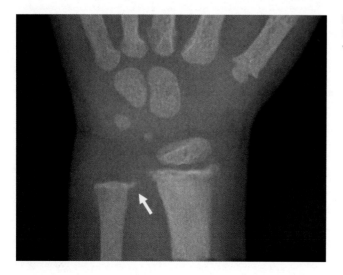

Fig. 5.180   Rickets and metabolic bone disease. Metaphyseal irregularity simulating a metaphyseal corner fracture (arrow) in a 3-year-old girl with resorptive metabolic bone disease of unclear etiology.

Table 5.99   Child abuse: specificity of fracture locations[72]

Specificity	Fracture
High	Classic metaphyseal lesion ▷ *Fig. 5.74, p. 545* ▷ *Fig. 5.75, p. 545* Rib fractures ▷ *Fig. 5.181* Scapular fractures Spinous process fractures Sternal fractures
Moderate	Multiple fractures (especially bilateral) Fractures of different ages Epiphyseal separation Vertebral body fractures and subluxations Digital fractures Complex skull fractures
Low	Subperiosteal new bone formation Clavicular fractures Long bone shaft fractures Linear skull fractures

Table 5.99 reproduced with permission from Kleinman PK. Diagnostic imaging of child abuse. 2nd ed. St. Louis: Mosby, 1989.

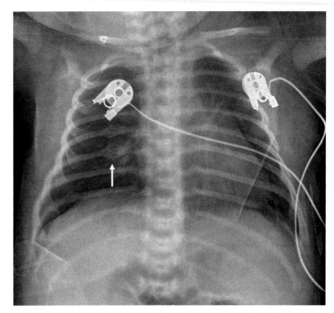

Fig. 5.181   Healing posterior rib fractures (arrow) in child abuse.

■ References

1. Restrepo CS, Martinez S, Lemos DF, et al. Imaging appearances of the sternum and sternoclavicular joints. Radiographics 2009;29:839–859
2. Yekeler E, Tunaci M, Tunaci A, Dursun M, Acunas G. Frequency of sternal variations and anomalies evaluated by MDCT. AJR Am J Roentgenol 2006;186:956–960
3. Jeung MY, Gangi A, Gasser B, et al. Imaging of chest wall disorders. Radiographics 1999;19:617–637
4. Edwards DK 3rd, Berry CC, Hilton SW. Trisomy 21 in newborn infants: chest radiographic diagnosis. Radiology 1988;167: 317–318
5. Levine MS, Borden S 4th, Gill FM. Sternal cupping: a new finding in childhood sickle cell anemia. Radiology 1982;142:367–370
6. Mehta AV, Chidambaram B, Suchedina AA, Garrett AR. Radiologic abnormalities of the sternum in Turner's syndrome. Chest 1993;104:1795–1799
7. Khanna G, Sato TS, Ferguson P. Imaging of chronic recurrent multifocal osteomyelitis. Radiographics 2009;29:1159–1177
8. Kimonis VE, Mehta SG, Digiovanna JJ, Bale SJ, Pastakia B. Radiological features in 82 patients with nevoid basal cell carcinoma (NBCC or Gorlin) syndrome. Genet Med 2004;6:495–502
9. Glass RB, Norton KI, Mitre SA, Kang E. Pediatric ribs: a spectrum of abnormalities. Radiographics 2002;22:87–104
10. Kumar R, Madewell JE, Swischuk LE, Lindell MM, David R. The clavicle: normal and abnormal. Radiographics 1989;9:677–706
11. Oestreich AE. The lateral clavicle hook-an acquired as well as a congenital anomaly. Pediatr Radiol 1981;11:147–150
12. Lachman R. Taybi and Lachman's radiology of syndromes, metabolic disorders and skeletal dysplasias. 5th ed. St. Louis: Mosby, 2006
13. OMIM: Online Mendelian Inheritance in Man Web site. Johns Hopkins University. http://www.ncbi.nlm.nih.gov/omim. Accessed July 2009
14. Waters PM, Smith GR, Jaramillo D. Glenohumeral deformity secondary to brachial plexus birth palsy. J Bone Joint Surg Am 1998;80:668–677
15. Wetherell RG, Amis AA, Heatley FW. Measurement of acetabular erosion. The effect of pelvic rotation on common landmarks. J Bone Joint Surg Br 1989;71:447–451
16. Paajanen H, Hermunen H, Karonen J. Pubic magnetic resonance imaging findings in surgically and conservatively treated athletes with osteitis pubis compared to asymptomatic athletes during heavy training. Am J Sports Med 2008;36: 117–121
17. Muecke EC, Currarino G, Currarino G. Congenital widening of the pubic symphysis: associated clinical disorders and roentgen anatomy of affected bony pelves. Am J Roentgenol Radium Ther Nucl Med 1968;103:179–185
18. Zook PD, Winter TC 3rd, Nyberg DA. Iliac angle as a marker for Down syndrome in second-trimester fetuses: CT measurement. Radiology 1999;211:447–451
19. Klein DM, Barbera C, Gray ST, Spero CR, Perrier G, Teicher JL. Sensitivity of objective parameters in the diagnosis of pediatric septic hips. Clin Orthop Relat Res 1997:153–159
20. Simmons BP, Southmayd WW, Riseborough EJ. Congenital radioulnar synostosis. J Hand Surg Am 1983;8:829–838
21. Steinberg ME, Steinberg DR. Classification systems for osteonecrosis: an overview. Orthop Clin North Am 2004;35:273–283, vii–viii
22. Laor T, Jaramillo D. MR imaging insights into skeletal maturation: what is normal? Radiology 2009;250:28–38
23. Gardner DJ, Azouz EM. Solitary lucent epiphyseal lesions in children. Skeletal Radiol 1988;17:497–504
24. Varich LJ, Laor T, Jaramillo D. Normal maturation of the distal femoral epiphyseal cartilage: age-related changes at MR imaging. Radiology 2000;214:705–709
25. Jaramillo D, Shapiro F, Hoffer FA, et al. Posttraumatic growth-plate abnormalities: MR imaging of bony-bridge formation in rabbits. Radiology 1990;175:767–773
26. Levesque M, Legmann P, Le Cloirec A, Deybach JC, Nordmann Y. Radiological features in congenital erythropoietic porphyria (Gunther's disease). Review of 3 cases. Pediatr Radiol 1988;18:62–66
27. Kleinman PK. Problems in the diagnosis of metaphyseal fractures. Pediatr Radiol 2008;38(Suppl 3):S388–S394
28. Kleinman PK. Diagnostic imaging of child abuse. 2nd ed. St. Louis: Mosby, 1989
29. Grayev AM, Boal DK, Wallach DM, Segal LS. Metaphyseal fractures mimicking abuse during treatment for clubfoot. Pediatr Radiol 2001;31:559–563
30. Kozlowski K, Sutcliffe J, Barylak A, et al. Hypophosphatasia. Review of 24 cases. Pediatr Radiol 1976;5:103–117
31. Goldfarb CA, Manske PR, Busa R, Mills J, Carter P, Ezaki M. Upper-extremity phocomelia reexamined: a longitudinal dysplasia. J Bone Joint Surg Am 2005;87:2639–2648
32. Le Goff C, Cormier-Daire V. Genetic and molecular aspects of acromelic dysplasia. Pediatr Endocrinol Rev 2009;6:418–423
33. Diren HB, Kutluk MT, Karabent A, Gocmen A, Adalioglu G, Kenanoglu A. Primary hypertrophic osteoarthropathy. Pediatr Radiol 1986;16:231–234

34. Cheema JI, Grissom LE, Harcke HT. Radiographic characteristics of lower-extremity bowing in children. Radiographics 2003;23:871–880

35. Nguyen ML, Jones NF. Undergrowth: brachydactyly. Hand Clin 2009;25:247–255

36. Temtamy SA, Aglan MS. Brachydactyly. Orphanet J Rare Dis 2008;3:15

37. Hussmann J, Russell RC, Kucan JO, Khardori R, Steinau HU. Soft-tissue calcifications: differential diagnosis and therapeutic approaches. Ann Plast Surg 1995;34:138–147

38. Wong KS, Chiu CH, Huang YC, Lin TY. Childhood and adolescent tuberculosis in northern Taiwan: an institutional experience during 1994–1999. Acta Paediatr 2001;90:943–947

39. Houser JR, Kan JH. Langerhans cell histiocytosis of the epiphysis. Pediatr Radiol 2008;38:351

40. Brien EW, Mirra JM, Ippolito V, Vaughan L. Clear-cell chondrosarcoma with elevated alkaline phosphatase, mistaken for osteosarcoma on biopsy. Skeletal Radiol 1996;25:770–774

41. Resnick D, Greenway G. Distal femoral cortical defects, irregularities, and excavations. Radiology 1982;143:345–354

42. Mar WA, Taljanovic MS, Bagatell R, et al. Update on imaging and treatment of Ewing sarcoma family tumors: what the radiologist needs to know. J Comput Assist Tomogr 2008;32:108–118

43. Gladish GW, Sabloff BM, Munden RF, Truong MT, Erasmus JJ, Chasen MH. Primary thoracic sarcomas. Radiographics 2002;22:621–637

44. Ablin DS, Azouz EM, Jain KA. Large intrathoracic tumors in children: imaging findings. AJR Am J Roentgenol 1995;165:925–934

45. Bonetumor.org Web site. bonetumor.org. Accessed July 30, 2009

46. Greenspan A, Jundt G, Remagen W. Differential diagnosis in orthopaedic oncology. 2nd ed. Philadelphia: Lippincott Williams & Wilkins, 2007

47. Moppett J, Oakhill A, Duncan AW. Second malignancies in children: the usual suspects? Eur J Radiol 2001;38:235–248

48. Gartner L, Pearce CJ, Saifuddin A. The role of the plain radiograph in the characterisation of soft tissue tumours. Skeletal Radiol 2009;38:549–558

49. Van Rijn RR, Wilde JC, Bras J, Oldenburger F, McHugh KM, Merks JH. Imaging findings in noncraniofacial childhood rhabdomyosarcoma. Pediatr Radiol 2008;38:617–634

50. Beall DP, Ly J, Bell JP, Parker EE, et al. Pediatric extraskeletal osteosarcoma. Pediatr Radiol 2008;38:579–582

51. McCarville MB, Kaste SC, Pappo AS. Soft-tissue malignancies in infancy. AJR Am J Roentgenol 1999;173:973–977

52. Garces-Inigo EF, Leung R, Sebire NJ, McHugh K. Extrarenal rhabdoid tumours outside the central nervous system in infancy. Pediatr Radiol 2009;39:817–822

53. Subbarao K. Periosteal reactions in pediatrics. Indian J Pediatr 1987;54:45–52

54. Makley JT, Dunn MJ. Prostaglandin synthesis by osteoid osteoma. Lancet 1982;2:42

55. Poznanski AK, Fernbach SK, Berry TE. Bone changes from prostaglandin therapy. Skeletal Radiol 1985;14:20–25

56. Shabshin N, Schweitzer ME, Morrison WB, Carrino JA, Keller MS, Grissom LE. High-signal T2 changes of the bone marrow of the foot and ankle in children: red marrow or traumatic changes? Pediatr Radiol 2006;36:670–676

57. Zubler V, Mengiardi B, Pfirrmann CW, et al. Bone marrow changes on STIR MR images of asymptomatic feet and ankles. Eur Radiol 2007;17:3066–3072

58. McQueen FM. Magnetic resonance imaging in early inflammatory arthritis: what is its role? Rheumatology (Oxford) 2000;39:700–706

59. Mora S, Gilsanz V. Establishment of peak bone mass. Endocrinol Metab Clin North Am 2003;32:39–63

60. Gilsanz V, Perez FJ, Campbell PP, Dorey FJ, Lee DC, Wren TA. Quantitative CT reference values for vertebral trabecular bone density in children and young adults. Radiology 2009;250:222–227

61. Cohen MM Jr. A comprehensive and critical assessment of overgrowth and overgrowth syndromes. Adv Hum Genet 1989;18: 181–303, 373–376

62. Green DM, Breslow NE, Breslow NE, Beckwith JB, Norkool P. Screening of children with hemihypertrophy, aniridia, and Beckwith-Wiedemann. Med Pediatr Oncol 1993;21:188–192

63. Goldman AB, Kaye JJ. Macrodystrophia lipomatosa: radiographic diagnosis. AJR Am J Roentgenol 1977;128:101–105

64. Spranger J. Radiologic nosology of bone dysplasias. Am J Med Genet 1989;34:96–104

65. Patel MD, Filly RA. Homozygous achondroplasia: US distinction between homozygous, heterozygous, and unaffected fetuses in the second trimester. Radiology 1995;196:541–545

66. Prosser I, Maguire S, Harrison SK, Mann M, Sibert JR, Kemp AM. How old is this fracture? Radiologic dating of fractures in children: a systematic review. AJR Am J Roentgenol 2005;184:1282–1286

67. Offiah A, van Rijn RR, Perez-Rossello JM, Kleinman PK. Skeletal imaging of child abuse (non-accidental injury). Pediatr Radiol 2009;39:461–470

68. O'Connor JF, Cohen J. Dating fractures. In: Kleinman PK, ed. Diagnostic imaging of child abuse. 2nd ed. St. Louis: Mosby, 1998:168–177

69. Brill PW, Winchester P, Kleinman PK. Differential diagnosis I: diseases simulating abuse. In: Kleinman PK, ed. Diagnostic imaging of child abuse. 2nd ed. St. Louis: Mosby, 1998:178–196

70. Keller KA, Barnes PD. Rickets vs. abuse: a national and international epidemic. Pediatr Radiol 2008;38:1210–1216

71. Slovis TL, Chapman S. Evaluating the data concerning vitamin D insufficiency/deficiency and child abuse. Pediatr Radiol 2008;38:1221–1224

72. Kleinman PK. Skeletal trauma: general considerations. In: Kleinman PK, ed. Diagnostic imaging of child abuse. 2nd ed. St. Louis: Mosby, 1998:168–177

6 Normal Values

Thorax, Mediastinum, Heart, and Great Vessels

The Abdomen and Gastrointestinal Tract

Urogenital Tract

Skull, Intracranial Space, and Vertebral Column

→

The Skeleton and Soft Tissues

The aim of this chapter is to present normal values in pediatric radiology that, in the view of the authors, are useful in daily practice. In order for these values to be easily implemented in daily practice, we primarily include studies that reported normal values for age, instead of normal values for height or weight. Whenever possible, gender differences and left-right differences were averaged and measurements were rounded off to the nearest millimeter.

For practical purpose, all volumes were (re)calculated using the formula for the volume of an ellipsoid because this is the default software application in most equipment. The list of normal values is not meant to be complete, but it should be used as a practical guideline in interpreting pediatric radiologic studies during daily routine. For detailed information, the reader is encouraged to read the original paper. This chapter follows the order of the chapters of the book.

For all reported normal values, a short excerpt of the materials and methods, related to data collection and subject numbers, is presented.

Thorax, Mediastinum, Heart, and Great Vessels

Tracheal Dimensions by CT[31]

■ Material and Methods

One hundred and thirty children (71 boys and 59 girls) who were referred for chest CT usually as part of a search for pulmonary metastases were included in this retrospective study (**Table 6.1**). Tracheal diameters and cross-sectional diameters were determined from each section (between vocal cords and carina) and averaged. Tracheal length was determined on the AP scout view and measured from the vocal cords to the carina (**Fig. 6.1**). There were no differences between boys and girls until age 14 to 16 years.

Table 6.1 Tracheal dimensions by CT[31]

Age (years)	Number	Tracheal dimensions (cm)			
		Length (SD)	AP diameter (SD)	Transverse diameter (SD)	Cross-sectional area (cm²)
0–2	13	5.4 (0.7)	0.5 (0.1)	0.6 (0.1)	0.28 (0.09)
2–4	15	6.4 (0.5)	0.7 (0.1)	0.8 (0.1)	0.48 (0.08)
4–6	8	7.2 (0.8)	0.8 (0.1)	0.9 (0.1)	0.58 (0.10)
6–8	11	8.2 (0.7)	0.9 (0.1)	0.9 (0.1)	0.69 (0.11)
8–10	11	8.8 (0.9)	1.0 (0.1)	1.1 (0.1)	0.89 (0.09)
10–12	8	10.0 (1.0)	1.2 (0.1)	1.2 (0.1)	1.10 (0.18)
12–14	15	10.8 (1.5)	1.3 (0.2)	1.3 (0.2)	1.39 (0.36)
14–16	12	11.8 (1.2)	1.4 (0.1)	1.4 (0.1)	1.62 (0.14)
16–18 (male)	13	12.4 (1.3)	1.6 (0.1)	1.6 (0.2)	2.01 (0.30)
16–18 (female)	13	12.2 (1.1)	1.4 (0.2)	1.4 (0.1)	1.54 (0.29)

SD, standard deviation.
Reproduced from Griscom NT, Wohl ME. Dimensions of the growing trachea related to age and gender. AJR Am J Roentgenol 1986;146:233–237. Reprinted with permission of American Journal of Roentgenology.

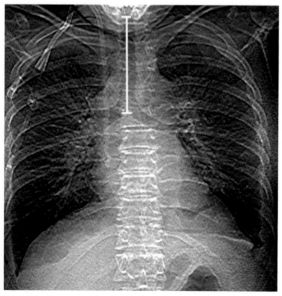 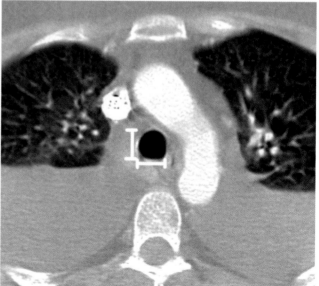

a   b

Fig. 6.1a, b Measurement of the length of the trachea on CT scanogram (**a**) and AP and lateral diameter on transverse CT slice (**b**).

The Volume of Lung Parenchyma as a Function of Age[32]

■ Material and Methods

A total of 1050 CT scans performed over a 3-year period were reported to be normal and were included in the retrospective study (**Fig. 6.2**). Distribution in age and sex is shown as a stack bar in the original paper, but actual numbers are not reported.

The window for volume assessment was set at −992 to −198 Hounsfield units.

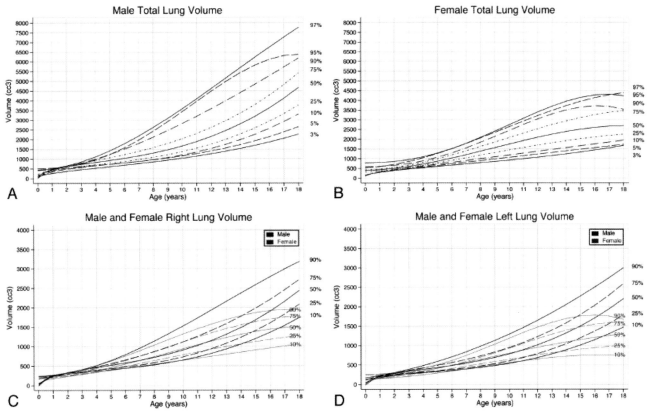

Fig. 6.2a–d Lung volume. (**a**) Smoothed data for total male lung volume as a function of age from birth to 18 years of age. (**b**) Smoothed data for total female lung volume as a function of age from birth to 18 years of age. (**c**) Smoothed data for right lung volume in male patients and female patients. (**d**) Smoothed data for left lung volume in male patients and female patients. (Reproduced with permission from Gollogly S, Smith JT, White SK, Firth S, White K. The volume of lung parenchyma as a function of age: a review of 1050 normal CT scans of the chest with three-dimensional volumetric reconstruction of the pulmonary system. Spine [Phila Pa 1976] 2004;29:2061–2066, with permission from Wolters Kluwer Health.)

Thymus Size from 0 to 2 Years of Age[33]

■ Material and Methods

Mediastinal ultrasonography was performed in 151 infants (79 boys and 72 girls; **Table 6.2**). All children were healthy and had no stress factors affecting their thymic size. The maximum transverse diameter, right lobe AP, and left lobe AP were assessed. Perpendicular to the transverse plane, the longest craniocaudal dimension (length) was assessed. The thymic index was calculated by multiplying the transverse diameter by the largest sagittal area (**Fig. 6.3**).

Table 6.2   Thymus size from 0 to 2 years of age[33]

Age (months)	Number of cases	Thymic dimensions (cm)				
		Transverse (mm)	AP right (mm)	AP left (mm)	Length (mm)	Thymic index (cm³)
Premature	20	2.9. (0.3)*	1.5 (3.7)	1.5 (0.3)	3.1 (0.4)	11.9 (3.9)
0–1	25	3.3 (0.3)	1.6 (0.3)	1.8 (0.3)	3.6 (0.3)	18.1 (6.7)
1–2	21	3.6 (0.6)	1.9 (0.3)	2.0 (0.3)	3.9 (0.4)	25.4 (9.4)
2–3	11	3.7 (0.5)	1.9 (0.3)	2.1 (0.3)	3.8 (0.3)	22.3 (6.9)
3–4	15	3.8 (0.4)	1.9 (0.5)	2.2 (0.6)	4.0 (0.4)	26.8 (10.3)
4–5	7	4.0 (0.6)	2.0 (0.6)	2.2 (0.4)	4.1 (0.3)	29.7 (17.6)
5–6	8	3.9 (0.2)	1.9 (0.4)	2.3 (0.3)	4.0 (0.2)	24.2 (9.3)
6–8	8	3.6 (0.5)	1.8 (0.4)	1.9 (0.5)	3.6 (0.6)	22.2 (8.9)
8–10	14	3.7 (0.5)	1.7 (0.5)	1.9 (0.5)	3.7 (0.4)	21.5 (6.8)
10–12	5	3.7 (0.5)	1.9 (0.6)	1.8 (0.5)	3.6 (0.2)	23.2 (7.2)
12–18	7	2.8 (0.5)	1.2 (0.5)	1.4 (0.4)	3.2 (0.9)	17.2 (6.4)
18–24	10	3.3 (0.4)	1.2 (0.4)	1.2 (0.3)	3.4 (0.7)	15.4 (5.6)

*Standard deviation.

Reproduced with permission of American Institute of Ultrasound in Medicine - AIUM from Yekeler E, Tambag A, Tunaci A, et al. Analysis of the thymus in 151 healthy infants from 0 to 2 years of age. J Ultrasound Med 2004;23:1321–1326; permission conveyed through Copyright Clearance Center, Inc.

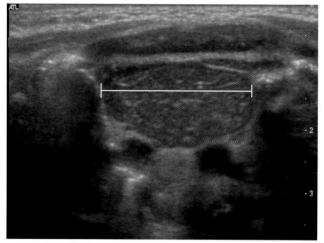 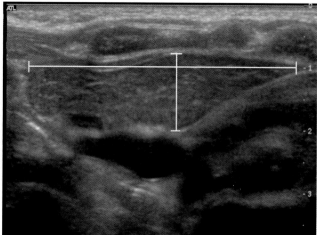

Fig. 6.3a, b   Thymus. Maximal transverse diameter (**a**) and largest sagittal area (**b**).

Adenoid Pad[9]

■ Material and Methods

The size of the adenoid pad (**Table 6.3**) was assessed on a mid-sagittal MRI slice in 189 patients (77 male and 112 female); of the total study population, 61 were younger than 20 years (sex differentiation in the subpopulation was not presented). The thickness of the adenoid pad was measured along a line through the pharyngeal tubercle constructed perpendicular to the anterior clival surface (**Fig. 6.4**).

Table 6.3   Adenoid pad

Age (years)	Adenoid size		
	Number of controls	Mean thickness in mm (SD)	Range
0–3	20	11.9 (3.5)	4.7–18.0
4–6	11	13.3 (5.0)	5.6–23.8
7–10	11	14.6 (4.5)	6.6–22.2
11–15	13	14.4 (2.9)	10.0–18.8
16–20	6	11.4 (4.1)	3.7–15.6

SD, standard deviation.
Reproduced from Vogler RC, Ii FJ, Pilgram TK. Age-specific size of the normal adenoid pad on magnetic resonance imaging. Clin Otolaryngol Allied Sci 2000;25:392–395, with permission from John Wiley and Sons.

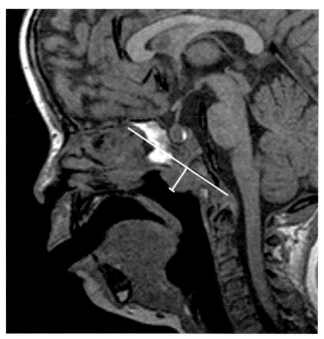

Fig. 6.4   Measurement of adenoid perpendicular to the anterior clival line in a 3-year-old boy.

The Abdomen and Gastrointestinal Tract

Liver Length in Premature Infants and Neonates[10]

■ Material and Methods

This was a US study in 261 healthy newborn infants. Craniocaudal dimension of the liver on the midclavicular line was determined with ultrasonography (**Table 6.4**).

Table 6.4   Liver length in premature infants and neonates[10]

GA (weeks)	Liver length in midclavicular line (cm)		
	Number of patients	Mean length (±1 SD)	Min-max
24–31	29	3.7 (0.7)	2.8–5.8
32–35	33	4.6 (0.7)	3.2–6.2
36–37	35	5.4 (0.6)	3.5–6.3
38–41	153	5.5 (0.8)	3.9–7.8

SD, standard deviation.
Reprinted from Soyupak SK, Narli N, Yapicioglu H, Satar M, Aksungur EH. Sonographic measurements of the liver, spleen and kidney dimensions in the healthy term and preterm newborns. Eur J Radiol 2002;43:73–78, with permission from Elsevier.

Liver Length in Children[11]

■ Material and Methods

This was a US study in 307 healthy children (**Table 6.5**). Craniocaudal dimension of the liver on the midclavicular line was determined with ultrasonography (**Fig. 6.5**).

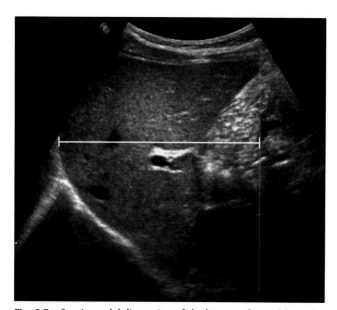

Fig. 6.5   Craniocaudal dimension of the liver on the midclavicular line was determined with ultrasonography.

Table 6.5   Liver length in children[11]

Age (years)	Liver length in midclavicular line (cm)		
	Number of patients	Mean (SD)	Limits of normal
0–0.25	53	6.4 (1.0)	4.0–9.0
0.25–0.5	40	7.3 (1.1)	4.5–9.5
0.5–0.75	20	7.9 (0.8)	6.0–10.0
1–2.5	18	8.5 (1.0)	6.5–10.5
3–5	27	8.6 (1.2)	6.5–11.5
5–7	30	10.0 (1.4)	7.0–12.5
7–9	38	10.5 (1.1)	7.5–13.0
9–11	30	10.5 (1.2)	7.5–13.5
11–13	16	11.5 (1.4)	8.5–14.0
13–15	23	11.8 (1.5)	8.5–14.0
15–17	12	12.1 (1.2)	9.5–14.5

SD, standard deviation.
Reproduced from Konus OL, Ozdemir A, Akkaya A, Erbas G, Celik H, Isik S. Normal liver, spleen, and kidney dimensions in neonates, infants, and children: evaluation with sonography. AJR Am J Roentgenol 1998;171:1693–1698. Reprinted with permission of American Journal of Roentgenology.

Liver Volume in Children[12]

■ Material and Methods

The CT study population consisted of 54 children and young adults (age range 10 days to 22 years) with no history of liver disease (**Table 6.6**). The volume was calculated as follows[1]: the edges of the liver were traced on each scan image and the area was calculated by computer[2]; the areas were summed and multiplied by the scan interval in centimeters (**Figs. 6.6** and **6.7**).

Table 6.6   Liver volume in children[12]

Age (years)	Liver volume	
	Volume cm³ (SD)	Volume/body weight cm³/kg (SD)
0–1	178 (82)	34 (6)
1–2	281 (52)	29 (5)
2–4	426 (95)	32 (6)
5–9	596 (218)	25 (4)
10–15	1024 (210)	24 (4)
≥16	1114 (193)	20 (3)

SD, standard deviation.
With kind permission from Springer Science + Business Media: Noda T, Todani T, Watanabe Y, Yamamoto S. Liver volume in children measured by computed tomography. Pediatr Radiol 1997;27:250–252.

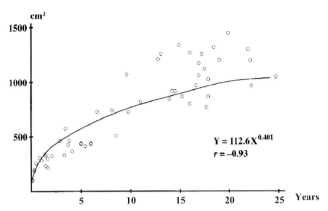

Fig. 6.6   Graphical representation of liver volume versus age. (With kind permission from Springer Science + Business Media: Noda T, Todani T, Watanabe Y, Yamamoto S. Liver volume in children measured by computed tomography. Pediatr Radiol 1997;27:250–252.)

Fig. 6.7   Tracing of the edges of the liver on transverse CT slices.

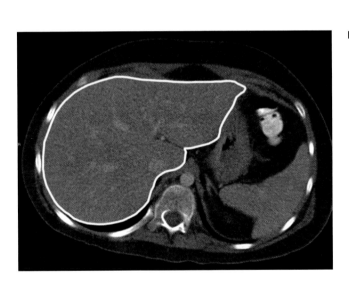

Common Bile Duct: Sonographic Dimensions[13]

■ Material and Methods

One hundred and seventy three consecutive children, referred for abdominal ultrasonography not related to hepatobiliary pathology (**Table 6.7**), were included in this study (100 boys and 73 girls), age range 1 day to 13 years (median age 5.0 years). The diameter of the common bile duct was ≤ 3.3 mm in all patients (**Fig. 6.8**).

Table 6.7 Common bile duct: sonographic dimensions[13]

	Diameter common bile duct (mm)	
Age (years)	Diameter	95% confidence interval
0	0.7	0.2–1.6
1	1.2	0.2–1.7
2	1.0	0.3–1.8
3	1.3	0.3–1.9
4	1.1	0.4–2.0
5	0.8	0.5–2.1
6	1.2	0.5–2.2
7	1.3	0.6–2.3
8	1.5	0.6–2.4
9	1.9	0.7–2.5
10	1.7	0.7–2.6
11	1.7	0.8–2.7
12	1.9	0.8–2.8

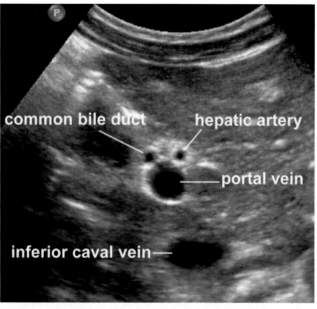

Fig. 6.8 Ultrasonographic image of common bile duct and surrounding anatomy.

Gallbladder Volume of Term and Preterm Infants[15]

■ Material and Methods

US gallbladder volume assessment (length × width × height × π/6) was performed in 50 preterm (mean GA 31.7 ± 2.5 weeks and mean birth weight 1556 ± 441 g) and 46 term infants (mean GA 38.3 ± 1.2 weeks and mean birth weight 3253 ± 440 g). Data were collected soon after delivery and at 6-hour fasting, and at 3-hour and 6-hour fasting following regular milk feeding (**Table 6.8**).

Table 6.8 Gallbladder volume of term and preterm infants[15]

	Gallbladder volume (mL)	
	Term neonates	Preterm neonates
Number of observations	46	50
At birth	1.1 (0.2–2.4)	0.7 (0.1–1.2)
6 hours after birth	1.0 (0.2–2.2)	0.7 (0.1–1.2)
After regular feeding		
Number of observations	46	294
3 hours fasting	0.08 (0–0.2)	0.08 (0–0.2)
6 hours fasting	0.7 (0.1–1.3)	0.3 (0.1–0.9)

Normal Portal Venous Diameter[14]

■ Material and Methods

One hundred and fifty children aged 0 to 16 years, without clinical evidence of liver or intestinal disease, referred for abdominal US were included in the study (**Fig. 6.9** and **Table 6.9**). The portal vein was visualized in the longitudinal axis from the splenomesenteric junction to the liver hilum. The greatest anteroposterior (AP) diameter was measured at the site where the hepatic artery crosses the portal vein (**Fig. 6.10**).

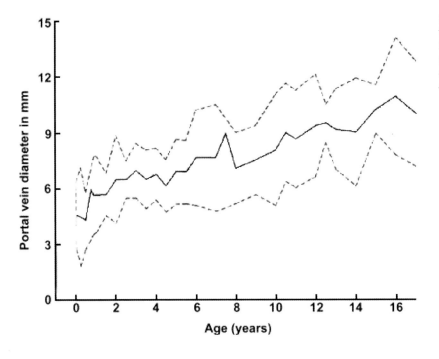

Fig. 6.9 Portal vein diameter in mm in relation to age (years). (With kind permission from Springer Science + Business Media: Patriquin HB, Perreault G, Grignon A, et al. Normal portal venous diameter in children. Pediatr Radiol 1990;20:451–453.)

Table 6.9 Normal portal venous diameter[14]

Age (years)	Portal venous diameter	
	Mean (mm)	Limits of error
0	4.5	3.0–6.3
1	5.7	3.6–7.8
2	6.5	4.2–8.8
3	7.0	5.5–8.5
4	6.8	5.5–8.2
5	7.0	5.2–8.7
6	7.7	5.0–10.3
7	7.7	4.8–10.6
8	7.2	5.3–9.0
9	7.6	5.7–9.5
10	8.2	5.0–11.3
11	8.7	6.1–11.3
12	9.5	6.7–12.1
13	9.2	6.9–11.4
14	9.0	6.2–12.0
15	10.2	9.0–11.5
16	11.0	7.8–14.2

Table created from data within and with kind permission from Springer Science + Business Media: Patriquin HB, Perreault G, Grignon A, et al. Normal portal venous diameter in children. Pediatr Radiol 1990;20:451–453.

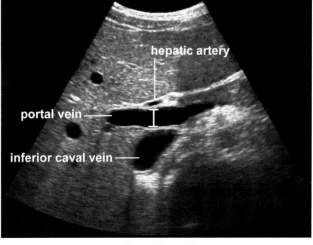

Fig. 6.10 Measurement of portal vein diameter.

Splenic Length in Premature Infants and Neonates[10]

■ Material and Methods

This was a US study in 261 healthy newborn infants (**Table 6.10**). Craniocaudal dimension of the spleen was determined with ultrasonography.

Table 6.10 Splenic length in premature infants and neonates[10]

GA (weeks)	Splenic length (cm)		
	Number of patients	Mean length (±1 SD)	Min-max
24–31	29	2.4 (0.4)	1.6–3.2
32–35	34	2.8 (0.5)	1.7–4.0
36–37	35	3.3 (0.4)	2.6–4.2
38–41	155	3.4 (0.5)	2.4–4.9

SD, standard deviation.
Reprinted from Soyupak SK, Narli N, Yapicioglu H, Satar M, Aksungur EH. Sonographic measurements of the liver, spleen and kidney dimensions in the healthy term and preterm newborns. Eur J Radiol 2002;43:73–78, with permission from Elsevier.

Splenic Length in Childhood[16]

■ Material and Methods

These US studies (**Table 6.11**) comprised 512 healthy children (238 boys and 274 girls) with ages ranging from 1 day (full-term neonate) to 17 years and 96 singleton premature infants with GAs from 25 to 35 weeks.[16] None of the children had a problem that could affect spleen size. Ultrasonography was performed using standard probes matched for age. The measurement of spleen length (**Fig. 6.11**) was the optically maximal distance (ideally at the hilum) on the longitudinal coronal view (between the most superomedial and the most inferolateral points).

Table 6.11 Splenic length in childhood[16]

Age and Sex	Number	Spleen length (cm)			Age and Sex	Number	Spleen length (cm)		
		Mean	SD	Min-max			Mean	SD	Min-max
0–3 mo					6–8 y				
F	22	4.4	0.57	3.2–5.5	F	25	8.2	0.99	6.6–10.0
M	35	4.6	0.84	2.8–6.8	M	26	8.9	0.91	7.4–10.5
3–6 mo					8–10 y				
F	6	5.2	0.47	4.5–5.6	F	26	8.7	0.92	6.4–10.5
M	10	5.8	0.65	4.9–7.0	M	15	9.0	1.02	7.4–11.2
6–12 mo					10–12 y				
F	15	6.3	0.68	5.1–7.5	F	34	9.1	1.09	6.8–11.4
M	12	6.4	0.78	5.4–7.4	M	19	9.8	1.05	7.3–11.3
1–2 y					12–14 y				
F	18	6.3	0.69	5.1–8.2	F	30	9.8	1.02	7.9–11.6
M	17	6.8	0.72	5.6–8.3	M	18	10.2	0.81	8.5–11.7
2–4 y					14–17 y				
F	24	7.5	0.83	5.7–8.9	F	13	10.3	0.69	8.7–11.0
M	22	7.6	1.07	5.9–9.9	M	13	10.7	0.90	9.5–12.5
4–6 y									
F	36	8.0	0.74	6.7–9.5					
M	18	8.1	1.01	6.4–9.9					

F, female; M, male; SD, standard deviation.
Permission to reuse from Megremis SD, Vlachonikolis IG, Tsilimigaki AM. Spleen length in childhood with US: normal values based on age, sex, and somatometric parameters. Radiology 2004;231:129–134. © Radiological Society of North America.

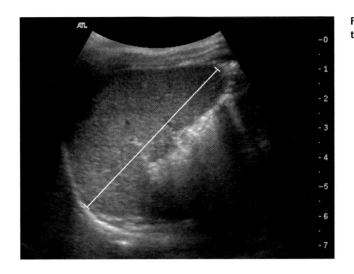

Fig. 6.11   Ultrasonographic measurement of maximal length of the spleen.

Normal Values of the Pancreas in Children[17]

■ Material and Methods

Two hundred and seventy-three patients (differentiation in sex not mentioned) were included in this retrospective ultrasonography study (**Table 6.12**). The maximum AP diameters of the head, body, and tail of the pancreas (**Fig. 6.12**) were measured on transverse/oblique images. Echogenicity was low in 27 (10%), isoechoic in 145 (53%), and high in 101 (37%).

Table 6.12   Normal values of the pancreas in children[17]

Age	Maximal AP diameter pancreas (SD)		
	Head	Body	Tail
Newborn infants	1.0 (0.4)	0.6 (0.2)	1.0 (0.4)
1 mo–1 y	1.5 (0.5)	0.8 (0.3)	1.2 (0.4)
1–5 y	1.7 (0.3)	1.0 (0.2)	1.8 (0.4)
5–10 y	1.6 (0.4)	1.0 (0.3)	1.8 (0.4)
10–19 y	2.0 (0.5)	1.1 (0.3)	2.0 (0.4)

SD, standard deviation.
Permission to reuse from Siegel MJ, Martin KW, Worthington JL. Normal and abnormal pancreas in children: US studies. Radiology 1987;165:15–18. © Radiological Society of North America.

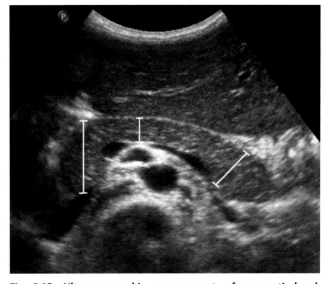

Fig. 6.12   Ultrasonographic measurements of pancreatic head, body, and tail.

Sonographic Bowel Wall Thickness[18]

■ Material and Methods

The study population consisted of 128 patients (57 male and 71 female); of this population, 86 were between the ages of 1 and 19 years (only data pertaining to this selection is presented) (**Table 6.13**). Bowel wall thickness was measured on transverse sections and comprised of mucosa, lamina propria, muscularis mucosa, submucosa, and muscularis propria (**Fig. 6.13**).

Table 6.13 Sonographic data on bowel wall thickness (mm)

Age (y)	Number	Small bowel wall thickness in mm (SD)			Colon wall thickness in mm (SD)		
		Jejunum	Ileum	Cecum	Ascending	Transverse	Descending
0–4	20	0.7 (0.1)	0.8 (0.1)	1.1 (0.2)	1.1 (0.2)	1.0 (0.2)	1.1 (0.2)
5–9	19	0.8 (0.1)	0.9 (0.1)	1.2 (0.1)	1.2 (0.2)	1.2 (0.2)	1.2 (0.2)
10–14	29	0.8 (0.1)	1.0 (0.2)	1.4 (0.2)	1.3 (0.3)	1.3 (0.3)	1.3 (0.2)
15–19	18	0.9 (0.1)	1.1 (0.1)	1.6 (0.2)	1.4 (0.2)	1.4 (0.2)	1.4 (0.2)

SD, standard deviation.

Reproduced with permission of American Institute for Ultrasound in Medicine - AIUM from Haber HP, Stern M. Intestinal ultrasonography in children and young adults: bowel wall thickness is age dependent. J Ultrasound Med 2000;19:315–321; permission conveyed through Copyright Clearance Center, Inc.

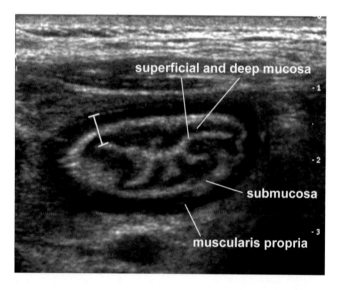

Fig. 6.13 Ultrasonographic measurement of wall thickness of terminal ileum in a 12-year-old boy with cystic fibrosis.

Normal Appendiceal Measurements[19]

■ Material and Methods

In this US study, 146 consecutive patients (62 boys and 84 girls; mean age, 7 years; age range, 2 to 15 years) were included (**Table 6.14**). Children with cystic fibrosis, acute abdominal pain, with previous appendectomy, and below the age of 2 years (because of difficulty in performing the examination) were excluded. In 120 children, the appendix was visualized (**Fig. 6.14**).

Table 6.14 Normal appendiceal measurements[19]

	Mean (SD)	Range	Mean +2SD
AP	3.9 (0.8)	2.1–6.4	5.5
Left-to-right	5.6 (1.1)	2.8–8.5	7.8
AP with compression	3.8 (0.9)	1.6–6.4	5.6
Left-to-right with compression	5.7 (1.1)	2.4–8.5	7.9
Mural thickness	1.8 (0.6)	1.1–2.7	3.0

SD, standard deviation.
Permission to reuse from Wiersma F, Sramek A, Holscher HC. US features of the normal appendix and surrounding area in children. Radiology 2005;235:1018–1022. © Radiological Society of North America.

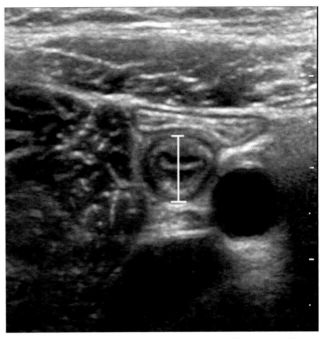

Fig. 6.14 Ultrasonographic AP measurement of the appendix.

Mesenteric Lymph Nodes in Children[20]

■ Material and Methods

In this retrospective study, 61 children (36 boys and 25 girls, mean age 10.7 years, range 1.1 to 17.3 years) underwent noncontrast abdominal CT examination for evaluation of suspected or known renal stones; abdominal lymph node size was evaluated (**Table 6.15**). Enlarged mesenteric lymph nodes (short axis > 5 mm) were found in 33 (54%) of the 61 children. The majority of the enlarged mesenteric lymph nodes were found in the right lower quadrant (88%). Based on their findings, the authors state that using a short-axis diameter of > 8 mm might be a more appropriate definition for mesenteric lymphadenopathy in children.

Table 6.15 False-positive rate for enlarged mesenteric lymph nodes with varying lymph node threshold size

Threshold size (mm)	Number enlarged lymph node(s)	False-positive (%)
≥ 5	33	54
> 6	18	30
> 7	8	13
> 8	3	5
> 9	3	5
> 10	0	0

With kind permission from Springer Science + Business Media: Karmazyn B, Werner EA, Rejaie B, Applegate KE. Mesenteric lymph nodes in children: what is normal? Pediatr Radiol 2005;35:774–777.

Urogenital Tract

Kidney Length in Premature Infants and Neonates[10]

■ Material and Methods

This was a US study in 261 healthy newborn infants (**Table 6.16**). Craniocaudal dimension of the kidneys was determined with ultrasonography (**Fig. 6.15**).

Table 6.16   Kidney length in premature infants and neonates[10]

GA (weeks)	Kidney length (cm)		
	Number of patients	Mean length (±1 SD)	Min-max
24–31	29	3.3 (0.4)	2.5–4.0
32–35	33	3.6 (0.4)	2.5–4.6
36–37	35	4.1 (0.4)	3.0–4.9
38–41	155	4.1 (0.4)	2.6–5.2

SD, standard deviation.
Table created from data within Soyupak SK, Narli N, Yapicioglu H, Satar M, Aksungur EH. Sonographic measurements of the liver, spleen and kidney dimensions in the healthy term and preterm newborns. Eur J Radiol 2002;43:73–78, with permission from Elsevier.

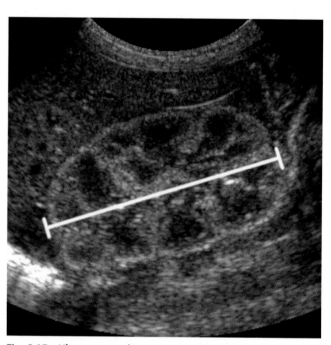

Fig. 6.15   Ultrasonographic measurement of the length of a neonatal kidney. Note the increased echogenicity of the renal parenchyma compared to liver parenchyma; this is normal at this age.

Kidney Length in Children[21]

■ Material and Methods

Two hundred and three patients were included in this ultrasonography study (**Table 6.17**). Patients were excluded if they had a history of malignancy, use of steroids, upper urinary tract abnormality, vesicoureteral reflux greater than grade I, urologic surgery, or if sonography of the kidney was regarded as abnormal. On average, the left kidney was 1.9 mm larger than the right kidney (**Fig. 6.16**).

Table 6.17   Kidney length in children[21]

Age	Renal length (cm)	
	Number	Renal length (SD)
0–1 wk	10	4.5 (0.3)
1 wk–4 mo	54	5.3 (0.7)
4–8 mo	20	6.2 (0.7)
8 mo–1 y	8	6.2 (0.6)
1–2 y	28	6.6 (0.5)
2–3 y	12	7.4 (0.5)
3–4 y	30	7.4 (0.6)
4–5 y	26	7.9 (0.5)
5–6 y	30	8.1 (0.5)
6–7 y	14	7.8 (0.7)
7–8 y	18	8.3 (0.5)
8–9 y	18	8.9 (0.9)
9–10 y	14	9.2 (0.9)
10–11 y	28	9.2 (0.8)
11–12 y	22	9.6 (0.6)
12–13 y	18	10.4 (0.9)
13–14 y	14	9.8 (0.8)
14–15 y	14	10.0 (0.6)
15–16 y	6	11.0 (0.8)
16–17 y	10	10.0 (0.9)
17–18 y	4	10.5 (0.3)
18–19 y	8	10.8 (1.1)

SD, standard deviation.
Reproduced from Rosenbaum DM, Korngold E, Teele RL. Sonographic assessment of renal length in normal children. AJR Am J Roentgenol 1984;142:467–469. Reprinted with permission of American Journal of Roentgenology.

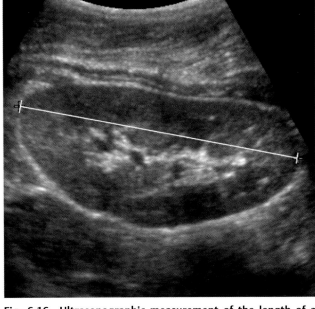

Fig. 6.16   Ultrasonographic measurement of the length of a kidney.

Kidney Volume[22]

■ Material and Methods

A total of 3376 children were recruited in this US study (**Table 6.18**). Kidney volume was calculated using the ellipsoid formula as length × width × depth × 0.523 (**Fig. 6.17**). In this study, the total renal volume was obtained by adding together both kidney volumes but without mentioning the separate values for the left and right kidney. The values in the above-mentioned table were obtained by dividing the total renal volume by 2.

Table 6.18   Kidney volume[22]

Age (years)	Number	Renal volume mL (SD)
0	99	15 (4)
0.25	81	22 (6)
0.5	121	28 (3)
1	111	31 (5)
2	87	37 (5)
3	135	45 (6)
4	115	51 (5)
5	109	56 (7)
6	173	162 (6)
7	142	68 (6)
8	127	76 (7)
9	147	82 (6)
10	125	87 (5)
11	104	94 (6)
12	90	101 (6)
13	87	108 (8)
14	90	113 (8)
15	85	118 (7)
16	50	126 (8)
17	41	131 (6)

SD, standard deviation.
Table created with data within and with kind permission from Springer Science + Business Media: Leung VY, Chu WC, Yeung CK, et al. Nomograms of total renal volume, urinary bladder volume and bladder wall thickness index in 3,376 children with a normal urinary tract. Pediatr Radiol 2007;37:181–188.

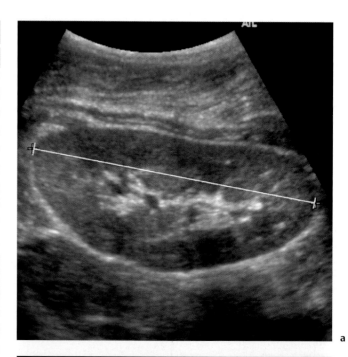

a

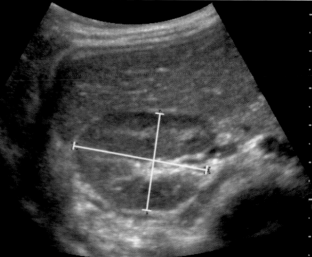

b

Fig. 6.17a, b   Ultrasonographic measurement of the length (a) and the width and depth (b) of a kidney.

Bladder Capacity[22]

■ Material and Methods

A total of 3376 children were recruited in this US study (**Table 6.19**). The bladder volume was calculated first by measuring the maximum length of the urinary bladder on the longitudinal scan, which was obtained from the neck to the fundus of the bladder. Depth was measured, perpendicular to the first plane at the level of the maximum area, in the midline from the anterior to posterior mucosal surface of the bladder (**Fig. 6.18**). The width was taken perpendicular to the depth at its midpoint. Bladder volume as presented in the table was recalculated from the data in this study using the equation for an ellipsoid: length × width × depth (in centimeters) × 0.523.

Table 6.19   Bladder capacity[22]

Age (years)	Bladder capacity in mL	
	Number	Volume (SD)
Newborn infants	99	34 (10)
1	111	80 (21)
2	87	110 (32)
3	135	136 (43)
4	115	173 (43)
5	109	205 (49)
6	173	235 (49)
7	142	273 (49)
8	127	299 (37)
9	147	334 (42)
10	125	363 (28)
11	104	396 (26)
12	90	433 (37)
13	87	465 (47)
14	90	497 (35)
15	85	524 (42)
16	50	551 (38)
17	41	585 (43)

SD, standard deviation.
The total number of patients does not add up to the total number of patients in this study because not all age subgroups were included in the table.
Table created with data within and with kind permission from Springer Science + Business Media: Leung VY, Chu WC, Yeung CK, et al. Nomograms of total renal volume, urinary bladder volume and bladder wall thickness index in 3,376 children with a normal urinary tract. Pediatr Radiol 2007;37:181–188.

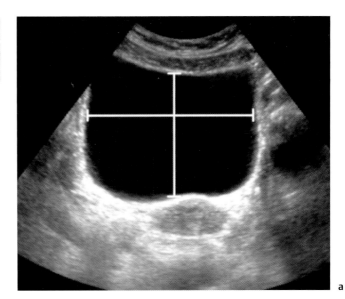

a

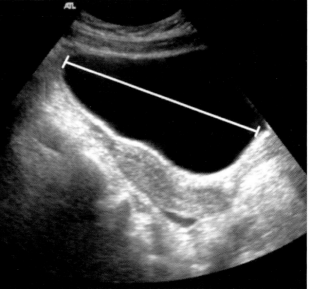

b

Fig. 6.18a, b   Bladder. (a) Transverse measurements. **(b)** Longitudinal measurement.

Bladder Wall Thickness[22]

■ Material and Methods

A total of 3376 children were recruited in this ultrasonographic study (**Table 6.20** and **Fig. 6.19**). Bladder wall thickness was only measured when the residual bladder volume was < 10% of the original volume. Bladder wall thickness was measured from a zoomed image of the transverse plane of the voided bladder at three points: anterolaterally, laterally, and posterolaterally (**Fig. 6.20**). The mean was taken for these three measurements.

Table 6.20   Bladder wall thickness[22]

| Age (years) | Bladder volume wall index (BVWI) in cm² | |
	Number	BVWI (SD)
Newborns	99	210 (88)
1	111	524 (154)
2	87	649 (250)
3	135	850 (292)
4	115	1045 (387)
5	109	1212 (399)
6	173	1410 (402)
7	142	1594 (397)
8	127	1774 (408)
9	147	1923 (436)
10	125	2106 (419)
11	104	2315 (460)
12	90	2492 (577)
13	87	2713 (541)
14	90	2958 (537)
15	85	3103 (435)
16	50	3322 (521)
17	41	3495 (503)

SD, standard deviation.
With kind permission from Springer Science + Business Media: Leung VY, Chu WC, Yeung CK, et al. Nomograms of total renal volume, urinary bladder volume and bladder wall thickness index in 3,376 children with a normal urinary tract. Pediatr Radiol 2007;37:181–188.

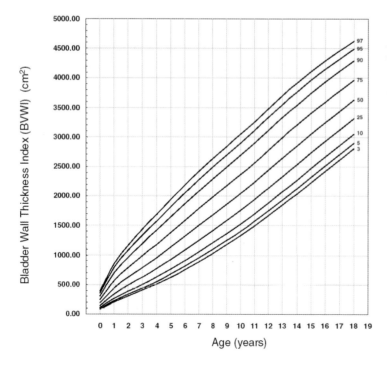

Fig. 6.19   Bladder volume wall thickness index (BVWI) (cm²) in relation to age (years). (With kind permission from Springer Science + Business Media: Leung VY, Chu WC, Yeung CK, et al. Nomograms of total renal volume, urinary bladder volume and bladder wall thickness index in 3,376 children with a normal urinary tract. Pediatr Radiol 2007;37:181–188.)

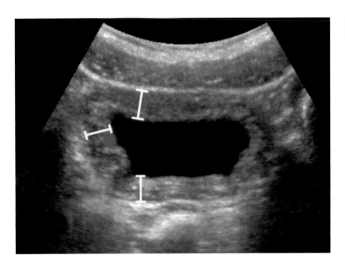

Fig. 6.20 Anterolateral, lateral, and posterolateral measurements of the bladder wall after voiding.

The bladder wall thickness depends on the degree of filling of the bladder *and* its capacity. Therefore, the bladder wall thickness was expressed as the "bladder volume wall thickness index" (BVWI):

$$\text{BVWI} = \frac{\text{Depth} \times \text{width} \times \text{length (cm)}}{\text{Average wall thickness (cm)}}$$

The total number of patients does not add up to the total number of patients in this study because not all age subgroups were included in the table.

Adrenal Gland Size[26]

■ Material and Methods

This was an US study of 92 infants (**Table 6.21**). The length of the gland was defined as the maximum cephalocaudal dimension (either coronal or sagittal plane; **Figs. 6.21** and **6.22**), the width was defined as the maximum thickness of one of the limbs.

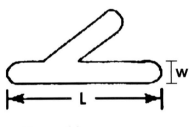

Coronal image

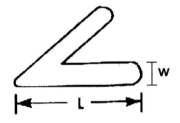

Sagittal image

Fig. 6.21 Coronal and sagittal schematics of measuring an adrenal gland. (Permission to reuse from Oppenheimer DA, Carroll BA, Yousem S. Sonography of the normal neonatal adrenal gland. Radiology 1983;146:157–160. © Radiological Society of North America).

Table 6.21 Adrenal gland size[26]

GA (weeks)	Dimensions adrenal gland in cm	
	Length (range)	Width (range)
25–30	1.2 (0.9–3.6)	0.3 (0.2–0.5)
31–35	1.4 (0.9–3.6)	0.3 (0.2–0.5)
36–40	1.7 (0.9–3.6)	0.3 (0.2–0.5)

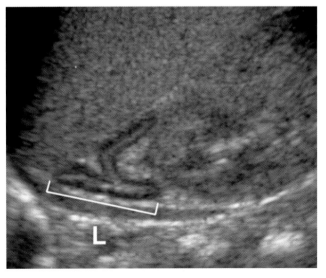

Fig. 6.22 Sagittal measurement of the adrenal gland.

Thickness of the Wall of the Collecting System[23]

■ Material and Methods

This was an ultrasonographic study of 48 renal collecting systems in 24 healthy children (age range 3 days to 12.6 years). The collecting system could be identified in all kidneys and its wall thickness varied between 0 (not visible) and 0.8 mm (**Fig. 6.23**).

Thickening of the wall ≥ 1 mm should be considered as pathologic and is caused by urinary tract infection, intermittent dilatation (e.g., vesicoureteric reflux), and dilatation in the recent past (**Fig. 6.24**).

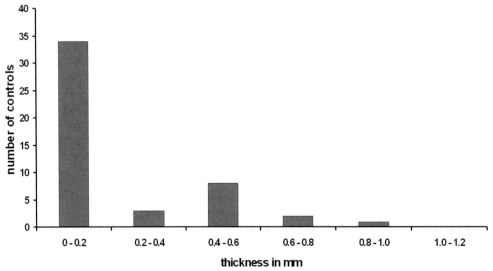

Fig. 6.23   Thickness of the wall of the renal collecting system. (With kind permission from Springer Science + Business Media. Robben SG, Boesten M, Linmans J, Lequin MH, Nijman RM. Significance of thickening of the wall of the renal collecting system in children: an ultrasound study. Pediatr Radiol 1999;29:736–740.)

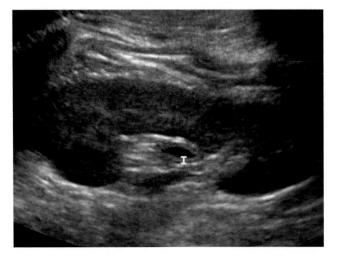

Fig. 6.24   Measurement of wall thickness of the renal pelvis.

Testicular Size[24]

■ Material and Methods

A total of 344 boys from different ethnic backgrounds were studied (**Table 6.22**). Testicular volume was calculated using the formula: length × width × height × 0.523. There were no differences between ethnic groups or between right and left testicle (**Fig. 6.25**).

Table 6.22   Testicular size[24]

Age	Testicular volume (mL) Mean (SD)
1 mo	0.30 (0.10)
3 mo	0.36 (0.10)
5 mo	0.39 (0.10)
7 mo	0.32 (0.10)
9 mo	0.31 (0.10)
11 mo	0.30 (0.10)
2 y	0.31 (0.10)
6 y	0.31 (0.10)

SD, standard deviation.
Table created from data within Kuijper EA, van Kooten J, Verbeke JI, van Rooijen M, Lambalk CB. Ultrasonographically measured testicular volumes in 0- to 6-year-old boys. Hum Reprod 2008;23:792–796, by permission of Oxford University Press.

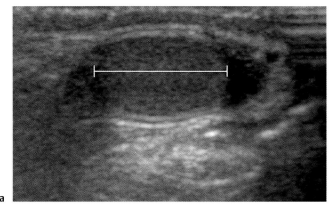 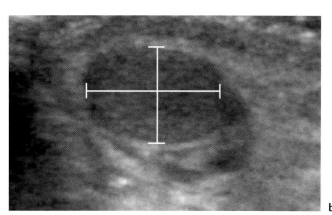

a   b

Fig. 6.25a, b   Ultrasonographic measurement of the length (a) and width and depth (b) of a testicle.

Uterine and Ovarian Volume[25]

■ Material and Methods

An ultrasonographic measurement of uterine and ovarian volume was performed in 178 healthy girls (**Table 6.23**). The volumes were calculated using the formula for an ellipsoid (longitudinal diameter × AP diameter × transverse diameter × 0.523; **Figs. 6.26** and **6.27**).

Table 6.23   Uterine and ovarian volume[25]

	Uterine and ovarian volume in mL (SD)			
Age[1]	Number	Uterus	Number	Ovary
0–1 mo	15	3.4 (1.2)	6	0.5 (0.4)
3 mo	7	0.9 (0.2)	4	0.4 (0.1)
1 y	19	1.0 (0.2)	6	0.5 (0.2)
3 y	26	1.0 (0.3)	17	0.7 (0.4)
5 y	26	1.0 (0.3)	13	0.7 (0.5)
7 y	28	0.9 (0.3)	15	0.8 (0.6)
9 y	18	1.3 (0.4)	12	0.6 (0.4)
11 y	16	1.9 (0.9)	10	1.3 (1.0)
13 y	8	11.0 (10.5)	8	3.7 (2.1)
15 y	15	21.2 (13.5)	9	6.7 (4.8)

SD, standard deviation.
With kind permission from Springer Science + Business Media: Haber HP, Mayer EI. Ultrasound evaluation of uterine and ovarian size from birth to puberty. Pediatr Radiol 1994;24:11–13.

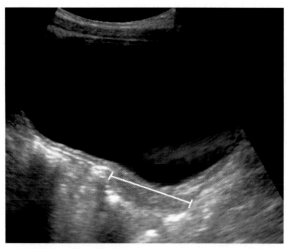
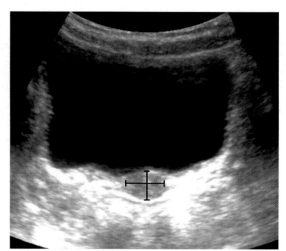

Fig. 6.26a, b   Sagittal (a) and transverse (b) uterine measurements.

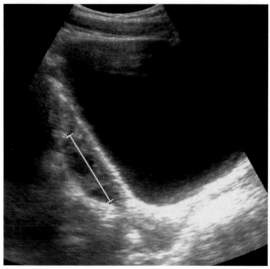
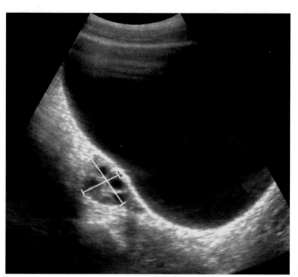

Fig. 6.27a, b   Sagittal (a) and transverse (b) ovarian measurements.

Skull, Intracranial Space, and Vertebral Column

Inner Ear Measurements[4]

■ Material and Methods

This was a computed tomography (CT) study of inner ear structures in 15 patients (children and adults) without hearing loss (**Table 6.24**). Measurements were taken from 1-mm transverse and coronal slices (**Fig. 6.28**). The measurements are valid for all ages because the inner ear structures do not change in size after birth.

Table 6.24   Inner ear measurements

Anatomical site	Inner ear measurements (mm)	
	Mean (SD)	Description of measurement
Transverse cuts		
SSCC: lumen	1.2 (0.1)	Canal lumen measured at maximum diameter of the turn
SSCC: bony island width	4.9 (0.4)	Bony island measured at maximum diameter of the turn
PSCC: lumen	1.3 (0.1)	Canal lumen measured 1–2 cuts up from inferior limb
LSCC: lumen	1.3 (0.1)	All measurements can be made on the same cut
LSCC: bony island	3.7 (0.4)	Measured from medial to lateral
Cochlea: lumen basal turn	2.2 (0.2)	Basal turn can easily be identified
Cochlea: length basal turn	8.6 (0.4)	Length and lumen often can be measured on the same cut
Vestibulum: length	5.8 (0.6)	Both measurements can be taken on the same cut, often
Vestibulum: width	3.4 (0.3)	The same cut as the LSCC
IAC: opening width	6.9 (1.4)	Measurements taken on the longest cut
IAC: length	11.1 (1.7)	
Coronal cuts		
Cochlea height	5.3 (0.5)	Measurement on cut with maximum height that includes basal and upper turn

IAC, internal auditory canal; LSCC, lateral semicircular canal; PSCC, posterior semicircular canal; SD, standard deviation; SSCC, superior semicircular canal.
Reprinted from Purcell D, Johnson J, Fischbein N, Lalwani AK. Establishment of normative cochlear and vestibular measurements to aid in the diagnosis of inner ear malformations. Otolaryngol Head Neck Surg 2003;128:78–87, with permission from Elsevier.

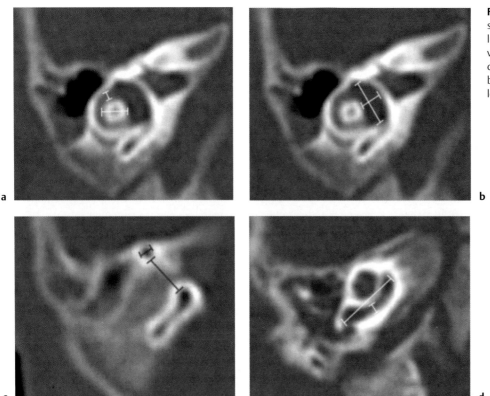

Fig. 6.28a–d　Inner ear. (a) Lateral semicircular canal (LSCC) transverse: lumen and bony island. **(b)** LSCC transverse: vestibulum. **(c)** Superior semicircular canal transverse: lumen and bony island. **(d)** Cochlea transverse: length and lumen of basal turn.

Ultrasonographic Measurements of the Premature Brain[5]

A US study of 1483 neonates (**Table 6.25**) with a gestational age (GA) range of 25 to 42 weeks (**Figs. 6.29** and **6.30**). The neonates were examined at day 3. All neonates with perinatal asphyxia, infection of the central nervous system, or intracranial hemorrhages of craniospinal malformation were excluded.

The anterior horn width and the ventriculo-hemispheric ratio were measured on the coronal view at the level of the foramen of Monro (**Figs. 6.31** and **6.32**).

Table 6.25　Ultrasonographic measurements of the premature brain

GA (weeks)	Anterior Horn Width (mm)		Ventriculo-Hemispheric Ratio
	No patients	Mean (P5–P95)	Mean (P5–P95)
26	7	1.1 (1.0–1.2)	0.28 (0.27–0.28)
28	25	1.2 (1.0–1.3)	0.28 0.27–0.28)
30	40	1.3 (1.1–1.4)	0.28 (0.27–0.28)
32	61	1.3 (1.2–1.6)	0.28 (0.27–0.29)
34	86	1.5 (1.4–1.8)	0.28 (0.28–0.29)
36	49	1.8 (1.6–2.1)	0.28 (0.27–0.29)
38	245	2.3 (1.8–2.6)	0.28 (0.27–0.29)
40	322	2.7 (2.2–3.0)	0.28 (0.28–0.29)
42	64	2.9 (2.7–3.1)	0.28 (0.28–0.29)

Table created from data within Sondhi V, Gupta G, Gupta PK, Patnaik SK, Tshering K. Establishment of nomograms and reference ranges for intra-cranial ventricular dimensions and ventriculo-hemispheric ratio in newborns by ultrasonography. Acta Paediatr 2008;97:738–744, with permission from John Wiley and Sons, Inc.

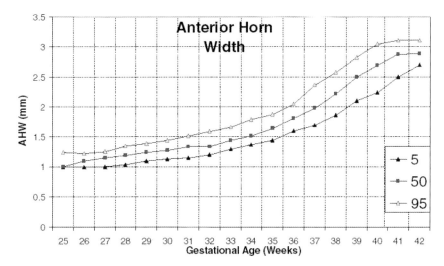

Fig. 6.29 Anterior horn width. (Reprinted from Sondhi V, Gupta G, Gupta PK, Patnaik SK, Tshering K. Establishment of nomograms and reference ranges for intra-cranial ventricular dimensions and ventriculo-hemispheric ratio in newborns by ultra-sonography. Acta Paediatr 2008;97:738–744, with permission from John Wiley and Sons, Inc.)

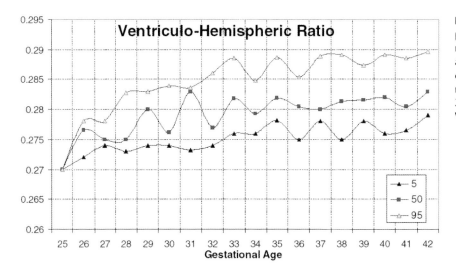

Fig. 6.30 Ventriculo-hemispheric ratio. (Reprinted from Sondhi V, Gupta G, Gupta PK, Patnaik SK, Tshering K. Establishment of nomograms and reference ranges for intra-cranial ventricular dimensions and ventriculo-hemispheric ratio in newborns by ultrasonography. Acta Paediatr 2008;97:738–744, with permission from John Wiley and Sons, Inc.)

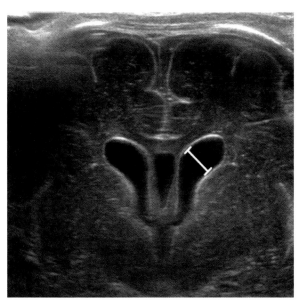

Fig. 6.31 Measurement of the anterior horn.

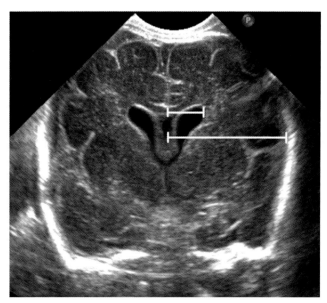

Fig. 6.32 Measurement of the ventriculo-hemispheric ratio.

Subarachnoid Space⁶

■ Material and Methods

The subarachnoid space was assessed using ultrasonography in 278 full-term healthy Chinese infants (**Table 6.26**). Measurements were taken in the coronal plane at the level of the foramen of Monro (**Figs. 6.33** and **6.34**).

The mean values in the table were calculated from the equations given in the article and the 95% confidence levels were derived from the graphs in the article.

Table 6.26   Subarachnoid space

| Age (weeks) | Subarachnoid space in mm (95th percentile) | | |
	CCW	SCW	IHW
0	2.4 (7.2)	2.2 (5.2)	2.9 (6.6)
4	3.2 (8.0)	2.7 (5.7)	3.4 (7.0)
8	3.8 (8.6)	3.1 (6.1)	3.8 (7.4)
12	4.3 (9.2)	3.4 (6.4)	4.1 (7.8)
16	4.8 (9.5)	3.6 (6.7)	4.4 (8.0)
20	5.1 (9.8)	3.8 (6.8)	4.6 (8.2)
24	5.2 (10.0)	3.9 (6.9)	4.7 (8.4)
28	5.3 (10.1)	3.9 (7.0)	4.8 (8.4)
32	5.2 (10.0)	3.9 (6.9)	4.8 (8.5)
36	5.1 (9.8)	3.8 (6.8)	4.8 (8.4)
40	4.8 (9.6)	3.6 (6.6)	4.6 (8.3)
44	4.4 (9.2)	3.3 (6.4)	4.5 (8.2)
48	3.8 (8.8)	3.0 (6.1)	4.2 (7.9)

CCW, craniocortical width; IHW, interhemispheric width; SCW, sinocortical width.
Table created from data within Lam WW, Ai VH, Wong V, Leong LL. Ultrasonographic measurement of subarachnoid space in normal infants and children. Pediatr Neurol 2001;25:380–384, with permission from Elsevier.

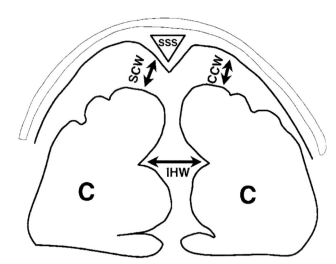

Fig. 6.33   Schematic coronal representation of the subarachnoid space at the level of the foramen of Monro. (Reprinted from Lam WW, Ai VH, Wong V, Leong LL. Ultrasonographic measurement of subarachnoid space in normal infants and children. Pediatr Neurol 2001;25:380–384, with permission from Elsevier.)
CCW   Craniocortical width
IHW   Interhemispherical width
SCW   Sinocortical width
SSS   Superior sagittal sinus

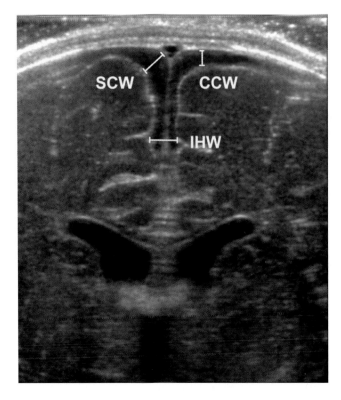

Fig. 6.34   Ultrasonographic coronal representation of the subarachnoid space at the level of the foramen of Monro.
CCW   Craniocortical width
IHW   Interhemispherical width
SCW   Sinocortical width

Pituitary Gland Dimensions[7,8]

■ Material and Methods

The height of the pituitary gland was measured in 60 children without hypothalamo-hypophyseal disease on sagittal midline T1 images (**Fig. 6.35**).[7]

The volumetric study consisted of 199 healthy pediatric patients (90 boys and 109 girls) with clinically normal pituitary function and no abnormal findings on routine magnetic reso-

nance imaging (MR) studies (**Table 6.27**). The volume of the normal pituitary gland in children and adolescents was measured by using three-dimensional MRI sequences with a section thickness of 0.6 to 0.75 mm. The volume of interest was determined by manual tracing with a mouse-guided cursor and processed using a workstation (**Fig. 6.35**).[8]

Table 6.27   Pituitary gland dimensions

		Pituitary gland dimensions in mm, resp. mm³		
	Age (years)	Height (range)[7]	Volume whole pituitary (SD)	Volume posterior pituitary (SD)[8]
Boys	0–1	3.8 (3.0–4.4)	148 (37)	31 (9)
	1–4	4.5 (4.0–5.0)	204 (54)	49 (16)
	5–9	5.1 (3.7–5.5)	336 (114)	61 (19)[2]
	10–14	5.3 (4.5–7.0)	567 (127)[1]	75 (20)
	15–19	6.5 (5.7–7.2)	655 (99)	76 (31)
Boys	0–1	3.6 (3.0–5.2)	133 (40)	27 (8)
	1–4	3.3 (3.0–4.0)	213 (44)	53 (23)
	5–9	4.3 (3.5–5.0)	310 (55)	72 (18)
	10–14	5.3 (4.5–6.5)	424 (110)	80 (18)
	15–19	5.7 (5.7–5.7)	586 (150)	90 (23)

SD, standard deviation.
Volume of whole pituitary gland includes both anterior *and* posterior pituitary gland.
Significant difference between boys and girls $p < 0.01$[1] and $p < 0.05$.[2]
Table created with data within and with kind permission from Springer Science + Business Media: Argyropoulou M, Perignon F, Brunelle F, Brauner R, Rappaport R. Height of normal pituitary gland as a function of age evaluated by magnetic resonance imaging in children. Pediatr Radiol 1991;21:247–249, and with permission of American Society of Neuoradiology from Takano K, Utsunomiya H, Ono H, Ohfu M, Okazaki M. Normal development of the pituitary gland: assessment with three-dimensional MR volumetry. AJNR Am J Neuroradiol 1999;20:312–315; permission conveyed through Copyright Clearance Center, Inc.

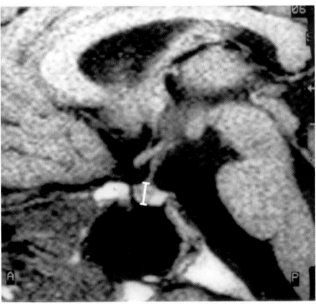
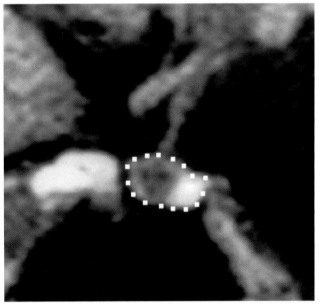

a   b

Fig. 6.35a, b   Pituitary gland. (a) Height of pituitary gland. **(b)** Volumetry of whole pituitary gland.

Thyroid Gland Volume[1–3]

■ Material and Methods

This was a US study of 100 English newborn infants in the first week of life,[3] a subset of iodine-sufficient European children from a study of 5709 children, aged 6 to 15 years,[1] and a subset of German children from a study of 252 children aged 2 to 4 years[2] (**Table 6.28**).

The volume of a thyroid lobe was (re)calculated by the formula of an ellipsoid (length × width × height × π/6). The thyroid volume was the sum of the volumes of both lobes. The volume of the isthmus was not included (**Fig. 6.36**).

Table 6.28 Thyroid gland volume

Age (years)	Thyroid volume (mL)			
	Number	Mean[2,3] or P50[1]	Upper limit (P97 or +SD)	
			Boys	Girls
Newborn infants	100	1.6	2.4	2.5
2	–	2.0	3.0	3.0
4	–	2.9	5.5	5.1
6	–	3.3	5.9	5.5
7	–	3.7	6.2	6.4
8	–	4.1	6.7	7.5
9	–	4.7	7.4	8.7
10	–	5.2	8.5	10.0
11	–	5.8	9.8	11.4
12	–	6.6	11.4	12.8
13	–	7.4	13.1	14.3
14	–	8.2	15.2	15.9
15	–	9.1	17.5	17.6

SD, standard deviation.
Table created from data within: Delange F, Benker G, Caron P, et al. Thyroid volume and urinary iodine in European schoolchildren: standardization of values for assessment of iodine deficiency. Eur J Endocrinol 1997;136:180–187. © Society of the European Journal of Endocrinology (1997). Reproduced kind permission of Georg Thieme Verlag: Menken KU, Engelhardt S, Olbricht T. [Thyroid gland volume and urinary iodine excretion in children 2–16 years of age]. Dtsch Med Wochenschr 1992;117:1047–1051. With permission from BMJ Publishing Group Ltd: Perry RJ, Hollman AS, Wood AM, Donaldson MD. Ultrasound of the thyroid gland in the newborn: normative data. Arch Dis Child Fetal Neonatal Ed 2002;87:F209–211.

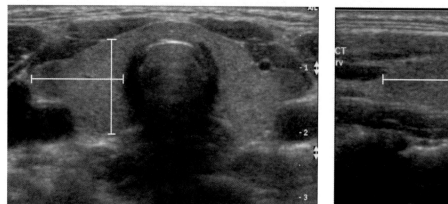
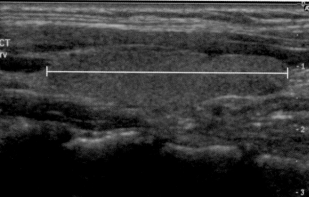

Fig. 6.36a, b Right thyroid lobe. Transverse (**a**) and sagittal (**b**) ultrasonographic measurements of the right thyroid lobe.

The Skeleton and Soft Tissues

Limb Bones Ratio[27]

■ Material and Methods

This was a radiographic study of middle and upper-middle class white children of northern European ancestry (**Table 6.29**). Length was measured parallel to the long axis of the most proximal edge of the diaphysis to the most distal edge of the diaphysis (**Fig. 6.37**). These ratios may be used to detect rhizomelic and mesomelic disorders.

Table 6.29   Limb bones ratio[27]

Bone ratio	Diaphyseal bone length ratios			
	Age (years)	Number	Mean	P_5–P_{95}
Radius/humerus	0.2–0.5	134	0.82	0.77–0.89
	0.5–1.0	132	0.79	0.74–0.85
	1.0–1.5	45	0.77	0.73–0.82
	1.5–2.0	123	0.76	0.72–0.80
	2.0–10.0	218	0.75	0.71–0.78
	10.0–15.0	170	0.75	0.71–0.78
Tibia/femur	0.2–0.5	133	0.81	0.75–0.87
	0.5–1.0	132	0.81	0.76–0.85
	1.0–1.5	45	0.81	0.78–0.83
	1.5–2.0	124	0.81	0.78–0.84
	2.0–10.0	218	0.81	0.78–0.85
	10.0–15.0	170	0.82	0.78–0.86
Humerus/femur	0.2–0.5	133	0.83	0.75–0.92
	0.5–1.0	132	0.79	0.73–0.83
	1.0–1.5	45	0.77	0.73–0.80
	1.5–2.0	124	0.76	0.73–0.80
	2.0–10.0	218	0.71	0.67–0.75
	10.0–15.0	170	0.69	0.65–0.72
Radius/tibia	0.2–0.5	134	0.84	0.77–0.94
	0.5–1.0	132	0.77	0.72–0.82
	1.0–1.5	45	0.74	0.69–0.78
	1.5–2.0	123	0.71	0.67–0.76
	2.0–10.0	218	0.65	0.61–0.70
	10.0–15.0	170	0.63	0.59–0.66

Permission to reuse from Robinow M, Chumlea WC. Standards for limb bone length ratios in children. Radiology 1982;143:433–436. © Radiological Society of North America.

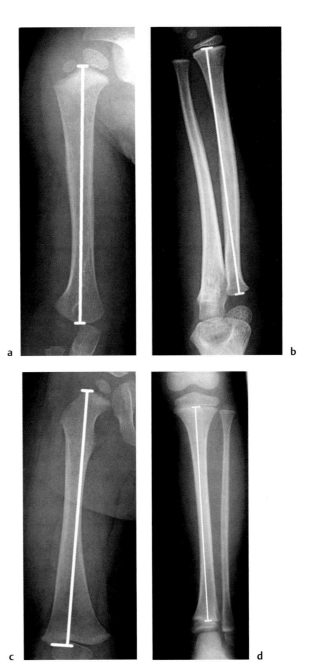

Fig. 6.37a–d Measurements of humerus (a), radius (b), femur (c), and tibia (d).

Anterior Hip Synovial Recess[28]

■ Material and Methods

This was a US study of 58 healthy children and 105 children with unilateral transient synovitis (age range 1.7 to 12.8 years; **Tables 6.30** and **6.31**). The children were examined in the supine position with hips in neutral position. An anterior approach along the long axis of the femoral neck was used. The anterior joint capsule was measured, including both of its components (the anterior and posterior layer;

Fig. 6.38). Also, the anterior contour of the joint capsule was evaluated.

There was no statistically significant correlation between age and thickness of the anterior joint capsule.

A difference of more than 2 mm between both hips was considered a sound threshold for pathology, and also an effusion of more than 2 mm was considered pathologic.

Table 6.30 Normal anterior joint capsule dimensions

Normal anterior joint capsule dimensions in mm			
	Number	Mean	SD
Anterior joint capsule	105	4.9	1.0
Anterior layer	83	2.5	0.6
Posterior layer	83	2.1	0.6

SD, standard deviation.
Permission to reuse from Robben SG, Lequin MH, Diepstraten AF, den Hollander JC, Entius CA, Meradji M. Anterior joint capsule of the normal hip and in children with transient synovitis: US study with anatomic and histologic correlation. Radiology 1999;210:499–507. © Radiological Society of North America.

Table 6.31 Shape of the border of the anterior joint capsule with unilateral transient synovitis

Shape of the border of the anterior joint capsule in 105 patients with unilateral transient synovitis		
	Asymptomatic hip	Transient synovitis hip
Convex	9	99
Straight	31	6
Concave	65	0

Permission to reuse from Robben SG, Lequin MH, Diepstraten AF, den Hollander JC, Entius CA, Meradji M. Anterior joint capsule of the normal hip and in children with transient synovitis: US study with anatomic and histologic correlation. Radiology 1999;210:499–507. © Radiological Society of North America.

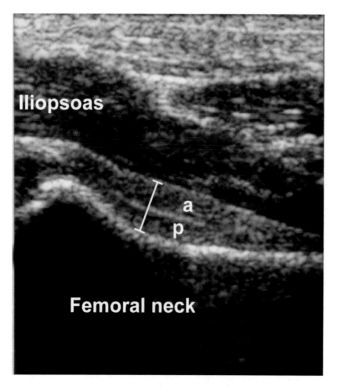

Fig. 6.38 Ultrasonographic measurement of the anterior joint capsule. Both anterior (a) and posterior (p) layer can be identified. (Permission to reuse from Robben SG, Lequin MH, Diepstraten AF, den Hollander JC, Entius CA, Meradji M. Anterior joint capsule of the normal hip and in children with transient synovitis: US study with anatomic and histologic correlation. Radiology 1999;210:499–507.© Radiological Society of North America).

Classification of Developmental Dysplasia of the Hip[29] (Fig. 6.39 and Table 6.32)

Type I: Mature centered hip joint. Well developed acetabular roof. Angular or slightly blunt bony rim.
Type II: Centered joint but deficiently developed acetabular roof. Rounded bony rim.

Type III: Decentered joint. Poorly developed acetabular roof. Flattened bony rim.

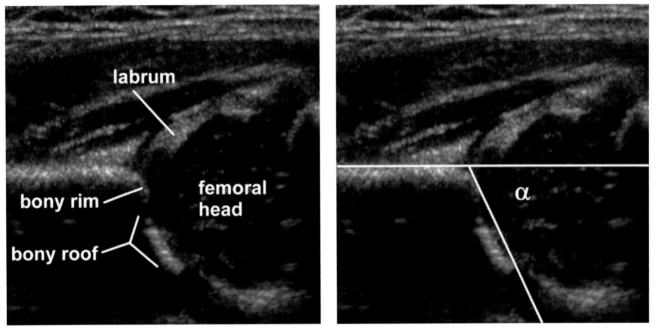

a   b

Fig. 6.39a, b   Normal ultrasonographic anatomy of the hip joint in the coronal plane. (a) Measurement of α angle. **(b)** Atlantoaxial interval.[30]

Table 6.32   Classification of developmental dysplasia of the hip

	Ultrasonographic parameters				
Type	*α -Angle/Bony roof*	*Bony rim*	*Cartilaginous roof*	*Age*	*Treatment*
Type I Mature hip	α ≥ 60 degrees adequate bony roof	Angular or slightly rounded	Covers femoral head	Any age	No
Type II a+ Immature but appropriate for age	α = 50–59 degrees adequate bony roof	Rounded	Covers femoral head	0–12 wk	No, but follow up
Type II a− Immature but inappropriate for age	α = 50–59 degrees deficient bony roof	Rounded	Covers femoral head	6–12 wk	Yes
Type II b Delay in development	α = 50–59 degrees deficient bony roof	Rounded	Covers femoral head	≥ 12 wk	Yes
Type II c Critical	α = 43–49 degrees very deficient bony roof	Rounded to flattened	Covers femoral head	Any age	Yes
Type D Decentering	α = 43–49 degrees very deficient bony roof	Rounded to flattened	Displaced	Any age	Yes
Type III Eccentric hip	α ≤ 43 degrees poor bony roof	Flattened	Displaced	Any age	Yes

From Graf R. Hip sonography: diagnosis and management of infant hip dysplasia. Berlin Heidelberg: Springer, 2006. With kind permission of Springer Science + Business Media.

■ Material and Methods

Computer-assisted digital measurements of atlantoaxial interval (ADI) in 101 children, aged 1 to 12 years, were obtained from lateral supine head-neutral radiographs (**Fig. 6.40**). First, a line was drawn from the inferior margin of the anterior arch of the atlas to the inferior margin of the posterior arch; the distance along this line between the posterior inferior margin of the anterior arch of the atlas and the anterior surface of the dens represented the ADI (**Fig. 6.41**). The maximum ADI value was found to be 3.5 mm.

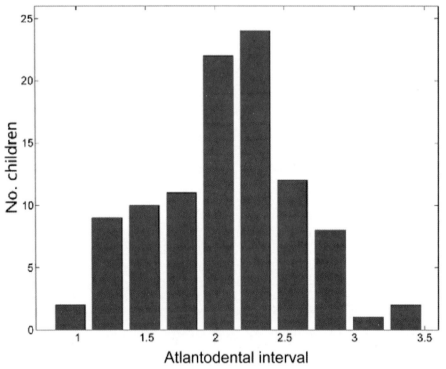

Fig. 6.40   Distribution of the atlantodental interval in 101 children aged 1 to 12 years. (Reproduced from Douglas TS, Sanders V, Machers S, Pitcher R, van As AB. Digital radiographic measurement of the atlantodental interval in children. J Pediatr Orthop 2007;27(1):23–26, with permission from Wolters Kluwer Health.)

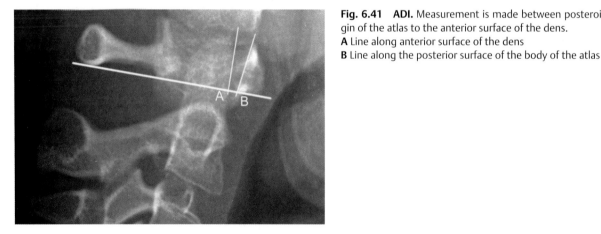

Fig. 6.41   ADI. Measurement is made between posteroinferior margin of the atlas to the anterior surface of the dens.
A Line along anterior surface of the dens
B Line along the posterior surface of the body of the atlas

■ References

1. Delange F, Benker G, Caron P, et al. Thyroid volume and urinary iodine in European schoolchildren: standardization of values for assessment of iodine deficiency. Eur J Endocrinol 1997;136: 180–187

2. Menken KU, Engelhardt S, Olbricht T. [Thyroid gland volume and urinary iodine excretion in children 2–16 years of age]. Dtsch Med Wochenschr 1992;117:1047–1051

3. Perry RJ, Hollman AS, Wood AM, Donaldson MD. Ultrasound of the thyroid gland in the newborn: normative data. Arch Dis Child Fetal Neonatal Ed 2002;87:F209–211

4. Purcell D, Johnson J, Fischbein N, Lalwani AK. Establishment of normative cochlear and vestibular measurements to aid in the diagnosis of inner ear malformations. Otolaryngol Head Neck Surg 2003;128:78–87

5. Sondhi V, Gupta G, Gupta PK, Patnaik SK, Tshering K. Establishment of nomograms and reference ranges for intra-cranial ventricular dimensions and ventriculo-hemispheric ratio in newborns by ultrasonography. Acta Paediatr 2008;97:738–744

6. Lam WW, Ai VH, Wong V, Leong LL. Ultrasonographic measurement of subarachnoid space in normal infants and children. Pediatr Neurol 2001;25:380–384

7. Argyropoulou M, Perignon F, Brunelle F, Brauner R, Rappaport R. Height of normal pituitary gland as a function of age evaluated by magnetic resonance imaging in children. Pediatr Radiol 1991;21:247–249

8. Takano K, Utsunomiya H, Ono H, Ohfu M, Okazaki M. Normal development of the pituitary gland: assessment with three-dimensional MR volumetry. AJNR Am J Neuroradiol 1999;20:312–315

9. Vogler RC, Ii FJ, Pilgram TK. Age-specific size of the normal adenoid pad on magnetic resonance imaging. Clin Otolaryngol Allied Sci 2000;25:392–395

10. Soyupak SK, Narli N, Yapicioglu H, Satar M, Aksungur EH. Sonographic measurements of the liver, spleen and kidney dimensions in the healthy term and preterm newborns. Eur J Radiol 2002;43:73–78

11. Konus OL, Ozdemir A, Akkaya A, Erbas G, Celik H, Isik S. Normal liver, spleen, and kidney dimensions in neonates, infants, and children: evaluation with sonography. AJR Am J Roentgenol 1998; 171:1693–1698

12. Noda T, Todani T, Watanabe Y, Yamamoto S. Liver volume in children measured by computed tomography. Pediatr Radiol 1997; 27:250–252

13. Hernanz-Schulman M, Ambrosino MM, Freeman PC, Quinn CB. Common bile duct in children: sonographic dimensions. Radiology 1995;195:193–195

14. Patriquin HB, Perreault G, Grignon A, et al. Normal portal venous diameter in children. Pediatr Radiol 1990;20:451–453

15. Ho ML, Chen JY, Ling UP, Su PH. Gallbladder volume and contractility in term and preterm neonates: normal values and clinical applications in ultrasonography. Acta Paediatr 1998;87: 799–804

16. Megremis SD, Vlachonikolis IG, Tsilimigaki AM. Spleen length in childhood with US: normal values based on age, sex, and somatometric parameters. Radiology 2004;231:129–134

17. Siegel MJ, Martin KW, Worthington JL. Normal and abnormal pancreas in children: US studies. Radiology 1987;165:15–18

18. Haber HP, Stern M. Intestinal ultrasonography in children and young adults: bowel wall thickness is age dependent. J Ultrasound Med 2000;19:315–321

19. Wiersma F, Sramek A, Holscher HC. US features of the normal appendix and surrounding area in children. Radiology 2005; 235:1018–1022

20. Karmazyn B, Werner EA, Rejaie B, Applegate KE. Mesenteric lymph nodes in children: what is normal? Pediatr Radiol 2005;35:774–777

21. Rosenbaum DM, Korngold E, Teele RL. Sonographic assessment of renal length in normal children. AJR Am J Roentgenol 1984;142:467–469

22. Leung VY, Chu WC, Yeung CK, et al. Nomograms of total renal volume, urinary bladder volume and bladder wall thickness index in 3,376 children with a normal urinary tract. Pediatr Radiol 2007;37:181–188

23. Robben SG, Boesten M, Linmans J, Lequin MH, Nijman RM. Significance of thickening of the wall of the renal collecting system in children: an ultrasound study. Pediatr Radiol 1999;29:736–740

24. Kuijper EA, van Kooten J, Verbeke JI, van Rooijen M, Lambalk CB. Ultrasonographically measured testicular volumes in 0- to 6-year-old boys. Hum Reprod 2008;23:792–796

25. Haber HP, Mayer EI. Ultrasound evaluation of uterine and ovarian size from birth to puberty. Pediatr Radiol 1994;24:11–13

26. Oppenheimer DA, Carroll BA, Yousem S. Sonography of the normal neonatal adrenal gland. Radiology 1983;146:157–160

27. Robinow M, Chumlea WC. Standards for limb bone length ratios in children. Radiology 1982;143:433–436

28. Robben SG, Lequin MH, Diepstraten AF, den Hollander JC, Entius CA, Meradji M. Anterior joint capsule of the normal hip and in children with transient synovitis: US study with anatomic and histologic correlation. Radiology 1999;210:499–507

29. Graf R. Hip sonography: diagnosis and management of infant hip dysplasia. Berlin Heidelberg: Springer, 2006

30. Douglas TS, Sanders V, Machers S, Pitcher R, van As AB. Digital radiographic measurement of the atlantodental interval in children. J Pediatr Orthop 2007;27:23–26

31. Griscom NT, Wohl ME. Dimensions of the growing trachea related to age and gender. AJR Am J Roentgenol 1986;146:233–237

32. Gollogly S, Smith JT, White SK, Firth S, White K. The volume of lung parenchyma as a function of age: a review of 1050 normal CT scans of the chest with three-dimensional volumetric reconstruction of the pulmonary system. Spine (Phila Pa 1976) 2004;29:2061–2066

33. Yekeler E, Tambag A, Tunaci A, et al. Analysis of the thymus in 151 healthy infants from 0 to 2 years of age. J Ultrasound Med 2004;23:1321–1326

Index

Page numbers in *italics* refer to illustrations